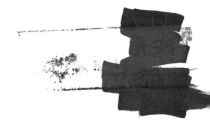

D1556235

Pediatric home care

10/14/97

PEDIATRIC HOME CARE

SECOND EDITION

Edited by

Wendy L. Votroubek, RN, MPH
Clinical Nurse Specialist
Pediatric Pulmonary Section
Department of Pediatrics
University Medical Center
Tucson, Arizona

Julie L. Townsend, RNC, MS
Instructor
University of Arizona
College of Nursing
Tucson, Arizona

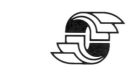

AN ASPEN PUBLICATION®
Aspen Publishers, Inc.
Gaithersburg, Maryland
1997

The authors have made every effort to ensure the accuracy of the information herein, particularly with regard to technique and procedure. However, appropriate information sources should be consulted, especially for new or unfamiliar procedures. It is the responsibility of every practitioner to evaluate the appropriateness of a particular opinion in the context of actual practical situations and with due consideration to new developments. Authors, editors, and the publisher cannot be held responsible for any typographical or other errors found in this manual.

Library of Congress Cataloging-in-Publication Data

Pediatric home care / edited by Wendy Votroubek and Julie Townsend.—2nd ed.
p.   cm.
Includes bibliographical references and index.
ISBN 0-8342-0884-9 (hardcover)
1. Pediatric nursing. 2. Chronically ill children—Home care.
I. Votroubek, Wendy L. II. Townsend, Julie.
[DNLM: 1. Pediatric Nursing. 2. Home Care Services—nurses' instruction
WY 159 P3695 1997]
RJ245.P384   1997
610.73'62—dc21
DNLM/DLC
for Library of Congress
97-18624
CIP

Aspen Publishers, Inc., grants permission for photocopying for limited personal or internal use. This consent does not extend to other kinds of copying, such as copying for general distribution, for advertising or promotional purposes, for creating new collective works, or for resale. For information, address Aspen Publishers, Inc., Permissions Department, 200 Orchard Ridge Drive, Suite 200, Gaithersburg, Maryland 20878.

Orders: (800) 638-8437
Customer Service: (800) 234-1660

About Aspen Publishers • For more than 35 years, Aspen has been a leading professional publisher in a variety of disciplines. Aspen's vast information resources are available in both print and electronic formats. We are committed to providing the highest quality information available in the most appropriate format for our customers. Visit Aspen's Internet site for more information resources, directories, articles, and a searchable version of Aspen's full catalog, including the most recent publications: **http://www.aspenpub.com**
Aspen Publishers, Inc. • The hallmark of quality in publishing
Member of the worldwide Wolters Kluwer group.

Editorial Resources: Ruth Bloom
Library of Congress Catalog Card Number: 97-18624
ISBN: 0-8342-0884-9

Printed in the United States of America

1 2 3 4 5

Table of Contents

Chapter 13—Care of the Child Post-Transplant **384**
Susan D. Wheeler and Christine Mudge

Chapter 14—Care of the Terminally Ill Child **412**
Belinda Barry Mitchell

Chapter 15—Cognitive Development **426**
Joanne K.H. Howard

Contributors

Jean Betschart, CRNP, MSN, MN, CDE
Pediatric Nurse Practitioner
Children's Hospital of Pittsburgh
Department of Nutrition, Endocrinology, and
   Metabolism
Pittsburgh, Pennsylvania

Angela Carlson, MS, PNP
Pediatric Nurse Practitioner
Division of Pediatric Neurosurgery
Children's Hospital at Strong Memorial
   Hospital
Rochester, New York

Jennifer Casteix, MS, CCC-SLP
Speech Language Pathologist
Outpatient Pediatric Therapies Department
Tucson Medical Center
Tucson, Arizona

M. Katharine Dolan, MSEd
Early Intervention Specialist
Katy, Texas

Lynn Feenan, RN, MSN
Clinical Nurse Specialist
Pediatric Pulmonary/Allergy
Children's Hospital at Dartmouth
Dartmouth-Hitchcock Medical Center
Lenanon, New Hampshire

**Mary Lou Fragomeni-Nuttall, MS,
   CCC-SLP**
Speech Language Pathologist
Outpatient Pediatric Therapies Department
Tucson Medical Center
Tucson, Arizona

Sharon Frierdich, RN, MS, CPNP, CPON
Clinical Nurse Specialist/Nurse Practitioner
Pediatric Hematology Oncology
University of Wisconsin
Children's Hospital
Madison, Wisconsin

Linda Gaudet, MSW
Psychotherapist
Private Practice
Sonora Behavioral Health Network
Tucson, Arizona

Anne Armstrong Griffin, RN, MS
Pediatric Clinical Nurse Specialist
Hemostasis/Thrombosis and Pediatric
   HIV Program
University of Wisconsin
Children's Hospital
Madison, Wisconsin

Joanne K.H. Howard, RN, PhD
Nurse Researcher Consultant
Spokane, Washington

Anne S. Klijanowicz, MS, PNP, CS
Senior Advanced Practice Nurse, Pediatrics
Associate Professor of Clinical Nursing
University of Rochester Medical Center
Rochester, New York

Janice C. Krueger, RN, MSN
Nephrology Clinical Nurse Specialist
Duke University Medical Center
Durham, North Carolina

Jill K. Martindale, PT
Pediatric Physical Therapist
Private Practice
Pueblo Pediatric Therapy
Tucson, Arizona

Barbara Masiulis, MS, RN, PNP
Pediatric Nurse Practitioner
Baltimore, Maryland

Kathleen Mauro, RN, PhD, CPNP
Clinical Instructor
College of Nursing
University of Arizona
Tucson, Arizona

Ruth Messinger, MSW
Coordinator of Social Work and Community
   Education
Strong Center for Developmental Disabilities
Department of Pediatrics
University of Rochester Medical Center
Children's Hospital at Strong Memorial
   Hospital
Rochester, New York

**Belinda Barry Mitchell, RN, MSN, PNP,
   FAAN**
formerly President and Chief Executive Officer
Children's Home Care
Los Angeles, California

Christine Mudge, RN, MS, PNP, CNN
Clinical Transplant Coordinator
Pediatric Liver Transplant Service
University of California at San Francisco
San Francisco, California

Nancy Harris Ossman, ORT/L
Pediatric and Adult Occupational
   Therapy
Private Practice
Tucson, Arizona

Christine O. Perreault, BSN, RN
Clinical Coordinator
School Health Program
The Children's Hospital
Denver, Colorado

Marsha S. Pulhamus, RN, MS, CNSN
Clinical Nurse Specialist
Nutrition Support Service
University of Rochester
Strong Memorial Hospital
Rochester, New York

Julie L. Townsend, RNC, MS
Instructor
University of Arizona
College of Nursing
Tucson, Arizona

Karen C. Uzark, RN, PNP, PhD
Nurse Practitioner
Children's Heart Institute
San Diego, California

Wendy L. Votroubek, RN, MPH
Clinical Nurse Specialist
Pediatric Pulmonary Section
Department of Pediatrics
University Medical Center
Tucson, Arizona

Susan D. Wheeler
Vice President of Operations
Biologic Health Resources
Santa Clara, California

Nancy Williams, MS, CCC
Speech Language Pathologist
Pueblo Pediatric Therapy
Tucson, Arizona

Foreword

Childhood ought to be full of exciting discoveries, unconditional love, and carefree days that stretch endlessly into the future. Unfortunately, for too many children, medical conditions limit life—in what they can do, in where they do it, and in how long they live. A growing number of people, however, believe that no human being—child or adult—should live without love, without family. These people are doing what they can to make sure that all children with disability or illness can receive care surrounded by family—and that means receiving care in their own homes.

Pediatric Home Care, Second Edition, addresses this concern. Its update this year is timely, with all the changes that are occurring in home care. Congress even touched on pediatric home care in its last session (the 104th), with the proposed "baby bill." This bill would have legislated home care for mothers who are sent home 24 hours after giving birth. The National Association for Home Care (NAHC) advocated strongly for this bill; although the home care component was left out of the bill that finally did pass, NAHC will continue to pursue similar bills. For 15 years, NAHC has been a strong proponent of home care, of course, but especially for those who are, in the words of Vice President Hubert Humphrey, "on the fringes of life"—including children who face problems in the dawn of life. NAHC will always advocate for home care for children who need it.

As recently as 25 years ago, the most chronically ill children could look forward to was an early death. Many of these children now survive to adulthood. Technology is responsible for an almost 50 percent reduction in infant mortality, resulting in populations of medically fragile children who depend on that technology. Approximately four million children are significantly disabled to the extent that normal childhood activities are interrupted. Many of these children do well because of advances in technology; however, they still need complex health care, often for the rest of their lives.

Such children were long thought to be happier in settings where they wouldn't face the rigors of daily life. They were protected and grew up unable to function in society. Because many of them required care beyond typical hospital, physician, and pharmaceutical care, they remained in an institutional setting; they had no satisfactory alternatives.

That's where home care comes in. It has finally become apparent that families are more than willing to bring their children home. Home care is in fact the preferred model for their care: this setting encourages family bonding, supports growth and development, and eliminates risks that institutional care poses.

Obviously, as children with disabilities and chronic illnesses live longer, their need for pediatric home care increases. Pediatric and perinatal services are emerging as two of the fastest growing segments of the home care market. And as children's needs and living arrangements and the reimbursement structure change, the challenge for home care is to be more creative. Thus, pediatric home care has evolved to include much more than traditional private duty and intermittent in-home models. Home care providers have, out of necessity, developed unique programs, including technology-dependent care, various therapies, maintenance care, and even foster care for these technology-dependent children. Their focus is on controlling quality, resources, and cost, and on providing continuity of service.

This evolution of medical technology for children with chronic health care needs has led to a parallel evolution in concepts, namely the evolution of care concept. Providers have switched their focus from the care of the defect or illness to care of the whole child and for the whole family.

This is the difference between pediatric and other types of home care. The family is the pivotal point for pediatric home care. Home care professionals take a total-person approach to pediatric care and, indeed, expand that approach to be a total-family approach. When a child is ill, the whole family is affected. Thus, the family must be taught how to deliver the appropriate care. This may be one of the greatest challenges in pediatric home care, a challenge providers rise to meet every day.

Research has demonstrated again and again that home visiting programs that focus on parent education, family support, and social and relationship skills effectively decrease the incidence of abuse and neglect. It stands to reason that these programs also effectively enhance the outcomes of the children, improving their lives. Using parent education and support as a primary means of intervention, home care programs can make a powerful difference.

With their development of new and innovative programs, home care providers show their commitment to the child and show that they recognize they have a commitment to the family as well. Home care providers do not shrink from such a challenge.

Pediatric home care providers face other challenges such as the following: inadequate or lack of Medicaid or private insurance reimburse-ment; the lack of social and emotional support for families; poor teaching; and the lack of continuity of treatment among key providers. There is not always "a clear pathway home"; money, resources, and time stand in the way of optimal care for children who are chronically ill or disabled.

The home care industry has an opportunity to provide leadership in pediatric care. It can redirect the nation's attention and resources toward positive long-term outcomes for children who are chronically ill. The nation must realize that a community focus—which means home care nurses—is a crucial component of the team that will make comprehensive services accessible and acceptable to vulnerable families. Home care must be recognized as the heart of any health care team.

To ensure that this is so, home care professionals must participate in planning, providing, and evaluating policies as well as care. Home care providers are partners in care, training families, and maximizing the children's integration into the community. This requires the least restrictive environment, which unquestionably is the home.

All children need the opportunity to explore, to play, to laugh, to be loved. Home care makes that opportunity a reality for those who might otherwise face lifelong limits. It gives them life beyond mere existence.

Pediatric Home Care, Second Edition, will be a valuable resource for providers and an invaluable source of information for the general public—including those members of Congress, NAHC, and the industry who seek to educate and influence. Having made the same commitment to helping these special children as providers have, NAHC further pledges to protect the interests of those who have dedicated their lives to making the lives of these special children better. There is no greater need, and no higher calling.

Val J. Halamandaris
President
National Association for Home Care
Washington, D.C.

Preface

This book is much more relevant and timely than when it was first published in 1990. Today, pediatric patients are leaving the hospital "sicker and quicker" than ever before. Students who graduate from colleges of nursing are finding it difficult to obtain jobs in hospitals. Consequently, schools of nursing are including more content in their curricula in the area of home health and community nursing. We envision this updated version to be a reference as well as perhaps a textbook as students venture or are pushed out into the community. This book is comprehensive, easy to use, and well organized.

New chapters have been added to this book to increase its relevance. It remains a valuable tool for discharge planners and case managers involved in the expanding field of home care. It may also be of interest to parents whose children are receiving care in the home. Home care is a competitive field; this book will be invaluable to agencies and hospitals developing home care programs.

This book is unique in several respects. It is a good reference for home care nurses because it provides technical guidance as well as theory. Each chapter includes valuable charts, care plans, and teaching tools. There is a wide variety of information on technology, social concerns, growth and development, and family interactions. The care plans are based on nursing diagnoses along with nursing objectives and interventions. The contributors and the editors are experienced in hospital care as well as home health care. We hope this updated version helps you in all of your efforts to provide quality care for these special children who need pediatric home care.

Acknowledgments

A book of this scope could not have been completed without the assistance and hard work of many colleagues, friends, and family members. Specifically, we would like to thank the many contributing authors for producing chapters that help share their expertise with the nursing profession. It was a delight to work with authors who were so dedicated, professional, and willing to give of themselves. We would also like to thank Mary Anne Langdon of Aspen Publishers, Inc., for her assistance, patience, and enthusiasm in helping us complete this manuscript.

We would also like to thank the authors of the first edition. Without their hard work, the second edition would not have been possible. We would like to thank those who provided various secretarial assistance from our respective work environments. We thank Val J. Halamandaris and his administrative assistant Tim Brown, for sharing with us their support and belief in pediatric home care by writing such a warm and comprehensive foreword. Heartfelt thanks to all of the pediatric patients and their families who have taught us so much and touched our lives.

Finally, we express special thanks to Catharine Drozdowski and Ward Townsend for their patience, support, love, and encouragement in helping us bring this book to fruition. Their moral support assisted us during those periods when it seemed this project would never end. Finally, we would like to thank each other for the gift of humor that was an important component of getting the job done!

CHAPTER 1

Discharge Planning: Transition to Home

Julie L. Townsend

Home care is an attempt to normalize the life of a child with special needs in a family and community setting to minimize the disruptive impact of the child's condition on the family (Wong 1991). The pediatric patient's growth and development also need to be maximized. Wong (1991) identifies that for home care to be successful, the family must want the child to be cared for at home. The family needs to be able to cope with all of the stresses and intrusions that occur during home care, and it must have the physical, emotional, educational, and social supports necessary to successfully care for the child at home.

Caring for a child at home provides a more natural and nurturing environment, improves physical functioning, encourages growth and development, ensconces the family as controller of care, helps to facilitate family cohesiveness, and usually reduces costs.

The success of the home care experience depends on a comprehensive plan of care, which begins with a thorough discharge plan initiated in the hospital by the primary care team in collaboration with the home care agency and/or the case manager. Even before the child's medical condition stabilizes in the hospital, discharge planning should be initiated.

The discharge planning must be tailored to meet the specific needs of the child and family. The discharge planning process includes the determination of the child's home care needs, the child and family's capacity for self-care, and an assessment of the living conditions. It may be necessary to counsel the child and family to help prepare them for home care. The goal of discharge planning is to ensure a smooth transition from hospital to home; however, it should be remembered that home care may not be feasible for every child and family (see Exhibit 1-1 for discharge criteria for appropriate pediatric home care candidates). Medical, social, or financial concerns may preclude home care as a realistic alternative. Alternatives should be discussed, and the parents should not be pressured into caring for their child at home.

In this chapter, the process involved in discharge planning for the pediatric patient and family is reviewed. The concept of case management as a method for coordinating services for the child requiring home care and his or her family and the essential components of the discharge planning process are discussed.

CASE MANAGEMENT

Case management is an important component of the discharge planning process because it offers service coordination to families. Case management as defined by the Center for Case Management (Zander 1987) is a clinical system that focuses on the accountability of an identified individual or group for coordinating a patient's care; insuring and facilitating the achievement of quality, clinical, and cost outcome negotiating; and procuring and coordinating services and

Exhibit 1–1 Discharge Criteria for Home Care

1. Medically stable child
2. Family willing and able to have child at home
3. Family motivated to gain skill for and knowledge of child's care
4. Adequate family support systems available
5. Financial support systems available
6. Residence structurally appropriate
7. Community resources available
8. Local medical supervision available
9. Trained home care providers available
10. Alternative method of care available should the home care experience prove unsatisfactory

Source: Adapted from Tucson's First Homebound Ventilator Child: Kim Nichols by P.A. McCoy and W.L. Votroubek, *Caring,* with permission of National Association for Home Care, © December 1986.

resources needed by the patient and family and intervening at key points.

Case managers may be employed by a payer source such as one affiliated with managed care. The source may be hospital- or community-based. The case manager may not even be a nurse. Currently, nurse case managers may be clinical specialists or pediatric nurse-practitioners and may have educational preparation ranging from an associate degree to an advanced degree specializing in case management. Historically, nurses in home care have assumed most of the responsibility for coordinating the management of the services. Some believe that case management should be independent of the reimbursement system.

The State of Michigan Department of Public Health has established a specialized home care program (SHCP) that emphasizes the needs of the child rather than cost savings. This SHCP was established in June 1988 to help families provide home care for children with complex

needs. Nurses with a minimum of a bachelor's degree and two years of pediatric clinical practice are qualified to become the case managers. Regardless of who provides the professional components of case management, the services should be family centered and responsive to the varying needs of the child and family (Gittler and Colton 1986).

Collaboration and coordination help the case manager to ensure the achievement of outcomes and a timely discharge from the hospital or program. The nurse case manager may also deliver direct services to the pediatric patient and his or her family. The nurse case manager must have current clinical skills, including current knowledge and practice in the areas of growth and development, specific nutritional needs, physical assessment skills, specific health care problems, and family theory.

The ultimate goal of case management should be for the family to assume the case management and advocacy roles for the child. The tools of the case manager may include the traditional care plan, critical pathways, or the care map, all of which are discussed in Chapter 2.

A case manager should be identified before the discharge process begins. It is important that a primary person be responsible for organizing and coordinating the discharge planning process. The importance of close coordination of financial management and clinical and social management cannot be overemphasized. The services of a case manager are extremely beneficial during the discharge planning process and the initial transition from hospital to home. As the family becomes more comfortable and established with providing care for the child, the role of the case manager changes. The family assumes the role of case manager, relying on the case manager for advice, guidance, and support.

DISCHARGE PLANNING

The goal of pediatric discharge planning is to facilitate a smooth and safe transition back to the community. The feasibility of home care depends on many factors. The American Academy of Pediatrics Task Force on Home Care (1984) identified several factors that should be considered when selecting candidates for home care. These include the following: patient factors (potential benefits and risks, and care needs), family factors (the presence of involved family members and an appropriate home setting, including, whenever possible, at least two knowledgeable family members), and community factors (medical, social, and educational supports). In addition, the most crucial factors in determining feasibility for home care are the child's disease process and medical stability.

The goal of the discharge plan is for the family and caregivers to become familiar with the child's needs and competent in caring for him or her. The needs of the entire family unit must be considered in comprehensive discharge planning. Clear expectations should be discussed with the parents regarding the child's needs at home, evaluation of the residence, accessibility of transportation, evaluation of existing community resources, and educational offerings in the community. Parents must identify what is realistic and workable in their home. The plan should include a system for managing emergencies, both medical and family, and a mechanism for providing continual social and emotional support to the family and child. It should also provide an appropriate alternative to home care, such as respite care or long-term placement. The discharge plan is continually evolving to meet the changing needs of the patient and family.

The discharge team should be multidisciplinary and include the family, nurses, and doctors, with collaboration and input from all the therapists who have been involved or will be involved with the care of the child. Parents must assume a variety of roles, including teacher, housekeeper, cook, chauffeur, and substitute playmate, among many others. Parents must become part-time nurses, case managers, and therapists. They must learn complicated new skills and procedures and a new vocabulary that includes medical, legal, and financial jargon. Involvement and

commitment of families can make home care work despite other drawbacks. Each member of the discharge team possesses special skills and knowledge to help facilitate a successful transition to the home.

A comprehensive discharge plan details outpatient care; medications; durable medical equipment; disposable medical supplies; transportation needs; adaptive equipment; therapies such as physical, speech, and occupational; counseling and social work nursing care; and respite plans. A large part of the population in pediatric home care was previously viewed as inappropriate for home care. Children in home care are sicker, require more support, and are medically more complex. An increasing number of these medically complex children have caregivers who are or were in complicated high-risk social situations. Therefore, these children will require more comprehensive discharge plans.

Hamilton and Vessey (1992) liken the discharge planning process to the nursing process. They identify the following four phases: assessment, planning, implementation, and evaluation. According to Wong (1991), discharge planning should consist of the following three phases: education and training of caregivers, a transition trial period, and final discharge to home. At least two people should be trained to care for the child. Training the caregivers in what to do in case of an emergency or equipment malfunction is important. If possible, the caregivers should be trained on the same type of equipment that will be used in the home. The transition period consists of the caregivers providing 24-hour care for the child under the supervision of the health care team in the hospital setting. It is helpful for parents to have calendars that include schedules, meetings, etc. Having parents stay overnight in the room empowers the parents and caregivers and helps them to feel competent with their ability to meet the child's needs. Usually, the patient and family are discharged directly home after the transition trial period. Written teaching plans should be sent home with the parents and caregivers to use as a reference. When the patient and family go home, the durable medical equipment, nursing care plan, follow-up appointments, and an emergency plan must all be functional.

Appropriateness for Home Care

The team should be aware of barriers that may affect successful discharge planning. An assessment should be done with the child and family to identify any problems pertaining to home care. This may, in part, be accomplished through a psychosocial assessment designed to assist the home care team in evaluating whether the decision for home care is appropriate.

Most families are eager to have their children return home. The complexities of daily care may usually be mastered by the family with time and appropriate teaching. No matter how comfortable the family may be with its roles, the development of stressors is inevitable once the child is at home. Many stressors are predictable; some are unique to the individual family. Examples of stressors include the following: (1) the issue of privacy with nurses in the home from 8 to 24 hours a day; (2) controlling, nurturing, and supporting the child while nurses provide hands-on care; and (3) turning a part of the home into a hospital room with equipment, alarms, and supplies.

Support Systems

One key to a successful outcome is the identification of support systems for the family. Each family should have an identified support system with which to share concerns about the impact of returning the child to the home. Initially, this will be the discharge planner. Other sources of support should be identified before the child is discharged home. Many families have found it helpful to share problems and concerns with parents who have experienced similar situations. Attention should be given to identifying temporary respite care services for families that do not have private-duty nurses available on a regular basis. This ensures that the family can obtain temporary relief from caregiving responsibilities. In addition, a variety of support services that the parents and caregivers may contact for information are included in the resources.

Funding Sources

The cost of home care may be a significant burden for a family. Although home care may be cost effective, many insurance companies that pay 100 percent of inpatient costs may pay only a partial percentage of home care costs. Uninsured costs of home care can financially overwhelm a family already burdened with nonreimbursable deductions such as insurance deductibles, traveling expenses during hospitalization, home renovations for the child, and increased utility bills after discharge (McCarthy 1986). The financial expenditures fall into the following three categories: medical, routine household, and extraordinary household.

Home care usually costs less than hospital care but is still relatively expensive. A report from the National Association of Children's Hospitals and Related Institutions, Inc. (1993) states that the trend in current reimbursement methodology by both private and government insurers is to use adult averages, therefore critically short-changing sick children. It is essential to determine if the child's insurance policy has a lifetime limit for reimbursement and the specific details of home care coverage under private and/ or public funding.

The system for financing home care is a mix of federal and state programs and private insurance companies (see Chapter 3). The complexity of the system may be particularly frustrating for parents with a child whose existence is dependent on specialized medical procedures and equipment as well as health care services. Although most families have a large portion of their medical care supported by a third-party payer, there are often large gaps in coverage that may cause severe financial burdens. In addition to insurance companies, other sources of revenue may include family income, supplemental health coverage, and community resources such as donations, contributions, and extended family support. An investigation of eligibility for federal, state, and local government funds should also be conducted under the direction of the discharge planner. Applications will need to be submitted by the parent or guardian of the child, after the funding sources have been identified. The processing of applications can take several weeks to several months.

Equipment and Supplies

There are several factors to consider when selecting equipment for home care. These include the child's safety needs, the availability and use of single items rather than kits to contain costs, comparison of cost with ease of use (for example, need for additional knowledge and skills, parents' ability to learn, and portability of equipment), and cost to rent versus cost to purchase.

Early identification of equipment and supply needs is an important factor in facilitating discharge. Preparation of equipment and supply lists must be completed before any type of funding package can be submitted. The cost and quality of items must be identified and should include (1) initial purchases, (2) monthly rental equipment, and (3) monthly supplies. Consider that most supplies for home care need to be clean but not sterile. Some items such as tracheostomy tubes and straight catheters can be reused at home, helping to decrease expenses.

Community suppliers must guarantee continuous availability, maintenance, and replacement of equipment. In addition, the durable medical equipment (DME) vendor should be able to provide all DME and disposable supplies. This will help prevent multiple contracts and the unnecessary complexity associated with coordinating requests through many different vendors. In addition, it is important that the DME vendor be available to service equipment malfunctions on a 24-hour basis. The DME company selected should have staff who have worked with children with complex care needs. The provider should assess the home to determine electrical, space, or other environmental needs. This should be accomplished before the child is discharged from the care facility.

Environmental Assessment

An environmental assessment should be conducted early in the discharge planning process to determine if the child's requirements necessitate structural modifications to the home. The home must meet local safety, sanitation, and building requirements and, depending on the child's condition, should be evaluated for adequacy of space, outlets, wiring, and accessibility for emergencies.

Changes in the home may be necessary to accommodate special medical equipment. These changes might include grounding all electrical outlets, building a ramp for accessibility, or weatherproofing or insulating the residence. Any room of the home may potentially be used as the child's room. The most important consideration is that the child not be isolated from the rest of the family. Storage space must be able to accommodate hourly, daily, and monthly supplies. A nightstand is helpful for storing equipment and supplies that are required within an 8-hour period. A large closet can be used to store equipment and supplies that are required during a 24-hour period (for example, diapers, scale, water bottles, and suction catheters). Items requiring bulk storage should be placed in the basement, garage, or other suitable area. There should be enough room to store up to one month's worth of supplies and equipment. Storage areas should be free of dampness, have moderate temperatures, and not contain toxic chemicals.

An electrician may be required to evaluate the structure for accommodation of electrical needs. This is particularly important if the child is ventilator dependent. There must be adequate power to maintain the equipment in addition to the household appliances. Spare fuses, if the family uses this type of circuit breaker, should always be available. The house should be equipped with a telephone and smoke alarms. A battery-powered floodlight and power failure alarm system should also be considered if the child is dependent on a ventilator.

Communication with Community Agencies

Community agencies include all resources and agencies that provide support to the family. Long-term home care should not be attempted if community services are not available to the child and family. These services would include public service agencies, home health care agencies (or available health care providers), respite care providers, and educational services.

Public service agencies play a vital role in ensuring safe care for the pediatric patient in the home. If the child is dependent on life-support equipment or has special needs that are affected by the use of public services, the following agencies should be notified before discharge: gas and electric companies, fire department, telephone company, ambulance service, snow removal service, and public works. Written notification should include a description of the child's diagnosis, age, medications, and the hospital identified for emergency transport. Notifying these agencies of the child's needs will help to facilitate a quick response in emergencies.

Nursing Care

Nursing care is the foundation of home care programs. It is not realistic to expect parents to care for their child indefinitely, 24 hours per day, seven days per week. The amount of assistance required is contingent on the dependency requirements of the child. Before discharge, the family and health care team should discuss the need for nursing care in the home. If nursing care is required, the family must select a method of providing that care. The family may have the option of choosing between independently hiring nursing staff or selecting a home care agency. Funding sources may place restrictions on the type of nursing service provided.

The home care agency recruits and selects nurses to work in the home. The agency may also identify a primary nurse for the child. This individual assumes the coordination of care for the child in the home and may also help order and inventory supplies, communicate changes in the care plan to other staff, and participate in training new staff as needed.

Parents often have many concerns and questions about selecting a home care agency. They frequently lack the necessary information required to determine if an agency is suitable for providing the care their child requires. A thorough examination of the agency should be completed before the agency is authorized to provide service. Considerations that parents should discuss with any prospective health care agency are identified in Exhibit 1–2.

Parents may also voice concerns regarding the competency of the agency's nursing staff. This may occur when parents are not consulted about the nursing personnel. Parental rights of approval and disapproval of personnel will help alleviate these concerns. Open communication between the agency and the parents and caregivers will help ensure a successful home care experience.

Educational provisions for the child requiring home care should not be neglected. Children requiring long-term, specialized home care will vary in their needs for educational services. Infants and small children may benefit from home-based intervention programs. Older children may need home school experiences or special education services. The case coordinator or the discharge planner should be in constant contact with school district personnel to inform them of the child's need for educational services and to plan strategies to fulfill this need. Further information on educational services is provided in Chapter 17.

Families will occasionally require temporary relief from caregiving responsibilities. Respite care services to provide that relief should be identified before discharge. This will help ensure that the child is able to remain in the home.

Exhibit 1–2 Considerations in Choosing an Agency

1. What type of experience does the agency have in caring for children with special needs?
2. How does the agency recruit qualified nurses?
3. Will the agency sign a contract/written agreement for care provision?*
4. Will the agency accept the insurance plan and do the paperwork required?*
5. What is the agency's policy for covering sick calls, vacations, and holidays?
6. Is the agency willing to send nurses to the hospital for training before discharge? (This service should be free of charge.)*
7. Does the agency have written standards of care for the pediatric population?
8. Is there a nursing supervisor available?
9. Will the nursing supervisor visit nurses in the home on a regular basis?*
10. Is the nursing supervisor available to assist with problems that might arise?*
11. Who is responsible for providing updated training needs for the nurses?
12. Does the agency provide other services?
13. What are the costs involved?*
14. Is someone available at the agency 24 hours a day?*
15. What if I (parent) don't like a nurse?
16. Am I (parent) allowed to interview a nurse?
17. What about lunch breaks? Do I (parent) provide coverage?
18. Do I (parent) stay at home while the nurse is there?

Source: The Family as Care Manager: Home Care Coordination for Medically Fragile Children by J. Kaufman and K. Lichtenstein. Prepared by Georgetown University Child Development Center, p. 12. 1985.

Discharge Teaching

Thorough teaching is essential. All caregivers, including home care nurses, should be instructed in every aspect of routine and emergency care. The teaching method should incorporate adult learning principles and should be geared toward the learning needs of the family and caregivers. Caregivers should be required to demonstrate all aspects of care before discharge. Teaching home care skills can be complex and demanding. The goals of discharge teaching are to validate mastery of tasks and ensure that parents and caregivers are able to function competently.

The written care plan serves as the basis for education of home care nurses and the patient's family. Education should begin early in the discharge planning process. Orientation to care should begin by teaching simple tasks, then progressing to more complex tasks. Mastery of tasks should be documented on separate teaching forms for each person who will provide care. This form should include a checklist of procedures that is marked by a team member (with date and initials) on the following four occasions: (1) when the procedure is discussed and demonstrated, (2) when the caregiver being trained performs a return demonstration of any skills, (3) when the caregiver being trained performs the procedure with assistance, and (4) when the caregiver performs the procedure independently. Procedures and skills may be practiced in a learning situation away from the child so that the caregiver can gain confidence in the use of equipment and supplies. All procedures need to be performed with the child before discharge.

Documentation of discharge teaching is extremely valuable. It provides a mechanism for hospital staff and the home care agency to review caregiver competencies and it identifies additional training needs. It is also important to note the degree of understanding and skill that the caregivers can verbalize. Exhibit 1–3 is an example of a teaching documentation form. Parents and caregivers must develop technical skills as well as good judgment.

The family and other caregivers must be carefully trained in all aspects of the child's care. Parents should be given progressive responsibility before their child's discharge. During this time, staff should offer assistance, advice, and support. Some programs strongly recommend contracting with parents and caregivers for them to attend a series of specific teaching sessions to accomplish discharge teaching. Parents and caregivers must demonstrate competence in operating equipment, performing procedures, and administering medicine. They must also learn to cope with emergencies. Educational efforts should include classroom exercises, hands-on training in the hospital, and postdischarge instruction.

Written discharge instructions should be developed and given to the parents and other caregivers before discharge. These instructions should include a summary of all aspects of the child's care, including steps of procedures, medication guidelines (for example, dose, route, and side effects), and equipment checklists. Information should be easy to read and understand. It is helpful if all necessary information is placed in a looseleaf notebook so that the information is in one place and is easily accessible. A family member or other caregiver should be des-

Exhibit 1–3 Sample Discharge Teaching Documentation Form

Patient's Name: _____

Name of Caregiver: _____

Instructions: Instructor should place date and initials into box under each column when task is completed.

Skills and Procedures	Discussion about Procedure by Instructor	Demonstration by Instructor	Return Demonstration by Caregiver	Review of Procedure Principles by Caregiver	Performed with Assistance	Performed Independently
Handwashing						
Suctioning						
Equipment Cleaning						
Medication Administration						
Chest Physical Therapy						
Tracheostomy Care						

Instructor: _____   Date Completed: _____

Name of Caregiver: _____   Date Completed: _____

ignated to maintain and update the manual for future teaching needs.

The home care agency must be completely familiar with the teaching instructions that occur in the hospital so that consistency can be maintained in the home environment. This can be accomplished by including the home care nurses in the discharge teaching sessions. This supervision will also help the parents feel more relaxed and comfortable with the staff providing care to their child.

Development of Discharge Plan

Caregiver readiness for discharge is an important component of the discharge plan. A rooming-in period provides an excellent method for assessing readiness. Before discharge, the parents or significant caregivers spend 24 to 72 hours in the hospital assuming full care for the child. This allows the parents or other caregivers to assume control of the child's care using the skills learned during discharge teaching, with assistance from professional staff as needed. Observation of the parents' or caregivers' skills during this period can help identify any additional preparation that may be needed. The nurse can also offer the family support and positive recognition for providing care.

The discharge planner should arrange for discharge transportation during this time. Arrange-ments should also be made for professional staff, if required, to accompany the child on the transport home. The DME vendor should be present on the day of discharge to assist with equipment assembly once the child has arrived home.

It is generally helpful for the child to be discharged during the early part of the week. This allows for availability of the discharge team to solve any minor problems that may arise.

Program Evaluation

Discharge planners, other health care professionals, and parents are responsible for evaluating all aspects of the discharge planning process. One effective method for program evaluation is to enclose an evaluation form in the initial correspondence to the parents. After discharge from the hospital, this form should be mailed back to the hospital, and information can then be shared with the staff. In addition, telephone calls during the first few weeks of home care can serve as an important method for gathering information during the evaluation process.

Program evaluation must be an ongoing process, with continuous evaluation of the home care program. A routine for coordinated review of the child's needs, how the family is managing, and other available findings can be useful in future endeavors of discharge planning.

REFERENCES

American Academy of Pediatrics Task Force on Home Care. 1984. Ad hoc task force on the home care of chronically ill infants and children: Guidelines for home care of infants, children, and adolescents with chronic disease. *Pediatrics* 74:434–36.

Gittler, J., and M. Colton. 1986. *Community-based case management programs for children with special health care needs.* U.S. Department of Health and Human Services Public Health Service, Washington, DC.

Hamilton, B., and J. Vessey. 1992. Pediatric discharge planning. *Pediatric Nursing* 18, no. 5:475–78.

McCarthy, M.F. 1986. A home discharge program for ventilator-assisted children. *Pediatric Nursing* 12:331–35.

National Association of Children's Hospitals and Related Institutions, Inc. 1993. Alexandria, VA: NACHRI.

Wong, D. 1991. Transition from hospital to home for children with complex medical care. *Journal of Pediatric Oncology Nursing* 8:3–9.

Zander, K. 1987. Nursing care management: A classic definition. *Center for Nursing Case Management* 2, no. 2:1–3.

BIBLIOGRAPHY

Davis, B.D., and S. Steele. 1991. Case management for young children with special health care needs. *Pediatric Nursing* 17:15–19.

Goodwin, D. 1992. Critical pathways in home healthcare. *Journal of Nursing Administration* 22, no. 2:35–40.

Haas, S., H. Gray, and B. McConnell. 1992. Parent-professional partnerships in caring for children with special health care needs. *Issues in Comprehensive Pediatric Nursing* 15:39–53.

Hill, D. 1993. Coordinating a multi-disciplinary discharge for the technology-dependent child based on parental needs. *Issues in Comprehensive Pediatric Nursing* 16:229–37.

Karr, J.P., P.D. Locke, and J. Leonard. 1993. Pediatric home care for kids. *Caring* 4:6–12.

Lewis, C.L., et al. 1992. Care management for children who are medically fragile/technology-dependent. *Issues in Comprehensive Pediatric Nursing* 15:73–91.

Maturen, V.L., and K. Zander. 1993. Outcomes management in a prospective pay system. *Caring* 4:46–53.

Richardson, M., et al. 1992. Establishment of a state-supported specialized home care program for children with complex health-care needs. *Issues in Comprehensive Pediatric Nursing* 15:93–122.

Task Force on Case Management in Nursing. 1988. *Nursing case management.* Kansas City, MO: American Nurses Association.

Weston, B.E., and J.A. Keefe. 1993. Pediatric home care and public policy. *Caring* 12:60–64.

CHAPTER 2

Assessment of the Child and Family

Julie L. Townsend

After the pediatric patient is discharged from the care facility, the pediatric home care nurse visits the home for the initial child and family assessment. The assessment process includes the pediatric health history and review of systems including analysis of any symptoms, the pediatric physical examination, and an environmental assessment. The information from the assessments forms the basis for identification of nursing diagnoses and development of the initial plan of care. This plan of care helps to continually monitor and evaluate the child's changing status.

The pediatric home care nurse needs to be aware of the uniqueness and differences when caring for pediatric patients. Many pediatric problems are congenital. These include cystic fibrosis, myelomeningocele, and various heart and kidney problems. The implications and ramifications for managing diseases that will probably last over a lifetime include the following: helping to prevent complications, encouraging normal growth and development, helping to foster family and community support, and being aware of educational and developmental needs. Being an advocate for the pediatric patient and family is another appropriate role for the home care nurse. There are some problems that are a direct result of child abuse, poor parenting, or inadequate parenting.

In pediatric home care, both the child and the family must be considered as the patient. The home care nurse needs to be aware of the developmental level of the child as well as the family and must also be aware of how illness and stress may affect the functioning of the child and family. It is extremely important for the home care nurse to be aware of the importance of the family to a successful outcome for the child.

INTERVIEWING

Interviewing the child and family is a complex process that requires skill in communication and interpersonal relationships. An attentive, nonjudgmental approach is essential for fostering an environment that allows the family to discuss concerns and problems openly.

An assessment of the family's knowledge and understanding of the child's diagnosis, including an understanding of medical terminology, is helpful in establishing a common ground. The family may not understand all of the medical terminology, especially if the child's problem has been recently diagnosed, and may not be able to provide accurate information. The home care nurse should clarify terminology and provide information to help the family gain an understanding of the child's illness. Some questions that seem important to the home care nurse may seem unnecessarily prying to the parents. This potential problem can usually be avoided by explaining the reasons for the question before asking it.

Information accuracy may be improved by interviewing the child without the parents being present. Whenever possible, the wishes of the child should be respected. If confidential information must be shared with the parents, the child should be informed of this need before discussing it with his or her parents.

Successful interviewing requires a combination of strategies to elicit pertinent information. Open-ended questions provide one effective approach. Questions such as "Can you tell me about your child's illness?" or "Can you describe your child's daily routine?" may help provide better information than objective questions.

Health History

Obtaining the health history is the first step in establishing and promoting a caring and therapeutic relationship among the child, parent or caregivers, the extended family, and the nurse. The interview should be a two-way process in which the nurse gathers information as well as provides information to the child and family. During this visit, the goals for the home care program and the expectations of the parents and child should be discussed. Boundaries of interaction regarding discipline and normal patterns of behaviors and any other significant concerns should be addressed.

Time management for the initial home visit can be a challenge, given the amount of information that must be gathered. The initial visit should be scheduled in advance for a convenient time and limited to one and a half to two hours. Longer periods may impinge on the family's routine and result in fatigue and frustration for the child and family. Information for the pediatric health history may be obtained directly or indirectly (Appendix 2–A).

The referral to the home care agency will probably include a great deal of information that may need to be verified or clarified by the nurse. The next part of the health history is the review of systems, which is done to gather information concerning any potential health problems.

PEDIATRIC PHYSICAL EXAMINATION

The physical examination is completed after the health history is taken and usually fol-lows a "head-to-toe" sequence. Age-specific approaches to the physical examination, including position, sequence, and preparation, are included in Appendix 2–B.

FAMILY ASSESSMENT

Caring for a child at home, especially a chronically or terminally ill child, can be psychologically challenging for the caregiver(s). In pediatric home care, the family must be taught how to care for the child, how to deal with the various systems, how to be an advocate for the child, perhaps how to supervise licensed or nonlicensed personnel, and a variety of other issues. The health history will usually give the nurse enough information for a basic family assessment.

ENVIRONMENTAL ASSESSMENT

The last assessment to be performed by the home care nurse is the environmental assessment (Appendix 2–C). The nurse can perform this assessment before the child is discharged from the care facility or when visiting the home after discharge. This information can often explain why the child has insect or rodent bites, reactive airway disease (from animal allergies), etc. If the home has no water, telephone, or electricity, referrals may be appropriate and necessary to facilitate the child's care and safety at home.

THE NURSING PROCESS

Knowledge is the home care professional's most powerful tool. Careful and meticulous data collection when combined with a sound knowledge base in normal growth and development will adequately prepare the nurse to plan the care for the child and the family. The nurse must analyze and synthesize the information that has been collected to identify the nursing diagnoses and develop an individualized plan of care. The nursing process helps to accomplish this through a systematic approach to analysis of the patient's health problems, and it allows for the development of a comprehensive treatment plan.

PLAN OF CARE TOOLS

Detailed plans, which outline specific interventions, are essential in establishing continuity for the many providers who come into contact with the patient and family. A detailed plan of care also assists in allaying caregivers' feelings of anxiety, insecurity, inadequacy, and apprehension. The plan should be well documented and easily understood, and a copy should be given to the family to keep in the home (Ahmann 1996) and should be updated regularly. A complete listing of services and providers to be used in the home, the funding sources, and lists of all equipment, supplies, and medications should be included in the plan.

The traditional care plan with its assessment, nursing diagnosis, goal setting, planning, and evaluation is one approach. There are several new tools that are being used in home care as an adjunct to, or in place of, the traditional care plan.

The Michigan Department of Public Health Division of Services for Crippled Children/ Children's Special Health Care Services uses a comprehensive plan of care (Richardson et al. 1992) to deal with children who require complex, technology-dependent care. This care plan stresses collaboration among the family, the professional, and a variety of community resources. The form has sections for review of systems, health patterns, and needed services. The comprehensive plan of care is signed by the professional, the caregiver, and the physician, signifying collaboration and agreement by all three.

Critical paths are another version of the nursing care plan that is sometimes used. Critical paths include the medical treatment regimen with the key incidents that must occur in a predictable and timely fashion. The key incidents of critical paths could include teaching, diet, medications, and usage of community resources. Using critical paths in home care gives the nurse a tool to help him or her plan and communicate the plan to patients and their families, physicians, and payer sources.

Another tool that case management and managed care providers have used is the CareMap system. The system includes a cause-and-effect grid that identifies outcomes as the result of actions plotted against a timeline. The four parts of the CareMap tool are a timeline, an index of problems with intermediate and outcome criteria, a critical path, and a variance record (Zander 1987).

DOCUMENTATION

Documentation of care delivered in the home has taken on greater significance because of the increased sophistication of technology used in the home, the increase in litigation, and closer scrutiny by payer sources. Documentation is a critical factor for home care agencies meeting state licensure and certification requirements. The clinical record serves a variety of purposes, including billing for services, maintaining continuity of care, collaborating with other professionals, and providing a basis for research and audits.

REFERENCES

Ahmann, E. 1996. *Home care for the high-risk infant.* Gaithersburg, MD: Aspen Publishers, Inc.

Richardson, M., et al. 1992. Establishment of a state-supported specialized home care program for children with complex health-care needs." *Issues in Comprehensive Pediatric Nursing* 15:93–122.

Zander, K. 1987. Nursing care management: A classic definition. *Center for Nursing Case Management.* 2, no. 2:1–3.

BIBLIOGRAPHY

Fields, A.I., et al. 1991. Outcome of home care for technology-dependent children: Success of an independent, community-based case management model. *Pediatric Pulmonology* 11:310–17.

Hamilton, B., and J. Vessey. 1992. Pediatric discharge planning. *Pediatric Nursing* 18, no. 5:475–78.

Jarvis, C. 1996. *Physical examination and health assessment.* Philadelphia, PA: W.B. Saunders Co.

Lewis, C.L., et al. 1992. Care management for children who are medically fragile/technology-dependent. *Issues in Comprehensive Pediatric Nursing* 15:73-91.

Maturen, V.L., and K. Zander. 1993. Outcomes management in a prospective pay system. *Caring* 4:46-53.

Whaley, L., and D. Wong, eds. 1995. *Whaley & Wong's nursing care of infants and children.* St. Louis, MO: Mosby.

Pediatric Health History

Name: _____   Nickname: _____

Age: _____ Sex: _____   Date of Birth: _____

Address: _____   Phone: _____

_____

Mother's Name: _____   Work Phone: _____

Father's Name: _____   Work Phone: _____

Parents living together: _____

PHYSICIANS

Doctor: _____   Phone: _____

_____   Phone: _____

Diagnosis: _____

_____

FAMILY AND HOME DATA

Family Members (list names and ages)

Mother _____   Age _____

Father _____   Age _____

Sibling _____   Age _____

Sibling _____   Age _____

Sibling _____   Age _____

Sibling _____   Age _____

Description of home and community (observation for safety, location of equipment, availability of telephone, transportation) _____

_____

Caregiver Skills and Family Adjustment

Growing confidence and competence _____

Generally comfortable in caregiver role, relaxed, seems confident _____

_____

Seems overwhelmed _____   Many questions _____

Lack of interest _____   Anxious _____

Parents' participation as caregivers:

Mother _____   Father _____

Siblings: Adjusting well _____   Not adjusting _____

Support systems (involvement with agencies) _____

_____

Comments: _____

_____

Family Health History

Source of information _____

Note the occurrence within the family of any of the following conditions: asthma/allergies, diabetes, heart disease, hypertension, renal disease, stroke, cancer, alcoholism, drug abuse, hearing/vision loss, mental illness, mental retardation, deaths, headaches, anemia

Mother _____

_____

Father _____

_____

Siblings _____

_____

Maternal grandmother _____

_____

Maternal grandfather _____

_____

Paternal grandmother _____

_____

Paternal grandfather _____

_____

PAST HEALTH HISTORY

Prenatal History

Age of mother _____ Gr _____ Para _____ AB _____

Prenatal care (frequency, source) _____

_____

Complications of pregnancy (infections, bleeding, etc.) _____

_____

Alcohol (frequency, amount) _____ Smoking (packs/day) _____

_____ Injury _____ Weight gain _____

Caffeine _____ Radiographs _____
Medications _____

Birth History

Hospital _____ Address _____
_____
Gestational age _____ Type of delivery _____ Length of labor _____
Labor: Spontaneous _____ Induced _____
Presentation: Vaginal _____ Breech _____ Vertex _____
Medications used _____
Apgars __/__ Birth weight _____ Length _____ Head circumference _____
Comments: _____
_____

Newborn History

(Place a check mark near applicable items and explain in comment section.)
Respiratory difficulties _____ Infections _____ Surgical procedures _____ Jaundice _____
Seizures _____ Anemia _____ Physical abnormalities _____ Feeding problems _____
Temperature instability _____
Length of hospitalization: Newborn nursery _____
Intermediate nursing _____ ICU _____
Comments: _____
_____
_____

Allergies

Foods _____
Medications _____
Other _____

Accidents

_____
_____

Illnesses

Measles _____   Rubella _____
Chickenpox_____   Mumps _____
Scarlet fever _____   Strep throat _____
Meningitis_____   Hepatitis _____
Pneumonia _____   Otitis _____
Tuberculosis _____   Abscesses _____

Febrile convulsions_____   Pertussis _____
Other _____
_____

Previous Hospitalizations

_____
_____
Brief history of the most recent hospitalization _____
_____

HEALTH MAINTENANCE

Immunizations

DT or DPT (circle) 1   2   3   Booster 1   2
TOPV   1   2   3   Booster 1   2
MMR _____
Tetanus _____ Booster _____
Tine test _____
Other _____
Reactions _____

Screening Procedures

Hct. _____ Hbg. _____ T.B. _____ Eye exam _____
Hearing exam _____ Dental exam (source and frequency) _____

DEVELOPMENTAL HISTORY

Reflexes (indicate presence with a check mark).
Moro _____ Stepping _____ Rooting _____ Sucking _____ Tonic Neck _____
Grasping _____ Blinking _____
Development milestones: (list age acquired)

Hold up head_____	Responds to name _____
Smiles responsively _____	Cruise _____
Roll prone to supine _____	Walk _____
Roll supine to prone _____	Babble _____
Voluntary grasp-release	First word _____
of toys _____	Finger feed _____
Sit alone _____	Cup drink _____
Four-point crawl _____	Spoon feed _____
Pull to stand _____	

PERSONAL HISTORY

Activities/hobbies/play/toys (note special security toy) _____
_____
_____

Caregiver's description of the child's usual personality (include how child usually expresses emotion)
_____
_____

Parent-child interactions _____
_____

Special fears/concerns of child _____
_____
_____

Peer relationships _____
_____
_____

Idiosyncratic behaviors or habits (for example, thumb sucking, nail biting, temper tantrums, head banging)
_____
_____

SCHOOL HISTORY

Does child attend school? _____ Name of school _____
Current grade _____ Address _____
Favorite subjects _____
_____

Least favorite subjects _____
_____

History of past performance _____
_____

General attitudes about school/career plans _____
_____

DAILY PATTERNS

Feeding Patterns

Bottle _____ Special nipple _____ Breast fed _____ Cup _____ Nasogastric tube _____
Gastrostomy _____
Appetite _____ Schedule _____
Type of formula (amount, frequency) _____
Juices (amount, frequency) _____
Concerns/problems _____
_____

Sleep Patterns

Sleep schedule (include naps) _____
Crib _____ Bed _____ Bedwetter _____ Climber _____ Pacifier _____

Bedtime routine and/or sleeping positions _____

Problems/concerns _____

Elimination Patterns

Toilet trained: Urine _____ Bowel _____ Cloth diapers _____ Disposable diapers _____
Training pants _____ Potty chair _____ Other _____
Urinary habits (frequency, amount, color, odor) _____
Bowel habits (frequency, type, color) _____
Word(s) for bowel movements _____ Urination _____
Problems/concerns _____

Special Needs for Activities of Daily Living

Crutches _____ Wheelchair _____ Braces _____
Other _____
Braces for teeth or other oral appliances _____

Glasses _____ Contacts _____ Hearing aid _____ Wig _____
Bathing (frequency, method) _____
Discipline _____

Self-care: Feeding _____   Bathing _____
Dressing _____   Toileting _____
Do you have any problems/concerns with managing your child in the home? _____

SPECIAL CARE NEEDS

Source of information _____
Parental description of child's medical problems _____

Equipment (type, location, arrangement, and prescribed settings) _____

Suppliers

Name _____ Phone _____
Name _____ Phone _____

Treatments

Name _____ Frequency _____ Schedule _____
Name _____ Frequency _____ Schedule _____

Medications

Name _____ Frequency _____ Schedule _____
Name _____ Frequency _____ Schedule _____

R.N. Signature _____ Date Completed _____

Age-Specific Approaches to the Physical Examination

INFANT

Position:
- in parent's lap

Preparation:
- completely undress the infant, if room warm
- leave infant's diaper on
- distract with toys to gain cooperation
- parents may help to restrain for examination of ears, etc.
- move smoothly and slowly
- speak calmly

Sequence:
- usual head to toe
- perform auscultation when quiet
- perform traumatic procedures or examine painful areas at the end

TODDLER

Position:
- in parent's lap or standing by parent

Preparation:
- remove toddler's outer clothing
- allow to play with equipment or other toys during exam
- restrain only when necessary
- explain what is being done
- use positive reinforcement

Sequence:
- introduce equipment slowly
- try to auscultate when quiet in a calm, gentle manner
- perform traumatic procedures or examine painful areas at the end

PRESCHOOL CHILD

Position:
- usually cooperative
- prefers standing or sitting
- parent close by

Preparation:
- ask to undress self
- allow child to keep underwear on
- allow to inspect equipment
- give choices when appropriate
- use short simple requests
- use positive reinforcement

Sequence:
- head to toe, if cooperative
- if uncooperative, proceed as with the toddler

SCHOOL-AGE CHILD

Position:
- prefers sitting
- cooperative usually

Source: Data from *Whaley & Wong's Nursing Care of Infants and Children*, 1995.

- younger child wants parent present
- older child may prefer privacy

Preparation:
- ask to undress self
- allow child to keep underwear on
- give child choice of gown
- explain purpose of examination
- teach as you do examination

Sequence:
- head to toe
- respect need for privacy
- examine genitalia last

ADOLESCENT

Position:
- same as for school-age child
- offer parent to be present

Preparation:
- allow to undress in private
- have patient put on gown
- explain purpose of examination
- teach as you do examination
- explain results
- emphasize normalcy
- be matter of fact, calm, and gentle

Sequence:
- same as for school-age child

Environmental Assessment

HOUSE:

- safety of structure
- plumbing
- electrical
- heating and cooling
- ventilation
- steps

FOOD:

- adequate storage
- adequate nutrition

CLEANLINESS:

- rodents
- insects
- pets
- cluttered or neat

FURNITURE:

- adequate and appropriate
- clean

TELEPHONE:

- absent or present
- if absent, a plan in case of an emergency

NEIGHBORHOOD:

- access to public transportation
- safe
- access to stores

TOYS:

- clean
- safe
- age-appropriate

CLOTHING:

- clean
- age-appropriate
- season-appropriate

CHAPTER 3

Financing Pediatric Home Care

Wendy L. Votroubek

Financing of pediatric home care can be considered a problem that results from success (Office of Technology Assessment 1987). The success is the technologic and medical science advancements that have dramatically increased survival rates for children who would not have survived even 20 years ago. The problem is that health care is experiencing a financial crisis, and funds available to finance long-term care are limited (Weston and Keefe 1993). Payment sources have not kept pace with the needs of children requiring long-term care, and their families face total health care costs significantly higher than what many people will pay in a lifetime.

Issues discussed in this chapter include costs of home care, methods of financing, and funding considerations or strategies before and during the duration of home care.

COSTS OF HOME CARE

Home care costs can be divided into two categories. Start-up costs, the first category, are one-time costs incurred before or at the time of discharge. They include the costs of home improvements, supplies and equipment, and caregiver training. The second category, ongoing costs, includes items such as supplies and services needed for the duration of home care. Some of the items included in this category are nursing care, therapies, and disposable equipment.

Start-Up Costs

A common start-up cost is financing of home improvements or modifications required to accommodate special equipment and/or nursing staff (Anguzza 1996). These modifications may include widened doorways and ramps, room additions or remodeling, wiring and other electrical work, and special needs such as electric generators. Occasionally, home modifications are not sufficient and the family may need to move to a home that is more suitable or closer to a medical facility.

Frequently, supplies and equipment are the largest component of the start-up costs. Equipment will be either rented or purchased, depending on the length of its use and/or insurance benefits.

The last component of start-up costs is family and caregiver training. The family must be trained to perform all aspects of the child's care even when professional home care is not deemed necessary. The amount of training depends on the diagnosis, the child's condition, and the family's ability to understand the components of the care. The family of a ventilator-dependent child, for example, will normally require at least two to three weeks of training by nursing and therapy staff and a rooming-in period (Baroni 1996).

Ongoing Costs

Ongoing medical supplies are the items the family purchases on a continuing basis to provide care for the child at home. These may include ventilator tubings, suction catheters, insulin syringes, central line supplies, formulas, and feeding bags. Some of the most costly ongoing supplies are probably incurred by children requiring total parenteral nutrition (TPN). This is because the individualized formulas require special handling and storage, and expensive components such as predigested fats, carbohydrates, protein solutions, vitamins, and minerals (Office of Technology Assessment 1987).

Certain funding sources may or may not pay for necessary ongoing medical supplies. For example, nutritional supplements that are taken either by gastrostomy or orally are not paid for unless they are the only source of nutrition. Other supplies will be covered as long as there is professional nursing care in the home. Families should review their insurance policies to determine the durable medical equipment and supplies coverage. If there is a choice of vendors, families should compare costs to obtain the best combination of price and service. Disease-specific organizations (for example, the Muscular Dystrophy Association) or community agencies will occasionally assist with the purchase or rental of various medical supplies.

Nursing is the most expensive component of ongoing home care costs. Paid nursing hours vary from 0 to 24 hours a day because in the home, unlike the hospital, they are determined by family factors in addition to medical factors (Leonard, Brust, and Sielaff 1991).The number of hours allotted to a family caring for a medically needy child at home is normally recommended by the physician and hospital discharge team and is based on the severity of the child's medical condition, the family's willingness and ability to provide care, and the availability of services (nurses) in the community (Keens et al.

1990; Mallory and Stillwell 1991). The final determining factors in many cases, however, are the family's funding policy and home care restrictions.

Home care costs can equal or exceed hospital costs if the child requires 24 hours a day of paid nursing care and the family is unable or unwilling to provide medical care (Borfitz 1993). As families increase their provision of nursing care, however, third-party payers increase their savings. It is not surprising then that nursing care in the home is directly related to the funding source benefits and not necessarily the amount of care the child requires to be safely cared for in the home.

Treatments performed by occupational, physical, or speech therapists form another major expense. Many funding sources will pay for these therapists if they are prescribed by a physician and there is an observable patient gain. If the funding sources will not pay for these therapists, state or local agencies or schools may provide care (see Chapters 18 and 19).

Outpatient costs, including physician and laboratory services, are also incurred on an ongoing basis. Outpatient care may include well child follow-up, including immunizations; management of the disease process, including specialty care; and laboratory tests, especially for children on TPN or chemotherapy. Follow-up care may also include the services of a dietitian for the child with nutritional needs.

Another cost that should be considered is that of respite care. Respite care will increase the total costs of home care, but it gives the family relief from ongoing nursing care and may allow them to care for the child at home for a longer period. Respite care may be paid for by third-party payers or, in some cases, by state or county funds. Often, though, funding is not available and the child is hospitalized, put in temporary foster care, or cared for by relatives.

METHOD OF FINANCING

The population of technology-dependent and medically needy children is relatively small but uses a large percentage of health care resources. The extent to which health care, including home care, is available for medically needy and technology-dependent children depends largely on the availability of financing. This availability can be broken down into the following three factors: (1) the degree to which this population is covered by private insurance or public health care programs, (2) whether the funding source covers home care for the population (for the technology-dependent child it is ideal to have long-term coverage), and (3) whether the home care benefits are sufficient to finance most of the medical needs of the child (Office of Technology Assessment 1987).

The various sources of financing for home care are private insurance, managed care plans, Medicaid, Department of Defense (Civilian Health and Medical Program of the Uniformed Services [Champus]), and other programs and services. In addition to describing what each program typically pays for, this chapter discusses the potential problems specific to each source of payment.

Private Insurance

In the past, private insurance was the main source of coverage for children with serious illnesses (Fox 1986). The number of individuals currently receiving their health care coverage through private insurance has declined significantly during the last 10 years. In fact, one source states that in 1994, private insurance represented only 5.5 percent of the reimbursement for home care costs (Mefford 1994).

Private insurance provides varying levels of service based on the needs and the premiums the clients are willing to pay. Coverage depends on the individual or group policy. The most extensive insurance benefit packages are provided through group policies. Some insurance policies (managed indemnity plans) operate as managed care policies with contracted providers for both inpatient and outpatient care. Not all policies, however, include home care benefits and often

the consumer is unaware of this lack of coverage until services are needed.

Although many privately insured chronically ill or disabled children have group policy coverage, the remaining percentage that have individual insurance policies are likely to have substandard coverage. The individual insurance for these children might include insurance with riders that exclude coverage for treatment of the child's specific preexisting condition and any isolated problems. The riders may be temporary or lifetime, depending on the severity and type of diagnosis.

The main features of insurance coverage that can affect long-term home care are lifetime maximums, stop-loss provisions, and covered or limited services. Insurance companies frequently have expanded home coverage benefits to include higher maximum lifetime benefits and annual catastrophic stop-loss provisions. On the other hand, many firms still have no provisions for home health care benefits and/or the home care coverage is not sufficient to meet the needs of a child requiring ongoing nursing care. In addition, some employers may have increased cost-sharing requirements, with resultant higher employee co-payments and deductibles. Undoubtedly, the cost-sharing requirements place a financial hardship on many families with children that require any additional care.

Individual benefits/case management is a program available through many insurers that recognizes the potential savings of home care and may assist the consumer in negotiating through the maze of available services. This program allows for reimbursement of a wide range of home and community-based services, provided that their total cost is less than that of hospitalization. The case manager, in many instances, is a registered nurse who assists the family and home care agency in providing effective services. Almost all large carriers offer this kind of benefit. It may be found under titles such as individual case management, large claims management, or medical care management.

Managed Care Plans

Managed care plans are another source of home care financing. One example, the health maintenance organization (HMO) is a licensed health insurance plan with a network of health care providers contracted to provide a comprehensive range of inpatient and outpatient services. It is a closed network, which means members of an HMO must access the services of the contracted providers to obtain the service paid for by the HMO (Balinsky and Blumengold 1995).

Preferred provider organizations (PPOs) are another example of managed care plans. These plans offer subscribers a choice of either in- or out-of-network providers. Members are given incentives to use network providers (for example, a lower co-payment and paperless claim submission) (Simione 1995).

Managed care plans use a variety of techniques to manage utilization and contain costs, including utilization review, case management, and the use of primary care physicians and gatekeepers. Managed care plans outline the specific care that is available for subscribers and provide significant financial incentives for patients to use low-cost providers and procedures. Inpatient care is provided through hospitals that have a contract with the plan; outpatient care is available through contracted physicians and therapists.

Home care is normally available through contracted home care agencies with varying limitations on the amount and type of nursing care provided. Because home care agencies and managed care organizations share the common goal to provide quality services and reduce the total cost of services, outpatient and home care services are tightly managed (Dodd and Coleman 1994). For example, depending on the local HMO contract, nursing visits may be the only type of nursing care available.

HMOs usually provide discharge coordinators at a local level, thus streamlining the process of providing payment for home care services. The case coordinator is in contact with the patient's physician, discharge planner, and family, and arranges home care according to contracted providers. Rarely will a cost analysis of services need to be provided. Authorization for services occurs at the time of referral, with issuance of an authorization number for the expected duration of treatment. Ongoing care is authorized at regular, scheduled intervals.

The primary advantages of coverage through an HMO are lower or predictable costs and ensured access to care. The family's indirect costs are lower than when using traditional insurance. The disadvantages are the limitations imposed by contractual providers and services. Occasionally, the mandated home care providers do not have the experience or expertise required to provide care for medically fragile children.

As mentioned previously, ongoing nursing care in the home may not be a covered benefit. Also, physical therapy and/or occupational therapy home care visits, beyond an acute episode of care, may not be covered benefits. Families then have some options to help ensure ongoing care in the home for their medically needy and technology-dependent children. These include financial eligibility for additional resources and/or letters written by the physician to the managed care plan's medical director stating both the medical needs of a child and the need for ongoing nursing care to facilitate a safe discharge home. A family may also consider hiring a lawyer and demanding safe care that is medically necessary, provided in appropriate amounts, and rendered at the most appropriate level (Dodd and Coleman 1994). The difficulty with the latter two options is that they require a significant amount of time and energy on the part of both the physician and the family.

Medicaid

Medicaid is the largest public sector financing program that involves children and accounts for approximately 25 percent of all home care revenues (Kinslow 1996). Medicaid provides health insurance to needy and low-income persons through state-administered programs that are funded with a mix of state and federal moneys. Medicaid is currently administered at the federal level by the Health Care Financing Administration (HCFA) and at the state level by a designated department, usually the public health or social service agency. Families who are eligible for Aid to Families with Dependent Children (AFDC); supplementary security income (SSI); Early and Periodic Screening, Diagnosis, and Treatment (EPSDT); and certain other services are automatically eligible for Medicaid (Kaufman 1991). The benefits vary from state to state, both in services provided and level of care provided to enable recipients to remain in their own homes or to provide a less costly alternative to institutional care (Mefford 1994).

In 1981, the Katie Beckett waiver was designed to provide a home care option to children not normally covered under Medicaid. Katie, a ventilator-assisted child from Iowa, was eligible for SSI and Medicaid while hospitalized but would lose her benefits once she returned home, even though she required nursing care at home. Through an exception to HCFA policy, Katie was allowed to keep her Medicaid benefits and return home. The rationale used for this decision was based on the fact that Medicaid-funded home care was less costly than the level of care required in the hospital (Leonard, Brust, and Sielaff 1991).

The HCFA has since been authorized to issue waivers known as home and community-based waivers to states that request them. These states may elect to expand coverage to include services beyond their state Medicaid plan for special populations and may disregard family income (Weston and Keefe 1993). To have a waiver approved, states must show that the care to be provided will be less expensive than the cost of providing either hospital or institutional care and that the child requires home care that otherwise would necessitate institutional placement.

The waivers designate specific target populations, broaden the usual income eligibility process, and expand the range of home- and community-based services available under the state's Medicaid plan. The individuals served under the waiver program must be from one of the following Medicaid target groups: aged, disabled, or both; mentally retarded, developmentally disabled, or both; or mentally ill. States can serve more than one group by having more than one waiver. Services allowed through the waiver program vary but usually include those services not typically covered under Medicaid, such as the following: private duty nursing at the child's home; medical supplies and equipment; case management services; transportation services; respite care; rehabilitation services; speech, hearing, and language disorder therapy; minor home modifications; and certain preventative services (Kaufman 1991). Any of these above-mentioned services are available to participating states within their waivers, provided that the services are less costly than inpatient care and hospitalization.

There are problems associated with the waiver system that limit the availability of home care services for technology-dependent or medically needy children. However, even with insufficient information available to providers and planners, restricted state moneys, and restrictive federal regulations, the waivers do provide alternative settings of care for children who would otherwise receive care in institutions.

The waiver system is not the only route to home care services through Medicaid. A few states use EPSDT to provide services to children who fall under the basic Medicaid program. Through federal Medicaid law, EPSDT is available to all categorically needy beneficiaries younger than 21 years. Program services include comprehensive health assessments; immunizations; vision, dental, and hearing care; and treatment for any conditions discovered by the assessment, whether or not that service is covered by the state plan. For example, if physical therapy services are needed, the state must reimburse providers for these services even if they are not routinely covered. This significantly broadens access to Medicaid financing for children with special needs (Weston and Keefe 1993).

In the future, the Medicaid program as we know it today will look drastically different. States will receive a lump sum from the federal government and will outline how they will run their own welfare/medical programs (Berke 1996). All mandatory eligibility groups, services, and current waiver programs will be eliminated and states will be free to choose whatever services they want to offer. States will have the opportunity to expand eligibility with the financing generated by cost savings from a statewide managed care delivery system. However, with a cap on federal spending, it will be difficult to provide services to the current group of eligible recipients, let alone expand the program (Kinslow 1996).

Because Medicaid funding is crucial to the operation of most home care agencies, the obstacles outlined previously will require intensive state-level action. Home health agencies will also need to stress that without home care, many Medicaid patients will be forced to remain in hospitals or institutions that cost substantially more than care at home (Hoffmann 1996).

Children with Special Health Care Needs

Children with Special Health Care Needs (CSHCN), formerly Crippled Children's Services, is the nation's oldest, most direct, and sustained effort for support of children with chronic health problems (Hobbs, Perrin, and Ireys 1985). Started in 1935, it was the only major public source of support (state and federal mix) until Medicaid and other programs were started in the 1960s. Maternal and child health block grants in 1981 (under the Omnibus Budget Reconciliation Act) removed federal requirements for state services with resultant individual state appropriations and a financing formula usually requiring states to match every federal dollar with three state dollars. The Maternal Child Health Services Block Grants consolidated all Title V programs into the state programs for CSHCN, Maternal and Child Health Services, and Women's, Infants' and Children's Program (WIC), the supplementary food program for women, infants, and children (Kaufman 1991, Weston and Keefe 1993).

CSHCN provides care primarily through specialty clinics as opposed to the Medicaid method of reimbursing for services provided. Fees charged are based on the family's size, income, and resources, with children of low-income families receiving services free of charge. Because eligibility, conditions, and services covered under Medicaid and CSHCN vary from state to state, a child may have access to excellent care in one area and limited care in another. One state may offer no services to a child with cancer and the reverse may be true in another state.

CSHCN services range from basic hospitalization and surgical care to supported clinics and special health teams. The major focus of CSHCN services is clinic based, but some home care services are available. Services include skilled nursing care, extended home care services, outpatient visits, medications, supplies, and equipment. Some states provide certain services such as case management to fill gaps not covered by Medicaid, other purchased equipment, special formulas, and medications. The wide discretion available in implementation of state-covered CSHCN services can dramatically impact the availability of home care options.

Department of Defense/CHAMPUS

The Department of Defense (DOD) directly provides or pays for medical care for active-duty and retired military personnel and their dependents. Care is provided through DOD hospitals and CHAMPUS, which pays for care that is not available at the military hospitals.

The DOD pays for long-term care through the regular home health benefits available through CHAMPUS, the Program for the Handicapped (PFTH), and the Home Health Care (HHC) Demonstration Project. The benefits of the regular home health care program include durable medical equipment, including ventilators; oxygen; parenteral and enteral nutrition therapies; physical therapy; skilled nursing care; and medications, medical supplies, and physician visits. Custodial care, however, is not paid for or provided. If a child is considered to be receiving custodial care, he or she is eligible for only a small part of the usual home benefits. The benefits available in this case include medications, medical supplies, and up to one hour of nursing care per day.

The PFTH is a CHAMPUS program for handicapped or mentally retarded dependents of active-duty personnel. To be eligible, persons must demonstrate that services from public programs or institutions are not available. This program requires prior approval for coverage of all supplies and services; the ceiling for benefits is $1,000 per month. The services covered include diagnostic tests, rehabilitation, durable medical equipment, disposable supplies, transportation, and in-home nursing care, and are restricted to exclude those children who require custodial care.

CHAMPUS' third program for providing home care is the HHC Demonstration Project. This program provides comprehensive home care services for technology-dependent children in lieu of hospitalization. Services include medical and skilled nursing care, home health aides, medications, durable medical equipment and supplies, therapies, and related services. CHAMPUS also has a catastrophic protection plan, which limits out-of-pocket expenditures to $1,000 per year. Both of these projects target but are not limited to children of active-duty personnel who are receiving inpatient hospital care. Custodial care is not provided through this program. CHAMPUS is currently being reorganized to provide more choices for active-duty military and their dependents. Families will be able to choose between the traditional CHAMPUS programs and those more similar to a traditional indemnity plan. The plans will vary slightly from state to state.

Disease-Oriented Voluntary Agencies

Disease-oriented voluntary agencies are a source of support for chronically ill children.

Assistance with hands-on home care service is usually not available, but some important services are available, including limited medical services, therapies, access to special equipment, transportation, community services, family education and support, political lobbying, and research. Agencies often focus on one disease or a group of associated diseases, such as muscular dystrophy, spina bifida, or cystic fibrosis.

The disease-oriented organizations occasionally may be a source of payment of last resort. Even then, the services provided would be family education and support. Many of these organizations have small budgets and have been faced with a decrease in amount of available moneys in the past few years.

Grassroots Funding

Grassroots fund-raising has been used by some families to help pay for the cost of home care. Local fund-raising may be successful for a specific piece of equipment; however, it is difficult to raise the funds necessary for ongoing nursing care. The methods include bake sales, raffles, media coverage, and specialty projects for ventilator-dependent children. Local groups will occasionally assist by donating time instead of money.

FINANCIAL CONSIDERATIONS

Financing must constantly be considered during provision of home care. A financial assessment is a major requisite for home care. This assessment should ensure the adequacy of funding and outline the family's financial responsibility. Assessments are then performed at regular intervals to monitor payment of services, evaluate the family's ability to pay out-of-pocket expenses, and determine if the funding source can continue payment.

In this section, information is provided to help the family find funding necessary for care. Much of this information is presented throughout this chapter, but the important points are summarized in the following list to provide a more concise reference to the financing issues associated with home care:

- Anticipate home care needs at the time of hospital admission. Home care is now considered an option for medically needy and technology-dependent children and children with acute or chronic health care problems who have traditionally been cared for in hospitals (for example, the newly diagnosed patient with diabetes). Physicians, discharge planners, and primary nurses should anticipate and plan home care for many of the children who are admitted to the pediatric unit.
- Determine home care benefits early in the child's hospitalization. Will the funding source pay for home care? What level of skill is required and/or provided? Does the state have a waiver program? If so, what are its limitations? Does the physician need to intervene with the funding source and outline home care needs? These questions must be addressed early in the child's hospitalization.
- Choose an appropriate home care agency. Does the funding source have a preferred home care agency? Does the home care agency have experience with providing care to pediatric patients? Does the agency have qualified caregivers on call 24 hours a day? If an agency has a proven track record, the discharge planner may need to advocate accordingly.
- Investigate thoroughly the various funding programs available to help finance home care. Insurance companies and managed care plans may have case managers to help provide home care for certain medically needy children. The discharge planner and/or home care agency should query the funding sources to determine the availability of this service. Discharge planners and families also need to be aware of the federal Consolidated Omnibus Reconciliation Act (COBRA). This allows persons to continue insurance coverage either through group membership or individual policy conversions at a reasonable premium. This is especially important for families in which one or both parents have changed jobs and/or insurance carriers.
- Check benefits thoroughly when negotiating a new insurance policy. The insurance benefits should be reviewed thoroughly, especially if a person has the option of choosing from more than one policy. The areas of consideration are immediate coverage at time of birth, duration of coverage after birth, conditions of policy renewal and cancellation, and total benefits. An insurance agent or financial planner may be needed to assist in the translation of various insurance policies.
- Be cost conscious, especially with suppliers and equipment. Equipment may be leased or purchased based on the child's prognosis and estimated length of equipment use. The funding source, durable medical equipment company, and family should negotiate rental or purchase prices. Supplies may often be reused, saving the family and the funding source money. A durable medical equipment company or home care agency should instruct the family regarding the cleaning and storage of the various reusable supplies.
- Documentation is essential in payment of home care services. Some funding sources will not pay for instruction or teaching of certain elements of care. Home care agencies need to communicate with funding sources to determine what services may be billed.
- Families unable to care for their children with special needs in the home setting should be aware of the other available options, including the following: medical foster care, skilled nursing facilities, and daytime facility-based care. Both medical foster care and skilled nursing facilities are appropriate for out-of-home respite care.

Children in daytime facility-based care are medically fragile and have families that must maintain employment or daytime responsibilities (Donaghby and Wright 1993; Samaripa 1990).

- Nurses and other professionals providing pediatric home care can and need to be a voice in the politic process. An ideal time to influence the process is during budget deliberations. Strategies must be planned early and organized well. There are many opportunities during the process to let legislators know how their votes will affect sick children (Weston and Keefe 1993).

- In the future, home care providers will have to be more flexible and creative to respond to the many changes that are occurring. Other programs will need to be explored such as respite services or programs that

have limited, if any, reimbursement from traditional sources. Alternative funding options and care centers such as the daytime facility-based care, as mentioned previously, will also need to be created to meet the expanding needs (Mefford 1994).

Funding for home care will continue to be an issue. Although home care represents only 2.6 percent of the total amount of health care expenditures, it is the fastest growing segment of the market (Mefford 1994). Billions of dollars are needed to help balance the federal budget, with the potential for massive cuts in existing programs. The financing of pediatric home care will undoubtedly remain a problem. The information presented here will assist those who are confronted with these issues and minimize the problems that arise from success (Office of Technology Assessment 1987).

REFERENCES

Anguzza, R.Z. 1996. Pediatric home ventilation. *Journal for Respiratory Care Practitioners,* December/January, 81-84.

Balinsky, W. and J.G. Blumengold. 1995. Home care's integration into managed care. *Caring,* June, 36–44.

Baroni, D.M. 1996. Home sweet home. *Journal for Respiratory Care Practitioners,* December/January: 87–90.

Berke, R.L. 1996. Democrats are fat, happy and adrift. *The New York Times: Week in Review,* August 4: sec. 4.

Borfitz, D. 1993. The home care alternative for ventilator-dependent patients. *The Journal for Respiratory Care Practitioners,* June/July, 20–34.

Dodd, K., and J.R. Coleman. 1994. Home care & managed care: Prospective partners. *Caring,* March, 68–71.

Donaghby, B., and A.J. Wright. 1993. New home care choices for children with special needs. *Caring,* December, 47–50.

Fox, H. 1986. *Private health insurance coverage of chronically ill children.* Washington, D.C.: Fox Health Policy Consultants.

Hobbs, N., J. Perrin, and H. Ireys. 1985. Patterns of paying for care. In *Chronically ill children and their families,* ed. N. Hobbs, J. Perrin, and H. Ireys. San Francisco: Jossey-Bass Publishers.

Hoffmann, N.E. 1996. Cost effectiveness is key to the future of Medicare and Medicaid. *Caring,* March, 5–8.

Kaufman, J. 1991. An overview of public sector financing for pediatric home care: Part 1. *Pediatric Nursing* 17 (May/June): 280–81.

Keens, T.G., et al. 1990. Home care for children with chronic respiratory failure. *Seminars in Respiratory Medicine* 11, no. 3:269–81.

Kinslow, M. 1996. Medicaid in 1996: Opportunities and challenges. *Caring,* March, 36–45.

Leonard, B.J., J.D. Brust, B.H. Sielaff. 1991. Determinants of home care nursing hours for technology assisted children. *Public Health Nursing* 8, no. 4:239–44.

Mallory, G.B., and P.C. Stillwell. 1991. The ventilator-dependent child: Issues in diagnosis and management. *Archives of Physical Medicine and Rehabilitation,* 72:43–55.

Mefford, J. 1994. Funding alternatives for home care agencies. *Caring,* April, 4–7, 58–60.

Office of Technology Assessment. 1987. Technology-dependent children: Hospital vs. home care—A technical memorandum. Washington, D.C.: U.S. Government Printing Office.

Samaripa, J. 1990. Kangaroo kids: Jumping into full-service pediatrics. *Homecare: The Business Newsmagazine of the Home Health Industry, a Miramar Publication.*

Simione, W. 1995. Capitation. *Caring,* June, 24–34.

Weston, B.E., and J.A. Keefe. 1993. Pediatric home care and public policy. *Caring,* 60–64.

CHAPTER 4

Care of the High-Risk Infant

Anne S. Klijanowicz

Advances in neonatal care have markedly improved the survival rate for all low–birth-weight and preterm infants. Generally accepted definitions to describe this high-risk population are provided in Table 4–1. Smaller, less mature infants with complex medical problems have increasingly been discharged from neonatal intensive care units to the home. For several reasons, these infants are at greater risk for developmental problems throughout infancy and early childhood (Hack et al. 1994). Parents and professional caretakers face many challenges in managing the medical conditions and optimizing the development of these special infants. This chapter addresses issues related to growth and development as well as special considerations for general infant care. Common medical conditions and their related management are described. Unique family issues are identified and resources are provided for parents and professional care providers. More extensive coverage of this important topic is found in a related text, *Home Care for the High-Risk Infant* (Ahmann 1996).

COMMON ISSUES IN GROWTH AND DEVELOPMENT

Nutrition and Growth

Growth patterns of the high-risk infant require careful monitoring. Parameters including weight, length, head circumference, and weight for length should be plotted at regular intervals on a standard growth chart using the infant's adjusted age. This adjustment should be continued until two or three years of age, at which point the difference is no longer significant (Bernbaum and Hoffman-Williamson 1991). Growth outcomes for high-risk infants are variable but usually deviate from expected norms. After an initial period of growth delay associated with the acute neonatal course, infants generally stabilize and then enter a period of accelerated growth. This catch-up growth usually occurs during the first two years of life, with maximal growth rates between 36 and 40 weeks after conception. Optimal nutritional intake is essential during this phase to maximize growth potential. Little catch-up growth occurs after three years chronologic age (Ross, Lipper, and Auld 1990). Table 4–2 summarizes growth patterns of concern in preterm infants. Such findings require further exploration of potential causes.

Breast milk is nutritionally well suited to the needs of preterm infants, providing, among other advantages, anti-infective factors and digestibility. Breast milk requires supplementation with human milk fortifier or preterm formulas until the infant reaches 2,000 grams in weight. Longer periods of supplementation are often required for infants with chronic illnesses. A daily multivitamin is required to achieve adequate vitamin and mineral intake. Detailed information about infant formulas is presented in Chapter 8. Bottle-fed infants may also require a

Table 4–1 Definitions of Terms Related to Prematurity

Term	Definition
Prematurity	Gestational age of less than 37 weeks
Low birth weight (LBW)	Birth weight less than 2,500 g
Very low birth weight (VLBW)	Birth weight less than 1,500 g
Extremely low birth weight (ELBW)	Birth weight less than 1,000 g
Small for gestational age (SGA)	Birth weight significantly less than expected for gestational age, indicating intrauterine growth retardation
Adjusted (corrected) age	Chronologic age minus the number of weeks born prematurely

multivitamin supplement if not consuming enough formula to meet the recommended daily allowance for vitamin requirements (Bernbaum and Hoffman-Williamson 1991).

Healthy, premature infants generally require 110 to 130 kcal/kg/day to achieve adequate growth. Chronically ill infants may need up to 200/kcal/kg/day (Ackerman 1994). Caloric intake should be gradually increased until weight gain is satisfactory. The most obvious way to accomplish this is to increase the volume and/or frequency of feedings, although this is not possible for some infants. Breastfeeding may be augmented through use of a supplemental nursing system. When necessary, the caloric content of feedings can be increased by concentrating formula or addition of carbohydrate or microlipid supplements. This should be done only after consultation with the infant's physician or nutritionist because caution is required to main-

Table 4–2 Growth Patterns in Preterm Infants

Parameter	Pattern
Weight	Failure to gain Decrease in weight Decrease in percentile for age
Length	Cessation of growth Decrease in percentile for age
Weight for length	Less than the 5th percentile Downward sloping curve
Head circumference	Measurement above the 95th percentile or increase greater than 1.75 cm/week[1] Measurement levels off at five to six months of age

[1] Hack, M., and A.A. Fanaroff. Growth Patterns in the ICN Graduate. In ed. R.A. Ballard. *Pediatric Care of the ICN Graduate*, Philadelphia, W.B. Saunders, 1988, pp. 33–39.

Source: Data from C. Lierman, Nutrition and Feeding of the Chronically Ill Infant, in *Home Care for the High-Risk Infant,* E. Ahmann, ed., pp.120–21, © 1996, Aspen Publishers, Inc.

tain the appropriate caloric distribution of nutrients and ensure maintenance fluid intake. Infants receiving higher osmolality feedings should be monitored closely for symptoms of intolerance, such as vomiting or diarrhea (Bernbaum and Hoffman-Williamson 1991). Tube feedings may be required for infants who are unable to take adequate calories by mouth. Refer to Chapter 8 for additional information about increasing caloric content and tube feedings.

It is recommended that low–birth-weight infants receive supplemental iron (2 mg/kg/day to a maximum of 15 mg/day) beginning at two months chronologic age (Committee on Nutrition 1993). This is usually provided in the form of iron-fortified formula, multivitamin with iron, or ferrous sulfate drops. Iron supplementation should continue until the infant is consuming enough iron-rich solid foods, usually for 6 to 12 months (Hagedorn and Gardner 1991). Solid foods can be introduced when developmentally appropriate, following recommendations for full-term infants, using adjusted age. High caloric, nutritious foods should be selected to supplement, not replace, high-caloric formula feedings (Ahmann 1996).

Feeding disorders are relatively common in preterm infants and often relate to a combination of physiologic, environmental, and behavioral factors. Infants should be assisted to develop regular schedules so that infants are fed when they are fully alert and give cues of being hungry. Environmental distractions should be reduced as much as possible (Wolff and Lierman 1994). Successful feeding is also facilitated by positioning the infant with the neck in a neutral midline position or slightly flexed. The feeder's thumb and finger can be used to provide jaw stabilization during bottle feeding to improve the infant's seal on the nipple. Effective sucking and a smooth suck-swallow-breathe pattern require a nipple of appropriate size, length, and consistency. A soft, small nipple is useful for a young infant with a weak suck. Older infants may do better with a more firm, crosscut nipple. Experimentation with various nipples is often required to meet the infant's needs (Lierman 1996). Con-

sultation with an infant-feeding specialist may be helpful when difficulties with feeding skills interfere with nutritional intake and growth. Parents require support and encouragement to deal with the stress, frustration, and anxiety that accompany feeding disorders and interfere with parent-infant bonding (Bernbaum and Hoffman-Williamson 1991). Additional suggestions for encouraging the development of infant-feeding skills are found in Chapter 18.

Development and Behavior

Premature infants lack neurologic maturation and typically display different developmental patterns than healthy, full-term infants. In addition, these infants are more likely to experience mild to moderate developmental problems. When assessing developmental progress, it is important to form expectations based on the infant's adjusted age. Even then, progress may be slow in the first year. Variations in the sequence of skill development and interest of infants are common. It is not unusual for preterm infants to demonstrate transient neuromuscular abnormalities, which usually disappear by 18 months of age (Bernbaum and Hoffman-Williamson 1991).

The home care nurse is in a unique position to contribute to developmental assessment through observation of the infant and family in their familiar setting. Observation should include the quality of muscle tone, noting any asymmetries or posturing as well as acquisition of fine motor and gross motor skills. The infant's ability to attend to tasks and adapt to new circumstances should also be evaluated. Behavioral issues such as irritability, impulsivity, and abnormalities of responsiveness should be noted. Interactions will be most successful when the infant demonstrates signs of readiness including relaxed muscle tone, flexion of extremities, and quiet, alert state. Such periods should gradually increase in frequency and duration as the infant matures (Bernbaum and Hoffman-Williamson 1991). Techniques for increasing periods of readiness and other management strategies are presented in Chapter 18.

Involvement of the family is absolutely key to maximizing infant development (Infant Health and Development Program 1990). The nurse should assess the family's knowledge of child development and its ability to provide adequate support to the infant. Parental expectations and concerns about infant development should be identified. The nurses should assist in explaining developmental needs to parents in ways that are meaningful based on the family's socio-economic and cultural framework (Huber, Holditch-Davis, and Brandon 1993). Parents require information about normal development in relation to their own infant's medical problems and need to be aware of the infant's strengths as well as areas of delay (Diehl, Moffitt, and Wade 1991). Medical jargon and the use of diagnostic labels should be avoided. The nurse should model and teach appropriate developmental stimulation activities to parents. Bonding and the development of trust can be facilitated by supporting parents in meeting their infant's needs and establishing regular routines. The nurse should help parents monitor the infant's tolerance for developmental stimulation and plan activities that ensure physiologic stability. Activities should be suggested that can easily be incorporated into daily routines such as feeding and diapering (Ahmann and Klockenbrink 1996). Finally, the nurse should help parents identify and access necessary developmental services for the infant. Recent legislation including Part H of Public Law (P.L.) 99-457, the Individuals with Disabilities Education Act (IDEA), has encouraged states to provide services for developmentally delayed or atrisk children from birth to three years of age. Admission criteria and processes vary somewhat by state. Available services including audiology, speech and language pathology, physical and occupational therapy, special education, psychological services, and parent/family training and counseling are provided, with certain exceptions, at no cost to the family (Stepanek 1996).

Vision

Preterm infants, especially those of very low birth weight, are at risk for severe visual impairment secondary to retinopathy of prematurity (ROP), a proliferative vascular disease of the retina, which, in severe cases, can lead to retinal detachment and blindness. Surgical intervention including cryotherapy or laser techniques may be indicated to control disease progression or to prevent or correct retinal attachment. Even in the absence of ROP, other ophthalmologic problems including strabismus and refractive errors occur with increased frequency in infants of very low birth weight (McGinnity and Bryars 1992). Most premature infants receive at least one ophthalmologic evaluation before discharge from the neonatal intensive care unit (NICU). The home care nurse should be aware of the results of such examinations and whether ophthalmologic follow-up is required. All preterm infants should be observed for major visual milestones, such as fixating and following, hand regard, and evidence of the development of eye-hand coordination (Schraeder 1996).

Hearing

The preterm infant's immature auditory system is at risk for damage by many stressors, including hypoxia, environmental noise, hyperbilirubinemia, infection, and ototoxic drugs (Bernbaum and Hoffman-Williamson 1991). Most preterm infants meet criteria for audiologic evaluation established by the Joint Committee on Infant Hearing (1994). Screening is usually by means of the brainstem auditory evoked response (BAER) and occurs before hospital discharge or before three months of age. The home care nurse should be aware of screening results and whether further evaluation or follow-up is indicated. Nursing assessment should include careful observation of the infant's response to sound and development of speech. Rescreening is indicated for certain infants and toddlers including those who require ototoxic medications or experience persistent otitis media with effusion for at least three months (Joint Committee on Infant Hearing 1994).

Speech and Language

Many factors place the preterm infant at risk for speech and language difficulties. Periods of inactivity, feeding disorders, and oral defensiveness predispose the infant to poor development of the muscles used in speech. Excessive environmental stimulation may create difficulties in learning to attend to relevant auditory and visual stimuli. In addition, the extensive attention that these infants often require reduces their need for expression (Jackson 1996). Exhibit 4–1 provides some specific suggestions that the nurse can use to stimulate language development during usual interactions with the infant. Further evaluation is indicated for infants and toddlers who fail to achieve age-adjusted language milestones. Chapter 17 provides more detailed information about communication intervention. Cognitive development is addressed in Chapter 15.

SPECIAL CONSIDERATIONS FOR USUAL INFANT CARE

Immunizations

The American Academy of Pediatrics recommends that preterm infants receive full doses of all immunizations at the same chronologic ages as recommended for full-term infants (Committee on Infectious Disease 1994). The same contraindications for pertussis vaccine in the full-term infant apply to premature infants. Oral polio vaccine is not administered to hospitalized infants or those with human immunodeficiency virus (HIV), acquired immune deficiency syndrome (AIDS), or with immunodeficient or HIV-positive household contacts. Inactivated polio vaccine (IPV) is given in these situations. High-risk infants such as those with bronchopulmonary dysplasia (BPD), symptomatic heart disease, or immunosuppression who are older

Exhibit 4–1 Interventions To Stimulate Language Development

1. Talk to the child often.
2. Talk to the child normally and use simple sentences.
3. Listen to what the child says.
4. Leave time for the child's response during conversations.
5. Encourage the child to use his or her voice to indicate wants and needs.
6. Tell the child what you are doing during all direct care. Name body parts during bathing and dressing.
7. Point out and name new and familiar objects and people in the child's environment.
8. Read age-appropriate books.
9. Watch age-appropriate, child-oriented television programs with the child (for example, *Mr. Rogers' Neighborhood*, *Sesame Street*).
10. Play social games such as peek-a-boo and pat-a-cake.
11. Encourage reciprocal vocal play. Play games that include sound imitations (for example, animal sounds, car sounds, sound-making toys).
12. Sing with and to the child. Listen to child-oriented audiotapes.
13. Include the child in normal family social activities like mealtimes.

Source: Reprinted with permission from *Pediatric Nursing*, Vol. 20, No. 2, p. 152, © Jannetti Publications, Inc.

than six months should receive influenza immunization. Family members and care providers, including home care nurses, should also be immunized against influenza. The nurse should be aware of the infant's immunization schedule and the usual effects of the vaccines.

Sleep

Immature sleep patterns are common in preterm infants. Neurologic immaturity and nutritional needs often rouse the infant every two hours until three or four months adjusted age. In addition, the infant may experience difficulty transitioning from the hospital to home environment. Lengthy sleep periods may not occur until six to eight months of age. Medication and treatment schedules should be arranged to minimize disruption of the nighttime hours for the infant and family (Ahmann 1996).

Irritability and Crying

Premature infants are more likely to demonstrate abnormal patterns of crying and irritability. In addition, the cry of the preterm infant is perceived as more irritable because of its higher frequency and more frequent pitch shifts (Bernbaum and Hoffman-Williamson 1991). Irritable crying is frustrating and worrisome for most parents. They may require assistance to understand their infant's temperament and support in developing effective calming strategies.

Travel

Because preterm infants are at risk for hypoventilation in a car seat, it is recommended that they be assessed using a pulse oximeter before discharge from the hospital (Willett et al. 1989). Special arrangements may be required for some very small infants (Committee on Injury and Poison Prevention and Committee on Fetus and Newborn 1991). Proper positioning can be ensured by placing blanket rolls on both sides of the infant's body for head and trunk support and between the crotch strap and the infant to reduce slouching. Necessary medical equipment should be secured with adjacent seat belts, wedged on the floor, or placed under the seats (Goldman, Goldman, and Hirata 1996). Travel should be minimized for infants at risk for respiratory compromise and care providers should be pre-

pared for potential emergencies. A small travel bag can be assembled with necessary equipment for travel. For infants requiring oxygen or ventilatory support, planning is necessary to ensure an adequate gas supply during travel and at the destination.

Safety

It is important that the home environment be safe for the preterm infant, family, and care providers. In addition to general safety precautions, specific issues related to home care equipment, supplies, and procedures should be addressed. Medications and syringes should be secured safely away from young children. Needles and contaminated materials require safe disposal. Control panels of ventilators, monitors, and other equipment should be covered with clear plastic panels or have dials taped so that children are unable to change equipment settings. Safety covers should be placed over electrical outlets when not in use. Unused equipment should be unplugged, and any wires should be stored out of reach. Extra tubing and long wires should be coiled and secured to prevent accidental strangulation of the technology-assisted infant during sleep. An inexpensive intercom or infant monitor can assist parents to hear equipment alarms at night (Ahmann 1996). Safety concerns related to specific types of equipment and procedures are reviewed in subsequent chapters.

Outcome

Definitive conclusions about the outcomes of morbidity and mortality for preterm infants are lacking because existing studies differ widely in identified populations, assessment techniques, definitions of handicapping conditions, and ages at which infants are studied (Bregman and Kimberlin 1993). Overall, survival has improved significantly over the last 15 years. Poor outcome is related to the associated complications of prematurity, the effects of which are often cumulative. Because the smallest infants have the most complications, the worst outcome is in the smallest infants (Goldman, Goldman, and Hirata 1996). Although the majority of low–birth-weight survivors experience positive outcomes, the rate of severe disabilities has been reported as 4.5 to 10 percent. Recent studies have also reported increasingly higher incidences of mild learning deficits interfering with school achievement for this population (Bernbaum and Hoffman-Williamson 1991). Home nursing care should be directed toward optimizing outcomes through careful attention to the complex medical and developmental concerns that these infants experience.

Family Issues

Parents of preterm infants experience a multitude of unique issues (Able-Boone and Stevens 1994). They are often unprepared for their new roles associated with the unexpected birth of their infant. Common emotions include guilt, anxiety, anger, and helplessness. Even with supportive care in the neonatal intensive care unit (NICU), many parents lack confidence in their ability to provide care and make decisions. The home care nurse should use every opportunity to assist parents in reestablishing their rightful role. Chapter 20 provides some specific recommendations for achieving this goal. Selected resources for parents are identified at the end of this chapter (see Appendix 4–A).

COMMON MEDICAL CONDITIONS

Gastroesophageal Reflux

Gastroesophageal reflux (GER) refers to the return flow of acidic gastric contents from the stomach into the esophagus, caused by an incompetent lower esophageal sphincter. Symptoms of GER include recurrent vomiting or gagging and discomfort associated with esophagitis. The condition is more common in premature infants and may lead to apnea, bradycardia, and aspiration pneumonia (Armentrout 1995). Management of GER is discussed in Chapter 8.

Ricketts

Preterm infants are at risk for the development of nutritional ricketts because almost all aspects of vitamin D metabolism are affected by the premature birth. Those infants with birth weights less than 1,000 grams are at greatest risk. Additional risk factors include long-term furosemide therapy, creating increased renal calcium losses and prolonged parental nutrition resulting in mineral deficiencies and/or liver dysfunction. Treatment of ricketts includes dietary supplementation and use of alternative diuretics such as spironolactone and hydrochlorothiazide when possible (Bernbaum and Hoffman-Williamson 1991).

Short Bowel Syndrome

Short bowel syndrome (SBS) refers to a constellation of signs and symptoms of malabsorption and malnutrition resulting from decreased intestinal length or function. The most common cause of SBS in preterm infants is necrotizing enterocolitis (NEC) requiring significant bowel resection (Huddleston 1996). Chapter 8 includes more extensive information about short bowel syndrome.

Inguinal Hernias

Inguinal hernias are more common in preterm infants, especially in those born at less than 32 weeks' gestation or weighing less than 1,250 grams. Surgical repair is indicated for inguinal hernias due to the risk of bowel incarceration. Because premature infants are at greater risk for apnea, anesthesia morbidity, and other postoperative complications, careful observation is required after surgery. Until surgical repair is accomplished, care providers should know how to reduce the hernia and be able to recognize signs of strangulation (Bernbaum and Hoffman-Williamson 1991).

Nephrocalcinosis

Infants of very low birth weight are at increased risk for developing renal calcification, or nephrocalcinosis. The incidence is notably increased in infants who require chronic administration of furosemide, which inhibits calcium reabsorption. Renal ultrasounds may be performed to monitor disease progress and screen for calculi (Greenough 1990). Furosemide is discontinued as soon as possible. Chlorothiazide, which decreases calcium excretion, may be added (Alpert, Allen, and Schidlow 1993). Infants with nephrocalcinosis should be observed for signs of renal stones including infection, obstruction, and irritability due to renal colic (Bernbaum and Hoffman-Williamson 1991).

Intraventricular Hemorrhage

Intraventricular hemorrhage (IVH) refers to bleeding that occurs in and around the brain. The immature brain of the preterm infant contains highly vascular areas that are poorly supported by tissue mass, predisposing to hemorrhage. The incidence of IVH is inversely related to age, occurring in approximately 40 percent of infants less than 32 weeks' gestation or less than 1,500 grams (Volpe 1995). IVH has been classified into four grades, with Grade IV being the most extensive. Serial ultrasound examinations are performed to document resolution of the hemorrhage and to detect anatomic sequelae such as hydrocephalus. Infants should also be monitored clinically for signs of increased intracranial pressure and delayed neurodevelopmental progress. Increased intracranial pressure may be manifested by unusual increase in head circumference or widely split sutures, full or tense anterior fontanelle, irritability or vomiting, alterations in baseline behavior and activity level, or downward deviation of the eyes (Bernbaum and Hoffman-Williamson 1991). Such symptoms require prompt medical evaluation.

Hydrocephalus

Hydrocephalus refers to an accumulation of cerebrospinal fluid (CSF) within the brain. In preterm infants, hydrocephalus may result from IVH. Temporary management of hydrocephalus may include medications that decrease the production of CSF or serial lumbar punctures to divert CSF. If these measures fail to control hydrocephalus, a permanent shunt is surgically implanted. Most commonly, a ventriculoperitoneal (VP) shunt is used to divert CSF from the ventricle to the peritoneal space (Bernbaum and Hoffman-Williamson 1991).

Infants with VP shunts require observation for symptoms of shunt malfunction, including obstruction and infection. Assessment of the infant should include level of orientation, alertness, and behavior and sleep patterns. Serial measurements of the head circumference should be recorded. The nurse should also palpate the anterior fontanelle for unusual fullness and the cranial suture lines for appreciable splitting or overlapping. The shunt insertion site, shunt tract, and abdominal incision site should be inspected. Unless specifically instructed by the neurosurgeon, the shunt reservoir should not be pumped. A complete assessment also includes observation of the infant's eye movements and monitoring of the bowel elimination pattern (Bird and Ahmann 1996). In addition to signs of increased intracranial pressure, complications may be indicated by fever, erythema, tenderness, or swelling along the shunt tract or abdominal tension and tenderness. These symptoms should be reported promptly to the infant's physician.

Bronchopulmonary Dysplasia

Definition

Bronchopulmonary dysplasia refers to a complex of pathologic changes in the lungs of affected infants, resulting in chronic respiratory disease. BPD occurs most frequently in preterm infants after treatment of respiratory distress syndrome. The disorder occurs occasionally in full-term infants after pneumonia, meconium aspiration syndrome, and other conditions that require treatment with mechanical ventilation and supplemental oxygen.

Incidence

The reported incidence of BPD varies with the characteristics of the population described and the diagnostic criteria used. The risk of BPD clearly increases with lower birth weight and gestational age (Parker, Lindstrom, and Cotton 1992). The impact of new therapies such as surfactant, steroids, and high-frequency ventilation is unclear. Although improved outcomes have been demonstrated, the overall incidence of BPD has not decreased primarily because of the survival of smaller infants (Abman and Groothius 1994).

Etiology

The BPD process begins with cellular injury to the immature lung caused by high-pressure ventilation and supplemental oxygen necessary to sustain life. Initial lung injury causes release of toxic oxidants and proteolytic enzymes that initiate a persistent inflammatory process, eventually leading to bronchiolar changes including edema, fibrosis, and smooth muscle hypertrophy (Rozycki and Kirkpatrick 1993). The development of BPD can be simplified by the following equation: immaturity + oxygen + pressure + time = BPD (Merritt, Northway, and Boynton 1988). Changes in lung function include decrease in lung compliance, increase in pulmonary resistance, and variable degrees of hypoxemia and hypercapnia (Ackerman 1994).

Clinical Manifestations

Infants with BPD demonstrate a range of respiratory symptoms including tachypnea, tachycardia, and retractions. Wheezing or prolonged exhalation is observed in some infants. Chest auscultation may reveal wheezes, crackles, or uneven air entry. Cyanosis and activity intolerance with feeding and handling are common findings (Harvey 1996). Extrapulmonary complications may include neurodevelopmental delay, feeding difficulties, and poor growth. Underlying pulmonary disease may also result in cor pulmonale, a cardiac condition in which the right ventricle becomes enlarged (Guidelines for Care of Children 1989).

Treatment

The natural course of BPD is one of gradual improvement for the majority of patients, within the first two years of life. The goals of treatment are to minimize lung damage, promote growth of new lung tissue, maintain oxygen saturation, and prevent complications (Guidelines for Care of Children, 1989). Treatment modalities include oxygen therapy, medications, and nutritional supplementation (discussed previously in this chapter and in Chapter 9). Some infants benefit from postural drainage and chest percussion (refer to Chapter 5). In severe cases, management requires tracheostomy and mechanical ventilation (refer to Chapter 5). Occupational, physical, and speech therapies are essential components of care for many infants (refer to Chapters 17 and 18).

Oxygen. Management of hypoxia is a cornerstone of therapy for BPD. The need for supplemental oxygen varies with the severity of lung dysfunction. Some parents are reluctant to use adequate oxygen, fearing that it may cause further injury to the lung. They require encouragement and explanation of its essential role in decreasing respiratory effort while maximizing nutrition and preventing or decreasing pulmonary hypertension. When indicated, oxygen is usually delivered using a nasal cannula. The infant's color and respiratory status should be observed carefully during periods of sleep and activity for any signs of inadequate oxygenation. A pulse oximeter is sometimes used in the home setting to adjust oxygen administration within prescribed guidelines. Once the infant is clinically stable and gaining weight, a gradual, stepwise weaning process is usually initiated by the physician. The home care nurse should be familiar with the weaning schedule, carefully assess the infant, and report any difficulties with the weaning process. During periods of illness, it may be necessary to increase the amount of supplemental oxygen or restart it temporarily if the infant has recently been weaned. Parents should receive anticipatory guidance so that they do not become overly discouraged if this occurs. The home care nurse should reinforce teaching about infant assessment and the proper use of oxygen equipment as well as assess the home environment for compliance with safety guidelines. More extensive information about oxygen therapy is found in Chapter 5.

Medications. Several medications are used to treat BPD (Table 4–3). Diuretics are used to correct fluid retention, prevent fluid overload, decrease pulmonary resistance, and increase pulmonary compliance (Brem 1992). Because of the potential for electrolyte imbalance associated with diuretic therapy, serum electrolytes are monitored at regular intervals. Supplementation may be required, usually with potassium chloride. Nutritional requirements must be balanced with fluid restriction to avoid overloading the cardiopulmonary system (Harvey 1996). Bronchodilators are used to relax airway smooth muscles, reducing the effects of bronchoconstriction. These drugs are often administered via nebulizer or by using a metered-dose inhaler with a spacer and mask. The nurse should be skilled in these methods of administration. Oral or inhaled corticosteroids may be used for their anti-inflammatory effect. Medication schedules should be tailored as much as possible to the family's daily schedule. A medication checklist can help eliminate errors such as missed or extra doses. When administering medications, the dose and concentration on each container should be compared with those prescribed (Page 1996). The home care nurse should review the purpose, dosage, and administration methods for each medication with the parents or significant caregiver. Side effects and safety issues regarding proper storage of medications should also be discussed. Side effects of medication treatment should be brought to the physician's attention immediately.

Infection Control

Infection is the major cause of rehospitalization, late morbidity, and mortality in infants with BPD (Cunningham, McMilan, and Gross 1991). Environmental exposures should be minimized by avoiding large crowds and individuals with upper respiratory infections. Other principles of infection control include good handwashing by all caretakers and proper cleaning of equipment (Ackerman 1994). The infant with BPD should be routinely observed for signs of infection and should undergo early evaluation and close follow-up for any respiratory illness.

Nursing Care

A nursing care plan for a child with BPD is included in Appendix 4–B.

CARDIORESPIRATORY MONITORING

High-risk infants may require cardiorespiratory monitoring for a variety of problems. Indications for monitoring are summarized in Exhibit 4–2. Cardiorespiratory monitors are sometimes used for other groups of infants, including those with less severe apparent life-threatening events (ALTEs), siblings of sudden infant death syndrome (SIDS) victims, infants with tracheostomies, preterm infants with serious residual problems, and infants of opiate- or cocaine-abusing mothers (National Institutes of Health 1987).

Definition of Terms

Apnea

Apnea refers to cessation of respiration. It may be central, when there is no chest movement and absence of respiratory effort; obstruc-

Table 4–3 Medications Used in the Management of BPD

Medication*	Use	Common Side Effects
Bronchodilators	For relief or prevention of bronchospasm (several bronchodilators may be used in combination)	
Xanthine derivatives (oral) Aminophylline (Somophyllin) Theophylline (TheoDur, Slo-phyllin, Slo-bid)		Irritability, insomnia, palpitations, tachycardia, nausea, vomiting, anorexia
Beta agonists (oral, inhaled) Metaproterenol (Alupent, Metaprel) Terbutaline (Brethine) Albuterol (Proventil, Ventolin)		Insomnia, nervousness, tremor, palpitations, tachycardia (all side effects are transient with inhaled preparations); oral preparations may aggravate gastroesophageal reflux
Anticholinergics (inhaled) Atropine Ipratropium bromide (Atrovent)	May be used in conjunction with or as a substitute for beta agonists	Dry mouth, may irritate cough (if inadvertently sprayed into eyes, may irritate eyes or have transient visual effects)
Corticosteroids (oral, inhaled) Prednisone (Liquid Pred) Prednisolone (Pediapred, Prelone) Dexamethasone (Decadron) Flunisolide (Aerobid) Triamcinolone (Azmacort) Beclomethasone (Beclovent, Vanceril)	Anti-inflammatory effects; decrease inflammation of airways	Irritability, hypertension, infection, growth alteration, gastric irritation; considerably fewer side effects with inhaled preparations
Cromolyn sodium (inhaled) (Intal)	Inhibits bronchoconstrictive reaction to inhaled antigens; attenuates bronchospasm caused by exercise, cold air, environmental pollutants	
Digitalis	For cor pulmonale complicating bronchopulmonary dysplasia	Fatigue, muscle weakness, agitation, anorexia, nausea, cardiotoxicity
Diuretics Furosemide (Lasix) Chlorothiazide (Diuril) Spironolactone (Aldactone)	For fluid retention with cor pulmonale	Dehydration, electrolyte imbalances

continues

Table 4–3 continued

Medication*	Use	Common Side Effects
Electrolytes	For electrolyte replacement during diuretic therapy, as indicated (sodium and potassium are those commonly required)	
Sodium		Gagging (because of taste), vomiting
Potassium		With overdosage leading to hyperkalemia, cardiotoxic effects, as well as nausea, vomiting, and abdominal pain

*For specifics on a particular medication or for a full range of side effects, contraindications, and drug interactions, consult the *Physicians' Desk Reference.*

Source: Adapted from D. Page, Home Care for the Infant with Respiratory Compromise, in *Home Care for the High-Risk Infant,* E. Ahmann, ed. p.176, © 1996, Aspen Publishers, Inc.

Exhibit 4–2 Indications for Cardiorespiratory Monitoring

1. Infants with one or more severe apparent life-threatening events (ALTE) requiring mouth-to-mouth resuscitation or vigorous stimulation.

2. Symptomatic preterm infants.

3. Siblings of two or more sudden infant death syndrome (SIDS) victims.

4. Infants with certain diseases such as hypoventilation.

Source: Data from National Institutes of Health: Consensus Development Conference on Infantile Apnea and Home Monitoring, *Pediatrics,* 1987, 79:2, pp. 292–99.

tive when chest wall effort is present but airflow is blocked; or mixed, when elements of both central and obstructive apnea are included. Brief (lasting 15 seconds or less) central apnea can be normal at all ages. Apnea is considered to be pathologic if it is prolonged (lasting 20 seconds or greater) or associated with cyanosis, marked pallor, hypotonia or bradycardia (National Institutes of Health 1987).

Apnea of Prematurity

Symptomatic preterm infants are those who continue to experience pathologic apnea when they are otherwise ready for discharge from the hospital. Apnea of prematurity should be distinguished from periodic breathing, a pattern in which there are three or more respiratory pauses with a duration greater than 3 seconds with less than 20 seconds of respiration between pauses. Periodic breathing is usually benign (National Institutes of Health 1987).

Apparent Life-Threatening Event

The terminology, ALTE, is used to describe an episode that is frightening to the observer and is characterized by some combination of apnea, color change, marked change in muscle tone, choking, or gagging. In many cases, an underlying cause such as gastroesophageal reflux, seizures, or infection can be identified. However, in approximately 50 percent of cases, the etiology of the ALTE episode cannot be determined (Brooks 1992).

Sudden Infant Death Syndrome

SIDS is defined as the sudden death of an infant, younger than one year, that remains unexplained after performance of a complete postmortem investigation, including an autopsy, examination of the death scene, and review of the case history (Willinger, James, and Catz 1991). The relationship between SIDS and apnea is unclear. Although SIDS has been reported in some infants who have experienced ALTEs, most SIDS infants had not been observed to experience ALTEs before the time of death (Brooks 1992). Although cardiopulmonary monitors can alert care providers to episodes of apnea or bradycardia, their role in SIDS prevention is questionable. SIDS risk can be decreased through proper positioning of the sleeping infant, elimination of passive smoking, and attention to crib and bedding safety (American Academy of Pediatrics Task Force on Infant Positioning and SIDS 1992; Herda 1992; Schoendorf and Kiely 1992). The nurse should follow the physician's recommendation regarding sleeping position for the high-risk infant.

Equipment

Various models of impedance monitors are used in the home setting. Respiration and heart rate are detected by use of disposable, adhesive electrodes or reusable electrodes that are held in place by a Velcro belt. Recent advances in computer technology have enhanced the capability of home monitors. Memory or documented monitors now use a microchip to record and store data that can be downloaded for interpretation by the physician. Event recordings are helpful in differentiating true from false alarms as well as determining monitor usage (Spitzer and Gibson 1992). Monitor settings vary with the infant's age and reason for monitoring. To avoid physiologic alarms, the bradycardia setting often requires adjustment as the infant ages.

Nursing Care

The nurse should serve as a role model for the family and reinforce discharge teaching concerning the use of the monitor, response to alarms, and recording of events. Clear parameters should be followed for when the monitor is to be used, generally during all sleep periods and whenever the infant is unobserved. The home environment should be assessed for safety. Easy access to the crib is essential, as is a stable location of the monitor. Households without a telephone should be assisted in obtaining one, or alternative arrangements must be made for accessing emergency services. Care providers must be able to hear the alarm and reach the infant within 10 seconds. Remote alarms or infant monitors can be used if necessary, but parents should understand that any activities that interfere with their ability to hear alarms must be avoided during periods of monitoring.

Information about the monitor should be reinforced including the function of lights, controls and alarms, placement of electrodes, connection of the infant to the monitor, and general care of the machine. All teaching should be consistent with information in the equipment manual.

Parents should be helped to distinguish false alarms from truly significant events. False alarms may result from loose leads, incorrectly placed electrodes, conduction problems, or monitor malfunction. Extra wires, electrodes, and a belt should be available so that parents can efficiently assume troubleshooting activities. Potential monitor problems and recommended actions are outlined in Table 4–4.

Electrode placement is important for proper monitor performance. The electrodes must make contact with the sides of the chest wall to sense the movement of breathing and should be placed symmetrically. Electrodes should be replaced as their attachment becomes less secure and should be repositioned at least every two to three days

Table 4–4 Apnea Monitor Troubleshooting Guide

Problem	Possible Causes	Possible Solutions
False apnea alarms—frequent apnea alarms when the infant is breathing normally.	Infant may be breathing shallowly.	Check electrode placement to be sure they are between the nipple and armpit.
	The belt may be too loose around the infant's chest.	Tighten the belt.
False slow heart rate alarms—frequent slow heart rate alarms when the infant has a heart rate above the limit set.	The electrodes may be dirty.	Clean the electrodes with mild soap and water.
	Infant may have lotion or powder on the skin under electrodes.	Cleanse the infant's skin with soap and water, rinse, and dry.
	Infant may have outgrown low heart rate limit settings.	Consult the infant's physician.
	The belt may be too loose around the infant's chest.	Tighten the belt.
Lead alarm indicates a disconnected or broken piece of equipment.	The belt may be too loose around the infant's chest.	Tighten the belt.
	Lead wires may be disconnected.	Check lead wires at electrode end and patient cable to be sure they are connected securely.
	The patient cable may be disconnected.	Check patient cable jack at the back of the monitor to be sure it is plugged in securely.
	Lead wires may be broken.	Replace lead wires.
	Electrodes may be old.	Replace the electrodes.
Battery alarm	The battery needs to be recharged.	Plug the battery charger into monitor and then into the house current.

Source: Reprinted by permission of Nellcor Puritan Bennett, Pleasanton, CA.

to prevent skin breakdown. Alternating disposable electrodes with use of a belt may also be helpful. The nurse should assess the area of electrode placement for skin irritation. If irritation does occur, it can be treated by thoroughly cleaning the area with mild soap and water and drying it carefully. The use of lotions or creams should be avoided.

All care providers should be confident in their ability to respond to monitor alarms. An organized sequence of activities is necessary including assessment, gentle stimulation, vigorous stimulation, and cardiopulmonary resuscitation (CPR). It is reassuring for parents to understand that CPR is seldom required, and that usually the sound of the alarm or gentle stimulation is all that is needed. Periodic review and practice are crucial for maintaining CPR skills. CPR guidelines should be posted at the infant's bedside.

Apnea or bradycardia events should be recorded in an organized manner. Standard forms are available and can be adapted for specific use. Care providers should record the type and length of the alarm, condition of the infant, and the intervention required. The form should also include space for recording relevant additional comments.

Parents should have 24-hour telephone access to the equipment vendor in case problems with the monitor arise and to the physician in case situations of medical concern occur. It is important that the physician be notified of alarms that are increasing in frequency or duration and of any alarm that requires vigorous stimulation or is of concern to the home care provider. The local rescue squad should be notified of the infant's special needs. Emergency telephone numbers and the home address with the closest major intersection or cross street should be posted near the home telephone(s). Plans should be established for safe transportation of the infant. Ideally, a second adult should be available to monitor and attend to the infant during transport.

The nurse should provide anticipatory guidance and support to help parents cope with the stresses of home monitoring. Disruption of family activities, social isolation, financial concerns, caretaker fatigue, and marital discord have been reported (Ahmann 1992). Parents should be encouraged to use available family and community supports. Individual parent contacts or parent groups may be helpful for some families. Often, other parents can provide unparalleled practical advice and support based on their successful experience with home monitoring.

Discontinuing the Monitor

The decision to discontinue the monitor is made by the physician based on the infant's clinical condition and reason for monitoring. It is helpful for parents to be aware of the criteria for discontinuation so that they can prepare for this occurrence. Even when it is medically appropriate to discontinue the monitor, parents may be reluctant to do so. Despite initial anxiety, most parents come to rely on the monitor as a source of security and safety. A weaning program allowing time to relinquish the monitor may be necessary. Caregivers should also be helped to recognize the infant's stable condition and to view the infant as no longer at risk.

REFERENCES

Able-Boone, H., and E. Stevens. 1994. After the intensive care nursery experience: Families' perceptions of their well-being. *Children's Health Care* 23:99–114.

Abman, S., and J. Groothius. 1994. Pathophysiology and treatment of BPD. *Pediatric Clinics of North America.* 41:277–314.

Ackerman, V.L. 1994. Bronchopulmonary dysplasia. In *Respiratory disease in children: Diagnosis and management,* ed. G. Loughlin and H. Eigen, 383–94. Baltimore, MD: Williams & Wilkins.

Ahmann, E. 1992. Family impact of home apnea monitoring: An overview of research and its clinical implications. *Pediatric Nursing* 18, no. 6:611–16.

Ahmann, E., ed. 1996. *Home care for the high-risk infant.* Gaithersburg, MD: Aspen Publishers, Inc.

Ahmann, E. and K. Klockenbrink. 1996. Developmental assessment and intervention in the home. In *Home care for the high-risk infant,* ed. E. Ahmann, 293–303. Gaithersburg, MD: Aspen Publishers, Inc.

Alpert, B., J. Allen, and D. Schidlow. 1993. Bronchopulmonary dysplasia. In *Pediatric respiratory disease: Diagnosis and treatment,* ed. B. Hillman, 440–56. Philadelphia: W.B. Saunders.

American Academy of Pediatrics Task Force on Infant Positioning and SIDS. 1992. Position statement: Positioning and SIDS. *Pediatrics* 89:1120–25.

Armentrout, D. 1995. Gastroesophageal reflux in infants. *The Nurse Practitioner* 20:54–63.

Bernbaum, J., and M. Hoffman-Williamson. 1991. *Primary care of the preterm infant.* St. Louis: C.V. Mosby.

Bird, B., and E. Ahmann. 1996. Home care of the infant and young child with hydrocephalus. In *Home care for the high-risk infant,* ed. E. Ahmann, 269–75. Gaithersburg, MD: Aspen Publishers, Inc.

Bregman, J., and L. Kimberlin. 1993. Developmental outcome in extremely premature infants. *Pediatric Clinics of North America* 40:937–53.

Brem, A. 1992. Electrolyte disorders associated with respiratory distress syndrome and bronchopulmonary dysplasia. *Clinics in Perinatology* 19:223–32.

Brooks, J. 1992. Apparent life threatening events and apnea of infancy. *Clinics in Perinatology* 19:809–32.

Committee on Infectious Disease. 1994. *Report of the Committee on Infectious Disease,* 23d ed. Elk Grove Village, IL: American Academy of Pediatrics.

Committee on Injury and Poison Prevention and Committee on Fetus and Newborn. 1991. Safe transportation of premature infants. *Pediatrics* 87:120–12.

Committee on Nutrition. 1993. *Pediatric nutrition handbook.* 3d ed. Elk Grove Village, IL: The American Academy of Pediatrics.

Cunningham, C., J. McMilan, and S. Gross. 1991. Rehospitalization for respiratory illness in infants of less than 32 weeks' gestation. *Pediatrics* 88:527–32.

Diehl, S.F., K.A. Moffitt, and S.M. Wade. 1991. Focus group interview with parents of children with medically complex needs: An intimate look at their perceptions and feelings. *Children's Health Care* 20:170–75.

Goldman, D., S. Goldman, and J. Hirata. 1996. Prematurity. In *Primary care of the child with a chronic condition,* ed. L.P. Jackson and J. Vessey, 650–70. St. Louis: Mosby-Year Book, Inc.

Greenough, A. 1990. Bronchopulmonary dysplasia: Early diagnosis, prophylaxis, and treatment. *Archives of Diseases in Children* 65:1082–88.

Guidelines for the care of children with chronic lung disease. 1989. *Pediatric Pulmonology.* Suppl. 3.

Hack, M., et al. 1994. School-age outcomes in children with birth weights under 750 gm. *New England Journal of Medicine* 331:753–59.

Hagedorn, M.I., and S.L. Gardner. 1991. Physiologic sequelae of prematurity: The nurse practitioner's role, part IV, anemia. *Journal of Pediatric Health Care* 5:3–10.

Harvey, K. 1996. Bronchopulmonary dysplasia. In *Primary care of the child with a chronic condition,* ed. L.P. Jackson and J. Vessey, 172–92. St. Louis: Mosby-Year Book, Inc.

Herda, J. 1992. Nursing interventions aimed at reducing risks of SIDS. *Pediatric Nursing* 18:531–33.

Huber, C., D. Holditch-Davis, and D. Brandon. 1993. High-risk preterm infants at 3 years of age: Parental response to the presence of developmental problems. *Children's Health Care* 22, no. 2:107–24.

Huddleston, K. 1996. Home care of the infant with short bowel syndrome requiring nutritional support. In *Home care for the high-risk infant,* ed. E. Ahmann, 149–61 Gaithersburg, MD: Aspen Publishers, Inc.

Infant Health and Development Program. 1990. Enhancing outcomes of low-birth weight, premature infants: A multisite, randomized trial. *JAMA* 263:3035–42.

Jackson, D. 1996. Speech and language development in the chronically ill preterm infant. In *Home care for the high-risk infant,* ed. E. Ahmann, 315–21. Gaithersburg, MD: Aspen Publishers, Inc.

Joint Committee on Infant Hearing. 1994. Joint Committee on Infant Hearing 1994 Position Statement. *Audiology Today* 6, no. 6:6–9.

Lierman, C. 1996. Nutrition and feeding of the chronically ill infant. In *Home care for the high-risk infant,* ed. E. Ahmann, 119–29. Gaithersburg, MD: Aspen Publishers, Inc.

McGinnity, F.G., and J.H. Bryars. 1992. Controlled study of ocular morbidity in school age children born at preterm. *British Journal of Ophthalmology* 6:520–24.

Merritt, A., W. Northway, and B. Boynton. 1988. *Bronchopulmonary dysplasia.* St. Louis: C.V. Mosby.

National Institutes of Health. 1987. National Institutes of Health Consensus Development Conference on Infantile Apnea and Home Monitoring, September 29 to October 1, 1986. *Pediatrics* 79: 292–99.

Page, D. 1996. Home care for the infant with respiratory compromise. In *Home care for the high-risk infant,* ed. E. Ahmann, 171–82. Gaithersburg, MD: Aspen Publishers, Inc.

Parker, R., D. Lindstrom, and R. Cotton. 1992. Improved survival accounts for most, but not all, of the increase in bronchopulmonary dysplasia. *Pediatrics* 90:663–68.

Ross, G., E.G. Lipper, and P.A.M. Auld. 1990. Growth achievement of very low birthweight premature children at school age. *Journal of Pediatrics* 117:307–09.

Rozycki, H., and B. Kirkpatrick. 1993. New developments in bronchopulmonary dysplasia. *Pediatric Annals* 22: 532–38.

Schoendorf, K., and J. Kiely. 1992. Relationship of sudden infant death syndrome to maternal smoking during and after pregnancy. *Pediatrics* 90:905–08.

Schraeder, B. 1996. Visual impairment in the preterm infant. In *Home care for the high-risk infant*, ed. E. Ahmann, 323–26. Gaithersburg, MD: Aspen Publishers, Inc.

Spitzer, A., and E. Gibson. 1992. Home monitoring. *Clinics in Perinatology* 19:907–26.

Stepanek, J. 1996. Early intervention services for the high-risk infant. In *Home care for the high-risk infant*, ed. E. Ahmann, 279–81. Gaithersburg, MD: Aspen Publishers, Inc.

Volpe, J. 1995. *Neurology of the newborn.* 3d ed. Philadelphia: W.B. Saunders.

Willett, L., et al. 1989. Ventilatory changes in convalescent infants positioned in car seats. *Journal of Pediatrics* 115: 451–55.

Willinger, M., L.S. James, and C. Catz. 1991. Defining the sudden infant death syndrome (SIDS): Deliberations of an expert panel convened by National Institutes of Child Health and Human Development. *Pediatric Pathology* 11:677–84.

Wolff, R.P., and C.J. Lierman. 1994. Management of behavioral feeding problems in young children. *Infants and Young Children* 7 no. 1:14–23.

BIBLIOGRAPHY

Friendly, D. 1994. Eye disorders. In *Neonatology: Pathophysiology and management of the newborn,* 4th ed., ed. G. Avery, M.A. Fletcher, and M. MacDonald, Philadelphia: J.B. Lippincott.

Resources for Parents and Professionals

Featherstone, H. 1990. *A difference in the family: Life with a disabled child.* New York: Penguin Viking.

Finston, P. 1990. *Parenting plus: Raising children with special health needs.* New York: Penguin Books USA.

Gotsch, G. 1994. *Breastfeeding pure and simple.* Schaumburg, Ill.: La Leche League.

Harrison, H., and A. Kosititsky. 1983. *The premature baby book: A parents' guide to coping and caring in the first years.* New York: St. Martin's Press.

Huggins, K. 1995. *The nursing mother's companion.* Boston: The Harvard Common Press.

Jason, J., and A. Van der Meer. 1989. *Parenting your premature baby.* New York: Henry Holt and Company.

Klein, S.D., and M.S. Schleifer. 1993. *It isn't fair! Siblings of children with disabilities.* Westport, Conn.: Bergin & Garvey.

Lawrence, R.A. 1994. *Breast feeding: A guide for the medical profession.* 4th ed. Toronto, Ontario, Canada: C.V. Mosby.

Miller, N.B. 1993. *Nobody's perfect: Living and growing with children who have special needs.* Baltimore, Md.: Paul H. Brookes Publishing.

Powell, T.H., and P.A. Gallagher. 1992. *Brothers & sisters: A special part of exceptional families.* 2d ed. Baltimore, Md.: Paul H. Brookes Publishing.

Segal, M. 1988. *In time and with love: Caring for the special needs baby.* New York: Newmarket Press.

Walker, M. 1989. *Breastfeeding your premature or special care baby: A practical guide for nursing the tiny baby.* Weston, Mass.: Lactation Associates.

Nursing Care Plan for a Child with Bronchopulmonary Dysplasia

Nursing Diagnosis/ Patient Problem	Defining Characteristics	Nursing Interventions	Expected Outcomes
1. Alteration in respiratory status related to impaired gas exchange	Signs of respiratory distress: • Tachypnea • Tachycardia • Paleness/ cyanosis • Diaphoresis • Irritability • Retractions • Nasal flaring • Wheezes, rhonchi, crackles • Hypoxia • Hypercapnia	Assess respiratory status frequently and at varying activity levels. Monitor oximetry as ordered. *Administer oxygen as ordered. *Perform chest percussion and postural drainage as needed. *Administer respiratory medications (bronchodilators, corticosteroids) as ordered. Reduce risk of infection: • Good handwashing • Avoid crowds • Avoid persons with respiratory illnesses • Caregivers receive influenza vaccine Avoid exposure to passive smoking and environmental irritants. Notify physician of any change from baseline respiratory status.	Patient is adequately oxygenated.

*Denotes nursing intervention requiring a physician's order.

Nursing Diagnosis/ Patient Problem	Defining Characteristics	Nursing Interventions	Expected Outcomes
2. Alteration in nutritional status: less than body requirements *Etiology:* Child has increased caloric needs and is unable to meet these secondary to: • Compromised respiratory status • Feeding aversions • Fluid restrictions • Gastroesophageal reflux	Inadequate weight gain for age (corrected for prematurity) Inability to take nourishment by mouth	*Obtain nutritional consultation. Weigh frequently, as ordered by physician. Monitor accurate intake and output. Maintain dietary record complete with symptoms of aversions or reflux and report to physician. *Establish hyperosmolar, calorie-dense feedings (maintaining fluid restriction as needed. Report compromised respiratory status during feedings. *Increase oxygen during feedings. If patient is unable to tolerate oral feedings, maintain feedings via gastrostomy, jejunostomy, or nasogastric tube. Maintain reflux precautions after feedings.	Patient has gradual, appropriate growth, concomitant with improved respiratory status. Patient is free from oral feeding aversions. Mealtime is positive experience for child and family.

*Denotes nursing intervention requiring a physician's order.

Nursing Diagnosis/ Patient Problem	Defining Characteristics	Nursing Interventions	Expected Outcomes
3. Alteration in respiratory status related to excess fluid volume	• Tachypnea • Cough • Labored respirations • Crackles • Decreased urine output • Edema	Assess for signs of respiratory distress due to fluid overload: • Monitor vital signs including blood pressure. • Auscultate breath sounds. • Report signs of respiratory distress. • Report edema. • Report increased oxygen requirement. Monitor intake and output every four to eight hours. Weigh daily (or more frequently if ordered). *Maintain fluid restriction. *Administer diuretics. *Administer potassium supplement. Assess for side effects of diuretics as needed.	Patient has appropriate ratio of fluid intake and urine output. Patient is without signs of respiratory distress. Patient has no untoward side effects from diuretics or electrolyte supplements.
4. Skin integrity: potential for impairment	Skin irritation from tape needed to secure tubes or leads: • Redness • Edema • Rash • Abrasions • Breakdown	Minimize amount of tape on skin. Minimize tension of tubes or lines. Rotate monitor lead or tape sites. When possible, tape onto something other than skin (e.g., another piece of tape, small gauze pad). Maintain clean, dry skin around tube sites. Maintain adequate nutritional state. *Apply antibiotic ointments or corticosteroid creams as ordered.	Patient has clear skin with no rashes, breakdown, or infection.

*Denotes nursing intervention requiring a physician's order.

Nursing Diagnosis/ Patient Problem	Defining Characteristics	Nursing Interventions	Expected Outcomes
5. Impaired growth and development: physical and psychosocial *Etiology:* • Isolation due to long-term and/or repeated hospital-izations • Immobility • Sensory depriva-tion and/or overload • Altered nutritional status • Decreased energy level from increased work of breathing • Repeated painful stimuli • Separation from parents • Inconsistent caregivers	Inability to maintain steady growth curve Inability to reach appropriate developmental milestones Inappropriate muscle tone—may be increased or decreased Irritability	Encourage parents to maintain active involvement in playful, stimulating activities. Maintain consistent caregivers. Maintain consistent daily schedule. *Provide organized program of develop-mental stimulation via occupational or physical therapy. Maintain record of developmental milestones.	Patient maintains steady, appropriate growth. Patient progresses through developmental milestones at appropriate pace (as outlined by developmental specialists). Patient achieves appropriate developmental milestones.

*Denotes nursing intervention requiring a physician's order.

Nursing Diagnosis/ Patient Problem	Defining Characteristics	Nursing Interventions	Expected Outcomes
6. Knowledge deficit related to • Pathophysiology of BPD • Treatment regimen • Signs and symptoms of infection, respiratory distress, fluid overload • Emergency management *Etiology:* • Inaccurate information given to family • No explanations given for rationale of treatments • Family unable to absorb all information at once	Verbalization of questions or problems regarding aspects of BPD and required interventions Inability to articulate rationale for treatment Inappropriate expectations of recovery from disease state Inability to independently care for child Lack of compliance with treatment regimen	Provide accurate information to parents using appropriate methods to promote learning. Reinforce all teaching frequently. Assess return demonstrations for accuracy. Encourage parents to keep journal of questions or concerns. Continually assess for further knowledge deficits. Assess reasons for noncompliance. Encourage follow-up with pulmonary center or physician knowledgeable in care of BPD.	Family verbalizes and demonstrates understanding of disease process and treatment regimen. Family forms trusting relationship with care providers and feels comfortable asking questions in future.

Nursing Diagnosis Patient Problem	Defining Characteristics	Nursing Interventions	Expected Outcomes
7. Coping: ineffective—family *Etiology:* • Chronicity of illness and very slow improvement of health status • Frequent hospitalizations • High care demands of patient • Isolation • Inability to appropriately bond with infant in neonatal period	Verbalization of inability to cope Infrequent visiting when child is hospitalized Role confusion Inability to meet basic care needs of child Inability to make decisions Chronic sadness, depression Anger Noncompliance with medical regimens	Determine etiology of ineffective coping and/or noncompliance. Assess coping mechanisms and encourage use of appropriate mechanisms. Determine alternative strategies for ineffective coping mechanisms. Encourage involvement with support groups or other families in similar situations whenever possible. Use resources such as social workers, family counselors, community aides, respite care, etc., as available and appropriate. Allow family opportunity to verbalize stress, frustration, fatigue, and anxiety.	Family: • Demonstrates decreased anxiety and stress. • Participates in caretaking activities. • Develops trusting relationship with care providers. • Describes role as parents. • Uses healthy, appropriate coping mechanisms.

Note: BPD, bronchopulmonary dysplasia.

CHAPTER 5

Alterations in Respiratory Function

Lynn Feenan and Wendy L. Votroubek

Respiratory illnesses are the number one reason for children and their families to seek care from a physician (Whaley and Wong 1993). With the increased survival rate, particularly for premature infants (Klaus and Fanaroff 1986), coupled with the improved ability to provide high-technology care in the home setting, there are more children with a variety of pulmonary disorders who are able to receive care in their home and school settings. These pulmonary treatments include new inhaler devices to increase efficacy of asthma medication, new airway clearance techniques to provide more independence for children with cystic fibrosis, oxygen equipment that allows for cost-effective delivery and mobility for children, home intravenous antibiotics through venous access devices that are easy to care for, and high-tech ventilator equipment that is less invasive and more portable than ever before.

This chapter reviews the newest home treatments available for children with asthma, cystic fibrosis, oxygen needs, tracheostomies, and ventilator dependence. Guidelines are presented for the care of these children. Home nursing care plans are also presented to outline important aspects of treatment that the home care nurse should consider when caring for a child with a chronic respiratory condition.

ASTHMA

Asthma morbidity and mortality are increasing (National Heart, Lung, and Blood Institute 1991). Asthma is the most common chronic illness in children, affecting nearly 10 percent of all children in the United States (Gergen, Mullally, and Evans 1988). It is also a costly disease, with an estimated $6.2 billion in costs related to the illness in 1990, and accounts for the most missed days of school for children between the ages of 5 and 17 years (Weissk, Gergen, and Hodgson 1992). In 1991, an expert panel of asthma health care professionals convened to develop guidelines for the definition and management of asthma in children and adults. According to that panel (National Heart, Lung, and Blood Institute 1991), asthma is defined as a chronic lung disease with the following three characteristics:

1. airway obstruction/narrowing that is reversible (but not completely so for some patients) either spontaneously or with treatment
2. airway inflammation
3. airway hyperresponsiveness to a variety of stimuli

It is important for families and patients to understand this definition so that they then understand the rationale for various methods of treatment.

A variety of risk factors are associated with a higher frequency of asthma in children (Smith 1993). Age, gender, race, and history of atopy are among these factors. For children younger than 10 years, asthma is more frequently diagnosed in boys. This preponderance lessens after the age of 10. Younger children are more at risk to be diagnosed with asthma, with 80 percent of children diagnosed before the age of 5 years. In the United States, asthma is more prevalent in African American children than in Caucasian children. Finally, children with asthma are more likely to have other allergies (allergic rhinitis or atopic dermatitis). A thorough history of these factors, family incidence of asthma or allergies, and clear description of symptoms are necessary to make the diagnosis, particularly in young children who cannot perform spirometry or airway challenges, which directly measure airway obstruction.

Triggers

It is also important to obtain a history of "triggers" related to asthma symptoms. Identification of a child's asthma triggers is not only important for diagnosis but also for treatment. Triggers can sometimes be avoided (for example, animal dander or environmental tobacco smoke), pretreated (for example, for exercise or cold air), or anticipated and treated early (for example, upper respiratory infections) (Exhibit 5–1). Family and patient education is vital in terms of understanding what the triggers are and how to either avoid or pretreat in anticipation of exposure to a trigger.

Viral upper respiratory infections (URIs) are one of the most common asthma precipitants in any age group but particularly in children (Pattemore, Johnston, and Bardin 1992). The most common of these are the respiratory syncytial virus, rhinovirus, influenza, and parainfluenza. These viruses increase inflammation in the airway, and the severity of the virus is directly related to the severity of the ensuing asthma. Although URIs are difficult to totally avoid, families can be instructed to limit exposure to infected individuals, practice good handwashing when a virus is in the household, and treat early with beta agonists and anti-inflammatories at the first sign of an infection.

Allergens (inhalant) become a more important factor in asthma after the age of two years (Zimmerman et al. 1988). Skin tests can be done when inhalant allergens are suspected to identify the specific allergen so that families can be taught environmental controls, avoidance, or decide on the option of immunotherapy. The dust mite is the major asthma-provoking allergen, followed by mold (*Alternaria*) and cat (Bush 1992). Environmental controls for dust mites include decreasing interior humidity (40–50 percent); encasing pillow, mattress, and box spring in airtight coverings; washing bedding on a weekly basis in hot water (greater than 130°F); and decreasing the number of "dust-catching" objects in the child's bedroom (for example, stuffed animals, collectible toys, venetian blinds, etc.).

Almost 90 percent of children with asthma experience some bronchospasm with exercise (Siegel and Rachelefsky 1985). Formal exercise testing can be done in the pulmonary function laboratory inducing measurable bronchospasm after exercise that brings the heart rate to 80 percent of maximum. A clear and recurrent history of asthma (outside of the laboratory) 10 to 15 minutes after the termination of vigorous exercise may also be enough for diagnosis. Frequently, a patient can be given a peak flow meter to measure airflow before and after exercise, aiding in the diagnosis. A drop in the peak expiratory flow rate (PEFR) of 10 to 20 percent is diagnostic of exercise-induced asthma (EIA). The etiology of EIA is linked to the temperature

---

Exhibit 5–1 Asthma Triggers

Viral upper respiratory infections
Allergens (dust, pollen, molds, foods)
Exercise
Irritants (tobacco smoke, paint fumes, aerosols)
Weather (cold air, humidity, sudden changes)
Gastroesophageal reflux
Emotional factors (crying, laughing, stress)
Drugs (aspirin, beta blockers)

and humidity of the airway. The exact mechanism is unknown but thought to be linked to airway water loss and temperature drop due to hyperventilation, triggering bronchoconstriction. Pretreatment with a bronchodilator (albuterol or cromolyn sodium) about 15 minutes before exercise can be adequate enough to manage EIA effectively. EIA should not be seen as a reason to restrict activity. Appropriate management is the goal of EIA therapy.

The most significant environmental irritant for children in general, and particularly children with asthma, is secondhand tobacco smoke (Halken et al. 1991). Increased coughing, wheezing, and bronchial hyperresponsiveness are associated with passive smoking. Approximately 20 percent of children experience exacerbation of asthma because of environmental tobacco smoke (U.S. Environmental Protection Agency 1992). Many families need education not only about the dangers of environmental tobacco smoke regarding their children's asthma, but also need encouragement to quit smoking and resources to support them in their efforts. Other irritants (for example, woodstove smoke, gas fumes, aerosols) should be assessed for and controlled when possible and necessary.

Asthma is often triggered by weather, particularly extremes in weather. Very cold air or very humid air can cause bronchospasm. Changes in pressure, like that which occurs in thunderstorms, can also trigger asthma. Pretreatment and avoidance (for example, staying inside) can be used as methods of management of weather-triggered asthma.

Gastroesophageal reflux and its connection to asthma is complex (Smith 1993). The mechanism is unknown but involves bronchial hyperreactivity. When it is suspected of being an asthma trigger it can be treated by a therapeutic trial of reflux medication.

Drug sensitivity, particularly to aspirin and other nonsteroidal anti-inflammatories, can cause bronchospasm. Oral challenges in a medically controlled environment can be used as a diagnostic test if the history is unclear. Avoidance of these medications is recommended. The use of a Medic-Alert identification bracelet or tag is also recommended for these patients.

Treatment

Asthma is a chronic disease with no cure. Asthma management encompasses both nonpharmacologic and pharmacologic treatments. Previously discussed methods of avoidance of some triggers or environmental controls of others are examples of management without medications. Allergen immunotherapy may be a consideration for some patients whose symptoms are not well controlled by these techniques or by medical management (for example, medications). It is a long-term commitment (three to five years) and requires patience and compliance on the part of the family and child. Education about the risks and benefits should take place before the mutual decision is made by the provider and the patient.

Medications

The medications used to control asthma treat airway obstruction, hyperresponsiveness, and inflammation and are divided into categories of either bronchodilators or anti-inflammatories. Not only must the correct medication be chosen, but it must be used correctly, delivered effectively, and assessed on a regular basis for its usefulness and ability to be adhered to properly. Dosage varies by product (Exhibit 5-2).

Bronchodilators (beta agonists, methylxanthines, anticholinergics) are medications that act directly on beta receptors in the airway to relax smooth muscle (National Heart, Lung, and Blood Institute 1991). They are taken orally or are inhaled. They include medications such as theophylline, albuterol, and ipratropium. Inhaled beta agonists are the medications of choice for the treatment of acute exacerbations of asthma and/or EIA. They are typically prescribed on an as-needed (prn) basis. When used for a prolonged period and on a regular basis, they have been shown to have diminished control over asthma (Sears et al. 1990). Inhaled beta agonists are preferred to the oral route because

Exhibit 5–2 Medications Used in Childhood Asthma

I. RESCUE MEDICATIONS (BRONCHODILATORS)

- work by opening air passages
- help stop attack once it has started
- best if used inhaled
- faster
- if using inhaled bronchodilator more than 4 times daily, a physician must be notified

A. Beta$_2$Agonists (side effects include shakiness, nervousness, dizziness)

Inhaled

Examples: Albuterol, metaproterenol, bitolterol, terbutaline, pirbuterol

Mode of administration
–Metered-dose inhaler (MDI)   2 puffs q 4–6 hours
–Nebulizer solution*   Albuterol 5 mg/mL; 0.1–0.15 mg/kg in 2 cc of saline
     q 4–6 hours, maximum 5.0 mg
     Metaproterenol 50 mg/mL; 0.25–0.50 mg/kg in 2 cc
     of saline q 4–6 hours, maximum 15.0 mg

Oral (not used for acute problems)

Liquids	Albuterol	0.1–0.15 mg/kg q 4–6 hours
	Metaproterenol	0.3–0.5 mg/kg q 4–6 hours
Tablets	Albuterol	2- or 4-mg tablet, q 4–6 hours
		4-mg sustained-release tablet q 12 hours
	Metaproterenol	10- or 20-mg tablet q 4–6 hours
	Terbutaline	2.5- or 5.0-mg tablet q 4–6 hours

B. Theophylline (Long-acting bronchodilators, work more slowly than short-acting. Side effects include headache, dizziness, nervousness, and nausea.)

Liquid
Tablets, capsules
Sustained-release tablets, capsules

Dosage to achieve serum concentration of 5–15 µg/mL

II. PREVENTATIVE MEDICATIONS (ANTI-INFLAMMATORIES)

- help prevent or reduce the underlying inflammation and swelling of air passages
- make air passages less twitchy and help prevent attacks
- won't stop attack once it has started

continues

Exhibit 5–2 continued

A. Corticosteroids

Most common steroids used for maintenance/prevention; must be used regularly to be effective

Inhaled[†] (side effects include hoarseness, dry mouth, fungal infections in mouth; patients must rinse mouth out after use)

Beclomethasone	42 at mcg/puff; two to four puffs bid–qid
Triamcinolone	100 mcg/puff; two to four puffs bid–qid
Flunisolide	250 mcg/puff; two to four puffs bid
Fluticasone	220,110 or 44 gg/puff; two to four puffs bid (depending on weight)

Oral[‡] (side effects include acne, weight gain, mood changes, stomach problems. Serious side effects may occur when used for long period or stopped abruptly without taper.) Medication is given for a few days when swelling, inflammation, and mucus are present.

Liquids	Prednisone	5 mg/5 cc
	Prednisolone	5 mg/5 cc
		15 mg/5 cc
Tablets	Prednisone	1, 2.5, 5, 10, 20, 25, 50 mg
	Prednisolone	5 mg
	Methylprednisolone	2, 4, 8, 16, 24, 32 mg

B. Nonsteroids

Reduce or prevent inflammatory changes in lungs by protecting the air passages from allergens (inflammatory mediators), have no bronchodilator effect. Can help prevent exercise-induced asthma.

Intal [cromolyn sodium (side effects rare)]

> MDI—800 mcg/puff; two puffs bid–qid
> Nebulizer solution—20 mg/2 mL ampule; 1 ampule bid–qid

Tilade (Nedocromil Sodium) (side effects rare)

> MDI—1.75 mg/puff; two puffs bid–qid

*Premixed solutions are available. It is suggested that the per/kg dosage recommendations be followed.
[†]Consider use of spacer devices to minimize local adverse effects.
[‡] "For acute exacerbations, doses of 1–2 mg/kg in single or divided doses are used initially and are then modified. Reassess in three days, because only a short burst may be needed. There is no need to taper a short (three- to five-day) course of therapy. If therapy extends beyond this period, it may be appropriate to taper the dosage. For chronic dosage, the lowest possible alternate-day A.M. dosage should be established.

Source: Adapted from Executive Summary: Guidelines for Diagnosis and Management of Asthma, National Heart, Lung, and Blood Institute, 1991.

they are delivered directly into the airway, thereby increasing effectiveness, having a faster onset of action, achieving desired effects at a lower dosage, and decreasing systemic side effects. The use of a spacer is always recommended when using a meter-dosed inhaler (MDI) for children.

Theophylline is the typical methylxanthine used to treat asthma. Its mechanism is not completely known but it works as a bronchodilator. Theophylline has been long used in the management of asthma and has been somewhat replaced by beta agonists. However, it can still be useful in the treatment of nocturnal asthma (in the sustained-release form) or in combination with beta agonists for additional bronchodilation (National Heart, Lung, and Blood Institute 1991).

Anti-inflammatory medications interrupt the cycle of airway inflammation during an acute exacerbation as well as have a prophylactic effect in chronic asthma management. Anti-inflammatories can be given orally, parenterally, or inhaled. They are both steroidal and nonsteroidal. They can be effective agents in treating both acute and chronic asthma symptoms. However, these medications are not "rescue drugs," in that they do not act rapidly. Some patients won't see effects of inhaled anti-inflammatories for up to four to six weeks. Patients should be educated about this timeline so that they do not get discouraged and abandon therapy because they have not noticed results in a short period.

Nonsteroidal anti-inflammatories include such medications as cromolyn (Intal) and nedocromil sodium (Tilade). These are used pro-phylactically for chronic airway inflammation. Cromolyn can also be useful in preventing acute symptoms seen in EIA. Both drugs are mast cell stabilizers, preventing the release of mediators that cause swelling in the airways. A great benefit of these drugs is that they have virtually no side effects, except a rare irritative cough. When used via MDI with a spacer device, they can be extremely preventive in controlling symptoms on a long-term basis.

Corticosteroids are currently the most effective agents in the treatment of chronic and acute symptoms. In the inhaled form, they have few local side effects—typically oral thrush, if the mouth is not rinsed after administration, dysphonia, and occasional irritative cough (Toogood 1990). Systemic absorption in the inhaled form is minimal (Kerrebijn 1990). There are many brands of inhaled steroids on the market, all of which are in MDI form, but they deliver varying amounts of different corticosteroids (Table 5–1). If an inhaled steroid is recommended for a very young child, it must be administered through an Aerochamber with mask, because a nebulized form does not exist for marketing. A spacer system is recommended for administration for all ages because it increases deposition in the lungs, decreases the sometimes bad taste, and decreases the potential side effect of candidiasis. The family and patient must be educated that an inhaled steroid is not only a treatment for symptoms but is also a preventative medication; therefore, the patient must be encouraged to adhere to the recommended daily dosage, even when feeling well.

Oral corticosteroids are most often used in short bursts (five to seven days) to treat an acute

Table 5–1 Inhaled Steroids

Generic Name	Brand Name	Mcg/puff
Beclomethasone	Vanceril/Beclovent	42 mcg/puff
Flunisolide	AeroBid/AeroBid M	250 mcg/puff
Fluticasone	Flovent	44 mcg/puff, 110 mcg/puff, 220 mcg/puff
Triamcinolone	Azmacort	100 mcg/puff

asthma exacerbation. The onset of action is within 3 hours, peaking at 8 to 12 hours (Smith 1993). The dose for such a burst is typically between 1 to 2 mg/kg/day, in divided bid doses. Adverse side effects of a short burst are rare but can include appetite increase, weight gain, mild cushingoid effects, fluid retention, and mood alterations (National Heart, Lung, and Blood Institute 1991). If a burst is less than 10 days in length, it can typically be stopped without the need for a taper. However, tapering of the dose can be done to decrease the side effects of abrupt withdrawal (Smith 1993). Children with more severe asthma may require longer-term therapy of oral steroids. If this is necessary, it is best to try to dose on an every-other-day basis to decrease side effects. Long-term side effects can include cataracts, osteoporosis, hypertension, impaired glucose metabolism, and immune compromise (National Heart, Lung, and Blood Institute 1991). Every effort should be made to reduce dependence on long-term corticosteroids, including the use of higher doses of inhaled steroids. Close follow-up and assessment for long-term side effects should occur on a regular basis in a clinic specializing in children with severe asthma.

Parenteral corticosteroids are used during acute asthma exacerbations that have not responded to standard oral or inhaled therapy. Parenteral administration needs to take place in the hospital setting where the child can be observed closely.

A new category of medication just approved by the Food and Drug Administration (FDA) for the treatment of asthma is the leukotriene antagonist and synthesis inhibitor. Leukotrienes are inflammatory mediators. Blocking their receptor sites and/or synthesis has been found to be effective in diminishing airway inflammation. Accolate is a new product on the market that is dosed at 20 mg twice a day. It has been found to be helpful as a preventative oral anti-inflammatory agent for some patients with asthma. Its use is limited at this time but it is approved for use in children 12 years and older.

Delivery Systems

Inhaled medications are either delivered through an MDI or an air compressor with updraft nebulizer. Proper administration of the drug must be taught and reviewed frequently. An estimation of between 12 and 89 percent (with an average of about 39 percent) of patients do not get good results from their medications because of poor technique administering the drug with an MDI (McFadden 1995). This particularly happens in the pediatric and geriatric populations.

The MDI is a portable device that can be easily carried in a backpack, fanny pack, or purse. It should always be used with a spacer to increase the delivery of the medication. Even with "perfect" technique only 20 percent of the medication inhaled directly from an MDI is deposited in the lungs with about 80 percent deposited in the mouth (Ahrens et al. 1995). Proper use of an inhaler is outlined in Exhibit 5–3. Spacer devices come in many shapes, sizes, and colors (Optihaler, InspirEase, Aerochamber with and without mask, EZ Spacer, etc.) (Figures 5–1 and 5–2). Again, the child and family need to be instructed about proper use of the unit, and this should be reviewed frequently. The device chosen should fit with the individual and family's lifestyle and needs.

Exhibit 5–3 Use of the Metered-Dose Inhaler

1. Remove cap and shake inhaler.
2. Tip head back to "sniffing position" (to open airway).
3. Exhale as much air as possible.
4. Position inhaler in mouth or (preferably) in the spacer unit.
5. Press once to activate inhaler.
6. Slowly inhale.
7. Hold breath to count of 10 seconds.
8. Wait 1 to 2 minutes and repeat procedure until all prescribed puffs are done.

If the child is too small, unable to coordinate the use of an MDI, or too ill to get benefit from the MDI (for example, has acute exacerbation with significant airway obstruction), then a por-

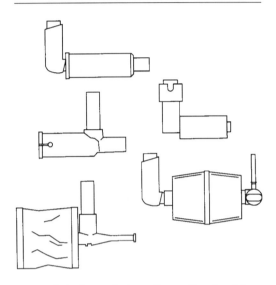

Figure 5–1 Spacer devices. *Source:* Reprinted from *Nurses: Partners in Asthma Care,* National Asthma Education and Prevention Program, National Heart, Lung, and Blood Institute, NIH Publication No. 95-3308, 1995.

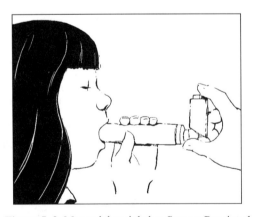

Figure 5–2 Metered dose inhaler. *Source:* Reprinted from Guidelines for Diagnosis and Management of Asthma, National Heart, Lung, and Blood Institute, 1994.

table air compressor with a small-volume nebulizer (SVN) can be used to deliver a beta agonist with or without cromolyn. Guidelines for the use of nebulizers in the home were recently developed to help in Medicare reimbursement (O'Donohue 1988). There are many air compressors and nebulizers (jet and ultrasonic) available on the market. The prescribing provider, with the help of the durable medical equipment (DME) vendor, should take into account such features as particle size delivered, portability, cost, speed of delivery, disposability, need for cleaning, and machine maintenance in choosing a system. The patient should ideally be instructed in the use, care, and troubleshooting of the machine by the DME vendor, preferably in person. The DME vendor should have a 24-hour number in case of emergencies.

Solutions used with the SVN vary from premixed vials to multidose bottles of medication mixed with bronchosaline for each treatment. The unit-dose vials are more expensive but are also more convenient and faster to prepare. Typically, children with asthma nebulize albuterol 0.25 to 0.5 cc in 2.5 cc of normal saline every four hours prn for symptoms. They can also be on a tid regimen inhaling 0.25 to 0.5 cc albuterol with 2 cc (20 mg) of cromolyn on a regular basis. The child may use a mouthpiece or mask for delivery and inhalation. Many children breathe directly from a piece of corrugated extension tubing. The child should be observed to make sure that he or she takes deep enough breaths from the nebulizer. Nose clips may be necessary to discourage nasal breathing during the treatment. The child's technique and the parents' knowledge of care of the compressor and nebulizer should be assessed regularly to ensure maximum benefit of delivery of the medication.

Peak Flow Meters

The PEFR measures the maximum airflow rate generated during a forced expiratory maneuver. It is measured in liters per second, and requires maximum effort and some practice on the part of the child for an accurate reading. It can provide the child, family, and provider with information regarding the presence or absence of airway obstruction in a simple, cost-effective, and quantitative way. The PEFR, when done correctly, correlates well with the FEV_1 on spirometry (National Heart, Lung, and Blood Institute 1991).

Handheld peak flow meters have been available for home monitoring for many years now. They can be helpful when used on a regular basis by a child with asthma, as long as the child is assessed to have good technique. Sporadic use or a "one-time" reading is not very helpful in making an assessment of airway obstruction. A child should use the peak flow meter when well, to establish a "personal best" range, and needs to use the meter regularly to allow for any accurate comparison of values. See Figure 5–3 for sample peak flow meters and Exhibit 5–4 on how to use a peak flow meter.

Daily monitoring of the PEFR is helpful in detecting early airway obstruction, in assessing circadian variations, and in providing objective criteria for planning and evaluating treatment (Quackenboss, Lebowitz, and Krzyzanowski 1991). The personal best value is usually obtained by taking AM and PM readings over one to two weeks (when healthy) and is the highest

Exhibit 5–4 How To Use a Peak Flow Meter

- Sit or stand up straight.
- Breathe in as much air as the lungs will hold.
- Place the mouthpiece of the flow meter in the mouth.
- Huff out as hard and as fast as you can. Give a short blow, not a slow one.
- Repeat the steps three times, using the highest of the three readings as the peak flow rate.

Source: Adapted from Executive Summary: Guidelines for Diagnosis and Management of Asthma, National Heart, Lung, and Blood Institute, 1991.

value achieved, usually in the evening. This provides a basis for comparison for that particular child. After that, at least daily readings should be done and written down, along with asthma symptoms, in an asthma diary (Exhibit 5–5). This can be used by the child, family, and provider to aid in the daily assessment of the child's asthma. An asthma diary with peak flow readings can also be a helpful tool for a school nurse to assess the child in school.

Zoning peak flow readings (Mendoza, Sander, and Scherrer 1988) can be useful in making assessments about home treatment, when to call the health care provider, and when to seek emergency care. Once the personal best value is established, the health care provider can establish zones for the patient and family to be aware of the following:

- The "green zone" (clear) is usually figured to be 80 to 100 percent of the personal best value. Asthma is in good control and no changes in therapy are necessary.
- The "yellow zone" (caution) is 50 to 80 percent of the personal best value. An asthma exacerbation may be present and a temporary increase in medication may be warranted. The physician or nurse can be called for advice.

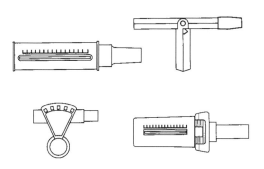

Figure 5–3 Peak flow meters. *Source:* Reprinted from *Nurses: Partners in Asthma Care,* National Asthma Education and Prevention Program, National Heart, Lung, and Blood Institute, NIH Publication No. 95-3308, 1995.

Exhibit 5–5 Pulmo-graph Daily Record Card

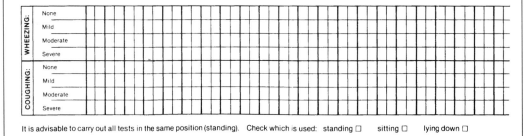

Courtesy of Vitalagraph, Lenoxa, Kansas.

- The "red zone" (danger) is less than 50 percent of the personal best. A bronchodilator should be administered immediately and consultation sought through the physician or nurse or an emergency room.

When a child is ill, PEFRs can be taken before and after a nebulizer or MDI dose of medication to evaluate the effectiveness of the treatment and the child's response to the drug. This can be particularly helpful to the clinician on the other end of the phone when making decisions about further treatment.

Asthma Education

The complexity of this disease and the need for the patient and family to be "in tune" with subtle changes in symptoms and level of illness warrant the need for concise and easy-to-understand education for the child, family, school personnel, and others involved in the child's care. Many asthma education programs exist and vary from informal teaching in the provider's office to the more formal, organized education programs offered by the American Lung Association ("Airwise"). Many health maintenance organizations are even beginning to offer asthma education programs to clients, as they understand the cost benefits of helping families understand prevention and early treatment strategies in the management of their children's asthma.

Whatever the program, it is necessary that the following content be considered and reviewed on a regular basis (usually yearly):

- definition
- pathophysiology
- signs and symptoms
- trigger identification, avoidance, and control
- treatment:
  - medications—uses, action, side effects, misuses
  - environmental controls
  - immunotherapy
- use of written guidelines for care
- use of asthma diaries
- use of inhalers, nebulizers, spacers
- use of daily peak flow meters and "zoning"
- evaluation and assessment skills
- family support
- communication with others (schools, babysitters, friends)
- feelings about asthma as chronic illness

Many organizations are prepared to furnish families with written pamphlets (for example, American Lung Association; Mothers of Asthmatics; American Academy of Asthma, Allergy & Immunology; see Appendix A) as well as support and to provide guidance in obtaining appropriate care and referral. Many instructional videotapes are also available for viewing at home or in the provider's office. All information given to parents should be explained, readable, and easy to understand. Providers giving out materials should know what the content is and be prepared and available to answer questions as needed. Finally, chapters of the American Lung Association throughout the country sponsor summer camps for children with asthma. These are typically one- to two-week camps that incorporate fun with asthma self-management skills.

The educational process should be a collaborative effort among family, child, and provider. Skills, such as MDI technique or the use of the peak flow meter, should be demonstrated by the provider with return demonstration from the child. Review of all content is often necessary, particularly because some education frequently takes place when the child is ill and the family is stressed. A patient/provider partnership that is set forth with mutual goals and objectives is often the most successful and reaps the most benefits regarding self-management skills.

CYSTIC FIBROSIS

Cystic fibrosis (CF) continues to be the number one genetic, autosomal recessive disease in the Caucasian population. It occurs in 2,500 to 3,000 live births (Davis, Drumm, and Konstan 1996). It is a clinical diagnosis that is constituted by an abnormal sweat chloride, pulmonary disease, and pancreatic insufficiency. The discovery of the CF gene on the long arm of chromosome 7 (Riordan et al. 1989) has led to further understanding about the etiology of the disease and possible future treatments. A protein, CFTR, accounts for the defective functioning of the chloride channel. This leads to inspissated mucus that clogs the lungs and pancreatic ducts and is clinically demonstrated by failure to thrive, nutritional deficiency, and recurrent lung infections leading to eventual scarring and respiratory insufficiency. The improved survival rate for patients with CF, with an average life span of 30 years (FitzSimmons 1995), has been the result of earlier diagnosis and more aggressive nutritional and pulmonary treatment. The advent of more available home care equipment, coupled with the current tenor of the health care system, has exponentially increased the number of CF patients who are cared for or care for themselves at home. Despite this, home care remains complex, stressful, and time consuming (Eiser et al. 1995). Therefore, careful medical and psychosocial assessment of the patient's and family's ability to carry through with home care plans is necessary before discharge.

Airway Clearance

Airway clearance remains a "constant" in day-to-day pulmonary therapy for the majority of patients with CF. The most widely used therapy over the years is chest physical therapy (CPT), which uses postural drainage, percussion, and vibration (Rochester and Goldberg 1980; Kirilloff et al. 1985) (Figure 5–4). In recent years, there have been more techniques available that enable individual patients to choose what works best for them. It is important to note that most patients receive some kind of airway clearance at least three to four times a day during hospitalization. When planning for home care, it should be emphasized that this frequency be adhered to as much as possible, particularly when coupled with home intravenous (IV) antibiotic treatment.

Adherence to CPT can be submaximal because of the time requirement, occasional discomfort, and the necessity of a care provider to do the therapy. Recent advances in techniques now allow patients to be more independent with airway clearance.

Positive expiratory pressure (PEP) masks are used to open obstructed airways by applying positive pressure to exhalation using a mask and one-way valve measuring 10 to 20 cm H_2O pressure. The pressure increases collateral ventilation in obstructed peripheral airways enhancing the likelihood of a productive cough (Groth et al. 1985; Andeson, Quis, and Kenni 1979; Hofmeyer, Webber, and Hodson 1986; Mahlmerster et al. 1991). PEP is often coupled with the forced expiration technique (FET) that uses two to three "huff" exhalations to clear central airways and has been observed to correlate with improved tracheobronchial clearance two to three hours after therapy (Mortensen et al. 1991). Children usually need to be older than five years to be able to coordinate the valve and the "huff" breaths appropriately.

Percussion and vibration vests use an air pulse generator and inflatable vest to oscillate the chest wall at high frequency. Studies have demonstrated increases in both mucus mobilization and spirometry results and have shown the vest to be as equally effective as CPT in improving weight gain, pulmonary function tests (PFTs), and sputum production and expectoration (Kluft et al. 1992; Warwick and Hansen 1991). Issues that must be taken into consideration before using the vest for home use include patient satisfaction (because it can be uncomfortable or claustrophobic for some patients) and funding sources. The vest is expensive and cost may be prohibitive if the patient does not have adequate insurance.

The Flutter valve is a handheld device (a hard plastic "pipe" with a metal ball bearing inside) that had been used in Europe for many years before its introduction to the United States in 1993. It facilitates mucus clearance by oscillating expiratory pressure and airflow that vibrates airway walls and loosens mucus. It also decreases the collapsibility of the airways and accelerates airflow to move mucus up through the airways. In an efficacy study by Konstan, Stem, and Doershuk (1994), the amount of sputum produced using the Flutter valve was three times that produced from voluntary coughing or postural drainage. The device is small, easily portable, relatively inexpensive (about $120, usually reimbursed by third-party providers), and simple to use (Figure 5–5). It requires initial instruction by a therapist, nurse, or physician and occasional review of technique, but can be used in children as young as four or five years. Once taught, the patient can be independent in airway clearance therapy.

Autogenic drainage (AD) is an independent-controlled breathing technique that allows the individual to achieve maximum airflow throughout the airways, enhancing mucus clearance. The following three phases are used with AD: unstick, collect, and evacuate (Chevailler 1984). The "unstick" phase involves a slow, deep inspiration through the nose with a two- to three-second breath hold and a passive expiration, keeping the glottis, throat, and mouth open. The expiratory force remains balanced to prevent airway collapsibility and obstruction. "Collecting" mucus is achieved by deeper inspiration and expiration. The longer the exhalation, the greater the distance the secretions are moved up the airways. Finally, the "evacuation" phase involves airflow from the middle of the inspiratory reserve capacity with small bursts of coughing, resulting in mucus expectoration. A treatment session can last anywhere from 20 to 40 minutes. This technique requires a considerable amount of teaching by a trained instructor as well as much patient practice that can be observed and

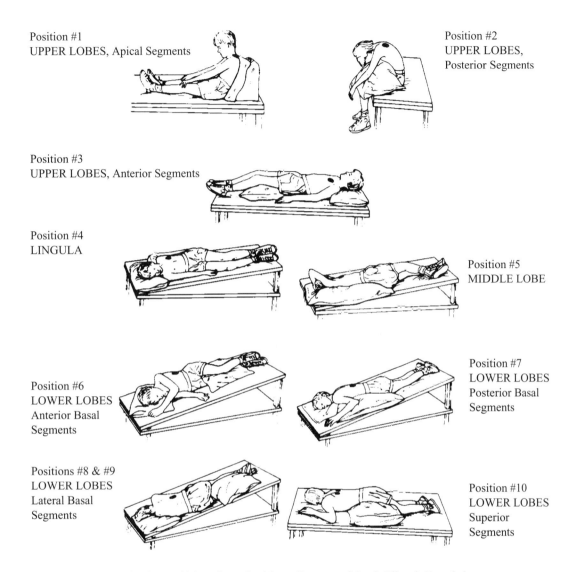

Position #1
UPPER LOBES, Apical Segments

Position #2
UPPER LOBES,
Posterior Segments

Position #3
UPPER LOBES, Anterior Segments

Position #4
LINGULA

Position #5
MIDDLE LOBE

Position #6
LOWER LOBES
Anterior Basal
Segments

Position #7
LOWER LOBES
Posterior Basal
Segments

Positions #8 & #9
LOWER LOBES
Lateral Basal
Segments

Position #10
LOWER LOBES
Superior
Segments

Figure 5–4 Summary of Bronchial Drainage Positions. Courtesy of Cystic Fibrosis Foundation.

assessed by the instructor. Videotapes and demonstrations by experienced patients can be helpful. This technique can be effective and the "technique of choice" for some patients and may never be mastered by others. It requires motivation and commitment on the part of the patient. When instructed properly, it can be used in patients as young as five years old.

Finally, daily exercise is encouraged for all patients with CF. It can be used alone as an air-

way clearance technique by some patients or in conjunction with the PEP or the Flutter valve (or other techniques) by other patients.

Home Antibiotics

Antibiotic treatment of common respiratory pathogens is a typical part of CF home care. Most older patients are maintained on oral prophylactic antibiotics, such as Bactrim, Ceclor, or

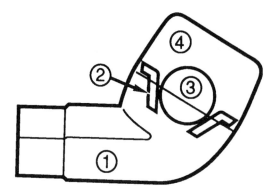

Figure 5–5 Flutter Valve for Airway Clearance. (1) Body, (2) Cone, (3) Steel ball, (4) Covering. *Source:* Reprinted with permission from Konstan, Stern, Doershut, *Journal of Pediatrics,* Vol. 124 No. 5, p. 690, © 1994 Mosby-Year Book, Inc.

dicloxacillin. In recent years, it has also become more common to treat *Pseudomonas aeruginosa* (PA) with an appropriate oral agent, Ciprofloxacin, or with aerosolized or IV antibiotics, such as gentamicin, tobramycin, ceftazidime, or aztreonam. Special considerations must be taken into account when prescribing either aerosolized or IV antibiotics.

Ramsey et al. (1993) have studied the safety and efficacy of aerosolized tobramycin in both low dose (80 mg bid) and high dose (600 mg bid or tid). Each was found to be both safe and efficacious in the control of PA. A higher dosage is thought to be more efficacious because more antibiotic is able to be transported through the thick mucous blanket that lines the airways of individuals with CF. The low-dose version can be administered through a typical air compressor and small-volume nebulizer with 2 mL of antibiotic added to 1 mL of normal saline. High-dose tobramycin must be administered through an ultrasonic nebulizer. The treatment typically takes about 30 minutes because of the large volume of liquid (30 mL) (Ramsey et al. 1993). To compromise, a current multicentered clinical trial is testing the safety and efficacy of a midrange dose of tobramycin (300 mg bid) through a small-volume nebulizer (Pari LC). Results

should be available by the end of 1997. Coly-Mycin is another aminoglycoside that is gaining popularity in its aerosolized form, particularly because of its diminished resistance pattern (Hoiby 1985).

Home IV antibiotic therapy for individuals with CF has been studied considerably (Hammond, Coldwell, and Campbell 1991; Bramwell et al. 1991; Pond et al. 1994; Kane et al. 1988; Donati, Guenette, and Auertach 1987). One must consider many aspects of this care before discharging a patient with a home care regimen, including the following: reliable IV access, funding coverage, family and patient education and readiness, necessary home care support (for example, home nursing care), appropriate electric and telephone access, and primary health care support, if necessary.

The use of intravenous antibiotics requires a reliable form of IV access. Some patients can use smaller peripheral vein catheters, but most require a device such as a midline catheter, a peripherally inserted central catheter, an implanted venous access device (Port-a-Cath®), or a central venous catheter (Hickman, Broviac, or Groshong) (see Chapter 8). Proper education regarding the maintenance and care of the device must be done before initiating home care. Sterility during access is vital to avoid septicemia. Proper care and flushing are necessary to maintain the device for either short-term treatment or long-term sporadic therapy.

There is a variety of home IV pumps available for infusion (Hammond, Coldwell, and Campbell 1991; Bramwell et al. 1991). The patient must be educated about the pump, including use and problem solving. The third-party reimbursers may dictate which pump is used by the patient and family, but it is the nurse's responsibility to assess the appropriateness of the pump, given the individual needs of the patient and family. Advocacy on behalf of the patient may be necessary.

Finally, it may be necessary to draw blood levels of certain antibiotics to determine adequacy of therapy. Erroneous sampling can be avoided using appropriate procedures (Fagerman 1994). It is typically not recommended to draw levels from a central catheter because that may yield false high levels. It is also important to time the levels correctly and to have prompt reporting so that appropriate therapeutic dosage decisions can be made.

Another aerosolized therapy for CF is the frequently used Pulmozyme (rhDNase) (Shak 1995). It is not an antibiotic, rather it is a mucolytic (that is, an enzyme that breaks down the viscosity of the mucus) that is typically aerosolized once a day (2.5 mg), though it is sometimes dosed bid for sicker patients. It requires administration on a daily basis to sustain a therapeutic effect. It must be administered by itself (that is, not mixed with any other drug) through one of the following three nebulizer systems: the Hudson T Updraft, the Marquest Acorn II, or the Pari LC nebulizer. Pulmozyme is an expensive therapy that has been shown to be effective in some patients. However, use of the drug should include close follow-up by the CF center to evaluate adherence to the treatment as well as improvement in the FEV_1.

Home Nutritional Therapy

An important aspect of CF therapy is nutritional management. Most (about 90 percent) individuals with CF experience some exocrine pancreatic insufficiency (Park and Grand 1981). Nutritional intervention is associated with improvement in growth (Hanning et al. 1993) and stabilization of pulmonary function (Levy et al. 1986). Dietary recommendations of at least 120 to 150 percent of the recommended daily allowance (RDA) are typically made including a high-calorie and high-protein diet (MacDonald 1996). Oral nutritional supplements are often used to boost caloric intake. Commercial high-calorie formulas (for example, Ensure, Scandishakes, Carnation Instant Breakfast) are sometimes recommended. Reimbursement for such products, however, can frequently be difficult, and cost may be prohibitive. In that case, families can often be instructed on how to make such formulas at home as well. Special cookbooks are available specifically for families of individuals with CF (Sondel and Hartmen, 1988).

Enzyme therapy is vital for those individuals with malabsorption. The use of such preparations, in combination with high-calorie and high-protein diets, has helped normalize growth and minimize malnutrition in CF patients (Shepard, Cooksley, and Cook 1980). Over the years, new preparations have been manufactured in enteric-coated and microtablet form. This has allowed for better absorption and utilization of the product and, therefore, better efficacy in the control of steatorrhea. Improved absorption lessens the burden of consuming large quantities of food and improves overall nutrition.

High-lipase products (Pancrease MT 16, Creon 20, Ultrase 20) can be useful in decreasing the number of enzymes required during a meal or snack but must be used with some caution. Case reports in 1994 linked very high lipase-dosed products with colonic strictures (Campbell, Forrest, and Musgrove 1994). Because of this, the Cystic Fibrosis Foundation created a consensus statement to recommend no greater than 2,500 units of lipase/kg of weight per meal. Dosages should be checked at least annually at a CF center by a CF nutritionist. If the patient continues to have problems with malabsorption despite high doses of enzymes, then counseling regarding the use of supplemental medication to increase the efficacy of the enzyme product should be provided by the individual's CF team.

Finally, despite the use of better enzyme preparations and high-caloric supplements, some patients still have difficulty maintaining and/or gaining weight. For those patients, nocturnal tube feedings via nasogastric, gastrostomy, or jejunostomy tube can help restore and maintain optimal growth (Steincamp and Hardt 1994; Levy et al. 1985). A thorough nutritional assessment must be done before making the decision in favor of this invasive nutritional intervention. It must be determined that the individual has, indeed, been unsuccessful with maximal noninvasive therapy before recommending tube feedings. It should also be determined that the individual and family have the resources and motivation to carry out the nightly home care tube feeding regimen, as well as the required daily care of the tube site, before recommending such therapy.

After the device (that is, G-tube/button or J-tube) is placed, the CF patient and his or her family must be educated about the use of the tube and the feeding regimen. Some patients may choose to insert a nasogastric tube nightly instead of having a semipermanent tube placed via surgery. Typically, the feedings are dripped in via feeding pump during sleep. The choice of appropriate formula should be made by the CF nutritionist in conjunction with the physician and family. Administration of pancreatic enzymes is usually required before the feeding begins and sometimes in the middle of the night, depending on the patient's needs and the formula chosen. The family should be educated about the mixing, administration, and storage of the formula; the use and problem solving of the feeding pump; and the care of the tube or button and site before discharge. Most families can manage the nighttime feedings independently, but may need to rely on home care nursing help in the event of a problem or mishap. At least a weekly assessment of the tube site is recommended to check for the possibility of local infection or excoriation. Weight checks are typically done at the regular CF center visits, but may be recommended more often for some individuals. This type of invasive nutritional therapy is sometimes used for the remainder of the patient's life. However, it can also be used to achieve a certain weight and health status. Once these are achieved and maintained, the decision to discontinue the feedings and remove the tube may be appropriate for some patients. Close follow-up with the CF center nutritionist is recommended throughout the therapy to guarantee maximum benefit with minimal effort and ease of care at home.

Summary

CF is the most common genetic disease present in the Caucasian population. It is a disease that requires occasional hospitalizations for treatment, particularly in the older adolescent and adult populations who tend to be more ill, but it is also a disease that is often managed almost entirely at home. Improvement in technologies now allows the administration of home IV antibiotics and enteral therapy for patients as well. It is vital, however, to properly assess an individual's and family's ability to handle that care at home and to provide them with the resources necessary to make that possible. This often requires the provider to advocate on the part of the family with the third-party reimburser. It is also necessary to maintain close follow-up with a certified CF center that offers an expert multidisciplinary team of health care providers who are specially trained to work with patients and families affected by CF.

OXYGEN THERAPY

Home supplemental oxygen therapy is used for a variety of pulmonary disorders including bronchopulmonary dysplasia (see Chapter 4), CF, and ventilator dependency. The type of oxygen system used in the home is based on dosage, mobility, safety, cost, patient's preference, duration of therapy, reimbursement constraints, and supplies available from the DME provider. The sources include gas, liquid, and concentrators. The home care nurse must be familiar with each of these sources of oxygen therapy, the portability and safety concerns of each source, and the various delivery methods used in the home.

Gas oxygen is provided in various sized cylinders made from aluminum or steel. Application is often limited to those patients needing a small amount of oxygen for less than 15 hours per day and/or limited mobility. E cylinders are used for portability in conjunction with a large tank or oxygen concentrator. These cylinders are awkward to transport, heavy (weighing more than 15 pounds empty), and must be secured in a wheeled cart or frame attached to the back of a wheelchair. They are unsuitable for a parent who must manage other young children in addition to an oxygen-dependent baby and difficult for the ambulatory oxygen-dependent person.

Oxygen tanks are an ideal backup system for an oxygen concentrator because they can be used in case of power outage. A bank of oxygen cylinders can be used for positive-pressure ventilators with a high gas requirement. They are useful in communities where liquid systems are unavailable or electric power unreliable and/or outlying areas where oxygen delivery is often infrequent. Safety considerations include damage to a tank or regulator that can result in sudden venting sufficient to propel it like a missile because of exceedingly high pressures (McDonald 1994). In addition, open flame or cigarette smoking should not occur near oxygen in the home because of danger of fire.

Oxygen concentrators are electrically powered devices that extract oxygen from room air and deliver it to the patient in concentrations between 93 and 95 percent. Concentrators generally provide only low-flow rates up to 2 to 3 L/min. They cannot be used with aerosol nebulizers or Venturi masks. Concentrators are rather large and bulky and not appropriate for portable use. If a concentrator is used, cylinder oxygen should be available in case of equipment malfunction, power failure, and portability.

Liquid oxygen is a low-pressure oxygen system that can be used with any low-flow oxygen delivery device. It is expensive, but it is the most cost-effective and convenient method for patients with low or moderate continuous flow needs (McPherson 1988). A typical stationary reservoir is capable of holding 40 pounds of oxygen and allows up to four days of continuous flow at 2 L/min. Because of the portability of the system through use of a relative lightweight reservoir (9–13 pounds), it is the system of choice for ambulatory patients. It does not, however, offer advantages for the homebound patient.

Pulsed systems that release short-pulse doses of oxygen at the beginning of the inspiratory cycle are also available (Barker 1994). They can be built into the oxygen reservoir or port-able unit or contained separately on a special belt pack (O'Donohue 1988). Oxygen use with demand systems may be as low as one-seventh that required with nasal prongs. These pulsed oxygen systems can provide substantial oxygen savings for patients and occasionally are used by both adolescents and adults with CF. Despite the cost

savings, some patients are bothered by the clicking noise that accompanies activation.

Oxygen delivery methods include tracheostomy mask, nasal cannulas, masks, and transtracheal catheters. Tracheostomy masks provide a humidified source of either room air or oxygen for a child with a tracheostomy. Potential problems exist if the mask becomes dislodged at night; occasionally, parents may have to put mittens (without a thumb) on the child to prevent removal.

Nasal cannulas are advantageous for oxygen-dependent patients of all ages because of minimal restrictions to visual or auditory stimulation and movement, an important consideration for infants and young children. A nasal cannula can be held in place with a headband, Velcro straps, tape, clear surgical adhesive dressing (for example, Opsite or Tegaderm), or mittens as mentioned previously. Special neonatal-pediatric cannulas are available for young children; makeshift cannulas can also be made by cutting off the nasal prongs, making a slit between the two holes, and positioning the slit below the nares. Flow meters with small calibrations are needed for young children because their flow rates are usually so much lower. The Timeter (Allied Health Care, St. Louis, Mo.) (0.1–1 L/min. $1/8$–3L/min; 25–200 cc min) or the Veriflow (Richmond, Calif.) ($1/8$–$3^1/2$ L/min; $1/32$–$1/2$ L/min) are available for regulation of very low flow rates (McDonald 1994). Nasal cannulas are appropriate for low-flow use only; they are not recommended for higher flows because of irritation and difficulty in maintaining oxygenation.

Oxygen masks are occasionally used in the home but are not typically used in the infant and pediatric patient. Masks interfere with eating and talking, require high-flow rates to achieve an acceptable level of oxygen; and may cause claustrophobia. Hoods or tents are rarely used in the home setting. Although tents permit greater freedom of movement for the child, they are usually frightening. They also usually require higher flow rates, which are a fire hazard.

Transtracheal oxygen therapy provides oxygen via a transtracheal catheter using the trachea as its own reservoir. Less oxygen is lost to ambient air, thus oxygenation can be achieved with a flow rate one-fourth to one-half that required with a standard nasal cannula, offering distinct advantages for the oxygen-dependent patient (D. Hill 1995; Yaeger 1994; Papeke-Benson 1992). The catheters, typically used for the adolescent or adult oxygen-dependent person, are inserted on the anterior chest and tunneled up to the trachea. Complications include the following: obstruction of the catheter from mucous balls, increased loss of catheter tract after catheter displacement; bronchospasm and hoarseness (Christopher et al. 1987). Patients with CF are usually considered poor candidates for transtracheal oxygen because of their copious sputum production.

CARE OF THE CHILD WITH A TRACHEOSTOMY

General Care Issues

Children receive tracheostomies for a variety of conditions including long-term ventilation. The underlying goal of a tracheostomy is the maintenance of the airway; thus, obstruction of the tracheostomy has the potential for being a life-threatening situation. Caregivers then must learn the different aspects of care of the child with a tracheostomy before discharge. In addition to cardiopulmonary resuscitation (CPR) and other emergency care, these components include the following: tracheostomy tube changes, stoma site care, safety concerns, use of resuscitation bag (if used), suctioning, humidification, and speech production. Both caregivers and home health nurses must be familiar with the various components of the tracheostomy care as well as the child's equipment before caring for the child in the home setting.

The type of tracheostomy tube used depends on the patient's circumstances. For children, the type or size of tube changes frequently because of growth in airway diameter, changes in ventilation needs, and development of granulation tissue (Mizmuri, Nelson, and Prentice 1994). The most commonly used tubes are PVC or Silastic

because they are soft and conform to the trachea (Figure 5–6). Although these tracheostornies are disposable, they may be rinsed, soaked in a half-strength hydrogen peroxide solution, rinsed again, and allowed to air dry to be reused.

Tracheostomy tubes can be either cuffed or uncuffed. Cuffless tracheostomy tubes are typically used for children and patients with neuromuscular problems. Cuffed tracheostomy tubes are rarely used in children younger than eight years because the cricoid cartilage is the narrowest part of the child's trachea and serves as a "natural cuff." Pediatric tracheostomy tubes with diameters of less than 5 mm usually provide an adequate seal for positive-pressure ventilation, at least initially (Persky 1985). The advantages of cuffless tubes are that they need to be changed less frequently and they rarely result in tracheal irritation. A cuffless tube is preferred in the home setting (Mizmuri, Nelson, and Prentice 1994).

Cuffed tracheostomy tubes are necessary when ventilation cannot be maintained in the presence of an air leak. Cuffed tubes seal the area between the outer cannula and the tracheal wall, thus protecting the lower airways (Figure 5–7). For this reason, they are also used to prevent aspiration in patients with swallowing difficulties. If cuffed tubes are used, the nurse must be familiar with the care issues to help prevent the risk of tracheal mucosal damage from excessive cuff pressure. These include either using a low pressure cuff tube or alternating periods of inflation and deflation to the trached wall, depending on patient condition and physician preference.

Pediatric tracheostomy tubes typically are more convenient because there is no inner canula because of the small size of the tracheostomy's diameter. Airway inner cannulas fit inside the outer cannula and facilitate airway maintenance because they can be easily removed and cleaned as needed (Exhibit 5–6). Because pediatric tracheostomies do not have inner cannulas and airway patency may be difficult to maintain, humidification and suctioning are important as well as frequent tube changes.

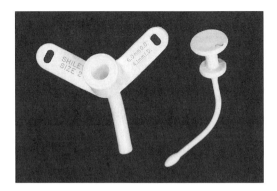

Figure 5–6 Pediatric Tracheostomy Tubes. Courtesy of Mallincroft, St. Louis, Missouri.

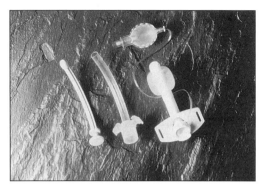

Figure 5–7 Tracheostomy Tube and Inner Cannula. Courtesy of Mallincroft, St. Louis, Missouri.

Tracheostomy tube changes are performed regularly to maintain airway patency, reduce incidence of infection, and prevent formation of tissue granulomas around the stoma. Frequency varies from three times weekly to once a month (Votroubek 1997). Regular and frequent changes give the family the ability and confidence to intervene if the tube comes out accidentally. Parents and other caregivers also need to be able to describe the sequence to follow if the tracheostomy tube is difficult to insert, which is a rare but life-threatening occurrence. The steps include the following: reposition the child's head, use one size smaller tracheostomy tube or use a suction catheter, and notify the physician and emergency services. Several helpful guidelines in the management of tracheostomy tube care are listed in Exhibit 5–7. The procedure for changing a tracheostomy tube is detailed in Exhibit 5–8.

Changing the tracheostomy tube can be an anxiety-provoking experience for parents. The home care nurse should be supportive to the parents during this procedure; however, parents should be encouraged to change the tube with the home care nurse assisting as necessary. This allows the parents to remain skilled in this procedure and offers confidence in any emergency situations.

In addition to tracheostomy tube changes, the emergency issues and safety concerns for the

Exhibit 5–6 Care of the Tracheostomy Tube Inner Cannula

Supplies

Clean bowl or paper cup
Pipe cleaner or small brush
Resuscitation bag (if needed)
Hydrogen peroxide
Distilled water

Procedure

1. Wash hands.
2. Prepare equipment; pour either full- or half-strength hydrogen peroxide into bowl.
3. Give three breaths with resuscitation bag if needed.
4. Remove inner cannula—soak in hydrogen peroxide.
5. Suction the outer cannula.
6. Clean inner cannula by gently scrubbing the inside and outside with pipe cleaner or brush.
7. Rinse under tap water, shake dry, and replace (make sure all hydrogen peroxide is removed before replacing because it can be irritating to the lungs).
8. Reinsert inner cannula and lock in place. (If needed, a temporary inner cannula or inner cannula from the spare tracheostomy tube can be used to maintain ventilation.)

Exhibit 5–7 Helpful Guidelines for Tracheostomy Tube Care

1. A small infant or child can be wrapped securely in a blanket (mummy wrap) to help prevent wiggling during tracheostomy tube changes.
2. A small towel may be rolled and placed under the shoulders of the child to facilitate exposure of the tracheostomy stoma during tracheostomy tube and/or tie changes.
3. If possible, do not change a tracheostomy tube alone. It is a good idea to have a second person to assist in steadying the child.
4. After cutting the tracheostomy ties, place thumb and index finger on wings of tracheostomy tube to steady while changing tubes and/or ties.
5. The child should be given three to five breaths with the Ambu bag (if dependent on ventilator) before removing the tube during tracheostomy changes. Oxygen should be used if ordered.
6. Depending on how long the child's stoma can be without a tracheostomy in place, stoma care can be performed during the tracheostomy change. Many times, a washcloth that is barely damp can be used to clean around the stoma and the skin around the back of the neck. Make sure it is completely dried before the new tracheostomy tubes are tied.
7. Tracheostomy ties should be placed on the new tube before insertion.
8. For tracheostomy care, sterile water or distilled bottled water can be used. To make sterile water, boil water for 5 to 10 minutes, let it cool, and then pour into containers. It is a good idea to keep the sterile water in the refrigerator; change water every three days.
9. Hydrogen peroxide may lose its cleaning power when exposed to air and light. If hydrogen peroxide and water are mixed and put into bowls each day for tracheostomy care, it is a good idea to change each day.
10. The suction machine collecting jars should be cleaned and dried at least every day. Mild household detergent (without lye) may be used. Rinse thoroughly after cleaning. The connecting tube may be cleaned the same way.
11. Tubing, glass, and plastic containers should be cleaned once a week. This can be done with Control III, vinegar solution (1 part vinegar to 3 parts water) or bleach solution (1 part bleach to 10 parts water).

child with a tracheostomy include the following: bleeding, symptoms of infections, difficulty inserting the tracheostomy tube, symptoms of respiratory distress, accidental decannulation, and tube occlusion. Infections will cause changes in odor and color of mucus. Physicians need to be notified if these persist for more than 24 hours. Blood-tinged mucus may indicate either trauma with tracheostomy change or frequent suctioning. Parents should notify the physician if bright red blood is suctioned from the tracheostomy. Bleeding, difficulty inserting a tracheostomy tube, or reduction in vocalization may indicate granuloma formation at the stoma. The child may then have a bronchoscopy so that the airway can be visualized before removal of potential scar tissue or granuloma.

Symptoms of respiratory distress include increased respiratory rate, increased work of breathing, and/or change in color (pale, dusky, blue). Parents should call 911 and go to the nearest emergency department if they notice these symptoms.

Accidental decannulation requires immediate tube placement. Because many infants and children with upper airway problems have little airway reserve, if replacement of the dislodged tube is impossible, a smaller-sized tube should be inserted. Life-threatening occlusion also requires immediate tube change. These occlusions

Exhibit 5–8 Tracheostomy Tube Change

Supplies

Tracheostomy tube (same size and size
  smaller)
Suction equipment
Tracheostomy ties
Scissors

Procedure

1. Wash hands and assemble equipment.
2. Check equipment. Make sure the inner and outer cannulas fit properly.
3. Secure tracheostomy ties through wings. Lubricate the end of the tracheostomy with water-soluble agent. Do not use petroleum jelly products.
4. Position the child to allow good exposure of the stoma.
5. If possible and/or necessary, suction the tracheostomy tube. The child may need to be given oxygen and three to five breaths with the resuscitation bag (if on ventilator) before removing the tube.
6. Hold old tracheostomy tube in place, cut ties with scissors, and pull out with slow steady motion.
7. Stoma care can be performed now following usual procedure or using a barely damp washcloth. This depends on medical stability, airway stability, and child's age.
8. Insert the obturator into inner cannula and hold in place with thumb. If inner cannula is used, keep it close by.
9. Standing at child's side, gently insert the tip of the new tracheostomy tube into the opening, following tract (first upward, then downward curved motion).
10. *QUICKLY* remove obturator while holding the tracheostomy tube in place.
11. Listen for air exchange. Suction if necessary.
12. If child is breathing well, fasten tracheostomy ties. Use one finger space at back of neck to ensure fit.
13. Insert inner cannula, if used.
14. Rinse tube and follow care instructions for reuse.

are apparent when the child displays symptoms of respiratory distress and a suction catheter cannot be passed to the end of the tube despite several attempts and saline instillation. This situation requires an immediate tube change.

Stoma Skin Care

The stoma site must be kept clean to prevent infections. Moisture and secretions can cause irritation and may lead to skin breakdown. Stoma care should be done at least twice a day to remove secretions from around the tube and to examine the appearance of the stoma. Cleaning should be done more frequently if an odor is present. The dressings, if used, should be changed at least twice daily and when they become soiled or dampened. Precut gauze dressings are available and convenient to use. Gauze sponges should never be used for tracheostomy dressings because filaments can easily be inhaled into the trachea. The procedure for daily stoma care is outlined in Exhibit 5–9.

All tracheostomy tubes must be secured to prevent accidental extubation, excessive movement, or misalignment. Changing tracheostomy ties should be a part of the routine care (Exhibit 5–10). There should always be a complete tracheostomy tube set at the patient's bedside for emergency replacement.

Suctioning

The purpose of suctioning is to remove secretions that accumulate in the lungs and large airways that cannot be coughed out. Suctioning of the tracheostomy tube should be done only when it is necessary. This is usually done in the early morning, before meals, and before going to bed. Too frequent suctioning causes increased sputum production. Clinical indications for suctioning include moist, noisy breathing; increased stridor and/or respiratory rate not caused by activity; frequent coughing; nasal flaring; restlessness, irritability, or crying; and color changes. The suction catheter should be inserted only to the end of the tracheostomy tube. Inserting the

Exhibit 5–9 Stoma Care

Supplies

Cotton tip applicators
Washcloth
Warm water
Hydrogen peroxide
Distilled or sterile water
Tracheostomy ties (if needing to be changed)
Ointment

Procedure

1. Wash hands and assemble equipment.
2. Use half-strength hydrogen peroxide to clean crusted areas (equal parts of hydrogen peroxide and water). Long-term use of hydrogen peroxide can cause irritation of the skin.
3. Using washcloth, barely moistened with warm water, clean around stoma, under the wings of tracheostomy tube, and under tracheostomy ties.
4. Use cotton tip applicators and/or dry washcloth to carefully wipe and dry.
5. Tracheostomy ties can be changed during stoma care.
6. Apply ointment as needed after skin is dry.

Exhibit 5–10 Changing Tracheostomy Ties

Supplies

Tracheostomy ties (length is to be at least twice as long as distance around neck, approximately 36 inches long, ends cut on diagonal)
Blunt-end scissors
Blanket roll
Extra tracheostomy tube

Procedure

1. Wash hands and assemble equipment.
2. Restrain child as needed and put blanket roll under shoulder to allow better visualization of tracheostomy tube.
3. Suction (as needed) before changing the ties.
4. If you have a helper, have him or her stabilize tracheostomy wings as close to the neck as possible; otherwise, with one hand, hold the wings yourself.
5. Cut the tracheostomy ties on one side while protecting the child's neck from scissors. Remove old ties without jarring tracheostomy tube.
6. Thread the new tie through the tab, pull half of the length through, bringing both ends around neck to the other side.
7. Cut the old tracheostomy ties from the other side and carefully remove.
8. Thread one free end of the new tie through the tab on the tracheostomy and gently hold the ends of the tie to align around the neck.
9. Carefully tighten the ties and start to tie a knot.
10. Check the ties for tightness, one finger should just fit underneath the ties.
11. Finish knot and cut ends to length of approximately one to two inches.

catheter past the end of the tracheostomy tube can cause increased secretions and, most important, injury to airway tissue (Votroubek 1997). The procedure and equipment for suctioning are outlined in Exhibit 5–11.

A bulb syringe can be used for suctioning the nose and mouth and also the tip of the tracheostomy tube when secretions are coughed up but cannot be cleared from the tube. Bulb syringes must be cleaned thoroughly every 24 hours. This can be done by filling the bulb with warm soapy water, letting it sit momentarily, and squeezing the water out of the bulb. This procedure should be repeated several times until the water returns clear.

A controversial issue is the reuse of suction catheters. Obviously, the major concern is fear of infection from the introduction of new or additional numbers of bacteria that could potentially lead to pneumonia. Some caregivers rinse the catheter after suctioning, changing suction catheters every 8 to 24 hours (Kuhn 1990). Others choose to soak or sterilize the catheters in

Exhibit 5–11 Suctioning the Tracheostomy Tube

Supplies

Suction machine with connecting tubing

Suction catheter kit

Clean container with lid for water

Saline unit dose vials (if needed for insertion into tracheostomy tube)

One of the following: saline, sterile water, or distilled water

Gloves: either sterile or disposable (optional)

Resuscitation bag (if needed)

Oxygen

Procedure

1. Assemble equipment.
2. Wash hands.
3. Open suction kit.
4. Pour saline or water into clean container.
5. Turn suction machine on. Suction pressure should not exceed 120 mm Hg and should be checked before suctioning.
6. Put on glove (if using).
7. Attach suction catheter to suction tubing making sure not to handle end of catheter.
8. Suction a small amount of water from the cup. This ensures that suction is working and catheter is lubricated.
9. Place prescribed amount of saline (from vials) into tracheostomy tube. This will help loosen secretions.
10. If ordered, administer 5 to 10 breaths with resuscitation bag at the prescribed oxygen concentration.
11. Insert catheter gently into the trachea. Do not insert past end of tracheostomy tube or until resistance is felt. (You may need to determine length of catheter insertion with an extra tracheostomy tube).
12. Put thumb over suction port to apply suction.
13. Withdraw suction catheter slowly. Suction should not last for more than five seconds.
14. Administer 5 to 10 breaths with resuscitation bag, if required.
15. Clear secretions from catheter by suctioning a small amount of sterile saline from container.
16. Listen to child's breathing; observe child's color; observe secretions in tubing. Repeat suctioning as needed.
17. When finished suctioning, clear suction tubing by suctioning the rest of the water from the sterile cup.
18. Either discard suction catheter (if symptoms of infection exist) or shake off excess water and wrap in towel or Ziploc bag until next suction.
19. One suction catheter can be used for 1 to 2 hours, or up to 24 hours, depending on frequency of use and recommendations from physicians and/or hospital. Each caregiver should use his or her own suction catheter.

bactericidal solution at the end of the day, rinse, and then reuse. No matter which standard is practiced, proper handwashing is necessary to avoid person-to-person or inanimate object-to-person contamination.

There is an ongoing controversy regarding clean (either nongloved, washed hands or gloved) and sterile-gloved suctioning technique. With clean suctioning, the disposable catheters are frequently reused. As long as the infant is not extremely young and not prone to frequent infections, the caregiver may prefer to use the simplest and least expensive method. If the child develops a respiratory infection, the caregiver should not reuse the suction catheters. Still another method uses "cath-n-sleeve" catheters. These catheters have a sleeve extending to about one inch beyond the catheter tip so caregivers can use bare hands while still maintaining sterile technique. The recommendation for clean versus sterile technique must be decided by the medical provider.

Secretions should be observed for color, consistency, and odor. Blood-tinged mucus could indicate that suctioning is being done too often. Infection will cause odor or color changes to the mucus. If this persists for more than 24 hours, the physician should be notified.

Communication

Communication is another important concern for the child with a tracheostomy. If the child is ventilator dependent, air leaks around the tracheostomy tube, permitting the patient to speak during inhalation. Speech will then occur when enough of the ventilator-delivered tidal volume has escaped around the tube and passes through the vocal cords. Speaking during inhalation is a problem and should be discouraged. If the child loses too much gas during inhalation, he or she will not be adequately ventilated while communicating verbally. The child must be taught to speak during exhalation; this may be done by playing games that encourage active oral exhalation such as blowing bubbles or pinwheels. If a cuffed tracheostomy tube is used, the tube cuff can be deflated and the patient is able to spontaneously breathe for a short while and protect his or her airway; otherwise, a fenestrated tracheostomy tube can be tried.

Fenestrated tracheostomy tubes allow the child to communicate. This is managed by an opening between the flange and the distal tip of the tube. Air flow passes through the opening during exhalation, allowing air to pass over the vocal cords for speech. To use this type of tube, the child must be able to breathe spontaneously or with minimal assistance. Another possibility is the placement of a Passy-Muir speaking valve either in the circuit or on the tracheostomy that allows the patient to speak during exhalation (DeVito and Olslund 1993; Passy 1986) (Figure 5–8). The Olympic Trach-Talk (Olympic Medical, Seattle, Washington) is also available for communication needs.

Humidification

Some form of humidification of inspired air is necessary for patients with a tracheostomy be-

cause the nose and mouth are bypassed. If the patient is ventilator dependent, the humidifier part of the ventilator circuit warms and moisturizes inspired air. If the patient is not being ventilated, other systems are needed, especially at night. Tracheostomy collars are available, but are difficult to use if the patient is not homebound. Vaporizers or room humidifiers may be acceptable but must be cleaned daily. Instillation of saline drops provides humidification when the patient is not at home. Another alternative is the artificial nose or in-line condenser, a corrugated filterlike device that fits snugly either over the end of the tracheostomy tube or inline between the exhalation valve and the patient. During exhalation, moisture from exhaled air condenses on the filter surface. During inhalation, air passes back through the moisture-laden filter and is warmed and humidified, replicating the natural function of the upper airway. Artificial noses are especially helpful for children with smaller tracheostomy tubes (Mallory and Stillwell 1991) (Figure 5–9).

Daily Care Issues

Daily care issues for the child with a tracheostomy at home include the following: bathing, feeding, playing, safety tips, baby-sitters, emergency awareness, and CPR. Depending on the age and size of the child, an apnea monitor is

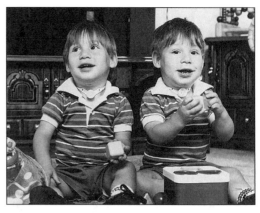

Figure 5–8 Passy Muir Speaking Valve. Courtesy of Passy-Muir Inc., Irvine, California.

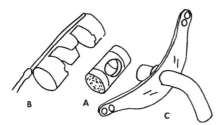

Figure 5–9 Artificial nose. **A.** Thermal humidifying unit, or artificial nose. **B.** Optional oxygen attachment. **C.** Tracheostomy tube, to which artificial nose attaches. Reprinted with permission from Turner, McDonald, and Larter, *Handbook of Adult and Pediatric Respiratory Home Care*, p. 289, © 1994, Mosby-Year Book, Inc.

also required (see Chapter 4). Caregivers should have a travel kit ready when the child is away from home, even for short trips (Exhibit 5–12). Portable suction devices, such as bulb syringes or DeLee mucus suction traps as well as battery-operated suction machines, should be included in the travel kit.

MECHANICAL VENTILATION

Increasingly, children requiring ventilation are being cared for in the home. Goals of long-term ventilatory support at home are the following: to optimize the child's quality of life, ensure medical safety of the child, use respiratory equipment safely and properly, and prevent or minimize complications. Discharge planning for the ventilated child, especially positive-pressure ventilation is a complex process taking two to four weeks in the best of circumstances (Kacmarek and Spearman 1986; Mallory and Stillwell 1991).

Children can be ventilated at home using a variety of assisted ventilation units. These include the following: the negative pressure ventilation systems, diaphragmatic pacing, continuous positive airway pressure with nasal mask, and positive-pressure ventilation with nasal mask or tracheostomy. The type of ventilation units used depends on diagnosis, pathology, and size of the child. Ventilation choices and home care issues are discussed in the following text.

Exhibit 5–12 Travel Kit ("Go Bag") for a Child with a Tracheostomy

1. Shoulder strap bag (many families use small diaper bag)
2. Suction machine (battery-operated ones are more flexible) with connecting tubing attached
3. Suction catheters (may also use DeLee suction traps)
4. Resuscitation bag (if needed)
5. Individual vials of normal saline
6. Tissues
7. Water in a screw-top bottle
8. Extra tracheostomy tube (sterile for emergency insertion) and one-size-smaller tracheostomy tube
9. Two small, tightly closed bowls filled with:
   a. half-strength hydrogen peroxide
   b. water
10. Pipe cleaners and Q-Tips (optional)
11. Gloves and/or hand cleaner (soap, wet wipes, etc.)
12. Tracheostomy adapter (if needed)
13. Ziploc bags
14. Quarter for telephone call

Negative Pressure Ventilation

Negative pressure ventilation (NPV) incorporates a vacuum source or bellows attached to a shell or tank that decreases the pressure surrounding the patient's chest and abdomen. This pressure change causes the diaphragm to descend and the thorax to increase in diameter, allowing air movement into lungs as in normal respiration (Blaufuss and Wallace 1987). The advantages of NPV devices are that they do not require an artificial airway in most patients and are easy to operate. Disadvantages include esophageal reflux, possibility of upper airway obstruction with obstructive sleep apnea, and the pooling of the blood supply in the abdominal area. Candidates for NPV must have a compliant chest wall to ensure ventilation and be medically stable to tolerate periods off the device. Many times, NPV is used for nighttime support only to stabilize respiratory reserve.

The chest shell (cuirass) ventilator uses a dome-shaped shell that fits over the patient's anterior chest and abdomen. Negative pressure is generated within the chest shell, expanding the chest. Cuirass ventilators can provide effective ventilation in older children and adolescents, many times without a tracheostomy. Infants and young children, however, may require a tracheostomy because of airway collapse during sleep (N.S. Hill 1994). Little advantage exists then for infants and young children, because the major benefit of negative pressure ventilation is that a tracheostomy may not be needed. In addition, the smallest commercial shell produced fits children approximately four years of age; therefore, this technique is not possible for children younger than four years.

Home care issues with the chest shell include portability, skin care, and comfort. Comfort is a concern because of the necessity for supine sleep position. In patients with gross deformities, irritation and skin sores can develop at point of sealing. Use of powder or cornstarch and a T-shirt worn under the shell may prevent irritation.

Another negative pressure device is the "raincoat" or wrap. It is essentially a poncho covering a shell-like grid placed on the patient's chest, encompassing either the entire body or only the upper body. Certain patients require the use of a back brace to help prevent a rocking motion of the grid. This device is uncomfortable because of the need to remain supine or reclining; thus, it is not usually appropriate for the pediatric patient.

The iron lung is a self-contained negative pressure ventilator. This "body tank" is an airtight cylinder that uses an electrically powered bellows system to produce negative pressure surrounding the entire body from neck to feet. The full-body chamber is not appropriate for most children or adolescents because patients can feel claustrophobic inside the tank. Nursing care is also made difficult because of patient accessibility. Battery capabilities are not available, and the weight makes the iron lung a permanent device.

Pneumobelts and rocking beds rely on mechanical movement of the diaphragm to aid in ventilation. The pneumobelt, a corsetlike belt attached to a positive pressure generator, allows the patient more freedom of movement but requires the patient to be in an upright position. It is used mainly as a daytime ventilatory aid during meals or wheelchair use. Rocking beds rely on motion to alternately apply and remove pressure on the diaphragm and assist ventilation. They do not require any invasive technology and are simple to operate and maintain. Present use, however, is limited. Disadvantages include size, patients not tolerating rocking motion, confinement, and disturbed sleep.

Diaphragmatic Pacing

Diaphragmatic pacing or bilateral pacing to the thoracic phrenic nerves is another method of supportive ventilation in pediatric patients. Used as an alternative or supplement to mechanical ventilation, pacing is appropriate in children with quadriplegia or inadequate central respiratory drive (central hypoventilation syndrome) (Keens et al. 1990).

Bilateral pacing to the thoracic phrenic nerves offers many advantages over traditional mechanical ventilation. Pacing promotes maximum independence and ability to perform age-appropriate activities for children requiring ventilatory support during the day. It is not uncommon for these patients to engage in various sports and hobbies. Exercise does need to be in moderation, though, because the pacer rate does not increase despite increased metabolic needs (Weese-Mayer et al. 1992). Children who are quadriplegic also enjoy it, allowing normalcy in the wheelchair without the need for a portable ventilator. Bilateral pacing in pediatric patients typically involves a minimum daytime use of 12 to 15 hours with additional ventilatory support by mechanical ventilation. Pacing can, however, provide overnight ventilation for patients needing only nighttime support, eliminating the need for mechanical ventilation (Moxham and Shneerson 1993).

Home care issues for children receiving diaphragmatic pacing include care of the pacer itself and a tracheostomy if mechanical ventilation is used at night. If so, a backup ventilator is required for patient support. Parents are instructed to examine the child's diaphragmatic excursion daily and follow a sequence of events in case of problems. These include replacing the battery and antenna and changing to the backup transmitter if problems occur. Families need to be aware of any potential problems with both the implanted or electrical components and understand the importance of daily monitoring (Votroubek 1995). It is important that physicians with considerable experience and substantial expertise work with the family.

Another pacing concern is the cost and limited availability of centers performing diaphragmatic pacing. Included in the cost are external components (transmitter and antennas), internal components (electrodes, receivers, and anodes), and a month-long intensive care hospitalization. Indirect costs to the family include batteries, transportation, and lodging at the appropriate center. When compared, however, to long-term home mechanical ventilation, the cost becomes negligible.

Noninvasive Positive-Pressure Ventilation

Noninvasive positive-pressure ventilation (NIPPV) is a method to provide positive-pressure ventilation without a tracheostomy (Meyer and Hill 1994). For certain patients who suffer from neuromuscular weakness or restrictive chest wall disease, this technique may provide better acceptance and comfort than the invasive technique. A tracheostomy may be necessary if the patient is unable to protect his or her airway or handle secretions (Leger 1994).

The three types of interfaces used for NIPPV are nasal mask, mouthpiece, and full face mask. Nasal masks may be appropriate for nighttime use but may require custom-molded masks for the pediatric patient. Irritation to the skin, nasal bridge, and mucous membranes may also occur. Mouthpieces with lip seal or custom orthodontic interface may be preferable for daytime use because they are not obtrusive and allow patients to talk and eat but still have assisted ventilation convenience. They may, however, pose a compliance issue for pediatric patients. Full face masks offer better leak control, but have poor tolerance, especially for long-term ventilation at home. Full face masks can also be expensive because they are custom-made and may require frequent adjustments in pediatric patients. No single mask or headgear matches the needs of all patients; it's usually best to try each type on patients to determine which is the easiest to use.

Care issues for patients with NIPPV include skin care, especially with poorly fitting nasal or face mask; gastrointestinal inflation, especially for patients on volume ventilation; and upper airway dryness. Patients also need to be assessed on a regular basis for worsening disease status and increased dependency on mechanical ventilation, necessitating either combined methods of NIPPV or tracheostomy ventilation (Branthwaite 1991).

Continuous Positive Airway Pressure

Continuous positive airway pressure (CPAP) is the application of positive pressure to the airways to prevent upper airway collapse. CPAP, used primarily for obstructive sleep apnea, is administered by a mask with a prescribed amount of resistance incorporated into the circuit. This results in continuous positive pressure against which the patient exhales (Kandall 1994). Bilevel positive airway pressure (BIPAP) is similar to CPAP with higher pressures applied during inspiration than expiration and a backup respiratory rate. It is indicated for patients who need additional respiratory support, have extended periods of apnea, or require higher levels of CPAP.

CPAP and BIPAP can be administered in the home with a tracheostomy or by a mask or nasal pillows held in place with head straps. Both masks and pillows are available in pediatric sizes, as well as nasal CPAP prongs, which may be appropriate for small infants. Custom-made masks derived from commercially available equipment can also be used. As in NIPPV, there is not one type of mask or headgear that is the best for patients. It is recommended that patients try each type to find the best fit.

Technical problems include mouth leaks, which may be remedied by use of chin strap, and nasal obstruction or nasal stuffiness especially during viral rhinitis, which can be treated with humidification and/or nasal decongestant spray. Some patients also complain of claustrophobic sensations, which can be avoided by use of the nasal pillows. Hand restraints may be needed with young children who resist mask administration and/or pull the mask off during sleep. Patient and family members need to be well versed in both technical and safety aspects of care before discharge.

Positive-Pressure Ventilation

The most commonly used approach for home mechanical ventilation is the positive-pressure ventilator. Parents, caregivers, and home care nurses need to be trained in ventilator management before discharge. The purpose of this section is to give the reader insight into routine home procedures for managing the ventilator. The ventilator selected for use in the home is dependent on the child's diagnosis, required oxygen concentration, daily requirements for mechanical ventilation, availability of equipment, and repair service (Kacmarek 1994). The ideal home ventilator is inexpensive, portable, small, and lightweight. Two mechanical ventilators commonly used in the home are the LP10 (Aequitron, Minneapolis, Minnesota) and the PLV100 (Lifecare, Phoenix, Arizona). These types of ventilators are relatively easy to operate, weigh less than 40 pounds, and can be battery operated, an important feature in allowing greater mobility in respiratory support in case of power failure (Lynch 1990).

One disadvantage in positive-pressure ventilation in the home is the requirement for an artificial airway or tracheostomy. Because the underlying goal of the tracheostomy is to provide an open airway, obstruction of the tracheostomy has the potential for being a life-threatening emergency. All caregivers then need to become expert in the management of the tracheostomy (see section, Care of the Child with a Tracheostomy).

Backup ventilator support must be available in the home. Patients who require 24-hour ventilation, those who tolerate only very short periods without ventilator support, or those who live a significant distance from a medical center need a second fully functional ventilator in the home.

Equipment and Supplies

Regular and systematic monitoring of ventilator equipment is essential for the safe delivery of care. Regular and frequent ventilator checks are mandatory, allowing for close follow-up of the child's respiratory status, as well as detection of mechanical flaws. Daily routines for equipment maintenance include ventilator checks, cleaning and changing the ventilator circuits, and cleaning the suction machine and resuscitation bag. Established routines for ventilator care at home are facilitated by the use of a ventilator activity list (Exhibit 5–13). Most manufacturers provide detailed troubleshooting guidelines. These guidelines list problems, possible causes, and corrective actions.

The most common nonmedical problems encountered with ventilator equipment include humidifier malfunction, electrical power failure, suction machine malfunction, frozen oxygen gauge, and holes in ventilator tubing. Consistent problems with the ventilator require the home care nurse to observe how the equipment is used, cleaning practices, and daily maintenance. This may help identify interventions to decrease problem areas.

The nurse also needs to be familiar with care of the child and ventilator in case of mechanical failure. If the ventilator power goes out while other household electrical equipment is still operating, the failure is in the ventilator. Either a

Exhibit 5–13 Activity List for Ventilator Home Care

Daily Activities

Stoma care:
- Change tracheostomy ties.
- Discard used suction catheters.
- Empty and clean suction bottle and rinse connecting tube.
- Replace tracheostomy care solutions.
- Check ventilator settings.
- Clean resuscitator bag and valve (if used). (This is typically changed every 24 to 48 hours, but two to three times a week is usually sufficient.)
- Clean ventilator circuits.
- Check oxygen level in tanks (can be done every two days).

Weekly Activities

Tracheostomy tube change:
- *Discard* suction machine connection tubing and *replace*.
- *Soak* suction equipment.
- Check inventory and order supplies.
- Thoroughly clean tracheostomy and ventilator care area.

circuit breaker or fuse has blown or the ventilator has a malfunction. Although ventilators have internal batteries, occasionally these batteries fail to take over. Anytime a mechanical failure occurs, the patient should be ventilated with the resuscitation bag or switched to the backup ventilator (if available) and the equipment vendor should be notified immediately. If the problem is a power failure, ensure that the ventilator is connected to the external battery and, if indicated, notify the power company. A flashlight should be kept near the ventilator in case of power outages (Mizmuri, Nelson, and Prentice 1994).

Some ventilator-assisted children require supplemental oxygen. If their oxygen needs are more than 21 percent, the oxygen system chosen for use in the home is based on the pressure input requirements of the ventilator, required flow rates, portability of oxygen system, and availability of supplier (see section, Oxygen Therapy).

All children receiving home mechanical ventilation via tracheostomy require a means for warming and humidifying inspired air to prevent drying and inspissation of tracheobronchial secretions, insensible water loss, and loss of body heat. The humidifier is the part of the ventilator circuit that warms and moisturizes inspired air during ventilation. Humidification can be provided by jet nebulizer, cascade, or regenerative humidifier. The purpose is to prevent drying of the tracheal secretions and insensible water loss. When the patient is not being ventilated or if additional humidification is needed during ventilation, another system such as warm or cool mist is useful. The type of humidifier should be selected and tested before the child's discharge. The nurse should be familiar with the system and symptoms of inadequate humidification including thicker secretions or occasionally blood-tinged sputum.

Monitors/Alarms

Some ventilators do not come equipped with the necessary monitors to ensure the child's safety. Additional monitoring equipment may be necessary. Minimally, the ventilator alarms should include patient disconnect, high- and low-pressure alarms, oxygen analyzer/monitor, and spirometers.

Equipment for the ventilator will need to be ordered periodically. It is helpful to take inventory of supplies weekly and order on a regular basis. Supplies required for home ventilation include tracheostomy supplies, ventilator circuits, and resuscitation bag. Ventilator circuits are typically changed every one to two days. Usually, two or three ventilator circuits are sufficient because the family and/or home care nurse will change and clean the circuits regularly. The circuits then are alternated and discarded monthly.

Travel

Children on ventilators are capable of returning to all aspects of community life; they attend regular classrooms in school (see Chapter 19), attend summer camps, and participate in many social activities with their friends (Gilgoff and Helgren 1992). This is because ventilators are portable, and mechanically operated wheelchairs with space available for mounting a battery-powered ventilator allow children flexibility. Trips away from home need to be carefully planned. Equipment needed for travel is similar to equipment needed at home. The home care nurse should plan for emergencies during travel and prepare equipment accordingly.

NURSING CARE PLANS IN THE HOME

This section provides some general guidelines for nursing care of children with CF, bronchopulmonary dysplasia (BPD), asthma, tracheostomies, and ventilator dependency. It is important to remember that the needs of the child and family will vary greatly from case to case. Information from the facility referring the child is vital in constructing specific, individual care plans. It is likely that parents have been instructed to some extent on providing medical and nursing care for their child. They, along with the primary and/or specialty care providers, should be used as resources. This will ensure and maintain consistent, safe, effective, and individualized care.

A broad range of skills is required to care for children with alterations in respiratory function. In addition to clinical skills, the home care nurse must be able to assess family coping ability, parental stress, self-esteem (child and parents), need for privacy and control, general health maintenance, and enmeshment of child, family, community, and primary, secondary, and tertiary health care providers. Effective intervention is based on a sound understanding of these concepts. These areas are addressed in this section. General nursing diagnosis and patient outcomes that apply to all four previously mentioned disease states are outlined. The care plans in Appendixes 5–A through 5–D address specific problems of each disease entity.

Alterations in Respiratory Function

This broad category includes impaired gas exchange, ineffective airway clearance, and/or ineffective breathing patterns. The goal of care is to maintain optimal respiratory function with proper gas exchange, effective respiratory patterns, and adequate airway clearance. Assessment of the child's respiratory status must be continuous because of the dynamic state of these diseases. This begins by establishing the child's baseline. For example, it is often common for children with CF to have a cough. Breathing patterns may be solely the result of the cycle of the mechanical ventilator and may, therefore, appear to be different from "normal" respiratory excursions. This baseline should allow the home care nurse to make a thorough respiratory assessment of the child within the first few minutes of the visit. This should include inspection for the following signs of respiratory distress: a tense, drawn, or worried facial expression; nasal flaring; chest retractions; shortness of breath that gets progressively worse; inability to catch breath or struggle to catch breath; difficulty walking or talking; and changes in skin color. The family needs to notify the physician and have the child go to the hospital if any of these symptoms of respiratory distress exist.

Notation of sputum color, consistency, odor, and amount can be of great importance in detecting a potential infection. A change in the child's cough should also be noted during the assessment. A recent history noted from either the previous shift's nurse, the parent, or the child will be necessary to determine the significance of any changes that may be observed during the examination.

Auscultation is another important part of the initial respiratory assessment. The presence of any adventitious sounds is significant in the final evaluation of the child's respiratory status. Complete thoracic auscultation with a reliable stethoscope is often the best way to identify potential alterations in gas exchange or airway clearance. Precise terminology is less important than recognition of an abnormal sound that is not a part of the child's baseline assessment. The location of the sound and the point at which it occurs in the respiratory cycle are both important. For example, a "crackle" noted in the right upper lobe during both inspiration and expiration or "wheezes" found bilaterally on expiration are important data that can help determine the action required in a given situation.

The initial respiratory assessment is the basis for determining the care plan for the day. If there is no alteration from the child's previous condition, then the nurse can proceed with specific daily treatments and interventions as outlined in the general nursing care plan. If an alteration in any respiratory parameter is noted, it may mandate changes to the care plan for that day. For example, if the child with a tracheostomy or with CF has an increased cough or has lungs that sound congested, he or she may benefit from extra chest physiotherapy, extra suctioning, and perhaps a consultation with the physician regarding a potential infection. If the child with asthma is noted to be more dyspneic or wheezy, he or she may require an additional dose from an MDI or small-volume nebulizer.

The initial respiratory assessment of the infant with a pulmonary disorder is the standard used to identify complications or improvements in the child's status. This information allows caregivers to detect, respond to, and prevent progression of complications and to note positive response to therapy leading toward an improvement in the child's status.

Alterations in Nutrition: Less Than Body Requirements

Nutritional deficits can be observed in varying degrees in children with alterations in respiratory status. The desired patient outcome is adequate nutritional intake that supports proper growth and development. In some instances, this is crucial to the ultimate resolution of the pulmonary ailment. The child with CF must maintain adequate nutrition to ward off impending pulmonary infections; yet, at the same time, the pulmonary disease increases the difficulty of maintaining adequate caloric intake for growth and healing. Compounding the problem is the need for increased calories.

Infants who have had recurrent oral intubations, oral or nasopharyngeal suctioning, or sucking deprivation secondary to their critical illness as a neonate may have developed a feeding aversion (see Chapter 4). Such children may require feeding from a nonoral route. These sites include gastrostomy, jejunostomy, or nasogastric tube. The home care nurse must be knowledgeable in the care of such tubes (see Chapter 8). Tubes should be patent at all times. This can be achieved by administering a small (10–30 mL) water flush after each feeding or medication. Some tubes require routine changes to maintain patency and to avoid deterioration. Parents should be observed and/or aided during the process of changing the feeding tube while they check for placement and patency and during daily use. A child with a nasogastric tube will need more frequent tube changes (that is, every two to three days) than a child with a gastrostomy tube, who needs a tube change every four to eight weeks. The discharging health care team should recommend a tube replacement schedule.

Providing adequate nutritional intake for the infant with a chronic pulmonary disorder can often be a challenging task. Parents need encouragement and positive feedback. Consultations with appropriate health care professionals, including counselors and/or social workers, may help those families frustrated by what is often perceived as the most difficult aspect of care.

Skin Integrity and the Potential for Impairment

There are several factors involved that can contribute to the development of skin difficulties. The first is the child's chronic condition, often complicated by an impaired nutritional state. Second, the child may require additional apparatus that impairs skin integrity. Oxygen nasal cannulas, tracheostomy tubes and ties, gastrostomy tubes, and/or monitor leads are all potential harbingers to skin irritation or breakdown. In addition, the underlying disease state may cause skin problems. For example, the child with asthma may also present with atopic dermatitis or the infant with CF may have perineal breakdown from frequent, malabsorbed stools. Finally, various treatments such as antibiotics or mist to a tracheostomy may cause skin irritation, rashes, or breakdown. The skin must be thoroughly examined on a routine basis to ensure that the child has intact skin free of breakdown or areas of infection.

Tubes that need to be held in place should, whenever possible, be taped onto something other than the skin itself (for example, a small piece of gauze, another piece of tape). This minimizes the number of times tape is put on and pulled off the skin itself. For example, placing two thin strips of adhesive tape on the cheeks of a child requiring oxygen via nasal cannulas allows the oxygen tubing to be taped onto the tape, which can stay in place for days. Rotation of tape, monitor leads, and tracheostomy tie knots will also decrease irritation. Thorough cleansing and drying of areas of potential skin breakdown are also crucial. A hair dryer set on low/cool can help dry areas of skin that are difficult to reach (for example, the back of an infant's neck) without causing abrasion from rubbing with a towel. Finally, when an area of skin breakdown is noted, the physician should be notified. Antibiotic creams and ointments or hydrocortisone cream might be useful treatment but should not be used without a physician's or nurse specialist's recommendation.

Impaired Growth and Development

Impaired growth and development can include both physical and psychosocial aspects. The desired patient outcome is normal growth and development. Inadequate nutritional intake is the precipitant of impaired physical growth and development. (Children with CF are often thinner and smaller than their peers.) Adolescents with CF also tend to enter puberty later, delaying the onset of secondary sexual characteristics. Children with severe asthma may be smaller in stature if they have required long-term corticosteroid therapy. The etiology of the impaired physical growth must be identified and efforts made to correct it whenever possible. For example, if the problem is inadequate caloric intake, then a nutritional plan to increase calories is appropriate. If the child with CF has significant malabsorption, then measures should be taken to correct it. Accurate records should be kept at specific intervals to plot the child's true physical growth. These data will help physicians and nutritionists plan future interventions.

Delayed psychosocial growth and development can result from isolation if the child has had long or frequent hospitalizations and dissociation from peers and family. Children on ventilators or with tracheostomies are often less mobile than their peers, decreasing their opportunities to play, explore, and interact appropriately for their age group. The signs and symptoms of delay can be obvious or may be manifested in more covert ways. Caregivers should be alert to the signs of chronic anxiety, irritability, and depression, which can be manifestations of the frustrations that often accompany isolation. Many times, child psychologists or other health care workers skilled in the care of these problems should be consulted.

Identification of developmental delays requires formulation of a plan of care. A written care plan should be completed before discharge so that family, home care nurses, school personnel, and home care physical and occupational therapists can partake in a program appropriate for that child's developmental stimulation. If developmental delays are detected during home care, the care plan should be developed in conjunction with the referring medical center. A physical or occupational therapy consultation will help quantify and qualify the delay. Interventions that involve family participation should then be identified. Involving the family augments therapy for both the child and family by allowing them time together (see Chapter 18).

Knowledge Deficit

Knowledge deficit related to the disease process and necessary treatment regimens is a common problem recognized by home care nurses. It is hoped that the parents and the child have been educated before the child's discharge. However, it must be recognized that hospitalization is a stressful period and a certain disruption. Many times, the patient and caregivers will not be able to integrate all components of the patient's care they have been taught. It is crucial to assess a family's level of knowledge regarding the disease and treatment interventions. This is especially true because families and patients are often expected to be independent in carrying out the entire treatment regimen at some point. Accurate assessment must be based on education received before discharge.

Once an accurate assessment has been made, the obvious intervention is to educate the family or patient in any areas of which they have deficient knowledge. Communication with the discharging facility will ensure that consistent teaching is being conducted. Consistency in teaching will help assimilate information as well as decrease confusion and frustration.

Parents or patients should be encouraged to ask questions and write down questions for later discussion. Many families and patients find the use of a journal invaluable for keeping track of day-to-day changes, assessments, occurrences, and questions. Some tertiary care settings provide families with records to facilitate follow-up visits and future hospitalizations.

Ineffective Coping

Ineffective coping can be manifested by recognition and verbalization of the inability to cope, role confusion, inability to make decisions or ask for help, and inappropriate use of defense mechanisms. Ineffective coping will affect the patient and family's ability to comply with any part of the home care plans and therapeutic regimens. Contributing factors can be pathophysiologic, situational, and maturational. The home care nurse must be aware of the signs of ineffective coping and must use assessment skills to ascertain the degree of impact on the family's ability to care for the child. Patient outcomes include recognition of ineffective coping strategies, facilitation of support and guidance in stressful situations, and patient and family use of appropriate, effective coping strategies.

Home care is more cost effective than hospital care, and the impact of chronic hospitalization and separation is often devastating to both the child and family. Sending the child home will not solve all problems. Many times, it may precipitate new stressors and challenges for the family to cope with (Quint et al. 1990; Wegener and Aday 1989). Once home, the multiple sources of support in the hospital are no longer available and the family is left with the overwhelming responsibility of caring for the child day to day, month to month, year to year. Families should know that the hospital and home care team are available for support and it should be clear whom to call with questions or concerns (Lobosco et al. 1991).

Nursing care in the home is a mechanism that promotes effective coping. It prevents parent "burnout" from shouldering the burden of 24-hour nursing care. It allows the parents time to truly "parent" rather than consistently tend to medical, technical, or nursing needs of the child. Home nursing should also allow the parents time away from the child to spend as a couple or to spend with other children. Siblings must be recognized for their importance as members of the family. Nurses in the home can also affect family coping strategies by being an educational resource. Often, families experience stress because they feel unknowledgeable regarding aspects of their children's care. The home care nurse can reinforce education and promote self-assurance for parents.

Home nursing care often promotes great relief for families but can also be a source of stress. Suddenly, families have strangers in the home.

Issues of privacy, independence, and role confusion surface. Parents often feel awkward disagreeing in front of the nurse. They may avoid disciplining their children for fear of being seen or heard and judged incorrectly. They may not trust the nurses. They may resent such an intrusion, although it is obviously necessary and helpful to them. Home care nurses must be aware and sensitive to these issues. Frequent care meetings can help keep communication lines open and lead to strategies for coping with the presence of nurses in the home. Ineffective coping can be an ongoing, fluctuating problem for children and families impacted by chronic illness. Recognition and assessment of the problem and contributing factors are the first steps toward resolution. Providing support, facilitating communication, and encouraging appropriate coping strategies will serve to maintain effective stress management and coping abilities for these children and families facing countless, yet surmountable, odds. (Also, see Chapter 20 for a further discussion of parents' perspective on home care.)

REFERENCES

Ahrens, R., et al. 1995. Choosing the metered dose inhaler, spacer, or holding chamber that matches the patient's needs: Evidence that the specific drug being delivered is an important consideration. *Journal of Allergy and Clinical Immunology* 96:278–83.

Andeson, J.B., I. Quis, and T. Kenni. 1979. Recruiting collapsed lung through channels with positive end expiratory pressure. *Scandinavian Journal of Respiratory Disease* 60: 260–66.

Barker, A.F. 1994. Oxygen conserving methods for adults. *Chest* 105, no. l: 248–52.

Blaufuss, J.A., and C.J. Wallace. 1987. Negative pressure ventilators: Clinical application and nursing care. *Critical Care Nursing* 9–14.

Bramwell, E.C., et al. 1991. Home treatment of patients with cystic fibrosis using the "intermate": The first year's experience. *Journal of Advanced Nursing* 22:1063–67.

Branthwaite, M.A. 1991. Non-invasive and domiciliary ventilation: Positive pressure techniques. *Thorax* 46: 208–12.

Bush, A.K. 1992. The role of allergens in asthma. *Chest* 101:3785–805.

Campbell, C.A., J. Forrest, and C. Musgrove. 1994. High strength pancreatic enzyme supplements and large bowel stricture in cystic fibrosis. *Lancet* 343:109–10.

Chevailler, J. 1984. Autogenic drainage. In *Cystic fibrosis: Horizons*, ed. D. Lawson. Chichester, MA: John Wiley.

Christopher, K.L., et al. 1987. A program for transtracheal oxygen delivery. *Annals of Internal Medicine* 107: 802–08.

Davis, P., M. Drumm, and M. Konstan. 1996. Cystic fibrosis. *American Journal of Respiratory and Critical Care Medicine* 154:1229–56.

DeVito, A. and L. Olslund. 1993. Using the Passy-Muir tracheostomy valve. *Perspectives in Respiratory Nursing,* March, 6–8.

Donati, M.A., G. Guenette, and H. Auertach. 1987. Prospective controlled study of home and hospital therapy of cystic fibrosis pulmonary disease. *Journal of Pediatrics* 111:28–33.

Eiser, C., et al. 1995. Routine stresses in caring for a child with cystic fibrosis. *Journal of Psychosomatic Research* 39: 641–46.

Fagerman, K.E. 1994. Erroneous tobramycin sampling in home intravenous therapy avoidable with modified blood draw. *Journal of Intravenous Nursing* 17, no. 3:135–37.

FitzSimmons, S. 1995. Cystic fibrosis registry. Bethesda, MD: Cystic Fibrosis Foundation.

Gergen, P.J., D.I. Mullally, and R. Evans. 1988. National survey of prevalence of asthma among children in the United States. *Pediatrics* 81:1–7.

Gilgoff, I.S. and J. Helgren. 1992. Planning an outing from hospital for ventilator-dependent children. *Development Medicine and Child Neurology* 34:904–10.

Groth, S., et al. 1985. Positive expiratory pressure physiotherapy improves ventilation and reduces volume of tapped gas in cystic fibrosis. *Bulletin European Physiopathology Respiratory* 21:339–43.

Halken, S., et al. 1991. Recurrent wheezing in relation to environmental risk factors in infancy. *Allergy* 46:507–14.

Hammond, U., S. Coldwell, and P.W. Campbell. 1991. Cystic fibrosis, intravenous antibiotics and home therapy. *Journal of Pediatric Health Care* 5:24–30.

Hanning, R.M., et al. 1993. Relationships among nutritional status and skeletal and respiratory muscle function in cystic fibrosis: Does early dietary supplementation make a difference? *American Journal of Clinical Nutrition* 57:580–87.

Hill, D. 1995. Transtrachael oxygen: Setting up a home care program. *Caring,* May, 44–47.

Hill, N.S. 1994. Use of negative pressure ventilation, rocking beds, and pnuemobelts. *Respiratory Care* 39: 532–49.

Hofmeyer, J.L., B.A. Webber, and M.E. Hodson. 1986. Evaluation of positive expiratory pressure as an adjunct to chest physiotherapy in the treatment of cystic fibrosis. *Thorax* 41:951–54.

Hoiby, N. 1985. Isolation and treatment of cystic fibrosis patients with lung infections caused by *Pseudomonas (Burkholderia)* cepacia and multiresistant *Pseudomonas aeruginosa. Netherlands Journal of Medicine* 46, no. 6: 280–87.

Kacmarek, R.M. 1994. Home mechanical ventilatory assistance for infants. *Respiratory Care* 39:550–65.

Kacmarek, R.M., and C.B. Spearman. 1986. Equipment used for ventilatory support in the home. *Respiratory Care* 31:311–28.

Kandall, K. 1994. Respiratory therapy devices. In *Handbook of adult and pediatric respiratory home care,* ed. J. Turner, G. McDonald, and N. Larter. St. Louis: Mosby-Year Book.

Kane, R.E., et al. 1988. Cost savings and economic considerations using home intravenous antibiotic therapy for cystic fibrosis patients. *Pediatric Pulmonology* 4: 84–89.

Keens, T.G., et al. 1990. Home care for children with chronic respiratory failure. *Seminars in Respiratory Medicine* 11: 269–81.

Kerrebijn, K.F. 1990. Use of topical corticosteroids in the treatment of childhood asthma. *American Review of Respiratory Disease* 141:577–81.

Kirilloff, L.H., et al. 1985. Does chest physical therapy work? *Chest* 88:436–44.

Klaus, M.H., and A.A. Fanaroff, eds. 1986. *Care of the high risk neonate.* Philadelphia: W.B. Saunders.

Kluft, J., et al. 1992. Comparison of bronchial drainage treatments by sputum quantity. *Pediatric Pulmonology.* L4-suppl. 2:299.

Konstan, M.W., R.C. Stem, and C.F. Doershuk. 1994. Efficacy of the flutter device for airway mucus clearance in patients with cystic fibrosis. *Journal of Pediatrics* 124: 689–93.

Kuhn, S. 1990. *Tracheostomy home care for children.* 3d ed. Los Angeles: Department of Nursing, Children's Hospital of Los Angeles.

Leger, P. 1994. Noninvasive positive pressure ventilation at home. *Respiratory Care* 39:501–09.

Levy, L., et al. 1986. Prognostic factors associated with patient survival during nutritional rehabilitation in malnourished children and adolescents with cystic fibrosis. *Pediatric Gastroenterology and Nutrition* 5:97–102.

Levy, L.D., et al. 1985. Effects of longterm nutritional rehabilitation on body composition and clinical status in malnourished children and adolescents with cystic fibrosis. *Journal of Pediatrics* 107:225–40.

Lobosco, A.F., et al. 1991. Local coalitions for coordinating services to children dependent on technology and their families. *Children's Health Care* 20:75–86.

Lynch, M. 1990. Home care of the ventilator-dependent child. *Children's Health Care* 19:169–73.

MacDonald, A. 1996. Nutritional management of cystic fibrosis. *Archives of Disease in Childhood* 74, no. 1: 81–87.

Mahlmerster, M.J., et al. 1991. Positive expiratory pressure mask therapy: Theoretical and practical considerations and a review of the literature. *Respiratory Care* 36: 1218–29.

Mallory, G.B., and P.C. Stillwell. 1991. Home ventilator-dependent child: Issues in diagnosis and management. *Archives in Physical Medicine Rehabilitation* 72:43–55.

McDonald, G. 1994. In-home oxygen therapy. In *Handbook of adult and pediatric respiratory home care,* ed. J. Turner, G. McDonald, and N. Larter. St. Louis: Mosby-Year Book.

McFadden, E.R. 1995. Improper patient techniques with metered dose inhalers: Clinical consequences and solutions to misuse. *Journal of Allergy and Clinical Immunology* 96:278–83.

McPherson, S.P. 1988. *Respiratory home care equipment.* Dubuque, IA: Kendall/Hunt Publishing Company.

Mendoza, G.R., N. Sander, and A. Scherrer. 1988. *A user's guide to peak flow monitoring.* Fairfax, VA: Mothers of Asthmatics, Inc.

Meyer, T.J., and N.S. Hill. 1994. Noninvasive positive pressure ventilation to treat respiratory failure. *Annals of Internal Medicine* 120:760–70.

Mizmuri, N., E. Nelson, and W. Prentice. 1994. Mechanical ventilation in the home. In *Handbook of adult and pediatric respiratory home care,* ed. J. Turner, G. McDonald, and N. Larter. St. Louis: Mosby-Year Book.

Mortensen, J., et al. 1991. The effects of postural drainage and positive expiratory pressure physiotherapy on tracheobronchial clearance in cystic fibrosis. *Chest* 100: 1350–57.

Moxham, J. and J.M. Shneerson. 1993. Diaphragmatic pacing. *American Review of Respiratory Disease* 148: 533–36.

National Heart, Lung, and Blood Institute. Executive Summary: Guidelines for the diagnosis and management of asthma: National Asthma Education Program Expert

Panel report. 1991. *Journal of Allergy and Clinical Immunology* 88:425–534.

O'Donohue, W.J. 1988. Guidelines for the use of nebulizers in the home and at domiciliary sites. *Chest* 109:814–20.

Papeke-Benson, K. 1992. Transtracheal oxygen therapy. *International Association of Cystic Fibrosis Adults (IACFA)*, November, 11–13.

Park, R.W., and R.J. Grand. 1981. Gastrointestinal manifestations of cystic fibrosis. *Gastroenterology* 81:1143–61.

Passy, V. 1986. Passy-Muir tracheostomy speaking valve. *Otolaryngology—Head and Neck Surgury* 95:274–84.

Pattemore, P.K., S.L. Johnston, and P.G. Bardin. 1992. Viruses as precipitants of asthma symptoms. *Clinical and Experimental Allergy* 22:325–36.

Persky, M. 1985. Airway management and post inhalation sequelae. In *Critical care pediatrics*, ed. S. Zimmerman and J. Gilden. Philadelphia: W.B. Saunders.

Pond, M.N., et al. 1994. Home versus hospital intravenous antibiotic therapy in the treatment of young adults with cystic fibrosis. *European Respiratory Journal* 7:1640–44.

Quackenboss, J.J., M.D. Lebowitz, and M. Krzyzanowski. 1991. The normal range of diurnal changes in peak expiratory flow rates: Relationship to symptoms and respiratory disease. *American Review of Respiratory Disease* 143:323–30.

Quint, R.D., et al. 1990. Home care for ventilator-dependent children. *American Journal of Diseases of Children* 144: 1238–41.

Ramsey, B.W., et al. 1993. Efficacy of aerosolized tobramycin in patients with cystic fibrosis. *New England Journal Medicine* 328:1740–46.

Riordan, J., et al. 1989. Identification of the cystic fibrosis gene: cloning and characterization of complementary DNA. *Science* 245:1066–73.

Rochester, D.F., and S.K. Goldberg. 1980. Techniques of respiratory physical therapy. *American Review of Respiratory Disease* 122, no. 2:133–46.

Sears, M.R., et al. 1990. Regular inhaled beta-agonist treatment in bronchial asthma. *Lancet* 336:1391–96.

Shak, S. 1995. Aerosolized recombinant human DNase for the treatment of cystic fibrosis. *Chest* 107:655–705.

Shepard, R.W., W.G.E. Cooksley, and W.D.D.Cook. 1980. Improved growth and clinical nutritional and respiratory changes in response to nutritional therapy in cystic fibrosis. *Journal of Pediatrics* 97:351–57.

Siegel, S.C., and G.S. Rachelefsky. 1985. Asthma in infants and children. *Journal of Allergy and Clinical Immunology* 76:1–15.

Smith, L. 1993. Childhood asthma: Diagnosis and treatment. *Current Problems in Pediatrics* 23, no. 7:271-305.

Sondel, S., and L. Hartmen. 1988. *A way of life: Cystic fibrosis nutrition handbook and cookbook.* Madison, WI: University of Wisconsin Hospital and Clinics.

Steincamp, G., and H. Hardt. 1994. Improvement of nutritional status and lung function after longterm nocturnal gastrostomy feedings in cystic fibrosis. *Journal of Pediatrics* 124:244–29.

Toogood, J.H. 1990. Complications of topical steroid therapy for asthma. *American Review of Respiratory Disease* 141:S89–S96.

U.S. Environmental Protection Agency. 1992. *Respiratory health effects of passive smoking: Lung cancer and other disorders.* EPA/600/6-90/006F. Washington, D.C.: Office of Health and Environment Assessment.

Votroubek, W.L. 1995. Home mechanical ventilation: What are the options? *Home Health Care Practice* 7:21–26.

Votroubek, W.L. 1997. Issues in home care. In *Pediatric respiratory medicine,* ed. L. Landau and L. Taussig. St. Louis, MO: Mosby-Year Book.

Warwick, W.T., and J.G. Hansen. 1991. The long term effect of high frequency chest compression on pulmonary function on patients with cystic fibrosis. *Pediatric Pulmonology* 11:265–71.

Weese-Mayer, D.E., et al. 1992. Diaphragm pacing in infants and children. *Journal of Pediatrics* 120:1–8.

Wegener, D.H., and L.A. Aday. 1989. Home care for ventilator-assisted children: Predicting family stress. *Pediatric Nursing* 15:371–76.

Weissk, K.B., P.J. Gergen, T.A. Hodgson. 1992. An economic evaluation of asthma in the United States. *New England Journal of Medicine* 326:862–66.

Whaley, L., and D. Wong, eds. 1993. *Essentials of pediatric nursing.* St. Louis: C.V. Mosby.

Yaeger, E.S. 1994. Oxygen therapy using pulse and continual flow with a transtracheal catheter and nasal cannula. *Chest* 106:854–60.

Zimmerman, B., et al. 1988. Allergy in asthma: The dose relationship of allergy to severity of childhood asthma. *Journal of Allergy and Clinical Immunology* 81:63–70.

BIBLIOGRAPHY

Leger, P., et al. 1989. Home positive pressure ventilation via nasal mask for patients with neuromuscular weakness or restrictive lung or chest-wall disease. *Respiratory Care* 34:73–79.

Pfister, S.M. 1995. Home oxygen therapy: Indications, administration, recertification, and patient education. *Nurse Practitioner* 20, no. 7:44, 47–52, 54–56.

Nursing Care Plan for a Child with Asthma

Nursing Diagnosis/ Patient Problem	Defining Characteristics	Nursing Interventions	Expected Outcomes
1. Alteration in respiratory status: ineffective airway clearance and gas exchange *Etiology:* • bronchoconstriction or spasm • Increased mucus production • Airway inflammation • Environmental "triggers" or allergens	Signs of respiratory distress: • Abnormal breath sounds (wheezes, crackles) • Cough • Tachypnea • Dyspnea • Anxiety • Irritability • Cyanosis	Assess respiratory status frequently during respiratory distress (every 15 minutes). Assess peak flow measurements if PF meter is used. *Administer medications as prescribed: prn bronchodilators, anti-inflammatories Use spacers with metered-dose inhalers Remove or avoid environmental allergens or "triggers" when possible. Assess for side effects of beta agonists, corticosteroids, etc. Assess MDI and/or nebulizer technique to ensure proper administration of medication. Remain calm and be supportive and reassuring during crisis.	Patient is free from respiratory distress. Patient is free from side effects of asthma medications.

*Denotes nursing intervention requiring a physician's order.

Nursing Diagnosis/ Patient Problem	Defining Characteristics	Nursing Interventions	Expected Outcomes
2. Anxiety related to ineffective gas exchange *Etiology:* • Actual or perceived threat to biological integrity • Acute change in health status	Restlessness Irritability Tension Fear Nervousness Increased respiratory distress	Stay with child during acute asthma attack. Maintain calm, quiet environment when possible. Allow patient to assume comfortable position. Reassure patient and family. Encourage use of relaxation techniques if familiar to child.	Patient and family demonstrate decreased anxiety during acute onset of symptoms.
3. Knowledge deficit related to • Pathophysiology of disease • Treatment regimen • Proper use of MDIs and medications • Environmental "triggers" and allergens • Use of peak flow meter • Keeping track of symptoms in asthma diary	Verbalization of questions, concerns, fears, misconceptions related to asthma and prescribed treatment Inability to verbalize rationale for medications Inability to demonstrate proper use of MDIs, nebulizers, spacers, or peak flow meters Noncompliance with treatment regimen Environmental "triggers" and allergens still present in home	Reinforce proper use of equipment and medications. MDIs: • Exhale. • Tilt neck to straighten airway. • Inhale puff. • Hold breath 10 seconds. • Exhale. • Wait 1 minute and repeat second puff. *Use holding chambers/ spacers for ease and effectiveness of administration. Assist family in finding ways to avoid or control environmental "triggers" or allergens. Reinforce signs and symptoms of respiratory distress and medication toxicity/side effects. Encourage follow-up for further education and reinforcement of teaching.	Patient and family are knowledgeable about disease process, treatment regimen, and environmental triggers to avoid. Patient and family can verbalize appropriate treatment regimen and demonstrate proper use of MDI, nebulizer, and/or oxygen.

*Denotes nursing intervention requiring a physician's order.

Nursing Diagnosis/ Patient Problem	Defining Characteristics	Nursing Interventions	Expected Outcomes
4. Coping: ineffective—patient and family *Etiology:* • Chronicity of illness • Ever-present possibility of acute onset of symptoms	Use BPD care plan.	Use BPD care plan.	Patient and family use appropriate coping mechanisms. Patient and family form trusting relationship with health care providers. Patient and family use support resources as appropriate.

Note: MDI, metered-dose inhaler; BPD, bronchopulmonary dysplasia; PF, peak flow.

Nursing Care Plan for a Child with Cystic Fibrosis

Nursing Diagnosis/ Patient Problem	Defining Characteristics	Nursing Interventions	Expected Outcomes
1. Alteration in coping related to chronic illness (patient and family) *Etiology:* • Recurrent, frequent pulmonary exacerbations and/or hospitalizations • Significant change in lifestyle with progressiveness of disease and time-consuming treatment regimens • Shortened life span related to prognosis	Demonstration of feelings of anxiety, fear, sadness, depression Inappropriate coping mechanisms Noncompliance to treatments	Encourage verbalization of feelings. Assess coping mechanisms and encourage use of appropriate mechanisms. Assess reasons for noncompliance. Encourage involvement with support groups if available. Use resources such as social workers, counseling, community aide, hospice, etc., as appropriate. Check with CF center or CF Foundation re further suggestions of sources of support. Provide information re more aesthetically pleasing devices (e.g., internal venous access device vs. Hickman, gastrostomy button vs. nasogastric tube) to maintain positive body image. Encourage verbalization of feelings of sexuality, body image, peer relationships. Encourage independence with treatments.	Patient and family: • Demonstrate decreased anxiety, fear, and/or sadness. • Develop trusting relationship with caregivers. • Use healthy, appropriate coping behaviors.

Nursing Diagnosis/ Patient Problem	Defining Characteristics	Nursing Interventions	Expected Outcomes
2. Knowledge deficit related to • Pathophysiology of CF • Treatment regimen • Signs and symptoms of infections	Inaccurate compliance to treatment regimen Inability to articulate rationale for treatments Verbalization of problems or questions regarding CF and/or treatment interventions	Assess reasons for inaccurate treatment or noncompliance. If knowledge deficit, then provide information to patient and family. Contact CF center or CF Foundation for more in-depth information. Arrange and/or encourage follow-up care with CF center. Encourage parents and patient to write down further questions. Reinforce all education prn. Assess on continual basis for further knowledge deficit.	Patient and family demonstrate and verbalize understanding of the disease process and treatment regimen. Patient and family feel comfortable asking questions and will admit knowledge deficit in future.
3. Alteration in skin integrity *Etiology:* • Frequent malabsorbed stooling in infants • Rectal prolapse (from malabsorption and frequent stooling) • Stoma sites of various catheters: Hickman, gastrostomy tubes, jejunostomy tubes	Excoriation in perineal area of infant Prolapse of rectal mucosa through anus Signs of infection or irritation at catheter insertion site (edema erythema, drainage, tenderness)	*Administer pancreatic enzymes as ordered. Change soiled diapers frequently. Apply protective layer of ointment (Desitin, Vaseline, etc.) to buttocks. Notify physician of rectal prolapse. Frequently assess catheter insertion sites for signs of infection. *Provide catheter site care as outlined by physician.	Patient has decreased stooling with minimal skin irritation and no rectal prolapse. Catheter insertion site is clean with no signs of infection.

*Denotes nursing intervention requiring a physician's order.

Nursing Diagnosis/ Patient Problem	Defining Characteristics	Nursing Interventions	Expected Outcomes
4. Self-concept: disturbance in role performance, body image, and self-esteem *Etiology:* • Physical changes from cystic fibrosis: clubbing, cachexia, cyanosis, barrel chest • Activity intolerance	Change in social involvement— resistance to interact with peers Verbalization of • Negative body image • Fear of rejection • Feelings of helplessness, hopelessness, sadness, depression Noncompliance or uninvolvement with treatment regimen	Educate parents and preadolescents for likelihood of delayed maturation and physical changes accompanying CF. Relay sense of acceptance for the patient, despite physical appearance. Encourage interaction with other CF patients as source of support. Encourage interaction with peers. Provide privacy whenever possible for chest physiotherapy, coughing and expectoration, and elimination.	Patient has positive feelings of self and body demonstrated by independence, motivation, participation in care, and verbalization of self-acceptance.
5. Alteration in respiratory status related to ineffective airway clearance and impaired gas exchange *Etiology:* • Unusually thick, tenacious respiratory secretions • Frequent respiratory infections • Eventual lung scarring and fibrosis	Increased cough from baseline Increased production of mucus Change in thickness or color of respiratory secretions Dyspnea Tachypnea Hemoptysis Chest pain	Encourage and/or perform airway clearance technique before meals and at bedtime (two to four times daily). *Administer medications as ordered (antibiotics IV, PO, or aerosolized bronchdilators, corticosteroids). Encourage hydration to decrease viscosity of secretions. *Administer oxygen as ordered and needed. Assess for further deterioration of respiratory status and notify physician of significant changes.	Patient has decreased cough and sputnum production, no fever, and no hemoptysis, tachypnea, chest pain, or adventitious breath sounds.

*Denotes nursing intervention requiring a physician's order.

Nursing Diagnosis/ Patient Problem	Defining Characteristics	Nursing Interventions	Expected Outcomes
		If hemoptysis, estimate volume; notify physician; transport to emergency department or physician's office if greater than two tablespoons.	
6. Alteration in nutrition: less than body requirements *Etiology:* • Malabsorption of nutrients fats/ proteins/fat-soluble vitamins • Decreased appetite secondary to infection • Emesis secondary to coughing	Frequent loose, foul-smelling bulky stools Inconsistent or inadequate weight gain Weight loss Abdominal pain and cramping Emesis after cough Increased signs of respiratory tract infections	*Administer supplemental pancreatic enzymes before or scattered throughout meals and snacks. *Administer supplemental vitamins (multivitamin, water-soluble vitamin E, vitamin K) Monitor stooling pattern Report significant changes to CF team for possible alteration of enzyme dose. Encourage diet high in proteins and calories. Monitor weight gain or loss pattern. *Treat symptoms of respiratory tract infection if present. Administer airway clearance technique *before* meals. Encourage smaller, more frequent feedings if emesis with cough. *Administer supplemental nutrition as ordered.	Patient maintains or gains weight as outlined by physician. Enzyme supplementation is adequate to control malabsorption. Patient is in well-nourished state.

*Denotes nursing intervention requiring a physician's order.

Note: PO, by mouth; IV, intravenous; CF, cystic fibrosis.

Nursing Care Plan for a Child with a Tracheostomy

Nursing Diagnosis/ Patient Problem	Defining Characteristics	Nursing Interventions	Expected Outcomes
1. Alteration in respiratory status: ineffective airway clearance *Etiology:* • Potential for airway obstruction due to ineffective cough, thick secretions, or mucus plugging	Signs of respiratory distress: • Adventitious breath sounds • Change in secretions: –Amount –Thickness –Color change • Increased cough • Tachypnea • Cyanosis • Retractions • Nasal flaring • Dyspnea	Encourage coughing to clear airway. Suction tracheostomy tube *when needed* (avoid excess suctioning). Suction length of tracheostomy tube *only:* if unable to clear airway, *then* deep suction beyond end of tube. *Provide continuous humidified air or oxygen to tracheostomy tube via air compressor or heat/ moisture exchanges ("artificial noses"). Instill drops of sterile normal saline as needed, to loosen secretions.	Patient has a clear airway. Patient and family are able to recognize signs of potential airway obstruction and to provide necessary intervention.
2. Impaired skin integrity: *Etiology:* • Tracheostomy stoma, tracheostomy ties, secretions, humidity	Moisture from secretions and humidity Mechanical irritation from pressure of tracheostomy ties, humidity mask, and/or tubing Presence of excoria-	Assess every 8 hours for areas of pressure or skin breakdown. Change tracheostomy ties and pad at least once a day and prn for moistness or loose-ness. *Clean stoma with half-	Patient has intact skin without break-down or signs of infections.

*Denotes nursing intervention requiring a physician's order.

Nursing Diagnosis/ Patient Problem	Defining Characteristics	Nursing Interventions	Expected Outcomes
	tion, rash, pressure sites	strength hydrogen peroxide and rinse with water at least twice a day and prn. Dry stoma area and area under ties *thoroughly*. (Hair dryer on cool setting can be helpful to dry hard-to-reach areas on side or back of neck.) Rotate knot of tracheostomy ties to avoid consistent area of pressure. Pad area of humidity mask if resting against chin. *Humidity setting should be 30–40 mm H$_2$O (to avoid excess moisture to skin). If rash is present, call physician for advice.	
3. Injury: potential for • Hypo-oxygenation • Tracheal mucosa irritation, tracheal stenosis, tracheitis • Decannulation *Etiology:* • Excessive or deep suctioning • Insecure tracheostomy ties • Mechanical irritation from movement of tube	Cyanosis: • Intolerance of suctioning procedure • Microatelectasis	*Hand ventilate with oxygen or room air before and after suctioning (*required* for mechanically ventilated patient). Apply suction on withdrawal of catheter only. Limit suctioning to 5–10 seconds. Use proper-sized suction catheter. Check breath sounds before and after suctioning.	Patient is without injury secondary to tracheostomy: • No respiratory distress • No tracheal irritation • Secure tracheostomy tube

*Denotes nursing intervention requiring a physician's order.

Nursing Diagnosis/ Patient Problem	Defining Characteristics	Nursing Interventions	Expected Outcomes
	Bleeding during or after suctioning • Presence of granulation tissue (internally viewed only via bronchoscopy) • Difficulty replacing tracheostomy tube during routine change • Excessive secretions (secondary to excessive suctioning)	Suction only when child cannot clear secretions independently. Suction only length of tracheostomy tube (if unable to clear airway, *then* deep suction). Report bleeding or difficulty changing tube to physician. Report presence of external granulation.	
	Displaced tracheostomy tube • Loosened ties • Signs of respiratory distress	Assess adequate gas exchange through tracheostomy tube at least every 8 hours. Change tracheostomy ties at least once a day and more often if wet, loose, soiled. Ties should be one fingerbreadth loose. Tie-changing procedure should be performed by two persons unless emergency. Emergency kit (extra tube, ties, scissors, suction catheter, saline) should *always* be within reach in case of obstruction or decannulation.	

Nursing Diagnosis/ Patient Problem	Defining Characteristics	Nursing Interventions	Expected Outcomes
4. Ineffective communication related to tracheostomy *Etiology:* • Patient is unable to effectively verbally communicate to caregivers, family, and peers because tracheostomy bypasses vocal cord vibration necessary for speech.	Ineffective attempts at communication Unwillingness to use alternative modes of communication other than vocal speech Family or patient: • Frustration • Anger • Sadness • Depression	*Speech therapy consultation should be made for inpatient and outpatient therapy (infancy to adolescence). *Tracheostomy tube can be "downsized" to allow for air movement around tube and vocalization as well as using devices such as Passy Muir speaking valve. *Encourage use of alternative modes of communication (sign language, communication board, mouthed speech, computer/robotic speech). Assess patient's and family's adaptation to method of communication. Assess coping skills related to communication. Reinforce recommendations from speech therapist.	Patient is able to effectively communicate with family, peers, and caregivers. Patient and family are satisfied with mode of communication.
5. Knowledge deficit related to tracheostomy care Etiology: • Family, patient, or designated caregiver is unable to safely, independently care for child	Questions regarding tracheostomy care/procedures Verbalization of problems, fears, misconceptions, and hesitation to care for child with tracheostomy Noncompliance with care regimen	Thorough discharge teaching should be carried out by referring facilty before discharge. Reinforcement of teaching to be done by home nurses (consistent with teaching done by referring facility).	Patient is safely cared for at all times by knowledgeable caregiver. Caregivers demonstrate ability to properly carry out care regimen. Patient and family feel comfortable asking questions

*Denotes nursing intervention requiring a physician's order.

Nursing Diagnosis/ Patient Problem	Defining Characteristics	Nursing Interventions	Expected Outcomes
based on knowledge deficit.	Inability to independently care for child Inaccurate return-demonstrations of cares	Ensure that *anyone* responsible for child's care is *thoroughly* educated (for example, baby-sitters, other family members, school personnel) regarding tracheostomy care. Community agencies, emergency personnel, electricity and phone companies, and local hospital emerency department personnel are notified of presence of tracheostomized child in community. Encourage follow-up with pulmonary center/ referral facilty. Contact facility with any questions/concerns.	and will admit knowledge deficit in future.
6. Coping: ineffective—patient and family *Etiology:* • Changes in body integrity • High care needs of patient • Frequent hospitalizations • Inability to vocalize • Isolation	Verbalization of inability to cope Role confusion Inability to meet basic care needs Inability to make decisions Noncompliance with medical regimens	Determine etiology of ineffective coping and noncompliance. Assess coping mechanisms and encourage use of appropriate mechanisms. Determine alternative strategies for ineffective coping mechanisms. Encourage involvement with support groups if available. Use resources such as social workers, counselors, community aides, hospice, respite care as available and appropriate. Allow patient and family opportunity to verbalize stress, frustration, fatigue, and anxiety.	Patient and family: • Demonstrate decreased anxiety, fear, and stress. • Develop trusting relationship with caregivers. • Use healthy, appropriate coping behaviors.

Nursing Care Plan for a Child with Ventilator Dependency

Nursing Diagnosis/ Patient Problem	Defining Characteristics	Nursing Interventions[*]	Expected Outcomes
1. Alteration in respiratory status: ineffective breathing patterns *Etiology:* • Neuromuscular impairment • Loss of functional lung tissue • Fatigue, anxiety • Central nervous system impairment	Signs of respiratory distess: • Shortness of breath • Dyssynchrony with ventilator • Use of accessory muscles • Retractions • Nasal flaring	Check all ventilator settings and connections. Correct any problems. Monitor effects of any ventilator setting changes Provide emotional support during periods of anxiety. Teach relaxation techniques used at times of anxiety. Show patient how to become synchronous with ventilator. Optimize patient's position to faciltate use of diaphragm and to maintain open airway.	Patient has no signs of respiratory distress. Patient is able to initiate relaxation techniques to decrease anxiety. Patient can describe optimal position of effective breathing.
2. Alterations in respiratory status: ineffective airway clearance *Etiology:* • Excessive, thick secretions	Change in secretions: • Color • Amount • Consistency • Odor Signs of respiratory distress: • Cyanosis	Monitor for signs of ineffective airway. Encourage coughing when possible. Suction tracheostomy tube as needed. Notify physician of signs of infecion.	Patient has open airway and can clear secretions either by cough or by suctioning. Patient has no signs of respiratory distress.

[*]See Appendix 5–C, Nursing Care Plan for a Child with a Tracheostomy.

Nursing Diagnosis/ Patient Problem	Defining Characteristics	Nursing Interventions*	Expected Outcomes
• Ineffective cough due to weakness/ fatigue • Bronchoconstriction • Infection • Immobility	• Tachypnea • Dyspnea • Retractions or flaring • Diaphoresis • Tachycardia Temperature elevation Difficulty suctioning secretions Intermittent elevated peak inspiratory pressures or "high pressure" alarms on ventilator Restlessness, anxiety	†Administer antibiotics or bronchodilators as ordered. Provide adequate humidification to airway. Provide adequate hydration. Initiate chest physiotherapy to aid airway clearance.	Patient has no signs of infection. Patient is adequately hydrated and humidified to keep secretions loose and manageable.
3. Altered respiratory status: impaired gas exchange *Etiology:* • Loss of functional lung tissue • Neuromuscular impairment • Central nervous system impairment • Increased secretions • Anxiety or fear • Fatigue	Signs of respiratory distress: • Tachypnea • Dyspnea • Cyanosis • Tachycardia Change in mental status Somnolence Headaches Night sweats Disorientation in morning Diaphoresis	Monitor for signs of respiratory distress. Monitor ventilator settings and functions. Check for disorientation or change in mental status after naps or in morning. Maintain clear airway. Observe for change in sleep patterns due to CO_2 retention.	Patient is without respiratory distress. Patient shows no signs of hypoxia or hypercarbia. Patient maintains adequate gas exchange with properly functioning ventilator.
4. Immobility: impaired *Etiology:* • Physical limitation due to attachment of ventilator	Muscle atrophy or decreased muscle tone Limited range of motion Dyspnea or fatigue with exertion Anxiety	Ensure use of portable mechanical ventilator whenever possible. Ensure use of wheelchair with mount for ventilator to increase mobility. Encourage use of	Patient is as independently mobile as possible. Patient is able to maintain optimal position or can direct others to do so.

†Denotes nursing intervention requiring a physician's order.

*See Appendix 5–C, Nursing Care Plan for a Child with a Tracheostomy.

Nursing Diagnosis/ Patient Problem	Defining Characteristics	Nursing Interventions*	Expected Outcomes
• Neuromuscular impairment	Anger Depression	adaptive devices to operate wheelchair (for example, P-switch, "sip and puff" device). Maintain daily range of motion exercises. †Initiate physical therapy referral if needed. Follow physical therapy recommendations for mobility exercises. Observe for signs of respiratory distress with exertion/exercise. Position and reposition patient frequently for optimal use of extremities.	Patient maintains baseline range of motion when-ever possible.
5. Impaired verbal communication *Etiology:* • Tracheostomy tube • Mechanical ventilator	Impaired ability to phonate: • Anger • Depression • Anxiety • Frustration	†Provide periods of phonation via cuff deflation and increas-ed volumes whenever possible and if tolerated. Provide alternate methods of communi-cation (for example, paper and pencil, letter board, picture board, computer, sign language). †Consult with speech therapist regarding use of adaptive communi-cation devices.	Patient is able to adequately communicate using most appropriate method for him or her. Patient demonstrates decreased frustra-tion when com-municating.

†Denotes nursing intervention requiring a physician's order.

*See Appendix 5–C, Nursing Care Plan for a Child with a Tracheostomy.

Nursing Diagnosis/ Patient Problem	Defining Characteristics	Nursing Interventions[*]	Expected Outcomes
6. Coping: ineffective—patient and family *Etiology:* • Changes in body integrity • Changes in lifestyle • 24-hour care/ supervision of patient demands • Social isolation • Loss of independence • Loss of privacy • Prolonged hospitalization • Unsatisfactory support systems • Exhaustion	Verbalization of inability to cope Role confusion Inability to meet needs of patient, family, or self Inability to follow suggested treatment regimen Inability to make decisions Chronic sadness or depression Anger Hopelessness/ helplessness expressed by patient or family Fatigue or exhaustion	Assess causative or contributing factors for ineffective coping. Assess use of coping mechanisms: encourage those that are appropriate and discourage those that are inappropriate. Offer anticipatory guidance and problem-solving techniques. Encourage use of relaxation techniques or stress-reducing activities. Allow as much independence and privacy as possible. Maintain consultation with social worker or counselor on ongoing basis. Encourage *all* family members (including siblings and involved extended family members) to seek support that they feel is appropriate and comfortable for them. Allow patient and family time to verbalize concerns, sorrows, feelings, and issues.	Patient and family: • Demonstrate and use approprite coping mechanisms. • Demonstrate ability to care for patient and self. • Demonstrate trusting relationship with professional (nurse, social worker, counselor, teacher). • Verbalize anxieties and fears. • Problem solve situations that are anxiety producing. • Have as much independence and privacy as is possible and safe.
7. Knowledge deficit related to • Care of tracheostomy • Care of ventilator • Medications	Verbalization of questions or deficiency in knowledge of skills Inability for correct	Provide individualized teaching plan to patient and family. Provide accurate information at rate appropriate to promote learning.	Patient and family are able to participate accurately and independently in all dimensions of care.

[*]See Appendix 5–C, Nursing Care Plan for a Child with a Tracheostomy.

Nursing Diagnosis/ Patient Problem	Defining Characteristics	Nursing Interventions[*]	Expected Outcomes
• Treatment schedule • Equipment care and cleaning • Signs of respiratory distress *Etiology:* • Inaccurate information given to family • Patient and family unable to absorb all information required due to volume of information, shock, and inability to cope • Ineffective or incomplete education	Inability for correct return-demonstration of skills Inaccurate compliance with specified treatment Inability to articulate rationale for treatment	Reinforce all teaching on regular basis. Encourage practice of all skills, particularly those needed in an emergency situation. Assess return-demonstrations for accuracy of skills. Consult tertiary care center or discharging facility for questions regarding routines of care and specifics of what family was taught. Provide inservice education to home nursing staff on regular basis regarding care of tracheostomy, ventilator and emergency procedures (use tertiary care center prn). Ensure that *all* care providers are educated in *all* aspects of care before independently caring for child.	Care providers can describe and demonstrate accurate skills required for care. Patient is, *at all times*, with knowledgeable care provider trained in all aspects of care. Family feels comfortable asking questions about care. Family trusts all care providers.

[*]See Appendix 5–C, Nursing Care Plan for a Child with a Tracheostomy.

CHAPTER 6

Alterations in Neurologic Function

Barbara Masiulis and Angela Carlson

Children with neurologic disorders or neurologic sequelae from serious injuries present multiple challenges for the home health care nurse. As the focus of specialty health care further evolves to outpatient/home care management, the home health care nurse takes on multiple roles in the delivery of comprehensive care to children with neurologic impairments. These roles include case management, direct care delivery, education, and providing family support.

Delivery of effective home care to this population requires an understanding of the neurologic impairments and their current management. It is the goal of this chapter to provide the home health care nurse with a beginning knowledge of common pediatric neurologic disorders such as seizures, head injuries, and spinal cord injuries. The etiology of these disorders, pathophysiology, current medical management, long-term care needs, and patient education needs are addressed.

SEIZURE DISORDERS

Seizures are a common pediatric health concern, presenting with various symptoms and degrees of severity. A seizure is a symptom of central nervous system dysfunction and results from an abnormal discharge of neurons. Epilepsy (seizure disorder) is a tendency toward recurrent, paroxysmal episodes of excessive neuronal excitation with resulting alteration in motor function, sensation, autonomic behavior, or consciousness (Barry and Teixeira 1983).

There are numerous causes of seizures, but in more than 50 percent of children, the cause is unknown or idiopathic (Vining and Freeman 1986). Children with a family history of seizures have a greater incidence of seizures than the rest of the population.

Seizures can result from a number of acute conditions such as fever, meningitis, chemical imbalances (for example, hypocalcemia, hypoglycemia, and hyponatremia), substance abuse, and tumors. Epilepsy can be acquired from brain injury due to hypoxia, trauma, infection, and metabolic imbalances. Seizures may be associated with congenital defects, inborn errors of metabolism, and neurocutaneous disorders (such as neurofibromatosis and tuberous sclerosis) (Roddy and McBride 1992). There are a number of precipitating factors in children with a tendency toward seizures. These include emotional stress, fever, infection, illness, fatigue, and sleep deprivation (Ferry , Banner, and Wolf 1986).

Seizure activity develops from a group of abnormally hyperactive and hypersensitive neurons that become an epileptogenic focus (Hickey 1992). The epileptogenic focus exhibits electrical excitability—firing discharges intermittently, often in bursts. These abnormal discharges may follow three different pathways in the brain and occur as various seizure types. A discharge may be focal or limited to one area of the brain or may originate in the brain stem and generalize throughout the brain or arise in one area and then become generalized. These varying pathways distinguish the two major groups of seizure types as focal seizures (including focal with secondary generalization) and primary generalized seizures.

The clinical features of seizures vary depending on the location of the abnormal discharge in the brain. Features of an epileptic event can include motor changes, alterations in level of consciousness, sensory symptoms, hallucinations, and autonomic symptoms. The various seizure types are presented in Table 6–1 according to the current classification of seizure types.

Medical Interventions

Medical interventions during the acute phase of seizure management include identifying an event as a seizure, controlling or terminating the

Table 6–1 Seizure Types

Type	Description
Partial	
Simple	Motor, sensory or autonomic; without alteration in consciousness
Complex partial	Motor, sensory, somatosensory autonomic and psychic with alteration in consciousness
Partial with secondary generalization	Begins as partial and progresses to generalized
Primary generalized	
Absence	Brief interruption of consciousness, with staring, often with mild jerks of eyelids
Atypical absence	Absence with automatism (for example, lip smacking)
Myoclonic	Quick symmetrical jerk or muscle contractions, includes infantile spasms
Clonic	Repetitive muscle jerking
Tonic	Stiffening of muscles, child falls usually, sudden loss of postural tone
Atonic/akinetic	Sudden loss of postural, child may fall
Tonic-clonic	Rigidity phase (sometimes with a scream), followed by clonic jerking, limpness, stupor, postictal sleep
Neonatal seizures	Five types including the following: • subtle eye movements, blinking, sucking; pedaling of legs, apnea • tonic, extension of limbs • multifocal, clonic activity that migrates • focal clonic, localized jerking • myoclonic, flexion jerks of upper or lower extremities
Febrile seizures	Seizures occurring with fever without intracranial infection or acute neurologic illness. Simple or complex, ages three months to five years
Pseudoseizures	Dramatic seizurelike activity without epileptogenic basis

Source: Reprinted with permission from M.J. Kolodgie, Home Care Management of the Child with Infantile Spasms, *Pediatric Nursing,* Vol. 20, No. 3, pg. 270–273, © 1994, Jannetti Publications, Inc.

seizure activity, and identifying a cause for the event. If a child presents acutely in the emergency room seizing, management focuses on stabilizing basic life-sustaining systems and terminating the seizure activity. Once the child is stabilized, the focus becomes establishing the event as seizure and identifying the seizure type. This is critical for planning the appropriate treatment; antiepileptic agents vary in their effectiveness by seizure type.

A comprehensive health history, which includes a detailed seizure event assessment is taken (Exhibit 6–1) and a detailed neurologic examination is performed. The history and examination will determine the extent of a laboratory test and diagnostic procedures pursued. A laboratory test after an initial seizure can assess complete blood count, serum electrolytes, blood glucose, calcium, magnesium, blood urea nitrogen, and urine. Electroencephalography (EEG) is critical in supporting the identification of the event as a seizure and the seizure type. Neuroimaging studies such as magnetic resonance imaging (MRI) or computed tomography (CT) are ordered for children with focal neurologic findings or with intractable seizures.

Once the diagnosis of a seizure disorder and type of seizure is made, the appropriate treatment plan is established. The goal of seizure management is to reduce or control recurrence of seizures with minimal side effects and help the child live as normal a life as possible. Treatment includes starting the child on an antiepileptic drug most appropriate for the seizure type and at the lowest therapeutic dose. The most commonly used antiepileptic drugs and their side effects are reviewed in Table 6–2. The goal of medication treatment is monotherapy to avoid possible toxicity of polytherapy. If adequate control is not obtained with one agent, a second may be added. Long-term follow-up includes ongoing assessment of seizure frequency, monitoring for drug side effects, and maintaining medications at therapeutic levels. Noncompliance with medications is one of the most common causes of recurrent seizures. Therapy is continued until the child is seizure-free for two years and has a nonepileptiform EEG.

In children with intractable or difficult-to-control seizures, epilepsy surgery or the ketogenic diet may be options. The ketogenic diet is composed of a high ratio of fat to protein and carbohydrate and may be beneficial, especially in reducing myoclonic and akinetic seizures (Freeman, Kelly, and Freeman 1994). The diet is begun in the hospital with a period of starvation to establish ketosis. Once established, ketosis is maintained on a diet primarily consisting of fat calories, usually a 4:1 ratio of fat to carbohydrates and proteins. This dietary management is complex and requires close follow-up and exact family compliance. Advances have been made in the surgical treatment of intractable epilepsies, particularly focal epilepsy in which an epileptogenic area can be identified for removal (Pilcher et al. 1992). Children discharged after epilepsy surgery are monitored for seizure recurrence and for surgical complications.

Exhibit 6–1 Seizure Assessment

- Description of specific clinical behaviors (for example, any impairment of consciousness, any unusual motor activity, eye movements)
- Progression of seizure
- Typical onset (for example, any aura or warning, focal activity)
- Frequency, pattern of occurence
- Duration
- Precipitating factors

Source: Adapted from M.J. Kolodgie, "Home Care Management of the Child with Infantile Spasms," *Pediatric Nursing*, 20(3), pp. 270–73, © 1994.

Teaching Issues before Discharge

Discharge planning for the child with a seizure disorder begins at the time of diagnosis or upon admission for an acute event. The teaching plan should be individualized based on the com-

Table 6–2 Antiepileptic Agents

Trade/Generic	Indications	Dosage (mg/kg/day)	Therapeutic Levels ($\mu g/ml$)	Side Effects
Tegretol/ carbamazepine	Partial, secondary generalized	5–25 5–10 (monotherapy)	4–12	Drowsiness, blurry vision, diplopia, nausea, ataxia, allergic rash, leukopenia, dry mouth, abnormal liver function
Depakene/ valproic acid	Primary generalized, absence, myoclonic, akinetic, infantile spasms, some partial	10–30 20–50 (infants and polytherapy)	50–100	Nausea, tremor, weight gain, hair loss, pancreatitis thrombocytope- nia, hepatic failure, sedation
Dilantin/phenytoin	Partial, secondary generalized, primary generalized	5–7	10–20	Dizziness, ataxia, nystagmus, gingival hyperpla- sia, hirsutism, lethargy, nausea, rickets, blood dyscrasias, psychomotor slowing, rashes, coarse features
Phenobarbital	Neonatal, febrile, partial, secondary generalized, primary generalized, akinetic	3–5 (<25 kg) 2–3 (25-50 kg) 1–2 (>50 kg)	10–40	Sedation, inatten- tion, hyperactivity, cognitive impair- ment, rare hypersensitivity reactions
Zarontin/ethosux- imide	Absence, myoclonic, akinetic	15–40	40–100	Nausea, abdominal discomfort, hiccups, drowsi- ness, dystonias, blood dyscrasias, behavioral problems

continues

Table 6–2 continued

Trade/Generic	Indications	Dosage (mg/kg/day)	Therapeutic Levels (μg/ml)	Side Effects
Mysoline/ primidone	Partial, secondary generalized, primary generalized	5–10	5–12 (check phenobarbital level also)	Sedation, irritability, psychomotor slowing, ataxia, rare hypersensitivity reactions
Clonopin/ clonazepam	Absence, primary generalized, infantile spasms	0.01–0.2	Usually not helpful	Sedation, hyperactivity, inattention, ataxia, aggressiveness, tolerance, withdrawal seizures, increased salivation
Diamox/ acetazolamide	Partial, absence, myoclonic, akinetic	10–20	Usually not helpful	Diuresis, sedation, paresthesias, rashes, hyperpnea
Tranxene/ clorazepate	Primary generalized, myoclonic, akinetic		Usually not helpful	Drowsiness, lethargy, tolerance
Valium/diazepam	Status epilepticus	0.12–0.8, divided q6–8h		Drowsiness, lethargy, ataxia, respiratory depression, nausea
Lamictal/ lamotrigine	Primary generalized (atypical absence seizures, tonic-clonic)		Therapeutic levels to be identified	Ataxia, dizziness, diplopia, fatigue, headache, drowsiness, rash (increased risk when given with valproate), Stevens-Johnson syndrome
Neurontin/ gabapentin	Partial (refractory)	30–60 mg, maximum daily dose 4,800 mg		Dizziness, lightheadedness, blurred vision, headache, rash

continues

Table 6–2 continued

Trade/Generic	Indications	Dosage (mg/kg/day)	Therapeutic Levels (µg/ml)	Side Effects
Felbatol/felbamate	Refractory partial seizures, generalized	15–45	Therapeutic levels to be identified	Nausea, double vision, anorexia, headache, insomnia, aplastic anemia, hepatic failure
Ativan/lorazepam	Status epilepticus, seizure clusters	0.1	Usually not helpful	Drowsiness, respiratory depression

plexity of the child's seizure disorder, the treatment plan developed, and the unique needs of the child and his or her family. The educational needs of the family include gaining an understanding of the disorder, the treatment plan, and safety issues and addressing the psychosocial issues related to seizure disorders (Appendix 6–A).

The child's caregivers should be knowledgeable about seizures, their presentation, and precipitating factors. Parents become the key managers of their child's disorder at the onset and they face many challenges with this role . Great fear and stress are associated with seizures, and parental concerns exist about the impact of seizures on their child and the potential recurrence of episodes. The family will be better prepared to manage their child's medical needs with a solid understanding of the nature of seizures and with reassurance. Improved understanding will lead to greater compliance with the treatment plan.

To monitor the effectiveness of the treatment plan, families should keep a seizure record that documents the frequency of events, the time of day an event occurred, any precipitating factors, length of the event, and a description of the event. An accurate seizure history will help to optimize the treatment plan.

To prevent possible injury or secondary injury from seizure events, training in first aid for seizures needs to be provided. Exhibit 6–2 describes first aid for the major seizure types. Families will have concerns about when to call for emergency care or to seek medical care for events. An individualized plan should be developed by the multidisciplinary team and family, based on the unique nature of the child's seizure disorder. Parents also need to understand that seizures may impact their child's daily activities and that it is important to encourage their child to live as normal a life as possible. For example, older children and teens should be encouraged to shower instead of taking a bath. All aspects of the child's life need to be addressed, including the child's reentry into school. The school nurse needs to understand the child's seizure disorder, treatment plan, and first aid needs and share that information with the school staff. Developmentally appropriate presentations on seizures to classmates can reduce prejudice, fear, and anxiety of all involved.

The usual treatment of seizures requires compliance with an antiepileptic medication program. Families need to obtain information on their child's particular medication, its potential side effects, and the long-term monitoring required for safe administration of the medication.

Exhibit 6–2 First Aid during Seizure Activity

Generalized Seizures

- If the child has an aura, have him or her lie down.
- Loosen any tight clothing around the neck.
- Prevent the child from hitting sharp or hard objects.
- Turn the child on his or her side to allow drainage of oral secretions.
- Allow the seizure to end without interference.
- If breathing is obstructed at the end of episode, reinstate ventilation by checking the airway.
- Help to reorient the child.

Partial Seizures

- Allow seizure to progress without interference or trying to restrain child.
- Observe child carefully to prevent any injuries.
- Help to reorient the child.

Exhibit 6–3 Side Effects of ACTH Therapy

Expected Effects

Mild hypertension
Cushingoid features
Irritability
Increased appetite
Weight gain
Fatigue
Facial acne

Adverse Effects

Hypertension >10 mm Hg above normal
Glucosuria >1+2 consecutive readings
Infection
Fever
Vomiting/electrolyte disturbance
Irregular respiration
Sudden change in seizure activity
Sudden behavioral change
Delays in development

Source: Reprinted with permission from M.J. Kolodgie, Home Care Management of the Child with Infantile Spasms, *Pediatric Nursing,* Vol. 20, No. 3, pp. 270–73, © 1994, Jannetti Publications, Inc.

In some situations, parents may need to administer antiepileptics emergently to control acute seizures at home. Benzodiazepines, such as diazepam or lorazepam, may be given rectally. Parents can be taught to administer medication rectally.

A complex treatment plan is developed for the infant with spasms discharged on ACTHCAR Gel injection. Adrenocorticotropic hormone (ACTH) is a corticosteriod that is helpful in controlling infantile spasms but has multiple potential side effects, including possible delays in development (Exhibit 6–3). During this hospitalization, parents are taught to give injections, to monitor for side effects (for example, to check urine for glucose), and to monitor the infant's response to treatment (Kolodgie 1994).

Another complex discharge plan is devised for the child placed on the ketogenic diet. A multidisciplinary team (physician, nurse, nurse-practitioner, social worker, and nutritionist) develops a teaching plan for parents, which presents various aspects of the diet, monitoring for side effects, and monitoring for metabolic and neurologic responses to the diet. For example, parents are taught to check urine for ketones.

The teaching plan for the child with seizures includes addressing the developmental needs of the child and family and the psychosocial impact of the diagnosis on the family. Having an understanding of normal developmental milestones helps parents better address their child's needs. Parents will experience multiple feelings and emotions as they learn to cope with the disorder. The fear and anxiety associated with seizures as well as the loss of control and change in self-image have a tremendous impact on the child and the family unit. Anticipatory guidance with the challenges facing families can help mobilize effective coping mechanisms. Providing information regarding community support groups and the Epilepsy Foundation of America can be helpful (see resources in Appendix A at the end of this book).

HEAD INJURY

Head injury refers to a continuum of injuries that are the result of trauma to the cranial vault and its contents. It is the most prevalent neurologic problem requiring hospitalization for patients younger than 19 years (Menkes and Till 1995). It is two to three times more common in males. Children of lower socioeconomic classes are also at higher risk. Motor vehicle accidents are the most lethal and the most common source of head injury in the adolescent population. Falls are the least lethal and the most common source in younger children. Other causes of head injury are sporting accidents, assaults, and child abuse.

Head injury occurs in two phases. The primary injury occurs at the moment of impact and is related to the mechanical forces that cause bruising, laceration, or compression of the brain. Secondary injury is the sequelae of events triggered locally or systemically by the primary injury that result in additional injury to the brain. Head injuries are classified into two basic categories, open or closed, then further delineated by severity (mild, moderate, or severe). The Glasgow Coma Scale (GCS) is the standard tool used to define severity (Table 6–3). Open injury refers to injuries involving a fracture of the skull, in which a break in the barrier between the outside environment and the intracranial contents occurs, causing primarily focal damage. Closed injury is a blunt, nonpenetrating injury to the head. Diffuse damage occurs from coup and contrecoup injury to the brain, resulting in more severe global cerebral deficits and increased risk for permanent unconsciousness. The type and severity of injury significantly influence the child's prognosis. Advanced technology has increased survival rates. The "survivors" are often

Table 6–3 Glasgow Coma Scale (GCS)

Eye Opening (E)

Spontaneous	4
To Speech	3
To Pain	2
None	1

Motor Response (M)

Obeys	6
Localizes	5
Withdraws	4
Abnormal Flexion	3
Abnormal Extension	2
None	1

Verbal Response (V)

Oriented	5
Confused Conversation	4
Inappropriate Words	3
Incomprehensible Sounds	2
None	1

TOTAL SCORE = E + M + V

<8 = Severe, 9–12 = moderate, 13–15 = minor

those more severely affected. The majority of head injuries in children are, however, mild to moderate (Goldstein and Powers 1994).

Medical Interventions

Medical interventions during the acute phase of the injury focus on assessment of severity of the injury and implementing lifesaving measures. A detailed neurologic examination is conducted when the child's basic life-sustaining systems are stabilized. Rapid and accurate diagnoses are critical to preventing secondary brain injury. The GCS is also the most common tool used for assessment of neurologic status. A modified form is available for use with infants. The assigned score on the GCS is a reliable measure for predicting outcomes.

Most children with a head injury are experiencing multisystem trauma; however, the major concern is maintenance of intracranial pressure

(ICP) and cerebral perfusion. This is accomplished with some type of indwelling ICP measurement device, hyperventilation, fluid restriction, and diuretics. The child may eventually require placement of a ventriculoperitoneal (VP) shunt. Prophylaxis with anticonvulsants is common. During the acute phase of injury, other typical issues are management of respiratory, neurologic, cardiovascular, and musculoskeletal complications, as well as support for the family in crisis. Less acute concerns involve issues related to nutrition, bowel and bladder elimination, skin integrity, and infection. Neurodiagnostic tests routinely ordered for comprehensive assessment and management of the child with head injury include CT scan, MRI, EEG, and angiography.

Teaching Issues before Discharge

Discharge planning for the child with a severe head injury should begin upon admission to the intensive care unit. Individualized planning is possible when the acute phase of injury has passed and an accurate assessment of the child's needs can be realized. When the child's medical status has stabilized, he or she should be transferred to a neurorehabilitation center. The child with a severe head injury will have a vast array

of disabilities that are best managed by a specialized team. This team typically consists of a physician, nurse, physical therapist (PT), occupational therapist (OT), speech therapist (ST), neuropsychologist, teacher, and family. Table 6–4 provides a comprehensive list of potential sequelae for the neurologically impaired child. The majority of motor and sensory recovery occurs in the first year after the injury. The behavioral, cognitive, and psychosocial issues extend over years (Johnston and Gerring 1992).

The family should be knowledgeable about their child's new physical, behavioral, and cognitive needs and how to respond to them to optimize his or her outcome. Realistic short- and long-term goals need to be established. The focus is to improve function while preventing secondary sequelae. The family will be expected to provide physically and mentally challenging care each day. It should be assisted with reintegration of their severely disabled child into the home to minimize disruption of family dynamics. It is often helpful for families to have a one-to two-day trial at home before the official discharge date.

The parents' educational program is extensive because it reflects the broad spectrum of their child's disabilities. Maintenance of musculoskeletal function focuses on safe ambulation and

---

Table 6–4 Potential Sequelae of the Neurologically Impaired Child

Motor/Physical	Cognitive	Behavioral	Other
Various degrees of immobility	Attention issues	Impulsivity	Depression
Spasticity	Learning	Socially inappro-	Loss of self-esteem
Contractures	disabilities	priate behavior	Loss of indepen-
Scoliosis	Memory	Aggression	dence
Osteoporosis	impairment		Decreased life
Decubiti	Aphasia		expectancy
Impairment of vision or hearing	Dysarthria		
Bowel and/or bladder incontinence			
Loss of reproductive function			
Impairment of respiratory function			
Loss of gag reflex			
Inability to coordinate chewing and swallowing			

avoidance of contractures, scoliosis, and decubiti. The parents of children with open head injuries in particular should be aware of the risk of posttraumatic seizures and be prepared to provide first aid for seizures. Behavioral and cognitive issues are the most pervasive of residual affects and are the most challenging for the family. A thorough assessment and plan for management at home and in school should be completed. Alternative methods of communication should be initiated. Parents will need to learn how to safely implement an altered-route-of-feeding program. The risk for aspiration is greater for children with impaired coordination of mastication or gag reflex. Maintenance of adequate nutrition without obesity should be stressed.

Many community resources will be necessary to address the child's long-term needs. The family should be acquainted with the available nursing, PT, OT, educational, mental health, and financial services. Any necessary medical supplies (splints, hoyer bed) as well as modifications to the family's home for accessibility should be addressed and provided before discharge.

SPINAL CORD INJURY

Acquired spinal cord injury (SCI) in children is relatively uncommon. Only 1 to 3 percent of SCI occurs in patients younger than fifteen years (Flett 1992). It is more prevalent in males and during the summer months. When injury does occur, it is as devastating an injury as in the adult population—perhaps even more so because of the length of life span that remains and the significant impact on growth and development.

SCI occurs when there is acute trauma to the spinal cord, resulting in varying degrees of impairment of movement, sensation, respiratory function, and bowel and bladder control. The instant loss of function is the result of both anatomic alteration and impaired physiologic function of the spinal cord (Menkes and Till 1995). The extent of deficit resulting from the injury is directly related to the location of the spinal cord

injury where the trauma occurred (Table 6–5). Deficits are also related to the type of injury, either complete or incomplete (Table 6–6). Sensory changes provide a more accurate picture of the location of the injury than do motor changes. A diagnosis of paraplegia or quadriplegia is assigned based on the location of the injury (Table 6–5). The most common (27 percent) site of injury is the second cervical vertebra (Menkes and Till 1995). A predisposition to this level of injury is the result of anatomic and developmental characteristics of children. SCI is most likely the result of indirect and accidental hyperextension or hyperflexion that occurs in motor vehicle accidents. Other likely sources of injury are falls and sports-related injuries in which vertical compression occurs.

The initial flaccid paralysis, also termed spinal shock, is replaced with spasticity usually within one to six weeks after injury, but may occur up to seven months later. The largest proportion and most rapid return of functions will occur within the first six months after injury. Small gains in neurologic function will continue for one to two years.

Medical Interventions

Medical management for the child with SCI requires a multidisciplinary approach. The injury to the spinal cord has impacted several body systems, thus requiring comprehensive assessment and implementation of basic lifesaving measures. Respiratory support with mechanical ventilation is necessary for injuries at the C-4 level and higher. Once basic lifesaving measures are instituted, the focus of the acute phase of injury becomes identification of the level of injury via CT scan. Stabilization of the spinal cord to minimize and prevent further damage follows. Stabilization is usually achieved by surgical measures. Administration of methylprednisone within eight hours of injury is related to better neurologic outcomes (Menkes and Till 1995). Other management issues revolve around the dysfunction of secondarily impacted organ systems. These systems include cardiovascular, nu-

Table 6–5 Clinical Features Based on Level of Spinal Cord Injury

Level of Injury	Sensation	Motor Function	Respiratory	Bowel and Bladder	Functional Ability
C1-4	None from neck and below	QUADRIPLEGIA None from neck and below	Respiratory paralysis; requires tracheostomy and mechanical ventilation	No bowel or bladder control	Completely dependent for ADL
C5-6	Loss below the clavicle and down	QUADRIPLEGIA None below the shoulders	Sparing of diaphragmatic movements, but not intercostal muscles	No bowel or bladder control	Oral adaptive devices for feeding, writing, and control of wheelchair
C7-8	Loss below the clavicle and part of arms and hands	QUADRIPLEGIA Loss to trunk and below; parts of arms and hands	Same as above	No bowel or bladder control	Independent in most ADL; includes bowel, bladder, and wheelchair
T1-6	Loss of everything below the midchest area	PARAPLEGIA Loss from mid-chest and below	Same as above and some impairment of intercostal muscles	No bowel or bladder control	Independent in ADL; full-time employment possible
T6-12	Loss of everything below the waist	PARAPLEGIA Loss below the waist	No impairment	No bowel or bladder control	Same as previous. Increased truncal control and ease of wheelchair athletics.

Note: ADL, activities of daily living.

Source: Reprinted with permission from J.V. Hickey, *Neurological and Neurosurgical Nursing*, 3rd ed., p. 409, © 1992, J.B. Lippincott Company.

tritional, musculoskeletal, genitourinary, gastrointestinal, and integumentary systems. Psychological support for the patient with a newly diagnosed chronic disability and his or her family must also be provided.

A shift toward rehabilitation medicine occurs when the acute phase of injury management is complete. As with the children with head injuries, the child with SCI will experience better outcomes and shorter hospitalizations when

Table 6–6 General Terminology Related to Spinal Cord Injury

Type	Description
Quadriplegia	Refers to a lesion involving a cervical segment of the spinal cord that results in dysfunction of the respiratory system, both arms, both legs, bowel, and bladder.
Paraplegia	Refers to a lesion involving the thoracic, lumbar, or sacral segments of the spinal cord that results in dysfunction of both legs, bowel, and/or bladder.
Complete Lesion	Child will have total loss of sensation and voluntary muscle control below the level of the injury.
Incomplete Lesion	Child will have preservation of the sensation or motor conrol or both, below the level of the lesion.

Source: Reprinted with permission from J.V. Hickey, *Neurological and Neurosurgical Nursing,* 3rd ed., p. 405, © 1992, J.B. Lippincott Company.

placed in the care of a specialized rehabilitation facility (Hickey 1992). Transfer to a regional facility should be permitted when the child is medically stable.

Teaching Issues before Discharge

The general discharge planning and teaching needs for the child with a spinal cord injury and his or her family are similar to those of the child with a head injury. See Appendix 6–B for detailed care plans that address their complex needs. Both injuries cause significant impairment to the same functional areas—physical mobility, feeding, and bowel and bladder management. Children with SCI will require coordination of multiple community services. Adaptations to the home and vehicles will be necessary, as will various other physical adaptive equipment. Refer to the teaching section on head injury for discussion of issues of basic musculoskeletal function and nutrition. There are additional issues, specific to these children, that are addressed here.

The family will likely require additional education regarding medications that will be prescribed for treatment of spasticity and constipation (see Appendix 6–B and Tables 6–7 and 6–8). Before discharge, these children will have an established bowel and bladder program. The parents will be expected to either provide this care themselves or serve as a resource to their children who may be independent with this function. This is also the case with wheelchair to bed transfers and positioning techniques. The parents should know the triggers, signs and symptoms, and interventions for autonomic hyperreflexia, a life-threatening condition that occurs in children with an injury at T-6 or above. Some children will be discharged home with mechanical ventilation. Extensive teaching is required for the family in those circumstances. Children should receive a yearly influenza vaccination, particularly those who are respiratory-compromised.

All children need support for their psychosocial adjustment, self-esteem, and sexuality issues. One of the major tasks of adolescence is establishing sexual identity, so this will be a more critical issue for this age group. Factual information regarding anatomy, physiology, and psychology (Flett 1992) should be offered.

Table 6–7 Skeletal Muscle Relaxants Used for Treatment of Spasticity in Neurologically Impaired Children

Trade/Generic	Forms Available	Dosage	Side Effects
Atarax/hydroxyzine hydrochloride	Tabs (HCL): 10, 25, 50, 100 mg Caps (pamoate): 25, 50, 100 mg Syrup (HCL): 10 mg/5 mL Susp (pamoate): 25 mg/5 mL	2 mg/kg/24 hours, divided q6h	Drowsiness, dry mouth, decreased alertness, tremor
Valium/diazepam	Tabs: 2, 5, 10 mg Oral solution: 1, 5 mg/1 mL	0.12–0.8 mg/kg/24 hours, divided q6–8h	Drowsiness, lethargy, ataxia, nausea and vomiting, hypotension, respiratory depression
Dantrium/dantrolene sodium	Caps: 25, 50, 100 mg	> 5 years 0.5 mg/kg/dose, bid. Titrate slowly to max dose 3 mg/kg//dose, bid-qid	Weakness, drowsiness, diarrhea, hepatotoxicity, sweating, fever, change in sensorium, photosensitivity
Lioresal/baclofen	Tabs: 10, 20 mg	2–7 years 10–15 mg/24 hour, divided q8h, max dose 40 mg/day >8 years max 60 mg, divided q8h	Drowsiness, dizziness, weakness, nausea, urinary frequency

Table 6–8 Medications Used for Bowel Management in Neurologically Impaired Children

Trade/Generic	Forms Available	Dosage	Side Effects
Colace/docusate sodium	Solution: 10 mg/1 mL, 50 mg/1 mL Syrup: 20 mg/5 mL Tabs: 50, 100 mg Caps: 50, 100, 240, 250, 300 mg	<3 years: 10–40 mg/24 h, divided qd-qid 3–6 years: 20–60 mg/24 h, divided qd-qid 6–12 years: 40–120 mg/24 h, divided qd-qid >12 years: 50–500 mg/24 h, divided qd-qid	Rare give with liquids
Milk of magnesia/magnesium hydroxide	Suspension 8%; 5 mL = 13.7 mEq Mg Tabs: 325 mg	0.5 mL/kg/dose or 40 mg/kg/dose po prn	Hypermagnesemia, hypotension, respiratory depression

SUMMARY

Home health care for the child with an alteration in neurologic function as presented in this chapter centers on the goals of returning the child to an optimal state of neurologic functioning, preventing and identifying potential complications, and mobilizing coping mechanisms for the child and family. The key to achieving these goals and optimizing recovery is comprehensive and coordinated care. The home health care nurse is in a critical position to become the case manager and coordinate all aspects of the child's care or the rehabilitation program. Rehabilitation is a multiphasic process that is individualized to meet the unique needs of the child and his or her family.

Various disciplines may be required to meet the child's care needs and, together with the family, to develop a comprehensive care plan. Nursing care plans for children with neurologic alteration are outlined in Appendix 6–B.

REFERENCES

Barry, K., and S. Teixeira. 1983. The role of the nurse in the diagnostic classification and management of seizures. *Journal of Neurosurgical Nursing* 15:243–49.

Ferry, P., W. Banner, and R. Wolf. 1986. *Seizure disorders in children*. New York: J.B. Lippincott.

Flett, P.J. 1992. The rehabilitation of children with spinal cord injury. *Journal of Paediatric Child Health* 28: 141–46.

Freeman, J.M., M.T. Kelly, and J.B. Freeman. 1994. *The ketogenic diet*. New York: Demos.

Goldstein, B., and K.S. Powers. 1994. Head trauma in children. *Pediatrics in Review* 15, no. 6:213–19.

Hickey, J.V. 1992. *Neurological and neurosurgical nursing.* 3d ed. Philadelphia: J.B. Lippincott.

Johnston, M.V., and J.P. Gerring. 1992. Head trauma and its sequelae. *Pediatric Annals* 21:362–68.

Kolodgie, M.J. 1994. Home care management of the child with infantile spasms. *Pediatric Nursing* 20:270–73.

Menkes, J.H., and K. Till. 1995. Postnatal trauma and injuries by physical agents. In *Textbook of child neurology,* 5th ed. J.W. Pine, 557–97. Baltimore: Williams & Wilkins.

Pilcher, W.H., et al. 1992. Update in epilepsy part III: Surgical therapy of intractable epilepsy. *New York State Journal of Medicine* 92:92–6.

Roddy, S., and M. McBride. 1992. Seizure disorders. In *Primary pediatric care,* R.A. Hoekleman, et al., 1481–90. St. Louis: Mosby–Year Book.

Vining, E.P., and J.M. Freeman. 1986. Management of nonfebrile seizures. *Pediatrics in Review* 8, no. 6: 185–90.

BIBLIOGRAPHY

Byers, V.L. 1993. Novel antiepileptic drugs: Nursing implications. *Journal of Neuroscience Nursing* 25: 375–79.

Coon, N., R. Carter, G.G. Chan, eds. 1994. *Journal of Neuroscience Nursing.* St. Louis: Mosby.

Greene, M.G. and K. Johnson, eds. 1993. *The Harriet Lane handbook.* 13th ed. St. Louis: Mosby.

Reynolds, E. 1992. Controversies in caring for the child with a head injury. *The American Journal of Maternal Child Nursing* 17:246–51.

Nursing Care Plans for the Child with a Seizure Disorder

Diagnosis/ Problem	Defining Characteristics	Interventions	Expected Outcomes
Coping ineffective Patient and family R/T new onset chronic illness Ever-present unpredict- ability of seizures	Patient or family verbalizes difficulty coping Behavior consistent with anxiety, depression, or anger Social isolation Feelings of inadequacy	Assess and monitor anxiety level and responses. Allow and encourage patient and family to verbalize feelings. Allow participation in decision making. Reinforce child's self-esteem. Provide information on support group.	Patient and family use appropiate coping mechanisms. Patient and family form trusting relationship with health care provid-ers. Patient and family use support resources as appropiate.
Alteration in neurologic status R/T recurrent paroxysmal events defined as seizures	Signs of seizure activity • altered conscious-ness • altered motor, sensory, auto-nomic, or behav-ioral function • postictal symp-toms (headache, nausea, confusion, lethargy, Todd's paralysis)	Assess and monitor for S&S of seizures. Establish a seizure calender with the patient and family. Administer antiepileptics as prescribed daily, and prn antiepileptics as ordered and indicated. Assess for side effects of antiepileptics or ketoge-nic diet as ordered. Remain calm and reassur-ing during crisis. Instruct caregivers in assessing seizure characteristics.	Patient no longer has or has reduced frequency of seizures. Patient does not have side effects from seizure medication. Seizure emergencies will be identified and treated promptly without insult to child.

Diagnosis/ Problem	Defining Characteristics	Interventions	Expected Outcomes
Alteration in safety R/T high risk of injury with seizures	Musculoskeletal trauma from falls Head injuries from falls Oral tissue trauma from biting Bruising Respiratory distress from airway obstruction	Assess seizure type and identify risk related to nature of seizure. Instruct caregiver in first aid for seizures as described in Exhibit 6–2. Instruct family to remove harmful objects during seizures. Develop a plan for emergent or prolonged seizure activity with family and medical team. Help family identify possible seizure triggers.	Patient does not suffer from injury from seizures. Patient does not suffer from complications from seizure activity. Family uses appropriate first aid during events. Patient and family demonstrate decreased anxiety with acute events.
Knowledge deficit R/T New onset disorder Treatment regimen	Verbalization of questions, concerns, misconceptions related to seizures and prescribed treatment Inability to verbalize rationale for medication Noncompliance with treatment regimen	Instruct family in seizure disorders and S&S of seizure activity. Instruct family in administration of antiepileptics including action of medications and possible side effects. Develop plan with family for long-term monitoring of medication therapy. Encourage follow-up for further education and involvement with support groups.	Patient and family are knowledgeable about the disorder and treatment regimen. Patient and family are compliant with the treatment plan. Patient and family use available resources as necessary.
Alteration in nutrition R/T ketogenic diet (if ordered) R/T possible side effects of antiepileptics	Complications of ketogenic diet—weight loss/gain, hunger, thirst, sleepiness Side effects of some antiepileptics—nausea, vomiting, weight loss, weight gain	Assess intake as defined by ketogenic diet, monitor I & O. Assess metabolic and neurologic impact of diet: • Check ketones. • Monitor for hypoglycemia. • Weigh at same time	Patient will tolerate ketogenic diet with reduced seizure activity. Patient will not suffer from side effects from medications. Maintain appropriate growth pattern for age.

Diagnosis/ Problem	Defining Characteristics	Interventions	Expected Outcomes
		daily. • Monitor seizure record. Ensure that family has appropiate equipment and resources to follow diet. Consult with nutritionists prn. Monitor for side effects of antiepileptics. Check antiepileptic levels. Inform MD or NP of side effect occurrence. Encourage well-balanced dietary intake. Encourage snacks with medication.	

Note: R/T, related to; S&S, signs and symptoms; PRN, as needed; ICP, increased cranial pressure; DVT, deep venous thrombosis; vs, venous stasis; GT, gastrostomy tube; JT, jejunostomy tube; bid, twice a day; ROM, range of motion; SOB, shortness of breath; qd, everyday; BM, bowel movement; NG, nasogastric; cath, catheter or catheterized; I&O, intake and output; CPT, chest physiotherapy; MD, physician; NP, nurse practitioner.

Nursing Care Plans for the Neurologically Impaired Child

Diagnosis/ Problem	Defining Characteristics	Interventions	Expected Outcomes
Alteration in respiratory status R/T underlying neurologic disability	Signs of respiratory compromise: • Tachypnea • Tachycardia • Pallor/cyanosis • Adventitious breath sounds • Irritability/ restlessness • Nasal flaring/ retractions	Assess respiratory status q4h. Perform CPT with postural drainage q4h. Deep breathing and coughing q1–2h. Elevate HOB 30 degrees. Turn q2 hours to prevent stasis. Give adequate fluids to liquify secretions. Assess for S&S of respiratory infection. Administer oxygen and bronchodilators as ordered by MD or NP **Specific to ventilator-dependent patients:** Assess functioning of ventilator q8h. Tracheostomy care q4h using aseptic technique. Change tracheostomy ties at least daily. Change tracheostomy cannula q month Observe stoma for infection.	Patient will have patent airway and effective breathing pattern will be maintained. Patient will not have respiratory infection.

Diagnosis/ Problem	Defining Characteristics	Interventions	Expected Outcomes
Alteration in elimination, bowel, and/or bladder	Incontinence Constipation	**General** Provide perineal hygiene q4h. Monitor I & O q8h. Monitor volume, color, clarity, and odor of each void. **Bladder Program** Intermittent straight cath q4–8h using clean technique (patient, parent, or nurse). Clean catheter equipment with antiseptic solution and store in clean container after each use. Monitor residual urine q void. 2–3L of fluid qd unless restricted. Skeletal muscle relaxants as orderd by MD or NP **Bowel Program** Bowel evacuation at same time qd Glycerin suppository before BM. Maintain appropriate fiber intake in diet. Digital stimulation prn. Daily stool softener or laxative as ordered by MD or NP	Renal complications prevented Constipation/obstruction prevented Routine elimination program maintained Incontinence minimized
Alteration in nutrition R/T underlying neurologic disability	Altered route for intake (i.e., NG, GT, JT secondary to altered level of consciousness or impaired/absent gag reflex	Provide appropriate nutritional intake based on age, weight, and feeding route. Assess gag reflex before oral feedings. Weigh child at same time daily. Daily calorie count Monitor I & O. Nutritional consult prn	Adequate nutrition provided without complications of aspiration Maintains appropriate height and weight for age

Diagnosis/ Problem	Defining Characteristics	Interventions	Expected Outcomes
Coping: ineffective—patient and family R/T new onset chronic disability	Patient or family verbalizes difficulty coping Behavior consistent with depression or anger Inappropriate stage of grieving process Suicidal threats or attempts Social isolation	Allow and encourage patient and family to verbalize feelings. Monitor responses of patient and family to chronic disability and encourage appropriate coping mechanisms. Allow participation in decision making and care. Provide information regarding child's disability. Reinforce child's self-esteem. Provide social interaction and diversion. Encourage participation in related community supports and respite programs. Request consult to assist patient and/or family with coping prn.	Patient and family form trusting relationship with health care providers. Patient and family use appropriate coping mechanisms. Patient and family use support resources as appropriate.
Alteration in skin integrity, potential for injury	Skin irritation from tape, tracheostomy, and immobility • Redness • Inflammation • Abrasions • Decubitus	Daily bath Mouth and perineal care q4h Apply moisturizer to dry skin. Assess all areas of skin at least q8h, bony prominences and heels q2h. Turn and position q2h if bedridden. Shift weight q5–10 minutes in wheelchair. Maintain adequate nutritional status. **NG, GT, or JT:** Change dressings qd and wash with $^1/_2$ strength hydrogen peroxide.	Skin will remain intact. Skin will be free of infection.

Diagnosis/ Problem	Defining Characteristics	Interventions	Expected Outcomes
Alteration in neurologic status	Altered level of consciousness Alteration in motor and sensory function	Assess level of consciousness with GCS q8h. Assess motor/sensory status q8h. Assess tone q8h. Assess for S&S of increased ICP q8h. Assess for S&S of seizures. Recognize S&S of autonomic hyperreflexia and treat immediately.	Neurologic status will remain stable or improve. Seizures will be identified and treated promptly. Neurologic emergencies will be identified and treated promptly without further insult to child.
Alteration in sexual function	Neurosensory deficits to reproductive organs Inability to achieve or sustain an erection Loss of libido Unwilling or uninformed partner Altered sexual self-concept	Provide support to patient and partner. Provide factual information and encourage discussion. Refer to sexual counselor as appropriate.	Patient will adapt to limitations in sexual functioning.
Alteration in physical mobility, R/T paresis, paralysis, spasticity		Turn and position q2 h. Maintain appropriate body alignment; keep in neutral position to optimize function. Provide PRAM at least 4×/day Assess ROM of joints, muscle tone, and presence of atrophy during PRAM. Assess posture for signs of scoliosis. Control noxious stimuli that trigger muscle spasms. Apply orthopedic equipment (splints, slings, jackets) as ordered by MD.	Child will not have contractures. Spasticity and related pain will be minimized. Child will be as optimally independent within constraints of physical limitations.

Diagnosis/ Problem	Defining Characteristics	Interventions	Expected Outcomes
		Encourage independent ambulation with wheelchair. Encourage use of transfers using good body mechanics. Supported weight bearing at least bid for 30–60 minutes as tolerated Skeletal muscle relaxants as ordered by MD or NP Pain medication as ordered by MD or NP	
Potential alteration in cardiac status	Orthostatic hypotension Edema of extremities SOB R/T pulmonary emboli Pain, redness, and swelling in extremity, R/T DVT	Monitor VS q8h. Assess pedal pulses and capillary refill q4h. Measure lower extremities qd and report increases of 2 cm or greater to MD. Apply stockings or Ace wraps to legs qd; remove when supine. Elevate lower extremities when supine. Monitor for S&S of DVT.	Child will have adequate peripheral perfusion. Child will not develop dependent edema or DVT.
Self-care deficit R/T immobility	Inability to complete ADLs related to hygiene	Provide basic hygiene care. Provide dressing and grooming.	Basic self-care needs will be provided for by caregiver/nurse.

Note: R/T, related to; S&S, signs and symptoms; MD, physician; NP, nurse practitioner.

Source: Adapted from J.V. Hickey, *Neurological and Neurosurgical Nursing,* 3d ed., © 1992, J.B. Lippincott, and N. Coon, R. Carter, and G.G. Chan, *Neuroscience Nursing,* © 1994, Mosby.

CHAPTER 7

Alterations in Cardiac Function

Karen C. Uzark

Each year approximately 32,000 children enter the health care system in this country with a structural abnormality of the heart (Moller et al. 1994). Nearly one-third of all infants with congenital heart defects (2.6 per 1,000 live births) are born with a critical cardiac anomaly leading to cardiac catheterization, cardiac surgery, or death within the first year of life. During the past three decades, the prognosis for the majority of these infants has improved dramatically. At the present time, more than 95 percent of infants born with significant congenital heart disease are potentially amenable to some form of medical or surgical treatment (Emmanouilides et al. 1995). Referral from the pediatric cardiac center for home care services is often indicated to promote optimal health and functioning of children now surviving with congenital heart disease.

DISCHARGE PLANNING ISSUES

The diagnosis of significant congenital heart disease is often made soon after birth. The physiologic and psychological impacts of the infant's heart defect have important implications for discharge planning. Clearly, the individual infant's needs after discharge will be related to the physiologic consequences or clinical features of the specific cardiac defect and will be influenced by the parents' response to the cardiac diagnosis.

Impact of the Cardiac Diagnosis

The two cardinal signs of serious congenital heart disease are cyanosis and congestive heart failure.

Cyanotic Heart Disease

Cyanotic defects usually produce symptoms at birth or within the first months of life. Cyanosis is found in patients with cardiac lesions associated with significant obstruction to pulmonary blood flow or with mixing of the systemic and pulmonary blood through a right-to-left cardiac shunt. Heart defects resulting in cyanosis (Table 7–1) include tetralogy of Fallot, transposition of the great arteries, tricuspid atresia, total anomalous pulmonary venous connection, pulmonary atresia with intact ventricular septum, truncus arteriosus, and Ebstein's anomaly of the tricuspid valve. Tetralogy of Fallot and transposition of the great arteries are the most prevalent cyanotic defects and are discussed in greater detail.

In tetralogy of Fallot, the site of obstruction to pulmonary flow may involve the infundibulum of the right ventricle, the pulmonic valve, the annulus of the pulmonic valve, or the branches of the pulmonary artery. The degree of obstruction also varies, ranging from mild, allowing net left-to-right shunting through a large ventricular septal defect (pink tetralogy), to severe, as in

Table 7–1 Cyanotic Heart Defects

Defect	Anatomy	Surgical Management
Transposition of the great arteries	The aorta arises from the right ventricle and the pulmonary artery from the left ventricle	Arterial switch (Jatene) operation in neonatal period or intra-atrial baffle (Mustard or Senning procedure) later in infancy
Tetralogy of Fallot	Combination of four defects: (1) pulmonary stenosis, (2) ventricular septal defect, (3) overriding aorta, and (4) right ventricular hypertrophy	*Palliative:* Blalock-Taussig or other aortopulmonary shunts in infancy *Repair:* patch closure of VSD and resection of infundibular pulmonary stenosis ± pulmonary valvulotomy if necessary
Tricuspid atresia	Complete agenesis of the tricuspid valve with no direct communication between the right atrium and a hypoplastic right ventricle	*Palliative:* shunt (or pulmonary artery banding if increased pulmonary blood flow via a ventricular septal defect) *Repair:* pulmonary artery connected to right atrium (Fontan procedure)
Total anomalous pulmonary venous connection	Pulmonary veins do not enter the left atrium but are connected either directly or indirectly to the right atrium	*Repair:* pulmonary venous trunk connected to left atrium in infancy
Truncus arteriosus	Single arterial trunk forms the aorta and pulmonary artery, overriding the ventricles and receiving blood from them through a ventricular septal defect	*Repair:* closure of ventricular septal defect, removing the origin of the pulmonary arteries from the trunk, and connecting the pulmonary arteries to the right ventricle with a conduit in infancy
Pulmonary atresia with intact ventricular septum	Complete atresia of the pulmonary valve and varying degrees of hypoplasia of the right ventricle	*Palliative:* Blalock-Taussig shunt ± pulmonary valvulotomy *Repair:* right ventricular outflow tract reconstruction or Fontan procedure
Ebstein's anomaly of the tricuspid valve	Redundant tricuspid valve tissue with the septal and posterior leaflets displaced downward into the right ventricle for a variable distance	*Repair:* tricuspid valve replacement or modified tricuspid annuloplasty (Patients with less severe forms do not require surgery.)

Note: VSO, ventricular septal defect.

pulmonary atresia. The age at onset of the dominant symptom of cyanosis varies according to the degree of obstruction to pulmonary flow. A life-threatening symptom in children with tetralogy of Fallot is paroxysmal hyperpnea or hypoxic spells. A "spell" usually consists of an initial period of irritability or inconsolable crying, followed by paroxysms of hyperpnea, deep cyanosis, and decreased level of consciousness or sometimes convulsions. Hypoxic or "hypercyanotic" spells frequently occur early in the morning after awakening. It has been suggested that the spell occurs when a sudden spasm of the right ventricular outflow tract causes a rapid decrease in pulmonary blood flow (Zuberbuhler 1995). If a child has a history of spells, surgical palliation or correction is required on an urgent basis. The Blalock-Taussig shunt, a subclavian artery to pulmonary artery anastomosis, seems to be the preferred procedure for palliation in infants with tetralogy of Fallot and tricuspid atresia. Complete repair of tetralogy of Fallot is usually accomplished before the child enters school.

In transposition of the great arteries, the systemic and pulmonary circulations function in parallel; hence, the greatest portion of the output of each ventricle is recirculated to that ventricle. Prominent cyanosis is usually evident soon after birth because systemic arterial oxygen saturation is dependent on the relatively small amount of blood that is exchanged between the two circulations through a patent foramen ovale, an atrial septal defect, a ventricular septal defect, or a patent ductus arteriosus. Although the systemic arterial oxygen saturation is generally improved by balloon atrial (Rashkind) septostomy, the infant usually remains cyanotic until surgical correction is accomplished. This cyanosis increases with crying, bathing, cold temperatures, and exercise. Parents are often anxious about their infant's cyanosis and may be afraid to let the infant cry. An increase in cyanosis unrelated to activity, however, may be insidious and thus difficult for parents to notice. Before the mid-1980s, most centers used either the Mustard or Senning operation as definitive surgical treatment when the infant was 6 to 12 months old. These procedures provided redirection of systemic and pulmonary venous return using an intra-atrial baffle created from atrial septum (Senning) or pericardium (Mustard). After these surgical interventions, children were generally asymptomatic and appeared healthy. Some patients developed atrial arrhythmias after placement of intra-atrial baffles or later failure of the systemic right ventricle. With recognition of these long-term complications, currently the arterial switch operation during the first weeks of life is the preferred correction for transposition of the great arteries in many cardiac centers. This involves transection of the aorta and pulmonary artery with reanastomosis to the appropriate ventricle and transfer of the coronary arteries to the new aortic root.

The surgical management of the other cyanotic heart defects previously mentioned is summarized in Table 7–1. With hypoxia present before surgical correction of cyanotic heart defects, the requirement for increased oxygen-carrying capacity requires increased iron for hemoglobin. In general, the hemoglobin level in a moderately cyanotic patient should be above 15 to 16 g/dL, and a normal hemoglobin level indicates a "relative" anemia. In cyanotic children, anemia may cause increased dyspnea with decreased exercise tolerance, as well as increased frequency of hypoxic spells and the risk of cerebrovascular accident. With chronic arterial desaturation, however, red blood cell formation is stimulated and polycythemia results. As the central hematocrit reaches 65 to 70 percent (or hemoglobin near 20 g/dL), a marked increase in blood viscosity elevates peripheral vascular resistance and decreases oxygen delivery to the tissues. Children may complain of headaches, chest pain, fatigue, and muscle cramps and are also at increased risk of cerebrovascular accident. If the child with cyanotic heart disease and polycythemia becomes dehydrated, the hematocrit may increase sharply, increasing the risk of spontaneous cerebrovascular accident. Dental caries and periodontal disease are also more common in children with cyanotic heart disease, and there is increased risk of developing infective endocarditis, even after surgical repair.

Congestive Heart Failure

Acyanotic defects that cause congestive heart failure include those causing large left-to-right shunts and those causing severe obstruction of the left side of the heart or of the aorta. Heart defects that commonly result in congestive heart failure (Table 7–2) include ventricular septal defect, patent ductus arteriosus (especially in premature infants), complete atrioventricular septal defect (endocardial cushion defect), severe coarctation of the aorta, and hypoplastic left heart syndrome. Critical aortic stenosis in the neonate and total anomalous pulmonary venous connection with obstruction also cause congestive heart failure. In children with these congenital heart defects, heart failure is most likely to develop within the first weeks or months of life. With the exception of hypoplastic left heart syndrome, surgical repair in the first year of life generally relieves congestive heart failure symptoms. In some cardiac centers, neonates with hypoplastic left heart syndrome are palliated during the neonatal period using a Norwood procedure in which the main pulmonary artery is anastomosed to the aorta with creation of a systemic to pulmonary artery shunt, followed by a Fontan-type operation that creates an atriopulmonary connection. In children without structural heart defects, congestive heart failure may be due to cardiomyopathy.

Congestive heart failure is the failure of the cardiac output, because of the inadequacy of myocardial performance, to meet all the metabolic demands of the body. This state arises as a consequence of the excessive workload imposed on cardiac muscle by the structural defects. The principal manifestations of congestive heart failure are tachycardia, tachypnea, and dyspnea. The striking feature of congestive heart failure in the infant is a resting respiratory rate over 60 per minute and often as high as 100 to 120 breaths per minute, sometimes associated with nasal flaring, retractions, and even wheezing. Expiratory grunting may be noted in some infants. A

Table 7–2 Acyanotic Heart Defects Commonly Causing Congestive Heart Failure in Infancy

Defect	Description
Hypoplastic left heart syndrome	Aortic atresia and underdevelopment of the left ventricle, mitral valve, hypoplastic aortic arch, and/or coarctation
Coarctation of the aorta	Constriction of the aorta usually located slightly distal to the origin of the left subclavian artery
Ventricular septal defect	An abnormal opening between the right and left ventricle that may result in congestive heart failure if the left-to-right shunt is large
Atrioventricular septal defect (endocardial cushion defect)	A defect in the lower part of the atrial septum (ostium primum) and the membraneous ventricular septum and a single common atrioventricular valve
Patent ductus arteriosus	A connection between the pulmonary artery and the aorta that fails to close after birth, allowing increased blood flow to the lungs

chronic "hacking" cough secondary to congestion of bronchial mucosa may be present, as well as an increased frequency of respiratory infection. Increased sweating has been noted in infants with cardiac failure, probably reflecting increased activity of the autonomic nervous system in the presence of impaired myocardial performance. The sweating is usually found on the face, neck, and head and is not related to the environment. Pallor or peripheral cyanosis may also be present, even if the heart defect is not associated with intracardiac right-to-left shunting, and the infant in failure may appear grayish or more mottled, especially with crying or feeding. The infant may have trouble sucking, swallowing, and breathing simultaneously, needing to rest frequently during a feeding, and thus the feeding takes longer. Sometimes the infant falls asleep exhausted before the intake is adequate, and, in older infants, poor weight gain may be the most prominent and, for the parents, the most worrisome feature of heart failure. Facial edema is more common than peripheral edema in infants, whereas ascites and generalized anasarca are rare.

Psychosocial Responses

The diagnosis of significant congenital heart disease, often made soon after birth, is a traumatic emotional experience for parents. The initial reactions of the family to the child's defect have been described as acute fear and anxiety, immediate shock followed by mourning the loss of a healthy child, anger or resentfulness, and guilt over causing the child's heart defect. Because the exact cause of the child's defect is usually not known, parents tend to fantasize about the etiology. The initial diagnosis often represents a family crisis, and health care professionals play a key role in supporting parents during their emotional ordeal of accepting a child with congenital heart disease. Parents often do not appreciate the differences between congenital and acquired heart disease. Bergman and Stamm

(1967) found that two-thirds of the parents interviewed believed the child had the same type of heart disease encountered in adults. Related to this misconception, parents fear the child's sudden death from a "heart attack." Parental reactions to the diagnosis may also interfere with their ability to cooperate with the therapeutic regimen and even threaten their ability to provide optimal care for their child (Lobo 1992). The loss of self-esteem that may accompany having produced an infant with a cardiac defect hinders the attainment of the parenting role. Development of the parental role is influenced by characteristics of the infant such as physical appearance and behavior. The infant with heart disease may be cyanotic, small for gestational age, tire easily, or feed poorly. The infant's expected weight gain or motor development may not be achieved at a level sufficient to promote parental self-esteem. Also, when the child differs so greatly from expectations, parents may miscalculate the child's needs. One study confirmed that parents have negative feelings about their infant with congenital heart disease as well as various misconceptions, especially regarding cyanosis, sudden death, and vulnerability to infection, which may hinder optimal parenting behaviors (Uzark and White 1981). As the child grows, these emotional reactions often further interfere with the parents' ability to set limits for acceptable behavior and administer disciplinary measures that are necessary parental functions, regardless of whether the child has heart disease.

The impact of a child with a congenital heart defect is not limited to parents as individuals but also affects marital ties, sibling relationships, and the entire family as a unit. Before discharge from the hospital, it is essential to assess the family's stress level and coping strategies, their abilities or strengths, and their resources. Lewandowski (1980) has suggested some parameters for assessing possible coping strategies of parents of children with congenital heart defects requiring surgery. These include the following:

- parents' perception of the situation (realistic or distorted)
- available situational supports, such as parents' relationships with each other, other family members, and friends, hospital staff, and other possible support systems
- family's interaction with each other
- ways parents have coped with stress in the past
- decision-making abilities
- parents' interaction with others
- parents' interaction with child
- types of questions and repetition of questions
- types of concerns voiced or voicing no concerns
- verbalizations about own anxiety level, coping strategies
- brief attention span or inability to focus on any one thing
- amount of involvement in child's care that parents desire or accept
- parents' outward physical appearance
- nonverbal behaviors (restlessness, rocking, tightly clasped hands, rigid posture, wringing of hands, shaking, crying)
- somatic signs and symptoms (headache, gastrointestinal upset, frequent urination, backache)

Besides personal coping resources, it is also important to assess the family's social support network and potential financial needs. Parents need support from extended family members or mature friends who express not only emotional concern but also willingness to provide periodic assistance with child care. Community resources, including the local heart association, services for children with disabilities offered by individual states, parent support groups, school systems, and other agencies may offer valuable services to families of children with heart disease. Primary physicians and nurses play a critical role in offering meaningful support to parents and promoting comprehensive health care for these children. Unfortunately, the actual cardiac pathology may assume such overwhelming importance for health care professionals that anticipatory guidance regarding "normal" child behavior and needs is omitted, and even the administration of immunizations and adequate dental care have been found to be neglected (Uzark et al. 1983).

The responses of significant others to the diagnosis of heart disease can have lasting, deleterious effects on the child's psychosocial well-being. Studies have suggested that behavioral problems and poor adjustment of the child are more highly related to maternal attitudes (for example, anxiety, protectiveness, and overindulgence) and perceptions than to the severity of the heart disease (DeMaso et al. 1991). It seems that psychopathology derives not so much from the direct effects of the disease or the severity of the physical symptomatology as from life experiences associated with the diagnostic label of congenital heart disease. Even "successful" adults with congenital heart disease have excess psychological stress unrelated to the clinical severity of the original cardiac defect (Brandhagen, Feldt, and Williams 1991). In discharge planning, accurate information regarding the child's physical and emotional needs will facilitate the home care nurse's ability to promote the child's physical health and help prevent or reduce untoward psychosocial consequences of the cardiac diagnosis. To ensure optimal planning and care, all referrals from the pediatric cardiac center to the nursing agency should include the following: (1) discharge data regarding the child's pulse, respiratory rate, color, and weight; (2) assessment of the family's responses to the child's diagnosis and care and their existing resources; and (3) information regarding the patient's medications, diet, activity, any special treatments, and plans for medical follow-up.

TEACHING ISSUES BEFORE DISCHARGE

Because the child with congenital heart disease frequently does not have the defect surgically corrected at the time of diagnosis, parents require essential guidance and direction to provide optimal care for their child. Discharge preparation should generally include information regarding symptoms of cardiac distress, medications, diet-feeding, activity, and health maintenance needs. The family also needs support and encouragement to recognize and meet their own psychosocial needs.

Cardiac Distress

Parents should be taught symptoms of increasing cardiac distress so that these can be promptly reported and treated (O'Brien and Boisvert 1989). Because a paroxysmal hyperpneic attack or hypoxic spell can result in death of the infant with cyanotic heart disease, a spell or suspicion of spells should be reported to the cardiologist immediately. When the parent observes a hypoxic spell, as previously described, the child should be placed in the knee-chest position to attempt to alleviate the attack. A severe spell, however, may be relieved only by administration of oxygen and morphine or may even require surgical therapy.

Parents should also be aware of other signs of increasing cardiac distress that require less urgent therapy. Although increased cyanosis associated with crying, activity, and cold temperature is expected in infants with cyanotic heart defects, parents can observe increased cyanosis of lips or nailbeds at rest over time. Increasing symptoms of congestive heart failure may also occur over several days, not suddenly as parents sometimes anticipate. Parents should note increased perspiration unrelated to the environment, slower feeding or decreased oral intake, cough, edema, and decreased urinary output. The symptoms should be reported to the cardiologist or primary care physician, who may increase the child's medications. Positioning the child at a 45-degree angle can help alleviate the respiratory distress associated with congestive heart failure by decreasing the pressure of the viscera on the diaphragm. This can be accomplished by placing the child in an infant seat or

by elevating the head of the mattress. Older children may be more comfortable using several pillows. It is rarely necessary to keep oxygen in the home.

Medications

Cyanotic infants or children are often discharged with no medication regimen. An iron preparation may be prescribed to treat anemia, which frequently occurs in 4- to 24-month-old infants. (Besides the increased risks to the cyanotic child with anemia, anemia also increases the work of the heart and may aggravate congestive heart failure.) Treatment for anemia is usually administration of an oral form of ferrous sulfate—Fer-In-Sol drops (25 mg Fe/mL), Feosol elixir (8 mg Fe/mL), or tablets. The dose is carefully based on weight and should be given only for a prescribed length of time with periodic checking of hemoglobin or hematocrit levels. Administration between meals or with a vitamin C–fortified juice helps increase iron absorption. Parents should be aware of possible side effects of iron therapy, including temporary staining of the teeth, darker stool, and occasional constipation.

Digoxin is the most frequently used cardiac medication for the treatment of congestive heart failure. The primary action of digitalis is to improve the force of ventricular contractility. Digitalization is usually done in the hospital and children are sent home on maintenance doses. In children younger than 10 years, the daily maintenance dose is generally 0.01 to 0.015 mg/kg but is also individualized based on the patient's needs and serum digoxin levels. Premature infants and patients with impaired renal function should receive lower doses. Digoxin elixir contains 0.05 mg/mL and is usually administered every 12 hours. Digitalis toxicity does not occur often, especially because appropriate maintenance doses are generally established and monitored with serum digoxin levels. Toxicity should be considered, however, when observing decreased appetite, nausea, vomiting, bradycardia, and other arrhythmias. Hypokalemia may augment toxicity. Besides knowledge of the drug's dose, administration, and potential adverse effects, parents need information about what actions to take if the child vomits the medication, if the parents forget to give a medication dose as scheduled, if a child accidentally receives too much medication, or if there are questions or concerns. Instructions for parents regarding digoxin are presented in Exhibit 7–1. Written medication instructions are most helpful and should be reviewed with parents.

Diuretics are frequently also used to facilitate the removal of accumulated fluid and sodium when there is considerable pulmonary or

---

Exhibit 7–1 Information on Digoxin for Parents

Digoxin is a medicine frequently given to infants and children with heart disease when they have congestive heart failure or a very rapid heart rate. This heart failure developed because of a heart defect and does not mean that the heart will stop beating; it means that the heart muscle is weak and cannot pump as forcefully as it should. The action of digoxin is to slow and strengthen the pumping of the heart muscle.

Some guidelines for parents giving digoxin are presented below:

1. *How to give digoxin at home:* Digoxin should be given twice a day, morning and evening, at times you can easily remember. Draw up the digoxin liquid in the syringe or dropper provided. Check amount carefully. With infants it is easiest to then place the dropper in the child's mouth so that it rests halfway back on the tongue or the side. Then give the medication slowly, allowing the child time to swallow.
2. *If your child vomits the digoxin,* do *not* repeat that dose of medicine unless the child vomited immediately (within 5 minutes) after the digoxin was given *and* you are sure all the medicine has come up. If it has been more than 5 minutes, just give the normal dose of digoxin at the next *regular* time. Digoxin starts to be absorbed shortly after being given.
3. *If you forget to give the digoxin dose,* you may give it up to 2 hours later. If it is more than 2 hours late, just give the next dose at the regular time. It is important for your child to receive the digoxin every day.
4. *If your child becomes ill with severe loss of appetite or frequent vomiting or diarrhea for longer than 24 to 48 hours,* encourage ingestion of fluids, especially fruit juices, and contact the child's physician. Digoxin's effect on the heart can be changed by loss of body fluids and salt, especially potassium.
5. *If your child is absorbing too much digoxin (digoxin toxicity),* you may notice that the child's appetite is much less than normal, vomiting is frequent, or the heart rate is slower than usual or irregular. Call the child's physician or the Pediatric Cardiology Department (see below).
6. *If the child accidentally swallows too much digoxin,* call the physician or take the child to the nearest emergency department *immediately*. Digoxin should *always* be kept in a safe place, if possible in a locked cabinet, out of any child's reach.
7. The dosage of digoxin is increased as a child grows. Your child's present dose is _____ mL per day.

Should you have any questions or concerns, please feel free to call _____ and ask for a pediatric cardiology nurse, clinician, or any member of the cardiology staff. At night or on weekends, call the paging operator and ask for the pediatric cardiology fellow on call.

Source: Reprinted with permission from C.S. Mott Children's Hospital, University of Michigan, Ann Arbor, Michigan.

systemic edema associated with congestive heart failure. Commonly prescribed diuretics are furosemide (Lasix), chlorothiazide (Diuril), and spironolactone (Aldactone). Usual doses are presented in Table 7–3. Diuretics can produce electrolyte imbalance, the most serious being potassium depletion. In many instances, children who receive a potassium-wasting diuretic will also take a potassium-sparing diuretic, such as spironolactone, to offset excessive potassium loss. Excessive fluid loss and potassium depletion can occur when the child becomes ill with prolonged vomiting, diarrhea, poor fluid intake, and fever. Parents of children receiving diuretics should notify the physician if these symptoms appear and observe for signs of dehydration or electrolyte imbalance (dry lips, decreased urination, weakness, and lethargy).

More recently, systemic vasodilator drugs that serve to alter ventricular afterload have been used in infants and children who have not shown a satisfactory response to treatment with digitalis and diuretics. These vasodilator drugs, which include hydralazine (Apresoline), captopril (Capoten), and prazosin (Minipress), decrease the work of the heart by lowering the resistance to flow in the blood vessels of the body. Hydralazine is probably the most commonly prescribed arteriolar vasodilator (dose = 0.5 mg/kg/day orally every six to eight hours). Possible side effects include headache and dizziness.

Antibiotics should be prescribed for prophylaxis against bacterial endocarditis before any bacteremia-producing orodental, genitourinary, or gastrointestinal procedures or surgery. The American Heart Association has published recommendations for prophylaxis in the form of a card to be carried by parents or patients (Exhibit 7–2). Virtually all congenital heart disease requires prophylaxis, with the exception of atrial septal defect secundum, partial anomalous pulmonary venous return, and trivial pulmonary stenosis.

Diet/Feeding

Nutritional management of infants or children with uncorrected congenital heart disease can present a difficult challenge for parents and health care providers. Poor weight gain is especially common in infants with congestive heart failure, when fatigue and tachypnea interfere with adequate food intake. These infants should be fed more frequently—in early infancy, perhaps as often as every two hours during the day and every four hours at night. Prolonging the duration of each feeding beyond 30 minutes frustrates both parents and infants. Swallowing and breathing will be easier if the infant is held in a semiupright position for feeding, and frequent burping is helpful. When the infant is bottle fed, energy expenditure can also be reduced by using a soft nipple designed for premature infants or one that has a hole large enough to allow easy flow of the formula.

When the bottle-fed infant cannot take an adequate volume of formula, the health care professional may recommend increasing the caloric concentration. This may be accomplished by adding less water to formula concentrate (13 ounces of formula concentrate + 9 ounces of water = 24 calories/ounce) or adding caloric supplements such as Polycose, MCT Oil, or corn oil to the formulas or breast milk. Attention must be paid to water balance in high-density formulas, and infants may develop diarrhea or vomiting when the high-calorie formula is not tolerated. Low-sodium formulas are commercially available and may occasionally be used, but some are not palatable, provide too little sodium to satisfy growth requirements, or may be asso-

---

Table 7–3 Usual Pediatric Doses of Diuretics

Drug	Dose
Furosemide (Lasix)	1–2 mg/kg/dose
Chlorothiazide (Diuril)	20–30 mg/kg/day
Spironolactone (Aldactone)	2–3 mg/kg/day
Aldactazide (chlorothiazide + spironolactone)	2–3 mg/kg/day
Triamterene (Dyrenium)	3 mg/kg/day

Exhibit 7–2 Recommendations for Preventing Bacterial Endocarditis

---

FOR DENTAL/ORAL/UPPER RESPIRATORY TRACT PROCEDURES

I. Standard Regimen in Patients at Risk (includes those with prosthetic heart valves and other high-risk patients):

Amoxicillin 3.0 g orally 1 hour before procedure, then 1.5 g 6 hours after initial dose.*

For amoxicillin/penicillin–allergic patients:
Erythromycin ethylsuccinate 800 mg or erythromycin stearate 1.0 g orally 2 hours before a procedure, then one-half the dose 6 hours after the initial administration.*

—OR—

Clindamycin 300 mg orally 1 hour before a procedure and 150 mg 6 hours after inital dose.*

II. Alternate Prophylactic Regimens for Dental/Oral/Upper Respiratory Tract Procedures in Patients at Risk:

A. For patients unable to take oral medications:
Ampicillin 2.0 g IV (or IM) 30 minutes before procedure, then ampicillin 1.0 g IV (or IM) *OR* amoxicillin 1.5 g orally 6 hours after initial dose.*

—OR—

For ampicillin/amoxicillin/penicillin–allergic patients unable to take oral medications:
Clindamycin 300 mg IV 30 minutes before a procedure and 150 mg IV (or orally) 6 hours after initial dose.*

B. For patients considered to be at high risk who are not candidates for the standard regimen:
Ampicillin 2.0 g IV (or IM) plus gentamicin 1.5 mg/kg IV (or IM) (not to exceed 80 mg) 30 minutes before procedure, followed by amoxicillin 1.5 g orally 6 hours after the initial dose. Alternatively, the parenteral regimen may be repeated 8 hours after the initial dose.*

For amoxicillin/ampicillin/penicillin–allergic patients considered to be at high risk:
Vancomycin 1.0 g IV administered over 1 hour, starting 1 hour before the procedure. No repeat dose is necessary.*

FOR GENITOURINARY/GASTROINTESTINAL PROCEDURES

I. Standard Regimen:

Ampicillin 2.0 g IV (or IM) plus gentamicin 1.5 mg/kg IV (or IM) (not to exceed 80 mg) 30 minutes before procedure, followed by amoxicillin 1.5 g orally 6 hours after the initial dose. Alternatively, the parenteral regimen may be repeated once 8 hours after the initial dose.*

For amoxicillin/ampicillin/penicillin–allergic patients:
Vancomycin 1.0 g IV administered over 1 hour plus gentamicin 1.5 mg/kg IV (or IM) (not to exceed 80 mg) 1 hour before the procedure. May be repeated once 8 hours after initial dose.*

continues

Exhibit 7–2 continued

II. Alternate Oral Regimen for Low-Risk Patients:

Amoxicillin 3.0 g orally 1 hour before the procedure, then 1.5 g 6 hours after the initial dose.**

*Note: Initial pediatric dosages are listed below. Follow-up oral dose should be one-half the initial dose. Total pediatric dose should not exceed total adult dose.

Amoxicillin: †	50 mg/kg	Vancomycin:	20 mg/kg
Clindamycin:	10 mg/kg	Ampicillin:	50 mg/kg
Erythromycin ethylsuccinate		Gentamicin:	2.0 mg/kg
or stearate:	20 mg/kg		

†The following weight ranges may also be used for the initial pediatric dose of amoxicillin:
<15 kg (33 lb.), 750 mg
15–30 kg (33–66 lb.), 1,500 mg
>30 kg (66 lb.), 3,000 mg (full adult dose)

**Note: Initial pediatric dosages are listed below. Follow-up oral dose should be one-half the initial dose. Total pediatric dose should not exceed total adult dose.

Ampicillin:	50 mg/kg	Gentamicin	2.0 mg/kg
Amoxicillin	50 mg/kg	Vancomycin	20 mg/kg

Note: Antibiotic regimens used to prevent recurrences of acute rheumatic fever are inadequate for the prevention of bacterial endocarditis. In patients with markedly compromised renal function, it may be necessary to modify or omit the second dose of gentamicin or vancomycin. Intramuscular injections may be contraindicated in patients receiving anticoagulants.

Name: _____

needs protection from BACTERIAL ENDOCARDITIS
because of an existing HEART CONDITION

Diagnosis: _____

Prescribed by: _____

Date: _____

Note: IV, intravenous; IM, intramuscular.

Source: Adapted from Prevention of Bacterial Endocarditis:Recommendations by the American Heart Association. *Journal of the American Medical Association* 1990;264:2919–2922, © 1990 American Medical Association (also excerpted in *Journal of the American Dental Association* 1991;122:87–92). Please refer to these recommendations for more complete information as to which patients and which procedures require prophylaxis.

ciated with electrolyte disturbances. In pediatric cardiology, it is now common practice to promote caloric and protein intake without strict sodium and fluid restrictions, even if this means more rigorous diuretic therapy.

When the breast-fed infant does not grow well or tires quickly at the breast, the mother can pump her breasts and offer breast milk (with a calorie supplement) in a bottle for one or more feedings each day or after nursing. Breast milk is naturally lower in sodium than many commercial formulas and is easily digested. Many mothers who prefer breastfeeding become anxious about their inability to monitor/measure the infant's intake of breast milk. It is usually possible to work out an effective schedule that combines breast and bottle feeding, and mothers need to be supported in their decisions regarding feeding their infant. When faster respiratory rates interfere with the infant's ability to suck from the bottle or breast, it may be easier for the infant to take cereal or other food from a spoon. In this case, early introduction of solid foods may be suggested when the infant appears ready. Even if the infant or child seems to have an adequate caloric intake, children with heart defects may still have delayed growth during infancy and childhood because of reasons not yet fully understood. Heart surgery can result in catch-up growth, but again this is unpredictable. Parents need support for their persistent efforts to meet their child's nutritional needs.

As previously mentioned in the section on medications, children with congenital heart disease may also experience iron deficiency or potassium depletion. Infants can be fed iron-fortified formulas and cereals. Parents of children eating "table" foods should include foods high in iron and potassium, such as bananas and orange juice, in the daily diet of these children. Parents must be encouraged to prepare well-balanced meals to ensure adequate nutritional intake and discouraged from constantly urging their children to eat foods with little nutritional value because they want their child with heart disease to gain weight.

Activity

Children with most heart defects may lead normal, active lives. An infant should be allowed to cry, crawl, and walk. It is unnecessary to restrict the young child's activity in any way, as long as he or she is allowed to rest as desired. No matter how active these children may appear, they will rest or seek less active play if needed. Parents and professionals need to promote realistic developmental behaviors among young children with heart disease.

School-age children often will have already had successful surgical repair at an early age and should be permitted to participate in physical education classes and all recreational activities to their levels of tolerance. Activities will be restricted for six to eight weeks after surgery.

Some children are advised, based on cardiac status and diagnosis, to avoid participation in strenuous sports and highly competitive games because their pride may force them to continue beyond their physical capabilities. Older children with pulmonary artery hypertension and pulmonary vascular obstructive disease should avoid strenuous physical activity and competitive sports because such activity increases the pulmonary artery pressure and may accelerate the development of pulmonary vascular obstructive disease. Isometric activities (for example, weight lifting and gymnastics) are contraindicated in children with marked left-sided obstructive disease (for example, aortic stenosis and coarctation) or cardiomyopathy because such work tends to disproportionately increase systemic blood pressure relative to myocardial oxygen uptake. When the cardiac lesion tends to be progressive with age, as in aortic stenosis, aortic regurgitation, and mitral regurgitation, children should be encouraged to develop skill in activities and sports that they will be able to continue in adulthood. Acceptable activities may include swimming, golf, cycling, bowling, horseback riding, archery, and fishing. These children may often participate in less strenuous team games such as baseball, badminton, or volleyball. The American Heart Association (1986) has published recreational and occupational recommendations for young patients with heart disease, classified by diagnosis and severity. Unnecessary restrictions should not be imposed by parents, schools, community organizations, or health care professionals. A written recommendation from the pediatric cardiac center is helpful to the patient and community agencies.

Provision of written discharge instructions is always helpful and prevents confusion. The parents should also have a written schedule of follow-up appointments and a phone number available to notify the physician of problems or questions.

NURSING CARE PLANS IN THE HOME

When caring for the child with an alteration in cardiac function due to a congenital heart defect, the goals are the following: (1) to maintain optimal cardiac output and alleviate cardiac distress; (2) to prevent and identify potential complications; (3) to promote adequate nutritional intake and optimal growth; (4) to support the family's and child's effective coping with stress associated with the cardiac diagnosis and hospitalization experiences; and (5) to foster primary health care and the psychosocial development of the child with heart disease. Because corrective surgery is increasingly being performed at an earlier age, especially in symptomatic children, the nursing interventions to follow are primarily directed toward the infant or very young child who requires home care. Pertinent nursing implications for each goal are presented in Appendix 7–A).

Nursing Considerations To Maintain Adequate Cardiac Output and Alleviate Cardiac Distress

Assessment of the child's cardiovascular status is a vital component of the home care nurse's role. The assessment process not only provides ongoing evaluation of the efficacy of the therapeutic regimen after discharge to allow early identification of problems or increased needs, but also provides tremendous reassurance to parents regarding their child's health status. A careful history should include assessment of the child's respiratory status, feeding behavior, activity level, and color. Suggested questions to be addressed at each visit are presented in Exhibit 7–3. Key elements of the physical assessment include heart rate, respiratory rate, color of lips and mucous membranes and extremities, and weight changes (Kohr and O'Brien 1995). A

Exhibit 7–3 Questions for Parents of Infants with Symptomatic Cardiac Disease

- Does the infant consistently breathe rapidly even while at rest?
- Does the infant have retractions or nasal flaring with breathing?
- Does the infant appear to be working harder just to breathe?
- Does the infant tire easily with feedings?
- Does the infant have to rest frequently while feeding?
- How many ounces does the infant take each feeding? Over what length of time?
- Does the infant vomit frequently?
- Does the infant always seem to have a cold?
- Does the infant's color become increasingly blue, gray, or mottled with feeding, crying, or other forms of exertion?
- Is the infant unduly lethargic or unusually irritable?
- Does the infant respond appropriately, according to age, to stimuli in the environment?
- What new behaviors (milestones) has the infant accomplished?

persistent respiratory rate of more than 60 breaths per minute and a heart rate greater than 160 beats per minute in a quiet infant suggest cardiac distress and should be reported to the physician. The nurse who has not observed the child daily may also be able to detect any subtle changes in color. The home care nurse should note increased cyanosis of lips and mucous membranes or a generalized gray color in a child with congestive heart failure. Such findings may not be appreciated by parents and should be shared with the cardiologist. A weight gain in infants of 60 g or more per day may suggest fluid accumulation.

It is important to assess the parent's accuracy and confidence in administering medications. The amount and method of administration of every medication should be reviewed. An understanding of the medication's purpose may help facilitate compliance, and barriers to compliance should be identified. Barriers may be related to difficulty in administration (for example, measurement and taste), medication cost, scheduling problems, or anxiety regarding side effects. Recently, more cardiologists believe that asking parents to count the heart rate before giving the digoxin causes unnecessary anxiety. This practice has been abandoned by many cardiac centers, because serum levels are monitored and infants are likely to outgrow the dosage. The nurse, however, should report any arrhythmia or a significant decrease in heart rate and should be more suspicious of digitalis toxicity if there is a history suggesting possible potassium depletion.

Measures to reduce energy requirements or expenditure include maintaining a comfortable environmental temperature, positioning, and planning daily care to ensure adequate periods of rest. As previously mentioned, children with congestive heart failure are more comfortable in a semi-Fowler's position, elevated 45 degrees to 60 degrees. Hypoxic infants may breathe more comfortably in the knee-chest position. Smaller, more frequent feedings and other feeding practices discussed earlier in this chapter can reduce energy expenditure with feeding.

Nursing Considerations To Prevent or Identify Potential Complications of Heart Disease

For all children with hemodynamically significant congenital heart disease, anemia can result in increased symptoms. If the cyanotic child becomes anemic, the risk of cerebrovascular accident increases. Whole cow's milk and infant formulas not supplemented with iron cannot generally meet the increased iron needs of cyanotic infants. The total amount of iron available in breast milk, although efficiently absorbed, may also be insufficient. The nurse should be aware of the child's most recent hematocrit or hemoglobin level and periodically evaluate dietary intake. The nurse can provide parents with information concerning good food sources of iron. When an iron supplement is prescribed, the nurse should review the dose and method of administration with parents and can recommend measures to help increase iron absorption.

When the cyanotic child becomes dehydrated, the hematocrit or viscosity of the blood can increase sharply, potentially leading to thrombus formation and cerebrovascular accident. In patients receiving digoxin or diuretics, fluid and electrolyte imbalances associated with gastroenteritis could also be catastrophic. The nurse should emphasize the importance of adequate fluid intake to avoid these complications. In children with diarrhea or vomiting who cannot tolerate clear liquids or oral electrolyte solutions, intravenous fluids may be necessary to maintain hydration. Parents should be instructed to seek prompt medical attention for illnesses causing any degree of dehydration from fever, lack of intake, or increased fluid losses.

Respiratory infections are common in infants with large intracardiac left-to-right shunts and congestive failure. Exposure to persons with infections should be minimized, and parents should avoid taking young infants to crowded places where they are more likely to acquire contagious illnesses. Good handwashing by family members who are ill is important. The nurse should be sure that a thermometer is available in the home and that the parents can take the child's temperature properly. Fevers should be reported to the primary care physician, and infections should be treated with the appropriate antibiotic when an organism is isolated or strongly suspected. Antibiotics are not needed when the infection is viral, and when patients are maintained on chronic antibiotic therapy or receive frequent courses of broad-spectrum antibiotics, they may be at increased risk for infections from resistant organisms or fungi. (Some patients with congenital heart disease, however, have associated immunodeficiency syndromes such as asplenia and require daily antibiotic prophylaxis.)

Infective endocarditis (subacute bacterial endocarditis) is an infection of the valves or inner lining of the heart and is a potential sequela of bacteremia in the child with a cardiac defect.

Instruction in the use of prophylactic antibiotic therapy is essential and should be periodically reviewed. Amoxicillin should be administered 30 minutes to one hour before dental work or any surgical procedure is performed, including tonsillectomy or any manipulation of the urinary or intestinal tracts. A second dose is given six hours later. Good oral hygiene is also important for these children because dental caries may be an added source of bacteria. Symptoms and signs of endocarditis are somewhat nonspecific, and the onset is usually insidious. There is usually unexplained fever (may be low grade), and malaise and anorexia are commonly noted in children. Other signs may be petechiae, Janeway's spots (painless hemorrhagic areas on the palms and soles), or splinter hemorrhages (thin black lines) under the nails. Some children develop headaches or other neurologic symptoms. Blood cultures should be obtained from any child with unexplained fever.

Nursing Considerations To Promote Adequate Nutritional Intake and Optimal Growth

Adequate nutritional management requires careful assessment of the child's dietary intake and parental feeding practice at each home visit. If the infant is bottle fed, 24-hour formula intake and formula preparation methods should be reviewed. Infants with heart disease may require as much as 70 calories per pound (or 150 calories per kilogram) of body weight daily for growth. A desirable weight gain for young infants is 0.5 to 1 ounce per day. Weighing the child daily is not necessary and should be discouraged because fluctuations are common and influenced by nondietary factors. Periodic, perhaps weekly, weight checks by the home care nurse, however, can be helpful to assess growth (or identify excessive fluid accumulation).

Observation of infant feeding practices is especially important to identify potential measures to facilitate caloric intake or reduce energy expenditure. As previously discussed, the nurse may recommend holding the infant in a more upright position for feeding, more frequent burping, or a softer nipple. Changes in the caloric concentration of formulas should be instituted only if the physician recommends them. A guide for parents in feeding infants with congenital heart disease is available from the American Heart Association (1992) and most cardiac centers.

The nurse can assist the parents of older infants and children by analyzing a three-day dietary record to be certain that nutritional requirements are being met. The parents can be provided with appropriate information regarding foods high in sodium, potassium, or iron, as indicated by the specific child's needs. Parents should be encouraged to prepare well-balanced meals to ensure adequate nutritional intake.

Nutritional management of infants with uncorrected significant heart defects can present a tremendous challenge for parents and health care providers. It can be frustrating and disheartening for parents when their child fails to gain weight despite their persistent efforts. Parents can be reminded that some children with heart defects have slow weight gain, regardless of the feeding method or caloric intake. Feeding by nasogastric tube will be instituted if the infant is unable to consume enough food to meet nutritional requirements. In these instances, it is important for the nurse to review tube feeding procedures and to encourage parents to continue to provide their infants with satisfaction derived from sucking and caressing. The nurse can offer invaluable support to these parents who are diligently working to meet their child's nutritional needs.

Nursing Considerations To Support the Family and Child's Effective Coping with Stress Associated with the Cardiac Diagnosis and Hospitalization Experiences

The diagnosis of congenital heart disease has a significant emotional impact on the child and family. The nurse can support the parents during the initial period of grief or mourning and recognize the parents' limited ability to understand information regarding the cardiac diagnosis during this process. The nurse's sensitivity and warmth may enable the parents to express their reactions and emerge with a sense of reassurance or acceptance of their feelings of loss, denial, anger or resentfulness, and guilt. Furthermore, parents are able to assimilate only the information about their child for which they are emotionally prepared and they are often apt to exaggerate and misinterpret the physician's explanations. Parents seem to be primarily interested in two kinds of medical information—prognosis and surgery. It is important, therefore, to assess the family's and child's level of understanding and to explore the meaning of the child's diagnosis to the family. Parents appreciate receiving written information and may have questions at home related to information received at the cardiac center. They should be encouraged to contact the pediatric cardiology service with urgent questions and write down questions to be answered at their child's next clinic visit. Parents often cannot anticipate the meaning or implications of their infant's heart defect before the child's discharge from the hospital. In an effort to increase knowledge and promote a more positive, less anxious attitude among parents of newborns with serious congenital heart disease, a videotape titled "Your Baby with a Congenital Heart Defect" was developed at the University of Michigan and is used at some cardiac centers (Uzark and White 1981). In this videotape, three families relate common feelings, problems, and infant care experiences from their home settings. It is suggested that the videotape transmits information about infant behavior that may not be included in the usual course of discussion with hospital personnel. Parents need affirmation of their child's normal attributes and behaviors, and routine child care issues should be discussed, including bathing, feeding, elimination, sleep habits, and comfort measures in response to crying. The parents should be encouraged to treat the child in as normal a manner as possible. Parents also often need permission and considerable encouragement to meet their own needs for rest

and recreation and should recognize the special needs and concerns of the child's siblings.

The cardiac diagnosis, heart surgery, poor prognosis, or perceived extraordinary home care requirements may create significant stress in the family. This anxiety or stress can create a barrier that not only prevents parents from comprehending explanations but may even interfere with their ability to provide optimal care to the child. The home care nurse is in a unique position to assess concurrent stresses in the family outside the hospital environment. Some parameters for assessing parental coping behaviors are outlined earlier in this chapter. Recognizing the emotional stress involved in caring for a child with a heart defect and helping parents to express their feelings and manage their stress may enable parents to then direct their energies toward caring optimally and realistically for their child. The nurse can explore the personal and social supports the parents have, including the presence of other family members and friends, recreation and activities for stress management, finances, ability to find baby-sitters, and access to other support services. The nurse can observe and assess the supportiveness of interactions among family members and the use of the identified resources. Stress and perceived social isolation can sometimes be alleviated through parent groups, which have developed in many areas of the country. When such groups are not available or approachable, meeting another parent of a child with a similar problem in the community can often provide unequaled support to the new parent, and such empathetic information sharing seems to be readily received and valued. The home care nurse is often in a position to introduce parents directly or identify an appropriate parent through the cardiac center. Referral to the local heart association, services for children with disabilities offered by individual states, and other community agencies may also provide helpful resources.

Parents may experience loss of self-esteem and perceived helplessness in response to the birth of their infant with a heart defect. Clear affirmation of positive parenting behaviors and effective coping strategies not only reinforces these behaviors but can promote feelings of greater control and confidence. Most families are capable and resilient in handling even complex problems related to the child's cardiac diagnosis.

It is also essential to provide psychological support and information to the child and family to help them cope with the increased stress of hospitalization. Although surgical repair of serious heart defects is often now accomplished during infancy, some children will require later hospitalization for heart surgery or heart catheterization. Preexisting conditions that influence the child's response to hospitalization include the parents' attitudes toward the child's condition, the child's age or stage of development, and the child's unique past experiences with any aspect of health care. Based on the assessment of these and other factors, such as the child's knowledge and identified fears, an individualized teaching plan can be developed. Important nursing considerations include the following:

- involving the parents in assessment and preparation
- adapting information to the child's cognitive and psychosocial development levels
- responding to the child's fears and past experiences
- providing the parents and child with role information
- describing sensations at appropriate times
- answering questions simply and honestly

The communication of accurate information about the events of hospitalization can reduce stress. Several methods of preparation, including tours, books, and videotapes, may be necessary to effectively communicate information to children. Videotapes and films seem to be powerful and acceptable media for communicating supportive information to children. These educational aids are available through many cardiac centers or bookstores in the community. References for parents are listed in Exhibit 7–4.

Exhibit 7–4 References for Families

AHA Council of Cardiovascular Disease in the Young. *If Your Child Has a Congenital Heart Defect: A Guide for Parents. The Committee on Congenital Cardiac Defects.* Dallas, Tex.: American Heart Association, 1991.

American Heart Association San Francisco Chapter. *Caring for a Child with a Heart Condition.* San Francisco: American Heart Association, 1987.

Clark, E., C. Clark, and C. Neill. *The Heart of a Child: What Families Need To Know about Heart Disorders in Children.* Baltimore, Md.: The Johns Hopkins University Press, 1992.

Elder, V. *Cardiac Kids—A Book for Families Who Have Kids with Heart Disease.* Dayton, Ohio: Tender Hearts Publishing, 1994.

Friedman, J., and S. Allen. *Understanding Cardiac Catheterizations.* San Bruno, Calif.: Krames Communications, 1993.

Moller, J., W. Neal, and W. Hoffman. *A Parent's Guide to Heart Disorders.* Minneapolis: University of Minnesota Press, 1988.

Nursing Considerations To Foster Primary Health Care and the Psychosocial Development of the Child with Heart Disease

Although the provision of comprehensive health care is the goal for every child, the added burden of cardiac disease reinforces the concern for the primary and preventive health care needs of these children. The child's cardiac diagnosis, however, may interfere with the delivery of primary health care services because of lack of involvement by primary physicians, uncertainty regarding responsibility for certain aspects of care, or parental and provider anxiety or misconceptions. The presence of congenital heart disease is not a contraindication to administration of immunizations. The home care nurse should inquire about the child's immunization status and can facilitate communication among health care providers regarding the child's primary care needs. Parents should be assured that the chances of their child experiencing side effects will not be increased and encouraged to ensure that their child receives immunizations to minimize the incidence of devastating preventable diseases. Parents may need encouragement to consult the local physician for matters not related to the cardiac problem and may be apt to attribute any symptom to the child's cardiac condition. Parents may also not recognize their child's need for dental health services, in spite of the child's increased susceptibility to infective endocarditis when dental or periodontal disease is not controlled. Visits to the dentist should start by three years of age or sooner if dental caries are apparent. If a particular dentist is reluctant to treat the child with heart disease, referral should be made to another dentist or the cardiac center. The nurse should also educate or reinforce information regarding scrupulous dental hygiene, including frequent teeth brushings, reduction of cariogenic sugars in the diet, and use of appropriate fluoride supplements.

The cognitive development of children with congenital heart disease is usually within normal limits. Delayed development, particularly in gross motor milestones, has been attributed to congestive heart failure, decreased arterial oxygen saturation, and/or psychological and social factors (Aisenberg et al. 1982). Symptomatic infants may have limited energy for accomplishing gross motor tasks, but parents often tend to anticipate the infant's every need and to inhibit the child's developmental striving. Parents should be informed about expected developmental milestones so that they can recognize strengths and progress. The importance of a stimulating environment and of avoiding an overly protective or restrictive parental attitude at home should be emphasized. Professionals and parents need to promote realistic developmental behaviors among these children. The

home care nurse can assist the parents in fostering optimal development by encouraging parents to stimulate the infant toward feasible goals through specific age-appropriate activities such as placing the infant in a prone position to encourage motor development or allowing older infants to explore in a safe environment to encourage mobility instead of being held. Referral to a developmental stimulation or early intervention program may be appropriate in some instances.

Parents of a child with congenital heart disease may also tend to be overly permissive in the home, avoiding conflict and failing to establish consistent rules or limits for the child's behavior. When different expectations for behavior are expected for well siblings who also may receive less attention, sibling jealousy and resentment can create additional stress in the family. Siblings often can understand and accept some special needs if explanations are given. Anticipatory guidance regarding these known problem areas should be given to prevent potential behavior problems and to foster independence and feelings of self-confidence in the child with heart disease.

Surgical repair is now likely to be accomplished before school age, so that treatment does not interfere with school attendance and performance. Teachers and parents should not be overprotective and lower expectations but provide realistic optimal educational opportunities. Legislation exists (P.L. 92-112) to guarantee the availability of special education programming when it is needed, and early referral is important. Some children may need homebound teaching for a period because of illness or recovery from surgery. Education is extremely important to children with heart disease, especially when future occupational decisions may be affected by decreased physical endurance. Although the majority of patients with congenital heart disease are functionally normal, early vocational guidance is important to prevent occupational choices that are unreasonable in relation to the person's potential work capacity.

REFERENCES

Aisenberg, R., et al. 1982. Developmental delay in infants with congenital heart disease. *Pediatric Cardiology.* 3: 133.

American Heart Association. 1986. Recreational and occupational recommendations for young patients with heart disease. *Circulation* 74:1195A.

American Heart Association. 1992. *Feeding infants with congenital heart disease.* Dallas, TX: American Heart Association.

Bergman, A., and S. Stamm. 1967. The morbidity of cardiac nondisease in school children. *New England Journal of Medicine* 276:1008.

Brandhagen, D., R. Feldt, and D. Williams. 1991. Long-term psychologic implications of congenital heart disease: a 25-year follow-up. *Mayo Clinic Proceedings* 66: 474–79.

DeMaso, D., et al. 1991. The impact of maternal perceptions and medical severity on the adjustment of children with congenital heart disease. *Journal of Pediatric Psychology* 16:137–49.

Emmanouilides, G., et al. eds. 1995. *Moss and Adams heart disease in infants, children, and adolescents including the fetus and young adult.* Baltimore: Williams & Wilkins.

Kohr, L., and P. O'Brien. 1995. Current management of congestive heart failure in infants and children. *Nursing Clinics of North America* 30:261.

Lewandowski, L. 1980. Stress coping styles of parents of children undergoing open-heart surgery. *Critical Care Quarterly* 3:78–81.

Lobo, J. 1992. Parent-infant interaction during feeding when the infant has congenital heart disease. *Journal of Pediatric Nursing* 7, no. 2:97–105.

Moller, J., et al. 1994. Cardiovascular health and disease in children: Current status. *Circulation* 89:923–30.

O'Brien, P., and J. Boisvert. 1989. Discharge planning for children with heart disease. *Critical Care Nursing Clinics of North America* 1:297–305.

Uzark, K. and S. White. 1981. *Your baby with a congenital heart defect.* Ann Arbor: Biomedical Media Productions.

Uzark, K., et al. 1983. Primary preventive health care in children with heart disease. *Pediatric Cardiology* 4:259–64.

Uzark, K., et al. 1985. Use of videotapes to promote parenting of infants with serious congenital heart defects. *Pediatric Cardiology* 7:111–19.

Zuberbuhler, J. 1995. Tetralogy of Fallot. In *Heart disease in infants, children, and adolescents*, ed. G. Emmanouilides, et al. Baltimore: Williams & Wilkins.

Nursing Care Plans for Alterations in Cardiac Function

Nursing Diagnosis	Goals/Expected Outcomes	Interventions
Potential decreased cardiac output	Infant will maintain adequate cardiac output as evidenced by: Heart rate < _____ Respiratory rate < _____ Bilateral palpable and equal pulses Capillary refill ≤ 3 seconds Absence of edema without excess weight gain.	1. Assess vital signs—heart rate, respiratory rate, blood pressure. 2. Assess systemic perfusion including color of mucous membranes and nailbeds, quality of and intensity of peripheral pulses, and capillary refill time. 3. Weigh. Assess edema. 4. Diuretic and/or digoxin therapy as ordered.
Potential complications related to the following: anemia dehydration infection	Complications will be prevented/identified as evidenced by the following: Hb/Hct > _____ adequate fluid intake and urine output no fever, other signs of infection	1. Assess dietary intake. Administer iron supplement as ordered. 2. Assess intake and output, skin turgor. Evaluate gastrointestinal symptoms. 3. Assess parents' ability to measure child's temperature and identify signs of infection. Ensure good hygiene. Review instructions regarding endocarditis prophylaxis.

Nursing Diagnosis	Goals/Expected Outcomes	Interventions
Potential alteration in nutrition: less than body requirements related to poor intake.	Infant/child will have adequate nutritional intake to promote optimal growth.	1. Assess nutritional status, feeding patterns. 2. Monitor weight. 3. Institute small frequent feedings with caloric supplementation as needed. 4. Provide emotional support to parents.
Potential for ineffective family coping, related to the following: knowledge deficit fear and anxiety altered family routine	Family/patient will verbalize/ demonstrate effective coping with stress associated with cardiac diagnosis and/or hospitalization. Family will verbalize understanding of patient care.	1. Encourage verbalization of questions and feelings. 2. Identify coping resources. 3. Provide emotional support. 4. Assess parental knowledge regarding cardiac diagnosis, medications, and health care. Provide teaching. 5. Provide anticipatory guidance regarding child care needs. 6. Reinforce positive parenting behaviors. 7. Assist in preparation of child and family for hospitalization experiences.
Potential for lack of comprehensive health care services and delayed psychosocial development	Infant/child's primary health care needs are met as evidenced by immunization status and receipt of dental care. Family promotes infant's psychosocial development.	1. Coordinate care among health care providers. 2. Provide information regarding preventive health care needs. 3. Encourage developmental stimulation.

CHAPTER 8

Alterations in Metabolic Function

Marsha S. Pulhamus

Pediatric gastrointestinal disorders can often cause metabolic and nutritional abnormalities that can affect a child's growth and development, body image, and lifestyle. Because of the chronicity of gastrointestinal diseases and the need for frequent hospitalizations, the home care nurse is essential in providing a smooth transition to the home setting. This will include reinforcement of patient and family teaching that has been done in the hospital, ongoing nursing assessments, and reevaluations at home to ensure continued adaptation and improvement in the patient's condition. An overview of pediatric gastrointestinal diseases that the home care nurse may encounter is presented in this chapter. General guidelines for nursing care of these patients are presented and include growth and development issues, optimizing nutritional status, and identification and prevention of medical complications.

Nonorganic failure to thrive (NFTT) is not discussed in this chapter. Despite its frequency in the pediatric population and the need for strong home nursing support, the cause of NFTT is usually unrelated to disease and most often the result of psychosocial factors (Whaley and Wong 1995). Failure to thrive (FTT) is frequently seen. Although FTT has no universal definition, children present with failure to grow or gain weight. Typically, the child's weight (and sometimes height) falls below the fifth percentile when compared to an established growth curve (Whaley and Wong 1995; Barness 1993). Most FTT secondary to gastrointestinal disease is classified as organic failure to thrive (OFTT), because it is a result of a physical cause (Whaley and Wong 1995).

GASTROINTESTINAL DISORDERS

Inflammatory Bowel Disease

Inflammatory bowel disease (IBD) is the term used to designate ulcerative colitis (UC) and Crohn's disease (CD). Although ulcerative colitis and Crohn's disease are grouped under the classification of IBD because they have similar epidemiologic, immunologic, and clinical features, they are two distinct conditions with significant differences (Whaley and Wong 1995). Etiology of IBD is unknown, although there is evidence for multifactorial etiology and inherited predisposition (Walker et al. 1996; Whaley and Wong 1995). The incidence of CD is 4.8 per 100,000 in the United States and for UC 5.7 per 100,000 (Silverberg and Daum 1988).

Ulcerative colitis is an inflammatory disease of the mucosa and submucosa of the colon and rectum that involves a continuous segment of inflammation along the length of the involved bowel. Approximately 15 to 40 percent of patients present before age 20 years. The incidence of onset for UC is bimodal, with peaks in the second and third decades and again in the fourth and fifth decades (Walker et al. 1996). Signs and symptoms include abdominal pain with cramping, diarrhea, blood per rectum, anorexia, fever, and weight loss (Whaley and Wong 1995; Silverberg and Daum 1988). The first sign of UC may be growth failure, characterized by decreased linear growth velocity (Walker et al. 1996).

Crohn's disease may affect any segment of the gastrointestinal tract but usually involves the small intestine. CD does not usually involve a continuous segment of the intestine, and often the inflammation and ulcerations are patchy and transmural. The onset often occurs in late childhood or adolescence, with 20 percent of new patients presenting before age 12 years (Silverberg and Daum 1988). Signs and symptoms to be monitored include constant abdominal pain with cramping, nonbloody diarrhea, anorexia, fever, and growth failure. Mild gastrointestinal symptoms, poor growth, and extraintestinal manifestations may be present for several years before overt gastrointestinal symptoms are present. Extraintestinal manifestations can include erythema nodosum, large-joint arthritis, uveitis, mouth sores, liver disease, and renal calculi.

Medical Interventions

Medical management of IBD focuses on control of the inflammatory process to reduce or eliminate the symptoms, obtain long-term remission, and promote optimal nutritional status. Nutritional therapy is directed at providing a well-balanced, high-protein, high-calorie diet with multivitamin, iron, and folic acid supplements to meet the increased nutritional needs of IBD patients. There is little evidence that avoiding specific foods will influence the severity of disease. Patients may need to avoid lactose-containing foods during exacerbations, and high-fiber foods may produce symptoms and obstructions in children with intestinal strictures. Enteral formulas, given by mouth or by continuous nasogastric (NG) infusion, may be required to correct nutritional deficiencies and growth retardation when oral diet intake is insufficient.

Elemental formulas have been used to improve growth failure and significantly decrease disease activity in children with CD (Polk, Hattner, and Kerner 1992). Total parenteral nutrition (TPN) should be reserved for children with feeding intolerance produced by gastrointestinal (GI) symptoms or when obstructions or fistulas are present.

Corticosteroids are the most effective drugs for treating moderate to severe IBD. Generally, the steroid dose is decreased or discontinued as soon as possible to minimize side effects. The child must be observed closely during the steroid taper for recurrence of symptoms. Sulfasalazine is used in less severe cases and during remissions of IBD. Because this drug interferes with the absorption of folic acid, daily supplements are often prescribed. Side effects of sulfasalazine include allergic responses, headache, nausea, vomiting, neutropenia, and oligospermia. Sulfasalazine is a combination of 5-aminosalicylate and sulfapyridine. Because many of the side effects are primarily due to sulfapyridine, other nonabsorbable salicylate drugs without sulfapyridine, including olsalazine and mesalamine, may be used. Other immunosuppressive drugs, including 6-mercaptopurine, azathioprine, and cyclosporine A, have been used with success in selected populations. The major risk of these drugs is bone marrow suppression.

Surgery is indicated for UC when medical and nutritional therapies have failed. A total colectomy is considered curative. Surgical options include a total colectomy and ileostomy; or an ileoanal pull-through, which preserves the normal pathway for defecation. Crohn's disease respond poorly to surgery. Segmental intestinal resections are performed for small bowel obstructions or fistulas. Partial colonic resections are not curative in CD, because the disease often recurs.

Home care issues focus on the child's nutritional status, early recognition of gastrointestinal symptoms, ostomy care (if necessary), and psychological support. Refer to the nursing care plan presented in Appendix 8–A. Because of the chronic nature of this disease, many patients and families benefit from many of the services provided by organizations such as Crohn's and Colitis Foundation of America, Inc. (CCFA), and the United Ostomy Association.

Short Bowel Syndrome

Short bowel syndrome (SBS) exists when a patient has malabsorption as a result of a bowel resection. The etiology of the malabsorption is multifactorial including decreased mucosal surface area, bacterial overgrowth, bile acid deficiency, and dysmotility. The most common causes of SBS in children include congenital anomalies (jejunal and ileal atresia, gastroschisis), ischemia (necrotizing enterocolitis), trauma, or volvulus. Other causes include bowel resection due to long-segment Hirschsprung's disease, Crohn's disease, and omphalocele.

The prognosis for children with SBS has dramatically improved over the past 20 to 30 years, primarily from advances in parenteral and enteral feedings. Advances in TPN and long-term management have made it possible for children with under 15 cm of bowel, even in the absence of an ileocecal valve, to eventually become independent of TPN (Vanderhoof et al. 1992). The presence of the ileocecal valve improves the prognosis of patients with SBS. Its presence is important both for increasing transit time and for preventing colonic bacterial backwash into the small bowel. Patients still dependent on TPN four years after resection are unlikely to be weaned from TPN.

Medical Interventions

Nutritional support becomes the long-term focus of care for children with SBS. The management of SBS is a multistage process, beginning with TPN. During this initial phase, stabilization of fluids and electrolytes is a priority. The introduction of enteral feedings constitutes the second phase and is started as soon as fluid and electrolyte status has stabilized. Enteral feedings

are key in stimulating the adaptive response in the small intestine. The adaptation response is characterized by increased villus length and increased number of cells to gradually improve absorption of nutrients. Generally, a continuous infusion of elemental or semielemental formula via an NG or gastrostomy tube is recommended to maximize absorption. Small amounts of oral feedings should be started so that a child can learn to suck and swallow, and problems with oral hypersensitivity and food aversions can be avoided. As enteral feedings are gradually advanced, TPN can be decreased in terms of calories, fluids, and total hours of infusion per day. At this stage, plans should be made for discharge to home.

The final phase of nutritional support occurs when enteral feedings alone can maintain adequate growth and development. Risk of development of specific nutritional deficiencies are increatUd once TPN is discontinued. Malabsorption of fat-soluble vitamins and trace elements are common in SBS. Vitamin B_{12} and folate deficiencies often occur with ileal resection.

Management of SBS consists of treating or avoiding chronic complications such as nutritional deficiency states, bacterial overgrowth, diarrhea, TPN liver disease, and catheter-related problems. Although medical management is the primary treatment for SBS, additional surgery may be indicated. Intestinal lengthening, intestinal valve procedures to slow transit time, and intestinal tapering procedures for small bowel dilatation may be considered on an individual basis. Intestinal transplantation may be an effective treatment in the near future.

Home care issues focus on the child's nutritional and fluid and electrolyte status. Strong psychological support and reinforcement of patient and family teaching are paramount for successful home care. Refer to Appendix 8–B for the nursing care plan for SBS. Frequent rehospitalizations may be necessary, so ongoing communication between home care and hospital team members is essential. The Oley Foundation may be an excellent support for patients and families dealing with home TPN and total enteral nutrition (TEN).

Hirschsprung's Disease

Hirschsprung's disease is a congenital anomaly caused by the absence of nerve cells (ganglia) in the wall of the intestine. This results in mechanical obstruction from lack of peristalsis. The incidence is 1 in 5,000 live births. It is four times more common in males than females (Silverberg and Daum 1988; Whaley and Wong 1995). Hirschsprung's disease is associated with other anomalies, such as Down syndrome. It is limited to the rectum and sigmoid colon in 75 percent of cases, and only 8 percent of all cases involve the entire colon with or without the small bowel (Silverberg and Daum 1988; Walker et al. 1996).

Medical Interventions

Surgery is required for the vast majority of children with Hirschsprung's disease. Few can be managed medically with frequent enemas. Surgical treatment consists of primarily removing aganglionic bowel to relieve obstruction and allow the bowel to rest and resume normal caliber and tone. In most cases, this is accomplished in two stages. First, the aganglionic bowel is removed and a temporary ostomy is placed to relieve the obstruction. Usually, when the child weighs about 20 pounds, the second corrective surgery is planned. This pull-through procedure consists of "pulling" the end of functioning ganglionated bowel down through the muscular sleeve of the rectum. The colostomy is usually closed at this time.

Home care issues focus on the child's nutritional status and ostomy care. After colostomy closure, attention is focused on promotion of normal diet for age and bowel control. A minority of children are troubled with persistent constipation, encopresis, or persistent enterocolitis. Families should be made aware of the services of the American Pseudo-obstruction and Hirschsprung's Disease Society, Inc. (APHS) and the United Ostomy Association.

Biliary Atresia

Biliary atresia is characterized by destruction or absence of portions of the extrahepatic biliary system, which results in eventual ductal obstruction. The incidence of biliary atresia is between 1 in 10,000 and 1 in 25,000 live births (Whaley and Wong 1995). The exact etiology is unknown, although immune mechanisms or viral injury may be responsible. Untreated biliary atresia results in progressive cirrhosis and death in most children by two years of age.

Medical Interventions

The primary treatment of biliary atresia is a hepatic portoenterostomy (Kasai procedure), which involves forming a substitute duct from a segment of jejunum. Complications after the Kasai procedure include ascending cholangitis, cirrhosis, portal hypertension, and GI bleeding. Antibiotics are used prophylactically to minimize the risk of ascending cholangitis. Despite achievement of bile drainage in the majority of patients, many children will ultimately develop liver failure. Liver transplantation is the definitive treatment for biliary atresia.

Medical management of biliary atresia is mainly supportive. Nutritional support includes the use of high-calorie formulas containing medium-chain triglycerides that can be digested without bile (Pregestimil, Alimentum, and Portagen). The fat malabsorption due to the lack of bile requires supplementation of water-miscible forms of vitamins A, D, E, and K. Multivitamin and mineral supplements including iron, zinc, and selenium are usually required. Aggressive nutritional support using continuous tube feedings or TPN may be indicated with severe growth failure. Phenobarbital may be prescribed after the Kasai procedure to stimulate bile flow, and ursodeoxycholic acid may be used to decrease cholestasis and the intense pruritus from jaundice.

Home care issues include aggressive efforts to maintain nutritional status, early recognition of cholangitis, skin care measures to relieve pruritus, and psychological support. Constant attention to these details to optimize patients' health and growth increases their chances to survive long enough for a liver transplant. Families of children with liver disease can get support from the Children's Liver Foundation.

Gastroesophageal Reflux

Gastroesophageal reflux (GER) is defined as passive regurgitation or emesis. GER occurs occasionally in everyone, but 1 in 300 to 1 in 1,000 children have a significant or pathologic problem (Whaley and Wong 1995; Walker et al. 1996). GER most likely occurs during inappropriate relaxation of the lower esophageal sphincter. The exact cause is unknown. Clinical manifestations include poor weight gain, heme-positive emesis or stools, anemia, irritability or heartburn, gagging or choking with feedings, apnea, and recurrent pneumonia. GER is associated with asthma, cystic fibrosis, bronchopulmonary dysplasia, neurologic disorders, and children that undergo tracheoesophageal or esophageal atresia repairs.

Medical Interventions

Therapeutic management of GER depends on the severity and whether complications such as poor growth, esophagitis, or respiratory problems are present. For the majority of children with reflux, only conservative measures are indicated. Small, frequent feedings every two to three hours may decrease emesis. Occasionally, continuous NG feedings are indicated if severe emesis and growth failure are present. Thickened feedings and postprandial positioning in a prone position with the head elevated 30 degrees may be helpful.

Pharmacologic therapy is often used with more severe cases of GER. Antacids and/or histamine-receptor antagonists (H_2 blockers), such as cimetidine (Tagamet), ranitidine (Zantac), or famotidine (Pepcid), reduce the amount of stomach acid and may prevent esophagitis. Prokinetic medications that increase intestinal motility are also helpful in GER. Cisapride has fewer central

nervous system side effects compared to bethanechol (Urecholine) and metoclopramide (Reglan) and is the prokinetic drug of choice for GER. Surgical management is reserved for children with severe complications who have failed medical management. The surgery of choice is a Nissen fundoplication. The surgery involves a 360-degree wrap of the fundus of the stomach around the distal esophagus.

Home care issues include aggressive efforts to promote growth and the education of caregivers about medication administration, special feeding regimens, and, if necessary, postoperative care. Psychological support is often critical with this frustrating condition.

TEACHING ISSUES BEFORE DISCHARGE

Pediatric gastrointestinal disease affects children in all age groups. This wide age range requires the home care nurse to be knowledgeable about growth and development issues that arise from infancy through adolescence. The incorporation of each child's development needs in his or her individual nursing care plan is essential to provide a smooth transition into the home environment and optimize the child's recovery both medically and psychosocially.

The home care nurse also must be competent in nutrition and fluid and electrolyte assessment in this fragile population. Home care providers who work with these patients must be educated in parenteral and enteral nutrition, intravenous (IV) and enteral access devices, delivery systems, formula preparation, and potential complications with these therapies. In addition, the home care nurse must have a strong background in medication administration, postoperative care, and ostomy care. The proliferation of nutritional formulas, access devices, and infusion equipment makes it necessary for the home care nurse to maintain close communication with hospital personal and home care vendors to keep up to date with the many changes in therapy. Finally, the home care provider must be informed about the various resources in the community, the state, and available nationally that could be supportive to the patient and family.

NURSING CARE PLANS IN THE HOME

The goals in caring for the child with alterations in metabolic function are to (1) identify and promote developmental issues, (2) maintain optimal nutritional status, and (3) identify or prevent potential complications. The following discussion and the nursing care plans presented in Appendixes 8–A and 8–B will help the home care nurse develop individualized nursing care plans for home.

Nursing Considerations To Promote Understanding of Developmental Issues

The infant with a congenital anomaly or disability is at high risk for developmental delay due to prolonged hospitalization. The infant with gastrointestinal disease may be at risk for altered parental bonding due to the loss of the anticipated perfect infant, frequent separations during hospitalizations, and the need for parents to use alternative nutritional methods to nourish their child. Often, these infants have limited or no opportunities for oral feedings. The lack of oral stimulation during the critical period from 6 to 12 months of age can result in aversion to oral feedings. Pediatric nurses should be sensitive to the infant's need for early oral stimulation and the need for small tastes of formula and solids to avoid long-term feeding problems. When the infant is ready for home care, an assessment of the infant's developmental level and of parental bonding is required to determine if intervention is needed. Many of these high-risk infants can benefit from intensive home care services such as early intervention infant programs.

The toddler and preschool period centers around the child's increasing autonomy and his or her egocentric and magical thinking. These children often feel responsible for their illnesses or hospitalizations, so an accurate assessment of their understanding of the illness is critical. To maximize learning in children in this age group, events should be explained in terms of how they perceive it and frequent reinforcement that they are not responsible for the illness. It is always necessary to clarify and emphasize the concrete facts. This will lessen the powers of magical thinking and increase their sense of control. Their fear of body mutilation makes it essential that every invasive procedure should be explained carefully. Home care should include coordination with any preschool programs.

The school-age period is highlighted by children's increasing need for independence, peer relationships, and productivity. Hospitalization and chronic illness often lessen their feelings of power and control. Nurses who care for school-age children should allow them to make choices in their care whenever it is medically possible. The school-age child's increased reasoning ability and verbal expertise make teaching and planning for home care both challenging and rewarding. The child and family can be taught, using audiovisual aids, models, and written materials, to explain the altered anatomy, special diet requirements, and technology for care. Home care for this group should include close coordination with school administrators. The coordination should include preparation of the peer group and any special arrangements for administration of medications, feedings, ostomy, or emergency care. Mealtimes at home or school require special attention for children receiving special oral diets, tube feedings, or parenteral nutrition.

Adolescents are struggling for independence, control, and acceptance of their rapidly changing body image. Their ability to think abstractly, communicate well with others, and need for independence emphasizes the importance of including adolescents in decision making and teaching. They should participate in planning for their home care.

This could include the scheduling of tube feeding or TPN and diet modifications. The adolescent's primary concern with any treatment option will be its effect on body image and peer relationships. Psychological or social work needs should be identified before the discharge planning process. Adolescent support groups may be beneficial during hospitalization and at home. Sexuality is an issue that must be assessed and addressed on an individual basis.

Nursing Considerations To Promote Optimal Nutritional Status

Assessment of Nutritional Status

A nutritional assessment should be completed before the child's discharge home. It should include caloric and protein requirements, ideal body weight, and expected rate of growth. The home care nurse should know what the child needs to consume daily to promote weight gain. Specific volumes of formula should be provided for the infant and child requiring tube feedings. Sample menus with specific guidance related to the child's needs (especially for supplements) and preferences should be initiated when the child is discharged and continued throughout home care. Weight changes can be controlled by using the same scale, obtaining weights for infants who are not clothed, and always weighing before feeding and at the same time of day. Stoma bags should be empty before weighing. The infant's length and head circumference should be obtained on a monthly basis. A dietitian should be consulted if weight gain is not appropriate or if the family is having difficulty with food choices. Dietary requirements may change from those estimated at the time of discharge. Activity level, resolution of infection, and changes in corticosteroid dosing may all affect caloric and protein requirements.

Children with gastrointestinal disease should be assessed for physical signs and symptoms associated with nutrient deficiency. These children are prone to developing electrolyte, vitamin, and mineral deficiencies from inadequate intake, malabsorption, or excessive losses. The signs and symptoms listed in Table 8–1 are not usually apparent until there is significant nutrient deficiency. They should be brought to the attention of the physician as soon as they are identified.

Oral Alimentation

Oral alimentation is the preferred method of providing nutrition. Children with biliary atresia, gastroesophageal reflux, and Hirschsprung's disease can usually meet their growth requirements with adequate oral nutrition. Children with biliary atresia experience fat malabsorption and require a formula high in medium-chain triglycerides (MCT). Children or adolescents with IBD may require a lactose-free diet during mild exacerbations and a low-residue diet with intestinal strictures. Corticosteroid therapy, particularly during exacerabation, may make it difficult for patients to eat enough to meet their nutritional needs. Children with colostomies or ileostomies require attention to the mineral, electrolyte, and free water content of their formulas and/or oral diets to prevent sodium, magnesium, zinc, or potassium deficiencies. Tube feedings and/or parenteral nutrition are essential when nutritional requirements cannot be met orally. Either of these modalities can be delivered at night to avoid interference with normal activities.

Meeting nutritional requirements of children with gastrointestinal disease may require the use of both parenteral and enteral nutrition during exacerbation of their disease or when oral intake is inadequate. Delivery of parenteral or enteral nutrition requires that the parents and/or child perform all associated care in a meticulous and safe manner.

Enteral Formulas

There are a number of factors to be considered when selecting an enteral formula. They include the disease state, absorptive capacity of the intestine, age of the child, feeding tube diameter, placement, and cost. Enteral formulas are presented in Table 8–2. A wide selection of formulas is available based on the variation in formula requirements in different gastrointestinal disease processes, other medical conditions, and the child's individual requirements. Children with SBS may be on elemental or semielemental diets such as Pregestimil, Vivonex Pediatric, or

Table 8–1 Signs and Symptoms Suggestive of Nutritional Deficiencies

Clinical Signs	Suspect Nutrient	Supportive Objective Findings
EPITHELIAL		
Skin		
Xerosis, dry scaling	Essential fatty acids	Triene/tetraene ratio >0.4
Hyperkeratosis, plaques around hair follicles	Vitamin A	Decreased plasma retinol
Ecchymoses, petechiae	Vitamin K	Prolonged prothrombin time
	Vitamin C	Decreased serum ascorbic acid
Hair		
Easily plucked, dyspigmented, lackluster	Protein-calorie	Decreased total protein
		Decreased albumin
		Decreased transferrin
Nails		
Thin, spoon-shaped	Iron	Decreased serum iron
		Increased total iron-binding capacity (TIBC)
MUCOSAL		
Mouth, lips, and tongue	B vitamins	Decreased red blood cells (RBC)
Angular stomatitis (inflammation at corners of mouth)	B_2 (riboflavin)	glutathione reductase
		See above
Cheilosis (reddened lip with fissures at angles)	B_2	Decreased plasma pyridoxal phosphate
	B_6 (pyridoxine)	
		See above
Glossitis (inflammation of tongue)	B_6	See above
	B_2	Decreased plasma tryptophan/
	B_3 (niacin)	urinary N-methyl nicotinamide
		See above
Magenta tongue	B_2	See above
Edema of tongue, tongue fissures	B_3	
Gums		Decreased plasma ascorbic acid
Spongy, bleeding	Vitamin C	
OCULAR		
Pale conjunctiva secondary to anemia	Iron	See iron above
	Folic acid	Decreased serum folic acid, or decreased RBC folic acid
	Vitamin B_{12}	Decreased serum B_{12}
	Copper	Decreased serum copper
Bitot's spots (grayish, yellow, or white foamy spots on the whites of the eye)	Vitamin A	Decreased plasma retinol
Conjunctival or corneal xerosis, keratomalacia (softening of part or all of cornea)	Vitamin A	See Vitamin A above.

continues

Table 8–1 continued

Clinical Signs	Suspect Nutrient	Supportive Objective Findings
MUSCULOSKELETAL		
Craniotabes (Thinning of the inner table of the skull); palpable enlargement of costochondral junctions ("rachitic rosary"); thickening of wrists and ankles	Vitamin D	Bone films Decreased 25-OH-vit D Increased alkaline phosphatase Possible signs: decreased calcium, phosphorus
Scurvy (tenderness of extremities, hemorrhages under periosteum of long bones; enlargement of costochondral junction; cessation of osteogensis of long bones)	Vitamin C	Decreased serum ascorbic acid Long bone films
Skeletal lesions	Copper	Decreased serum copper Radiographic film changes similar to scurvy because copper is also essential for normal collagen formation
Muscle wasting prominence of body skeleton, poor muscle tone	Protein-calorie	Decreased serum proteins Decreased arm muscle circumference
GENERAL		
Edema	Protein	Decresed serum proteins
Pallor secondary to anemia	Vitamin E (in premature infants)	Decreased serum Vitamin E Increased peroxide hemolysis Evidence of hemolysis on blood smear
	Iron	Decreased serum iron, increased TIBC
	Folic acid	Decreased serum folic acid Macrocytosis on RBC smear
	Vitamin B_{12}	Decreased serum B_{12} Macrocytosis on RBC smear
	Copper	Decreased serum copper
INTERNAL SYSTEMS		
Nervous		
Mental confusion	Protein	Decreased protein, albumin, and transferrin
	Vitamin B_1 (thiamine)	Decreased RBC transketolase

continues

Table 8–1 continued

Clinical Signs	Suspect Nutrient	Supportive Objective Findings
Cardiovascular		
Beriberi (enlarged heart, congestive heart failure, tachycardia)	Vitamin B$_1$	Same as above
Tachycardia secondary to anemia	Iron Folic Acid Vitamin B$_{12}$ Copper Vitamin E (in premature infants)	See above
GASTROINTESTINAL		
Hepatomegaly	Protein-calorie	Decreased protein, albumin, and transferrin
GLANDULAR		
Thyroid enlargement	Iodine	Decreased serum iodine

Source: Reprinted with permission from J. A. Kerner, Jr., *Manual of Pediatric Parenteral Nutrition*, pp. 22–23, © 1983, John Wiley & Sons, Inc.

Peptamen Junior and then progress to an intact protein formula such as Pediasure or Kindercal. Children with biliary atresia require formula with a high percentage of fat as MCT Oil. Examples of these formulas include Portagen, Pregestimil, and Alimentum. Protein, carbohydrate, and fat modules may be used to increase the caloric and/or protein density of formulas (Table 8–2). Commercial formulas are recommended, especially for infants, because they provide a consistent nutrient profile and their low viscosity allows delivery through a small-bore tube. Home-prepared formulas can be delivered only via large-bore tube, and obtaining an optimal nutrient profile may be difficult. The use of noncommercial formulas is restricted to children with intact digestive and absorptive capabilities. GI complications associated with enteral feedings are listed in Exhibit 8–1.

Special formulas and supplements can be costly. If the formulas are not covered by insurance, the child may become eligible for the Women's, Infants', and Children's program (WIC). Many commercial companies are offering direct-purchase programs to reduce the cost to families. The recent development of generic formula products, if proven to be clinically equivalent, should decrease the cost to the consumer. Social workers may be helpful in locating additional funds from local organizations such as the Lions Club to purchase formula and/or enteral pump and supplies.

Tube Feeding Types and Routes

Nasogastric tubes are passed through the nose, down the esophagus, and into the stomach. The most common tubes are made of polyvinylchloride (PVC), polyurethane, or Silastic. The stiffer PVC tubes do not require a guide wire for insertion, but they will become brittle and sharp when subject to the low pH of the stomach. They should be changed every two to seven days. The softer tubes (polyurethane or Silastic), which require a guide wire for intuba-

Table 8–2 Enteral/Tube Feeding Formulas

Product Name	kcal/oz	Special Features/Comments
Infant formulas—Milk base		
Mature human milk	20	Normal infant feeding; low iron
Similac*	20/24	Normal infant feeding; 24 calories for fluid-sensitive infants.
Similac PM 60/40[†]	20	Infant formula with low electrolytes/mineral content including iron; indications renal conditions
Enfamil*	20/24	Normal infant feeding; 24 calories for fluid-sensitive infants
Infant formulas—Soy base		
Isomil[†]	20	Use for infants with cow milk protein and/or lactose intolerance.
Isomil SF[†]	20	Use for infants with cow milk protein, lactose, and/or sucrose intolerance; CHO is glucose polymers.
Isomil DF	20	Ready to feed; use for infants for short-term management of diarrhea; contains soy fiber; lactose free.
ProSobee[†]	20	Use for infants with cow milk protein, lactose, and/or sucrose intolerance; CHO is glucose polymers.
Specialized infant formulas		
Neocare[†]	22	Discharge formula for the premature infant up to 1 year of age; extra fortification of vitamins and minerals; easier to digest; contains 50% glucose polymers and 50% lactose; fat source is 50% MCT Oil.
Lactofree[†]	20	Lactose-free formula; protein source is cow's milk protein
Nutramigen[†]	20	Protein source is casein hydrolysate; hypoallergenic formula; lactose free; no MCT Oil.
Pregestimil[†]	20	Protein source is casein hydrolysate; CHO is lactose and sucrose free; fat source is 55% MCT Oil; hypoallergenic and malabsorption syndromes.
Alimentum	20	Ready to feed; protein source is casein hydrolysate; lactose free; fat source is 50% MCT Oil; hypoallergenic and malabsorption syndromes.
Portagen[†]	20	Protein source is cow's milk; low lactose; fat source is 88% MCT Oil; fat malabsorption syndromes.
Neocate[†]	20	Protein source is free amino acids; for infants with severe protein allergies.

continues

Table 8–2 continued

Product Name	kcal/oz	Special Features/Comments
Children's formulas (1–10 years)—Intact protein		
Whole cow's milk	20	Protein source is cow's milk; contains lactose; low in iron.
2 % milk	15.5	Protein source is cow's milk; contains lactose; lower in fat; low in iron.
Skim milk	11	Protein source is cow's milk; contains lactose; essentially no fat; low in iron.
Kindercal	30	Protein source is cow's milk; lactose free; fat source 20% MCT Oil; fortified with vitamins and minerals.
Nutren Junior	30	Protein source is cow's milk; lactose free; fat source is 25% MCT Oil; fortified with vitamins and minerals.
Pediasure	30	Protein source is cow's milk; lactose free; fat source is 20% MCT Oil; fortified with vitamins and minerals.
Children's formulas—Elemental/Semielemental		
Neocate 1+	30	Protein source is free amino acids; lactose free; fat source is 35% MCT; used for severe protein allergies and/or malabsorption.
Vivonex Pediatric	24	Protein source is free amino acids; lactose free; fat source is 68% MCT; used for severe protein allergies and/or malabsorption.
Peptamen Junior	30	Protein source is hydrolyzed whey; lactose free; fat source is 60% MCT; malabsorption syndromes.
Selected adult formulas—Oral supplements		
Ensure	30	Protein source is cow's milk; Ensure + is 45 cal/oz for fluid-restricted patients.
Sustacal	30	Protein source is cow's milk; Sustacal + is 45 cal/oz for fluid-restricted patients.
Resource	30	Protein source is cow's milk; Resource + is 45 cal/oz for fluid-restricted patients.
Carnation Instant Breakfast with whole milk	36	Protein source is cow's milk; contains lactose; high-caloric supplement.
Adult formulas—Standard tube feeding (intact protein)		
Isocal	30	Protein source is cow's milk; lactose free.
Osmolite	30	Protein source is cow's milk; lactose free.

Table 8–2 continued

Product Name	kcal/oz	Special Features/Comments
Magnacal Renal	60	Protein source is cow's milk; lactose free; calorically dense; for fluid-sensitive patients; low electrolyte and mineral content; used for renal conditions.
Jevity	30	Protein source is cow's milk; lactose free; contains soy fiber; some fat as MCT Oil.
Ultracal	30	Protein source is cow's milk; lactose free; contains soy/oat fiber; some fat as MCT Oil.
Adult formulas—Elemental/ semielemental		
Peptamen	30	Protein source is hydrolyzed whey; lactose free; fat source is 60% MCT; malabsorption syndromes.
Vital HN	30	Protein source is partially hydrolyzed whey and free animo acids; lactose free; low fat—9% of calories; used for fat malabsorption and impaired digestion.
Vivonex Plus	30	Protein source is free amino acids; lactose free; low fat—6% of calories; indications are for severe protein allergies, fat malabsorption, and impaired digestion
Criticare HN	30	Protein source is hydrolyzed casein; lactose free; low fat—4.5%; used for fat malabsorption and impaired digestion.
AlitraQ	30	Protein source is hydrolyzed whey and free amino acids; lactose free; low fat—13%; used for fat malabsorption and impaired digestion.
Modular products— Carbohydrates		
Polycose	23 cal/tbsp	CHO source is glucose polymers; add to liquids or solids to increase calories.
Moducal	30 cal/tbsp	CHO source is maltodextrins; add to liquids or solids to increase calories.
Modular products— Protein		
Promod	28 cal/scoop	Protein source is whey; 5 g of protein/scoop; protein supplement to increase protein and calories.
Propac	16 cal/tbsp	Protein source is whey; 3 g of protein/tbsp; indications same as Promod.

continues

Table 8–2 continued

Product Name	kcal/oz	Special Features/Comments
Modular products—Fat		
MCT Oil	7.6 cal/cc	Fat source is fractionated coconut oil; fat supplement to increase calories; used for fat malabsorption.
Microlipid	4.5 cal/cc	Fat source is safflower oil; used to increase calories.
Vegetable oil	8 cal/cc	Type of fat is dependent on source; inexpensive; used to increase calories.

Note: CHO, carbohydrate; MCT, medium-chain triglycerides.
*Both iron and low-iron formulations.
†Can be prepared to 24 cal/oz by adding less water to the liquid concentrate or powder.

tion, are recommended when the frequency of NG replacement is greater than one week.

Nasointestinal tubes are passed through the nose, down the esophagus, and into the duodenum or jejunum. They are appropriate if the child has poor gastric emptying, has difficulty with regurgitation, or is at high risk for aspiration of formula. Polyurethane or Silastic tubes are preferred for this route because they remain soft for long periods and are not likely to cause intestinal perforation.

Gastrostomy tubes are used in children who require gastric feeding for an extended period. A gastrostomy tube can be placed surgically or through a percutaneous endoscopy approach. The gastrostomy tube is held in place inside the stomach by either a balloon or mushroom-shaped valve. An outside securing mechanism is required to stop the gastrostomy tube from migrating into the stomach and causing a bowel obstruction. Gastrostomy tubes are typically made from either silicone or rubber.

The skin-level gastrostomy tube (gastrostomy button) is now available for children who require gastric feedings for extended periods. The advantage of the gastrostomy button is that it lies flat against the abdomen when it is not in use. The gastrostomy button usually replaces a standard gastrostomy once the fistulous tract is well established (after four to six weeks). A recent development by one manufacturer makes it pos-

sible to insert the button initially using the percutaneous endoscopy approach. The button consists of the following three parts: safety plug, shaft, and dome or balloon. The button has an antireflux valve that decreases the possibility of gastric contents refluxing out of the shaft and irritating the surrounding skin. The safety plug remains in place between feedings and eliminates the need for a clamp. Extension tubing is attached to the button to administer feedings and medications. The site should be observed closely for evidence of pressure necrosis. This can occur if the button is too small and must be closely monitored during periods of rapid weight gain.

A jejunostomy is the placement of a tube in the jejunum for feeding. It can be placed surgically or by using the percutaneous endoscopy technique. Jejunostomy tubes are placed when long-term intestinal feedings are needed. The indications for a jejunostomy are the same as those for a nasointestinal tube. The technique of placing a jejunal extension through a gastrostomy tube may be useful when aspiration of gastric feedings are a problem. General guidelines for gastrostomy and jejunostomy tube site care are presented in Exhibit 8–2.

Delivery Method

The common methods of delivering enteral formulas are continuous or intermittent (bolus)

Exhibit 8–1 Gastrointestinal Complications Associated with Enteral Nutrition and Tube Feeding

DIARRHEA

Diarrhea is commonly multifactorial and is often associated with medications and causes other than the formula. The true prevalence is unknown because of the variable definitions of diarrhea.

Common causes

- Medications—the following commonly cause diarrhea in tube-fed patients:
  –Antibiotics
  –Elixers containing sorbitol
  –Antacids containing magnesium
  –Magnesium oxide
  –Suspensions
   Phosphate solutions
   Potassium solutions
  –Laxatives
  –Medications with diarrhea as a side effect
- Infection (*Clostridium difficile*, cytomegalovirus)
- Malnutrition or prolonged bowel rest (due to decreased villi number and height)
- Hypoalbuminemia (due to edematous bowel and decreased absorptive surface)
- Fecal impaction
- Other disease states or consequences of treatment (for example, IBD, radiation enteritis)
- Formula intolerance (hypertonicity, high fat content, low residue or lack of fiber, rapid administration, or bacterial contamination if formula is contaminated with a GI pathogen)

Treatment

- Check for medications that may cause diarrhea.
- Check whether medication can be changed or route switch (for example, from elixir to suppository).
- Suggest sending stool for *C. difficile* (especially if patient is taking antibiotics) or other tests to rule out an infectious cause.
- Check for fecal impaction and suggest abdominal films.

- Administer antidiarrheals (loperamide hydrochloride [Imodium] or diphenoxylate hydrochloride and atropine [Lomotil] if an infectious cause is ruled out).
- Change to define diet or fiber-enriched formulas if malabsorption is suspected.

CONSTIPATION

Causes

- Inadequate hydration
- Long-term tube feedings without fiber
- Narcotics
- Chronic laxative abuse
- Impaction
- Obstruction

Treatment

- Assess normal stool pattern.
- Assess abdomen for distention and perform a digital examination for impaction.
- Consider a laxative or an enema.
- Ensure adequate hydration.
- Change to a fiber-enriched formula.

DELAYED GASTRIC EMPTYING

Risk factors

- Critical illness (atony may develop)
- Brittle diabetes (neuropathy slows gastric emptying)
- Head injury

Treatment

- Monitor for gastric distention (can measure abdominal girth).
- Monitor for gastric residuals every four to eight hours during continuous feedings or before each intermittent feeding.
- Suggest prokinetic agent (for example, metoclopramide, cisapride, or erythromycin) to increase gastric emptying.
- Slow feeding rate.
- Stop feedings if patient has continuing nausea or vomiting.

Note: IBD, inflammatory bowel disease; GI, gastrointestinal.

Source: Reprinted with permission from *Nutrition Support Nursing Curriculum*, 3rd edition, © 1996, American Society for Parenteral and Enteral Nutrition.

Exhibit 8–2 Gastrostomy/Jejunostomy Tube Site Care

Equipment

Soap and warm water
Washcloth and/or cotton tip applicators
Silver nitrate sticks (if needed)

Procedure

1. Wash hands.
2. Clean the tube site daily with a washcloth and/or cotton tip applicators and soap with warm water followed by warm-water rinse. Use a spiral pattern beginning next to stoma and working outward to skin around stoma.
3. Thoroughly pat dry.
4. Clean and dry outside of tube and any retention disks/rods present with soap and warm water followed by warm-water rinse.
5. For low-profile gastrostomies (buttons) or gastrostomy tubes with a retention rod or bolster, rotate 45 to 180 degrees once per day (check manufacturer's directions).
6. If hypertrophic granulation tissue is present, apply silver nitrate stick once per day to moist, reddened areas and allow to air dry.
7. Monitor the tube and site every day for breakage, signs of infection, or skin breakdown.

---

methods. The term intermittent feeding is more appropriate than bolus feeding because it indicates that all noncontinuous feedings should be given slowly. The gravity feeding method is used for intermittent feedings, using either a syringe or gravity feeding set.

Continuous delivery is required when enteral formula is delivered into the jejunum or duodenum or the child is intolerant of intermittent gastric feedings. An enteral pump is usually required when continuous feedings are necessary. Slow constant delivery of formula into the je-junum or duodenum is necessary to prevent "dumping syndrome" symptoms (for example, dizziness, tachycardia, diarrhea, and nausea). These symptoms result from the rapid movement of extracellular fluids into the bowel to dilute the hypertonic formula to an isotonic mixture. Circulating blood volume is decreased by this rapid fluid shift. Portable backpack pumps are available that allow continuous enteral pump feeding without severely limiting the child's activities when nocturnal cyclic feedings are not possible. (See Exhibit 8–3 for home delivery techniques.)

Total Parenteral Nutrition

TPN formulas are designed to meet individual requirements for calories, protein, vitamins, electrolytes, and minerals. Fat requirements are met through the use of lipid (fat) emulsions. The three-in-one delivery system that combines the TPN and lipid in one bag has become available for home use. Three-in-one solutions are not suitable for all patients. TPN solutions with high electrolyte and mineral content and certain amino acid preparation make these solutions unstable. Parenteral nutrition is usually provided in a cyclic fashion in the home setting. The child will generally receive the infusion over a 12- to 18-hour period at night. The cycle typically ends with a 1- to 2-hour taper period to prevent rebound hypoglycemia. The new ambulatory infusion pumps make it possible to program the child's TPN cycle and tapering period automatically. Suggested procedures for starting and discontinuing TPN are outlined in Exhibits 8–4 and 8–5.

These solutions are usually delivered to the home on a weekly to monthly schedule depending on the child's metabolic stability. Certain TPN additives have limited stability and must be added to the TPN daily. These may include multivitamins, vitamin K, iron, carnitine, and histamine-receptor antagonists (cimetidine, ranitidine, or famotidine). The TPN should be removed from the refrigerator about one-half hour before infusion, the additives should be added using strict aseptic technique, and the

Exhibit 8–3 Tube Feeding: Home Delivery Techniques

FORMULA AND DELIVERY SYSTEM

A. Formula Preparation

1. Labeling
   a. Check for match with your prescription. The same brand of formula may be available in different concentrations and with different additives.
   b. Check expiration date of formula.
2. Preparation and storage for formula requiring mixing
   a. Wash hands.
   b. Clean area and utensils and blender for mixing.
   c. Wipe top of container before opening.
   d. Measure exact amount of formula, liquid, and other additives. Mix well.
   e. Cover and refrigerate any unused formula. Use within 24 hours.
   f. Keep unmixed formula powder covered and in an airtight container.
3. Preparation of ready-mixed formula
   a. Wash hands.
   b. Rinse and wipe the top of the container.
   c. Shake formula before opening.
   d. Cover and refrigerate any unused formula.
   e. Ready-to-hang formula (formula in prefilled containers) should be labeled with date and time and used within 24 hours.

B. Tube Placement and Residual

1. Check for placement of tube.
   a. Wash hands.
   b. Before each feeding, place stethoscope below xiphoid process and instill 10 to 15 cc of air. For children weighing less than 10 kg, instill 1–2 cc of air. Listen for "whoosh" of air.
   c. Make tube with indelible ink marking or tape where it exits the nose or skin. If the mark disappears or comes out farther than ____*____ inches, the tube placement may need to be adjusted. Call your health care provider.
2. Check residual volumes before intermittent feedings or every 2 to 4 hours for continuous feedings.
   a. Residual volume ____*____mL or less, refeed.
   b. Residual volume ____*____mL or greater. May hold feeding. Refeed aspirate (if large amount of curdled formula or oral secretions, discard). Wait 30 to 60 minutes, then check residual again. If remains high, contact your health care provider.

C. Delivery of Formula

1. Equipment
   a. 60-cc catheter tip syringe
   b. Feeding bag and tubing
   c. Spike set (ready-to-hang formula)
   d. Pump
   e. Container for water
2. Wash hands.

continues

Exhibit 8–3 continued

  3. Place child in upright position; head should be raised 45 degrees or more.
  4. Intermittent drip feeding
   a. Connect syringe without plunger or feeding bag with filled tubing (to prevent excessive air into stomach) to clamped gastrostomy or nasogastric tube.
   b. Unclamp tube. Allow formula to flow into stomach by gravity over 20 to 60 minutes.
   c. Flush feeding tube with water, after completion of feeding and before and after administration of each medication.
   d. Rinse syringe/bag with water. Discard equipment every 24 hours.
  5. Continuous pump feeding
   a. Pour feeding into feeding bag for the enteral pump; make sure tubing is clamped. For RTF formula, completely pierce spike port on closed-system bottle with spike set. Close clamp on set before inverting the container.
   b. Clear air from tubing and connect to the feeding tube.
   c. Start enteral pump. Infuse formula at prescribed strength and rate.
   d. Discard feeding set and ready-to-hang bottle within 24 hours.
   e. Flush feeding tube with water at least every 4 hours, after feeding is complete, and before and after administration of each medication.
   f. Hang time is 4 to 8 hours at room temperature, except ready-to-hang formula, which is 24 hours.

*Contact your health care provider for specifics for each patient.

Note: RTF, ready-to-feed.

TPN solution should be mixed gently. Formula changes are usually required only to meet growth requirements or correct metabolic alterations.

Frequency of metabolic monitoring (weekly to monthly) is determined by the child's physiologic stability. Parents should be aware of possible metabolic alterations that might indicate the need for more frequent monitoring. Table 8–3 presents potential complications of home TPN.

There are several types of central venous catheters that are suitable for infusing home TPN. The most frequently used are the tunneled central venous catheters (Hickman or Broviac) (see Figure 8–1). This catheter is placed surgically and is tunneled under the skin before entering into the venous system. A Dacron cuff is positioned in the tunnel to permit the formation of fibrous adhesions around the cuff, thus reducing the risk of catheter dislodgement and decreasing the risk of infection from skin flora.

The Groshong catheter is also a tunneled central catheter. In addition to the previous description, it has two valves that are located adjacent to the closed distal tip of the catheter. The valves remain closed when the catheter is not in use. This eliminates the need for routine heparinization and reduces the risk of retrograde blood flow, air embolism, and catheter occlusion. This catheter is flushed with saline once a week when not in use.

Another option for infusion of home TPN is an implantable vascular access device (port) (Figure 8–2). It is a totally implantable vascular access device with a self-sealing infusion port that is attached to a Silastic catheter. It is designed to provide repeated IV access to the vascular system. The advantage of this catheter is that it is completely under the skin. This is an

Exhibit 8–4 Procedure for Starting TPN

Supplies

Alcohol swabs and/or povidone-iodine swabs

TPN bag (separate lipids if necessary)

Intravenous tubing(s)

Extension tubing (if needed)

Occluding or rubber-shod clamp (if not attached to catheter)

TPN additives, necessary syringes

Procedure

1. Remove TPN from refrigerator 30 minutes before infusion.
2. Examine solution for turbidity, precipitation, cloudiness.
3. Organize supplies.
4. Wash hands.
5. Wipe infusion port of TPN bag with 70% isopropyl alcohol swab.
6. Add vitamins and other necessary additives to TPN bag.
7. Check infusion pump(s) to make sure infusion program is correct (that is, proper volume, length of infusion, taper period).
8. Insert intravenous tubing (cassette) into TPN bag and fat emulsion (if necessary) and connect to intravenous pump(s).
9. Connect extension tubing if necessary.
10. Turn on pump and purge until all tubing is filled.
11. Place cap on intravenous tubing.
12. If needed, swab "Y" injection site closest to the patient's TPN line with povidone-iodine or alcohol swab. Insert lipid tubing into the "Y" insertion site.
13. Clamp catheter with occluding clamp.
14. Remove sterile cap on catheter.
15. Wipe hub with alcohol swab and attach intravenous tubing.
16. Release clamp.
17. Turn on pump. Check pump to make sure it is infusing properly.

Note: TPN, total parenteral nutrition.

Exhibit 8–5 Daily Discontinuation of TPN

Supplies

Heparin solution ____*____ units/mL

____*____ cc syringe

Needle or vial adapter (needleless system)

Occluding or rubber-shod clamp (if not attached to catheter)

70% isopropyl alcohol swab

Sterile catheter cap

Procedure

CATHETER MUST ALWAYS BE CLAMPED WHEN OPEN TO AIR.

1. Wash hands.
2. Wipe top of heparin solution with alcohol swab.
3. Check label on heparin solution vial; it should read heparin ____*____ units/mL.
4. Withdraw ____*____ mL of heparin solution into syringe.
5. Clamp catheter.
6. Turn off infusion pump(s).
7. Remove intravenous tubing from catheter.
8. Wipe catheter hub with alcohol swab.
9. Insert syringe into hub of catheter.
10. Release clamp.
11. Inject ____*____mL of heparin solution.
12. Clamp catheter while pushing in last 0.5 mL of heparin. This step is very important. You must push the heparin solution as you clamp the catheter.
13. Remove syringe; leave clamp on catheter.
14. Connect sterile catheter cap.
15. Tape catheter in comfortable position.

* Contact health care provider for specifics for each patient.

Note: TPN, total parenteral nutrition.

Table 8–3 Metabolic Complications of Home Parenteral Nutrition

Problems	Signs and Symptoms	Intervention	Prevention
Hyperglycemia (high blood sugar) is a complication of parenteral nutrition caused by too much glucose (sugar), in your blood. Because your parenteral nutrition has a high concentration of glucose, hyperglycemia can occur if your parenteral infusion is infused too rapidly, or if your pancreas does not produce enough insulin to prevent hyperglycemia.	Glucose (sugar) in your urine Feeling thirsty Increased urine output Increase in the number of times you urinate Feeling confused, uneasy, or woozy Feeling tired Feeling your heart pound in your chest	Call your health care provider and report your symptoms. Check your urine for sugar. Call your home care nurse if your pump is not working correctly.	Check your urine as directed for sugar. Check your pump during your infusion to make sure it is functioning properly. Follow up on all of your scheduled health care and laboratory appointments.
Hypoglycemia (low blood sugar) is a complication of parenteral nutrition caused by not enough glucose (sugar) in your blood. Because your parenteral nutrition has a high concentration of glucose, hypoglycemia can occur if your parenteral infusion is suddenly stopped. The tapering-off period during your parenteral nutrition infusion slowly lowers your blood glucose (sugar) levels. This gives your pancreas time to decrease insulin production and help prevent hypoglycemia. Longer tapering periods may be necessary for patients taking insulin or oral hypoglycemics.	Weakness Trembling Sweating/diaphoresis Headaches Chills Hunger Feeling nervous Blurred vision Nausea Feeling your "heart pound" Decreased levels of consciousness	Drink or eat something that is high in sugar, such as orange juice, hard candy, or tea with sugar, if allowed. Call your health care provider and report your symptoms. Call your home care nurse if your pump is not working correctly. If instructed, prepare to set up an infusion of dextrose 10 percent.	Infuse your TPN as scheduled. Keep your catheter and tubing free of kinks. Check pump during your infusion to make sure that it is functioning properly. Follow up on all of your scheduled health care and laboratory appointments.

continues

Table 8–3 continued

Problems	Signs and Symptoms	Intervention	Prevention
Dehydration can occur when your body does not receive enough fluids or when your body output increases (such as diarrhea, vomiting, etc.).	Feeling thirsty Tired, weak Dry tongue and mouth Decreased urine output Dizziness/light-headedness	Call your health care provider to report symptoms.	Report any diarrhea or vomiting. Take antinausea medication as directed. Take antidiarrhea medications as directed. Keep accurate intake and output records. Weigh yourself at the same time of day.
Fluid overload can occur if you receive too much fluid into your circulatory system (blood) or if fluid is infused too rapidly.	Edema (swelling) especially in face, eyes, hands, and feet Difficulty breathing and/or shortness of breath Cough	Call your emergency squad or 911 if you need immediate attention. Call your health care provider immediately and report your symptoms.	Notify your health care provider if you notice any swelling in your extremities or weight gain. Keep accurate intake and output records and review any changes with your health care provider. Weigh yourself at the same time of the day.
Electrolyte imbalances can occur if there is a change in your physical condition. Electrolyte imbances are difficult to pinpoint so call if you feel "different" or "unusual."	Cramps and muscle weakness Feeling tired Twitching Thirst Confusion	Call your health care provider and report your symptoms. Call your health care provider if you experience an increase in output, such as diarrhea or vomiting.	Infuse your TPN as directed. Follow up on all of your scheduled health care and laboratory appointments. Keep accurate input and output records and review any changes with your health care provider.

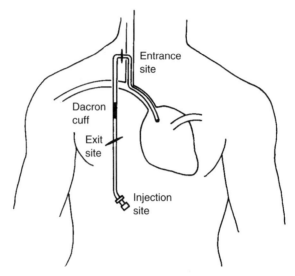

Figure 8–1 Tunneled central venous catheter.

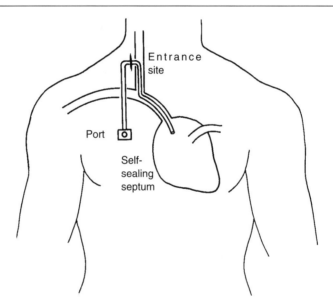

Figure 8–2 Implanted infusion port catheter.

important consideration for adolescents who want to limit their differences from their peers. The disadvantage is that it requires a needle puncture to access the system. A huber point needle is used to prevent coring of the self-sealing system.

The addition of the peripherally inserted central catheter (PICC) is an excellent option for children

Exhibit 8–6 Central Catheter Dressing Procedure

Supplies
  Nonsterile gloves
  Dressing change kit

Directions
1. Clean your workspace. Gather your supplies. Wash your hands.
2. Put on the mask or avoid speaking or coughing over the exit site.
3. Open the supplies using aseptic technique.
4. Put on nonsterile gloves and remove your old dressing. Avoid touching the catheter exit site.
5. Observe the exit site for the following:
   • redness
   • swelling
   • drainage
   • tenderness
6. Put on the sterile gloves.
7. Clean the catheter exit site with three hydrogen peroxide swabsticks. Use a circular motion, moving away from the catheter. Allow to dry.
8. Repeat the cleaning with the three povidone-iodine swabsticks. Allow to dry.
9. Squeeze a small amount of the antiseptic ointment onto exit site (omit this step as directed).
10. Cushion the catheter with gauze pads (omit this step as directed).
11. Apply the transparent dressing, touching only the nonsticky side. (You may want to remove the protective paper in the middle to make a window.) Do not stretch. Remove the paper border.
12. Secure the edges of the dressing with tape, as needed.
13. Tape the extra catheter tubing securely to your dressing or chest.

who require home TPN for a limited period (less than two months). This catheter is a long cut-to-fit intravenous catheter made of soft flexible material (silicone or soft polymers), which is inserted in one of the superficial veins of the peripheral vascular system and terminates in a deep peripheral or central vein (axillary or superior vena cava). This catheter does not require a surgical procedure, but is more cumbersome because it is inserted in the arm. A stretch gauze or spandex net dressing is necessary to protect and secure the line when the child is involved in strenuous activities, and the child should not lift more than 10 pounds with the catheter in place. It also requires more frequent flushes because of the narrow diameter of the lumen.

Strict aseptic technique is required to prevent catheter-related infections. Handwashing is critical before any care associated with the catheter. These catheters need sterile dressing changes from every day to biweekly depending on the child's immune status, newness of the catheter, and proximity of ostomy, fistulas, or wounds. The dressing should always be changed immediately if it becomes wet or soiled and after bathing or swimming. Extreme care must be taken for children who have an ostomy in addition to a central line to prevent cross contamination. See Exhibit 8–6 for a suggested dressing procedure for a central catheter.

The central line catheter must be heparinized (except the Groshong catheter) when not in use for continuous infusion. Correct flushing procedure for the central line catheter is critical to prevent occlusion. These catheters are made of Silastic or polymers, and the softness of this material allows blood to be aspirated into the lumen if it is clamped without continuing a gentle forward injection of a heparin solution (Exhibit 8–7).

It is important that the young child or infant be prevented from having direct access to the catheter. The child or infant should always wear clothing that minimizes access to the catheter. The catheter should be securely taped to avoid dislodgement. A clamp should be either attached to the catheter or available at all times. Caregivers should be aware that if a problem develops the catheter can easily be occluded by

Exhibit 8-7 Heparinization of Central Venous Catheter

Flushing Requirements:

1. If the child is receiving a continuous infusion into the catheter, no flush is required.
2. If the child is receiving an intermittent infusion (cyclic total parenteral nutrition, antibiotics), the catheter should be flushed with heparinized saline (dilution and volume as ordered by physician), at the conclusion of the infusion (except for Groshong tunneled central venous catheter—flush with 5 cc of saline).
3. If the child is not receiving any infusion through the catheter, the catheter must be flushed daily with heparinized saline (except for peripherally inserted central catheter (PICC)—flush every eight hours; Groshong tunneled central venous catheter—flush once a week with 5 cc saline; and implantable vascular access device (port)—flush every four weeks with heparinized saline).

Supplies:

Heparinized saline
Syringe
Needle or vial adapter (needleless system)
Occluding or rubber-shod clamp (if not attached to catheter)
70% isopropyl alcohol swab
Sterile catheter cap

Directions:

1. Wash hands thoroughly.
2. Draw up __*__ mL of heparinized saline using sterile technique.
3. Clamp the catheter.
4. Wipe catheter hub with alcohol swab.
5. Insert syringe into hub of catheter.
6. Inject __*__ mL of heparin solution.
7. Clamp the catheter while instilling the last 0.5 mL of heparinized saline. This creates positive pressure, which will prevent the backflow of blood into the tip of the catheter.
8. Connect sterile catheter cap.
9. Tape catheter in a comfortable position for the patient.

*Contact health care provider for specifics for each patient.

bending it rather than searching for a missing clamp.

Nursing Considerations for Identifying and Preventing Complications

Mechanical Complications—Enteral Nutrition

Mechanical complications associated with enteral nutrition are influenced by the size and position of the feeding tube. The use of soft small-bore nasogastric or nasointestinal feeding tubes has decreased the incidence of many mechanical problems associated with stiff wide-bore tubes. Fortunately, esophagitis, esophageal erosions and ulcers, nasal erosions and abscesses, nasopharyngeal discomfort, sinusitis, and hoarseness are rare with the fine-bore soft tube.

Tube migration is one of the most serious problems associated with small-bore feeding tubes. Tube misplacement is a result of deviation from the normal pathway, either by perforation of the esophagus or by misdirection into the larynx and bronchi. In conscious and alert patients, correct tube positioning can be assessed by aspirating gastric contents and auscultation. See Exhibit 8–3 for a description of these procedures. Nasogastric feeding tubes can be replaced at home if the caregivers have been properly trained in placement procedure. Nasointestinal tube replacement needs to be done in a hospital or clinic setting and needs radiologic verification to confirm placement. Radiologic verification needs to be done whenever there is doubt about proper feeding tube position.

Migration and catheter dislodgement can occur with gastrostomy or jejunostomy tubes. These can occur when the tubes are not adequately secured or with increased traction on the tube. Gastrostomies and jejunostomies should be marked with indelible ink or tape where they exit the skin to monitor for movement. External bolsters on gastrostomy tubes and sutures for jejunostomy tubes should be secure to prevent inward migration. Catheter dislodgement can occur with excessive tension on the tube or rupture of the balloon with certain types of gastrostomies. Gastrostomy tube migration inward can cause gastric outlet obstruction, which will result in poor gastric emptying and vomiting. Partial dislodgement of a gastrostomy or jejunostomy tube may result in inadvertent infusion of enteral feeding into the peritoneal cavity or subcutaneous tissues. Families should have a replacement tube at home that can be inserted into the stoma to prevent closure, in the case of tube dislodgement.

Unfortunately, occlusion of feeding tubes is a common problem. It is often related to inadequate flushing with feeding and medication administration, viscosity of the formula, and the size of the feeding tube. Prevention is the key to avoid this complication. The importance of flushing before and after each medication and the use of liquid or finely crushed tablets will decrease the incidence of clogging. Administration of water flushes after each intermittent feeding or every four hours with continuous feeding

is essential to lessen plugging. Avoiding use of viscous formulas with small-bore tubes will help prevent this problem. When obstruction of a feeding tube occurs, flushing the tube with warm water or trying to aspirate the clot may be helpful. A solution of meat tenderizer and warm water or Viokase powder and sodium bicarbonate tablet may dissolve the clot if it is from protein. A large syringe (greater than 30 mL) should be used to avoid excessive pressure and rupture of the feeding tube.

Mechanical Complications—TPN

The most common mechanical complications with TPN are related to the central line. Occlusion and/or catheter rupture of the central line can be prevented with correct flushing procedures. The family or caregivers should be instructed to call their health care providers immediately if the central line catheter becomes obstructed. The child will need to be taken to the hospital to have urokinase placed to dissolve the clot in the catheter. The effectiveness of the urokinase is diminished by the length of time the catheter remains obstructed.

Venous thrombosis is associated with long-term catheter placement. The cause is the development of fibrin and a sheath around the catheter. The increasing size of the thrombosis will obstruct the blood flow in the vein. The patient will experience swelling in the neck, chest, and arm on the same side the central catheter is placed. The physician should be notified immediately. The usual treatment of a venous thrombosis is catheter removal and short-term anticoagulation therapy. See Table 8–4 for complications of central venous catheters.

Metabolic Complications—TPN

Metabolic complications reported with home TPN are presented in Table 8–3. These metabolic complications may occur with either parenteral or enteral nutrition. The increased frequency of complications can occur with the addition or deletion of certain medications such as steroids, insulin, hypoglycemic agents, diuretics, and beta$_2$ blockers. Fluid assessments need

Table 8–4 Complications of Central Venous Catheters

Mechanical Complications

Problems	Cause	Action	Prevention
Blood backing up in the catheter	Connections are loose.	Clamp the catheter. Tighten connections. Repeat heparin flush.	Tighten cap or tubing connections. Tape all connections securely.
Resistance is felt when irrigating the catheter. A slow flow rate is noted during infusion. The pump alarms for no apparent reason.	Blood is clotted inside the catheter. The catheter is not properly heparin-ized. The solution is not infusing well.	DO NOT FORCE. Clamp the catheter. Call your health care provider.	Heparin-flush the catheter after each infusion. Maintain the infusion rate as ordered.
Crack in the catheter material; tear in the catheter material	Frequent manipula-tion of the catheter; use of unpadded tooth forceps. Leave the clamp on the catheter while trying to infuse.	DO NOT INFUSE. Immediately clamp your catheter between the crack and the exit site. Call your health care provider.	
Cough, shortness of breath, chest pain, loss of conscious-ness	Air has entered the circulatory system (air embolism).	Clamp your catheter. Call your physician or 911. Lie on your left side with your head lower than your feet.	Tape all connections securely. Always clamp the catheter before changing cap or intravenous tubing. Make sure all air is removed from intravenous tubing and syringes.
Tenderness, pain, or swelling in the neck or collarbone region; pain or swelling in the arm on the side where the catheter is placed; sluggish infusion flow	Vein irritation due to the presence of the catheter (venous thrombosis). The tip of the catheter may have flipped up toward the neck region.	Call your physician. Do not infuse until instructed to do so. The catheter may need to be replaced.	Flush catheter as directed.

continues

Table 8–4 continued

Infectious Complications

Problems	Cause	Action	Prevention
Drainage from the catheter exit site	Tension on the catheter. An early sign of infection.	Change the dressing more frequently to observe the site. Tape the catheter loop to the top of your dressing. Call your health care provider.	Tape the catheter loop to the top of the dressing. Clean the exit site as instructed.
Redness, swelling, or drainage at the catheter exit site. A temperature of greater than 100°F. Chills, sweating, fatigue, a positive urine test for sugar.	Signs of infection.	Write down your symptoms. Call your health care provider.	Always use aseptic technique when handling supplies and equipment.

to be monitored closely with children who are on only tube feeding or TPN for hydration. Close attention must be paid to children with increased ostomy or diarrhea losses, increased fluid losses during summer, and hypertonic formulas. Fluid overload can occur with excessive use of hypotonic or dilute formulas in cardiac and renal disease.

Managed care is moving more medical management to the outpatient arena. Many complications such as refeeding syndrome that were once seen only in the hospital can now occur at home. Refeeding syndrome can occur when a severely malnourished patient starts to receive feedings. It can occur within 1 to 10 days after feeding initiation. The signs and symptoms, as well as interventions, are included in Exhibit 8–8.

Infectious Complications—Enteral Nutrition

Contaminated formulas and aspiration pneumonia are the infectious complications most often associated with enteral feedings. The incidence of contaminated formula can be decreased by use of "ready-to-hang" formulas, commercially prepared formulas, and careful preparation technique when formula mixing is necessary. Good handwashing is essential when making formula and handling the delivery set. Opened cans and reconstituted formula can be refrigerated for 24 hours; formula hang time at room temperature is for approximately 4 to 8 hours, but the manufacturer's guidelines should be followed. Ready-to-hang formula can be safely infused over 24 hours. The home care nurse is in the best position to evaluate the family's ability to maintain the clean environment, techniques, and equipment necessary to prevent formula contamination

The child's potential risk factors for aspiration should be identified. They can include decreased cough or gag reflex, decreased gastric emptying, chronic gastric reflux, and tracheostomy. Children with potential risk factors should be monitored closely for signs and symptoms of aspiration. Signs and symptoms include tachypnea, tachycardia, fever, hypoxemia, cy-

Exhibit 8–8 Refeeding Syndrome

Refeeding syndrome can occur when feeding is initiated in a severely malnourished patient. Most notably, patients are at high risk of development of hypophosphatemia, hypokalemia, hypomagnesemia, altered glucose metabolism, and thiamine deficiency.

- **Hypophosphatemia:** One of the most life-threatening metabolic complications, hypophosphatemia is caused by depletion of total body phosphorus during starvation and increased cellular influx during refeeding. It can occur within 1 to 3 days after feedings are initiated and could occur up to 5 to 10 days after feedings are begun.
  - Signs and symptoms include the following: arrhythmias, congestive heart failure, sudden death, confusion, lethargy, paresthesia, seizures, weakness, acute respiratory failure, thrombocytopenia, hemorrhage, and white cell dysfunction.
- **Hypokalemia:** During starvation, serum potassium levels are usually maintained, even though total body potassium may be depleted. Upon refeeding, influx of potassium into newly formed cells occurs, and serum levels drop precipitously.
  - Signs and symptoms include the following: arrhythmias, cardiac arrest, inverted or flattened T waves, constipation, paralytic ileus, glucose intolerance, paresthesia, respiratory depression, weakness, paralysis, polyuria, and polydipsia.
- **Hypomagnesemia:** With refeeding, influx of magnesium occurs intracellularly, decreasing serum levels.
  - Signs and symptoms include the following: arrhythmias, torsades de pointes, anorexia, abdominal pain, mental confusion, seizures, tetany, weakness, paresthesia, and hyporeflexia.
- **Altered glucose metabolism:** During refeeding, the stimulus for gluconeogenesis in the previously starved patient is lost, which causes glucose intolerance. Overzealous use of glucose during refeeding can cause severe hyperglycemia and even lead to hyperosmolar nonketotic coma if not recognized early.
  - Signs and symtoms include the following: hyperglycemia, diuresis, thirst, altered mental status.
- **Thiamine deficiency:** Thiamine is an important coenzyme in carbohydrate metabolism, and it is theorized that refeeding carbohydrates to a severely malnourished patient may elicit symptoms of thiamine deficiency. Severe malnutrition results in baseline thiamine deficiency.
  - Signs and symptoms include the following: mental confusion, ataxia, muscle weakness, tachycardia, cardiomegaly, and coma.

INTERVENTIONS FOR REFEEDING

- Identify patients whose conditions make them most prone to development of the refeeding syndrome (those with chronic alcoholism, cancer cachexia, anorexia nervosa, marasmus, kwashiorkor, morbid obesity with massive weight loss, and prolonged fasting or prolonged intravenous hydration).
- Calculate calorie and protein requirements based on actual weight: it is suggested that feedings not be initiated at more than 1.2 times basal energy expenditure and that they be increased slowly over a period of five to seven days.
- Correct any electrolyte imbalances (that is, with intravenous supplementation) if possible, before beginning enteral nutrition, and monitor electrolyte (particularly phophorus, magnesium, and glucose) daily until stable.
- Monitor physiologic parameters for signs or symptoms of electrolyte disturbances (cardiac, respiratory, neuromuscular, and hematologic status and urinary output).

Source: Reprinted with permission from *Nutrition Support Nursing Curriculum*, 3rd Edition, © 1996, American Society for Parenteral and Enteral Nutrition.

anosis, wheezing and rales, and obvious stomach contents in pulmonary secretions or oropharynx. Preventive measures include administering postpyloric feedings to children at risk; monitoring for gastric distention, increased gastric residuals and/or gastrointestinal distress; and elevating the head of the bed 30 degrees to minimize reflux.

Local infection may occur at the gastrostomy or jejunostomy site if not kept clean and dry or if there is continuous drainage. Proper daily cleaning of the site and cauterization of granulation tissue with silver nitrate sticks when needed will prevent these complications (Exhibit 8–2). Irritation at the tube exit site can be relieved by use of a stoma wafer or other skin barriers, topical application of antacids, cholestyramine, and/or antibiotic ointments.

Infectious Complications—TPN

Infectious complications associated with TPN are related to the delivery system or the central line catheter. Proper handwashing technique is critical when dealing with solutions, tubing, catheter, and skin care.

Exhibit 8–6 reviews the central line dressing procedure and Table 8–4 presents signs and symptoms of catheter infections.

Medications

Medications used most commonly in children with gastrointestinal disease are discussed under the appropriate heading. Certain drugs can potentially affect the metabolic balance of a child on TPN or tube feedings. These medications are reviewed in the section, Metabolic Complications, in this chapter. Extreme care is necessary when administering medications via a feeding tube. Potential difficulties that may be encountered include altered absorption of the drug, gastrointestinal problems (for example, irritation and nausea), and clogging of the feeding tube with medication fragments. It is important to pay attention to whether the medication must be given only when a patient has an "empty stomach," especially with a child receiving continu-

ous feedings. Certain medications are incompatible with formulas such as most syrups (for example, cough syrups and cold preparations) because of their acidity and some antipsychotics (for example, chlorpromazine and thioridazine). Many medications are incompatible with each other; it is important not to combine medications and to flush with water between each medication administration. Medications that are hypertonic or are gastric irritants (for example, potassium chloride or sodium chloride) require dilution before administration. Common drugs that cause diarrhea in tube-fed patients are presented in Exhibit 8–1. With continuous feeding, higher doses of certain drugs (phenytoin, theophylline, and warfarin) may be necessary because of drug-nutrient interaction, unless feedings are withheld for one hour before and after drug administration. Time-released medication and sublingual or buccal tablets should not be crushed or given via a feeding tube. Medications that should not be given by a gastric feeding tube include enteric-coated pancreatic enzymes or medications that are acid labile and will be degraded by gastric acids. Consultation with a pharmacist is necessary when administering medications via a nasointestinal tube to ensure absorption or if any questions regarding drug-nutrient or drug-drug interactions exist.

Ostomy Care

The home care nurse should be familiar with and follow the ostomy care procedures taught to the parents and/or child during hospitalization. The enterostomal therapist should be consulted if there is difficulty with appliance fit, maintenance, or skin care.

Care of the colostomy and ileostomy sites is similar, with protection of the skin and prevention of dehydration being the primary requirements for nursing intervention. The infant or young child with a colostomy may not require an appliance; a small gauze pad kept in place by a diaper may be sufficient. The caustic nature and volume of an ileostomy requires the stoma to be bagged to prevent skin breakdown. An ostomy appliance should remain in place for at least 24 hours to decrease or prevent skin irritation. The stoma site should be cleansed well and dried, and then a skin preparation should be applied. A karaya product and/or stoma adhesive is then placed to prevent skin breakdown and promote adherence of the appliance. The correct size appliance is then secured.

REFERENCES

Barness, L.A., ed. 1993. *Pediatric nutrition handbook, American Academy of Pediatrics.* 3d ed. Elk Grove, IL: American Academy of Pediatrics.

Polk, D.B., J.A. Hattner, and J.A. Kerner. 1992. Improved growth and disease activity after intermittent administration of a defined formula diet in children with Crohn's disease. *Journal of Parenteral and Enteral Nutrition* 16:499–504.

Silverberg, M., and F. Daum, eds. 1988. *Textbook of pediatric gastroenterology.* 2d ed. Chicago: Year Book Medical Publishers, Inc.

Vanderhoof, J.A., et al. 1992. Short bowel syndrome. *Journal of Pediatric Gastroenterology and Nutrition* 14:359–70.

Whaley, L., and D. Wong, ed. 1995. *Whaley & Wong's nursing care of infant and children.* 5th ed. St. Louis, MO: Mosby.

Walker, W.A., et al., eds. 1996. *Pediatric gastrointestinal disease.* 2d ed. New York: Mosby–Year Book.

Nursing Care Plan for a Child with Inflammatory Bowel Disease

Nursing Diagnosis	Expected Outcomes	Nursing Interventions
1. Altered nutrition: less than body requirement related to poor oral intake, diarrhea	Patient demonstrates appropriate weight gain for age	Assessment/intervention • Nutritional consultation should be provided by referring facility. • Weigh daily to weekly per health care provider. • Check length every three months. Instruction • Instruct family in high-calorie and protein diet. • Instruct family in recording intake and output and adverse dietary reactions. • Instruct parents in procedure(s) for home enteral feedings or TPN if oral intake is inadequate. Evaluation • Evaluate growth progress by plotting length and height on standardized growth chart. • Evaluate nutritional regimen by reviewing intake and output (I & O) and adverse dietary reactions. • Evaluate family's response to teaching.
2. Potential for diarrhea related to exacerbation of disease	Patient demonstrates regularity in bowel pattern.	Assessment/intervention • Assess volume, type, frequency, color, and guaiac for each stool.

Nursing Diagnosis	*Expected Outcomes*	*Nursing Interventions*
		Instruction • Instruct family to recognize bowel pattern changes and abdominal pain or cramping and report to health care provider. Evaluation • Evaluate the effects of medication and dietary changes on bowel patterns.
3. Alteration in skin integrity related to presence of diarrhea, stoma	Patient demonstrates no erythema, rashes, edema, or tenderness at stoma or perianal area.	Assessment/intervention • Assess skin condition daily; record and report erythema, rashes, edema, and tenderness. • Expose erythematous area to air two to four times a day. • Treat rashes or skin breakdown with ointments or creams as prescribed by health care provider. Instruction • Instruct family in skin care measures. Evaluation • Evaluate response to skin care therapy.
4. Impaired growth and development related to the following: • poor growth • frequent exacerbation of disease • chronic disease • frequent absences from school and rehospitalizations	Patient progresses through developmental phases at appropriate pace.	Assessment/intervention • Use consistent schedule to meet the child's need for food, hygiene care, and rest. • Assess child's developmental level and, if necessary, involve child in early intervention program with necessary support services. Instruction • Instruct family in appropriate developmental milestones and ways to encourage child's developmental progress. Evaluation • Evaluate child's progress through developmental phases and redesign interventions as necessary.

Nursing Diagnosis	Expected Outcomes	Nursing Interventions
5. Knowledge deficit related to the following: • pathophysiology of disease • treatment of disease • special nutritional regimens • ostomy care (if needed)	Family and patient verbalize and demonstrate understanding of disease process, treatment regimen, specialized nutritional therapy, and ostomy care (if needed).	Assessment/intervention • Assess family's readiness to learn. • Use age-appropriate educational materials. • Encourage parent and child to keep a written log of questions and concerns. Instruction • Provide accurate information to patient and family at a rate appropriate to promote learning. • Reinforce teaching frequently, allowing ample time for questions. • Instruct family about the pathophysiology of disease, treatment, special nutritional regimens, and ostomy care (if needed). Evaluation • Frequently evaluate learning by return demonstrations, home visits, and follow-up with health care providers.
6. Coping: ineffective patient and family coping related to the following: • chronicity of illness • ever-present fear of onset of acute symptoms	Patient and family demonstrate decreased anxiety and stress. Patient and family develop a trusting relationship with health care providers. Patient and family demonstrate increased ability to care for child and increased involvement in health care plan. Patient and family use healthy, appropriate coping mechanism.	Assessment/intervention • Assess coping mechanism and encourage use of appropriate coping mechanism. • Involve patient and family in care planning and home care routines. • Allow family the opportunity to verbalize stresses, frustrations, fears, and fatigue. • Encourage involvement with support groups, social workers, family counselors, respite care, etc., as available and appropriate. Instruction • Instruct family in alternative strategies for ineffective coping mechanism. Evaluation • Evaluate coping mechanism and the family's ability to care for the patient and become involved in the health care plan.

Nursing Care Plan for a Child with Short Bowel Syndrome

Nursing Diagnosis	Expected Outcome	Nursing Interventions
1. Altered nutrition: less than body requirement related to increased loss from diarrhea, malabsorption	Patient demonstrates appropriate weight gain for age.	Assessment/evaluation • Nutritional consultation should be provided by referring facility. • Weigh daily to weekly per health care provider. • Check length every three months. Instruction • Instruct family in appropriate oral diet. • Instruct family in recording intake and output and any adverse dietary reactions. • Instruct family in procedures for home enteral feedings or total parenteral nutrition (TPN) as prescribed. Evaluation • Evaluate growth progress by plotting length and height on standardized growth chart. • Evaluate nutritional regimen by reviewing intake and output (I & O) and adverse dietary reactions. • Evaluate family's response to teaching.

Nursing Diagnosis	*Expected Outcomes*	*Nursing Interventions*
2. Potential fluid volume deficit related to the following: • liquid stools • intolerance of increased enteral feedings • insufficient free water	Child will maintain good hydration status.	Assessment/intervention • Assess for the following signs of dehydration: sudden weight loss, decreased skin turgor, dry mucous membranes, decreased urine output. • Document input and output including liquid stool. Instruction • Instruct family to accurately measure and document I & O. • Instruct family in the signs and symptoms of dehydration. Evaluation • Evaluate hydration status and report signs and symptoms of dehydration to health care provider.
3. Potential diarrhea related to short bowel syndrome, feeding regimen changes.	Child will maintain normal stool pattern as determined by health care provider.	See Appendix 8–A.
4. Altered skin integrity related to the presence of diarrhea, stoma(s).	Patient demonstrates no erythema, rashes, edema, or tenderness at stoma(s) or perianal area.	See Appendix 8–A.
5. Risk of infection related to central venous line, TPN infusions	Child will remain afebrile and free of infections.	Assessment/intervention • Keep sterile, occlusive dressing over exit site of central venous catheter. Change dressing at prescribed intervals. • Assess for the following signs of sepsis: fever, tachycardia, hypotension, lethargy, sudden glycosuria, and tachypnea. • Assess catheter exit site for the following signs of infection: tenderness, swelling, and drainage at exit site and along the length of the catheter.

Nursing Diagnosis	Expected Outcomes	Nursing Interventions
		Instruction • Instruct family in dressing change procedure and administration of TPN using sterile technique. • Instruct family in the signs and symptoms of sepsis and catheter exit site infection. Evaluation • Evaluate the family's ability to change catheter dressing and administer TPN using sterile technique. • Evaluate for signs of sepsis and catheter exit site infection and report to health care provider.
6. Knowledge deficit related to the following: • pathophysiology of disease • treatment of disease • special nutritional regimens that can include TPN and/or enteral feedings • ostomy care (if needed)	Family and patient verbalize and demonstrate understanding of disease process, treatment regimen, special nutritional therapy, and ostomy care (if needed).	Use inflammatory bowel disease care plan (Appendix 8–A).
7. Impaired growth and development related to the following: • poor growth • chronic disease • frequent absences from school and re-hospitalization • mobility restrictions • nonoral feeding methods for nutrition	Child progresses through developmental phases at an appropriate pace.	Assessment/intervention • Provide consistent schedule for meeting child's food, rest, and hygiene care. • Whenever medically feasible, allow small oral feedings to prevent food adversions. • For infants, use pacifier during gastrostomy tube feedings. • Use ambulatory pumps and nocturnal cycling of nutritional regimens to increase mobility and participation in normal activities.

Nursing Diagnosis	*Expected Outcomes*	*Nursing Interventions*
		• Assess developmental level and, if necessary, involve child in early intervention program with necessary support services. Instruction • Instruct family in appropriate developmental milestones and ways to encourage child's developmental progress. Evaluation • Evaluate child's progress through developmental phases and redesign interventions as necessary.
8. Coping: ineffective patient and family coping related to the following: • chronic disease • ever-present fear of onset of acute symp- toms	Patient and family demonstrate decreased anxiety and stress. Patient and family develop a trusting relationship with health care provider. Patient and family demonstrate increased ability to care for child and increased involve-ment in health care plan. Patient and family use healthy, appropriate coping mechanism.	See Appendix 8–A.

CHAPTER 9

Alterations in Endocrine Function

Jean Betschart

The endocrine system includes eight hormone-producing glands that exert influence on specific tissues or target organs. Hormones carried throughout the body by the circulatory system control and regulate growth and sexual development, metabolism, and physiologic stress response.

Endocrine dysfunctions in children can affect not only the child's general health and well-being but also impact both the family and community. Treatment is frequently lifelong and requires long-term follow-up. Treatment regimens can be as simple as swallowing a pill daily (such as treatment for primary hypothyroidism) or require major lifestyle changes (as in treatment for insulin-dependent diabetes). Goals of treatment are to correct the hormonal imbalance, maintain normal growth and development, prevent acute and chronic complications, promote optimal school performance, and assist the child and family in adjusting to the disease process and treatment regimen.

Home nursing care is directed toward achieving treatment plan goals through education, use of community resources, identification of problems, and development of strategies to cope with these problems. This chapter reviews the more common endocrine dysfunctions observed in children and addresses the role of the home care nurse in caring for the child and the family.

ALTERATION IN GROWTH: GROWTH HORMONE DEFICIENCY

Growth is an important indicator of a child's mental and physical health as well as the quality of the environment. Children with poor growth should be carefully monitored to assess genetic, prenatal, endocrine, nutritional, metabolic, psychological, and/or systemic chronic illness. All of these factors have profound influences on growth and development. The endocrine system influences growth through the activity of growth hormone and of other hormones, such as thyroxine, glucocorticoid, estrogen, and testosterone.

The general pattern of growth in children is relatively consistent. Growth in utero is strongly controlled by nutritional and other metabolic factors. By two or three years of age, children have established their own growth patterns based on their genetic potential. Standardized growth charts have been developed for plotting the child's growth against established norms.

Accurate measurement of height is essential in the assessment of growth. Supine length is the preferred position for measuring children younger than two years. The child is placed on an unyielding horizontal surface with the soles of the feet in a plane perpendicular to the body axis. The head is placed in the Frankfurt position, and a line drawn from the outer canthus of the eye to the external auditory meatus is placed perpendicular to the body axis. Children older than two years should be measured while standing against a wall with feet bare, medial malleoli touching, and the heels, buttocks, and shoulders in contact with the wall. With the head held in the Frankfurt position, a rigid, right-angled device is rested on the child's crown.

The height attained is plotted on the appropriate standardized growth chart for age and sex. Heights and weights should be carefully plotted at each well-child visit. The growth pattern usually establishes itself upon a certain percentile. When a child's growth chart indicates that growth is crossing over his or her usual percentile for growth, it should be cause for further assessment. A deviation in the established percentile channel or a decrease in growth rate or velocity signals the need for referral. The expected growth rate or growth velocity per year of the child's age is shown in Table 9–1. The referral is made to the child's primary health care provider or an endocrinologist. If growth hormone deficiency is not recognized early, there is greater risk of not reaching the genetically appropriate ultimate height. Growth hormone, therefore, should be introduced early and continued until epiphyseal plates are fused. Treatment in children whose parents are tall should not be delayed until the growth velocity is no longer normal (Blizzard and Johanson 1994).

Table 9–1 Growth Rates per Year of Age

Age	Growth Rate
0–6 months	16–17 cm
7–12 months	8 cm
13–24 months	10 cm
25–36 months	>8 cm
37–48 months	7 cm
4 years to puberty	5–6 cm

Source: Reprinted from *Clinical Pediatric and Adolescent Endocrinology* by S.A. Kaplan (Ed.), p. 3, with permission of W.B. Saunders Company, © 1982.

Nursing Care Plans in the Home

Potential for Knowledge Deficit Related to Administration of the Growth Hormone Preparation

Children with documented growth hormone deficiency are treated with synthetic growth hormone. The usual dose is 0.3 mg/kg/week. However, in children with chronic renal failure, or who are not growth hormone deficient, the dose may be 0.05 mg/kg/day (Blizzard and Johanson 1994). This medication is given subcutaneously on a daily basis. The dose is individualized to achieve maximum growth. To achieve this maximum growth, the growth hormone preparation is administered until growth is complete. It has been suggested that it is best to give growth hormone at night because it is more physiologic, but this has not been documented.

Education may include initial instruction on the administration of growth hormone or assessment of the child's or family's technique and their reeducation. Home care nurses can provide the initial instruction.

Growth hormone preparations are packaged as a powder and must be diluted with the accompanying diluent. The medications are obtained through the child's hospital or home care agencies designated by the manufacturers. However, now there is a preparation available that is already mixed (Genentech, Nutropin AQ, South San Francisco, California).

The manufacturers have patient education materials that can be helpful in the education process. The behavioral objectives for administration of the growth hormone are listed in Exhibit 9–1. The child's participation in the injections should be appropriate for developmental age. Adolescents wishing to take on more responsibility may administer their own injections. Educating the adolescent is indicated particularly for patients whose parents have had primary responsibility for the injections. Preschool- and school-age children can help to participate in their care by cleaning the site, helping to choose the spot, or just "holding still." Play

Exhibit 9–1 Behavioral Objectives for
Administration of Growth Hormone

1. State the rationale for receiving the growth hormone medication.
2. List equipment and materials needed.
3. Describe the care and storage of the needles, syringe, and growth hormone preparation.
4. State the schedule of administration.
5. Demonstrate understanding of the concept of sterility.
6. Demonstrate ability to correctly mix and draw up amount of growth hormone preparation.
7. Demonstrate ability to correctly inject the growth hormone preparation.
8. Identify sites for growth hormone injection.
9. Describe rationale for site rotation.
10. Demonstrate ability to record injection given and site used in logbook.
11. State resources to contact when questions or problems arise.
12. Identify follow-up plans.

therapy and a positive reinforcement system that includes praise and hugs can promote cooperative behavior. Parents are commonly anxious about giving their child injections and causing pain. Parental anxiety can be lessened by giving the parent an injection of normal saline before giving an injection to the child.

The average annual cost of growth hormone therapy is approximately $15,000. The cost may place financial burden on the family. Some states offer financial assistance through Children with Special Health Care Needs. The manufacturers also offer a program for financial assistance.

Potential for Disturbance in Self-Concept Related to Short Stature

School-age children and adolescents struggle to achieve a sense of identity and of belonging with a peer group. Children with growth delays are at risk for the development of disturbances in self-image. Compounding the problem is the possible accompanying delay in the development of secondary sexual characteristics. Assessment of the child and family's feelings about the growth delay and the child's self-image, relationships with peers, and performance in school should be regularly monitored, and the child and family should be referred for counseling as necessary.

Children with growth delays are frequently treated as if they are younger. Parents, family, teachers, and peers may need assistance in developing expectations and interactions appropriate for the child's age not stature. He or she may need assistance in developing realistic performance expectations in physical activities and athletics. Activities in which size is not of consideration should be encouraged. There are support groups affiliated with major centers that can be helpful, as well as local camping programs offered through the National Growth Foundation.

The child and family should be helped to be realistic in their expectations of the probable response to the treatment. If unrealistic expectations fail to materialize, the child and family may experience frustrations that interfere with psychological well-being.

ALTERATION IN WATER BALANCE: DIABETES INSIPIDUS

The diagnosis of diabetes insipidus includes disorders that are characterized by passing a large volume of dilute, sugar-free urine (Perheentupa and Czernichow 1994). Usually, there is an inability to concentrate urine resulting from a lack of antidiuretic hormone (ADH) or a poor response to ADH. Normally, ADH is synthesized by the hypothalamus and stored and released by the posterior pituitary. It increases permeability of the collecting tubules of water, promoting reabsorption of water.

The characteristic signs and symptoms of diabetes insipidus are polydipsia (with a preference for ice water), polyuria, nocturia, and enuresis. Constant thirst and frequent urination may interfere with play, school, sleep, and the intake of appropriate nutrients. When fluid is withheld and dehydration occurs, the child with diabetes insipidus will exhibit classic signs of dehydration, such as irritability, extreme thirst, poor skin turgor, dry mucous membranes, lethargy, and sunken eyes.

The clinical manifestations include increased 24-hour urine output, specific gravity below 1.005, serum osmolarity above 290 mOsm/kg, and mild hypernatremia above 145 mEq/L.

The three classifications of diabetes insipidus are (1) central, (2) nephrogenic, and (3) psychogenic. Central diabetes insipidus is caused by a deficiency in ADH. The major causes are trauma, tumors, infection, or surgical procedure, or it may be idiopathic. Signs of diabetes insipidus may be the presenting complaints of a child with an intracranial lesion. Nephrogenic diabetes insipidus results from renal insensitivity to ADH. This disorder can result from a variety of forms of chronic renal disease, from various drugs and toxins, and, in rare instances, from an X-linked inheritance pattern. Psychogenic diabetes insipidus, manifested by compulsive water drinking, is rare in children and is associated with a number of psychological disturbances.

Water deprivation tests and challenge with ADH are used to confirm the diagnosis. The goals of therapy are to obtain a normal water balance and diminish nocturia, polyuria, and polydipsia. Dietary sodium and protein restrictions and the use of chlorothiazide are helpful in reducing the polyuria associated with nephrogenic diabetes insipidus.

Desmopressin acetate (DDAVP) administered intranasally using a soft, calibrated plastic catheter is the drug of choice for the treatment of central diabetes insipidus. The usual dosage is 0.05 to 0.20 mL every 12 to 24 hours and is adjusted according to the child's pattern of response (McGee, Howie, and Dice 1994). In addition, there are several new forms of DDAVP administration including a nasal spray and an oral preparation. The nasal spray comes in 10-mL spray, so the dose cannot be adjusted based on body weight, which is problematic for use in

children. In those children receiving a single dose, the hormone is usually administered in the evening so that the polyuria and polydipsia do not interfere with sleep and school. Doses may need to be adjusted during periods of rhinitis (Perheentupa and Czernichow 1994).

Short periods of polyuria, polydipsia, and decreased urinary specific gravity (breakthrough) should occur 30 minutes to one hour before the administration of the next dose of DDAVP to prevent fluid intoxication. Older children usually can identify when breakthrough occurs. In infants and children who cannot make that determination, the assessment of specific gravity is essential.

Nursing Care Plans in the Home

Potential for Fluid Volume Deficit Related to Polyuria Secondary to Diabetes Insipidus

Assessment of the child's level of hydration aids in determining if the treatment plan is working. The history should include the following: intake, output, specific gravity, dose and timing of DDAVP, and the timing of any symptom breakthrough. Note changes in the child's behavior and school performance. Increased irritability and decreased attention span are frequently evident in children with poorly controlled diabetes insipidus. The physical assessment should include weight (particularly changes in weight over time); the integrity of the mucous membranes, skin, and extremities; and specific gravity. Rapid weight gain or loss, signs of dehydration, and breakthrough occurring more than one to two hours before the next dose should be communicated to the health care provider.

One important role of the home care nurse is to assess the method of administration of DDAVP because incorrectly administered DDAVP will cause increased polyuria and polydipsia. It must be administered with the child in a sitting position with the head hyperextended so the nasal bridge is flattened. The medication-filled catheter is inserted halfway up the nares. The other end is placed in the mouth and, with a quick puff, the medication is blown into the nares. Blowing too hard will blow the medication into the nasopharynx, and the DDAVP will be deactivated by the gastric juices. A bad taste in the mouth after administration indicates that the medication has entered the nasopharynx. The child must not sniff or blow the nose immediately after administration of the drug.

Potential for Knowledge Deficit Related to Disease, Administration of Medication, Signs and Symptoms of Dehydration or of Fluid Overload, and Prevention of Dehydration

It is important that the nurse assess the family's understanding of diabetes insipidus, ability to administer the DDAVP, and knowledge of the signs and symptoms of dehydration and fluid overload. The family's ability to measure specific gravity and to maintain the equipment must also be observed. When the refractometer is used to measure specific gravity, quality control testing with distilled water is essential to ensure that the readings are accurate.

The family must understand the potential for dehydration during illness. The absorption of DDAVP may be impaired when the mucous membranes become engorged because of a cold or allergic rhinitis. Vomiting and decreased fluid intake also place the child at risk. Dehydration generally will not occur as long as the child drinks sufficient amounts of fluid. Infants and children who do not have ready access to fluids are at greater risk. Instruct parents to contact their child's health care provider whenever persistent vomiting and decreased fluid intake occur. Hospitalization for intravenous administration of fluids may be necessary to ensure adequate hydration.

Alteration in Patterns of Urinary Elimination Related to Polyuria Secondary to Diabetes Insipidus

Polyuria frequently interferes with the child's play, sleep, and school performance. Bed-wet-

ting is distressing for the child and parents and can be reduced or eliminated with proper administration of DDAVP, timing of administration, and dosage. An increase in bed-wetting should be communicated to the health care provider.

For the school-age child, frequent trips to the rest room can lead to admonishment from the teacher and teasing from the other children. Education of school personnel and other students regarding the needs of a child with diabetes insipidus, such as the need for frequent trips to the rest room and water fountain, is helpful to the child who must cope with his or her illness in the school setting.

ALTERATION IN ADRENAL FUNCTION: ADRENAL INSUFFICIENCY

Deficient adrenal glucocorticoid and mineralocorticoid production results from dysfunction of the adrenal cortex, deficiency in production of adrenocorticotropic hormone (ACTH), or suppression of endogenous adrenal function due to exogenous glucocorticoid therapy.

Congenital adrenal hyperplasia is an autosomal recessive genetic disorder in the biosynthesis of cortisol due to a specific enzymatic defect. The most common form of this disorder is caused by overproduction of ACTH, leading to hyperplasia of the adrenal gland and excessive adrenal androgen secretion. This leads to prenatal virilization of the female (enlargement of the clitoris and fusing of the labia) and postnatal virilization of both female and male (enlargement of the clitoris or penis, development of pubic hair and acne, and acceleration of growth). Aldosterone deficiency may also be present, leading to low serum sodium levels, high serum potassium levels, and possible vascular collapse (New, Pang, and Levine 1985). Affected females are usually recognized at birth because of ambiguous genitalia. Affected males, who generally appear normal at birth, are often diagnosed at 7 to 14 days of age in adrenal crisis.

Adrenal insufficiency due to ACTH deficiency is generally caused by tumors, infections, cranial irradiation, or surgical procedures in the hypothalamus or pituitary region. Aldosterone secretion is normal.

The administration of glucocorticoid suppresses ACTH secretion and produces atrophy of the adrenal cortex. Glucocorticoid taken for more than two weeks at or above physiologic levels will suppress cortisol production. It may take 1 to 18 months for the function of the pituitary-adrenal axis to return to normal (Migeon and Lanes 1985).

Hydrocortisone is the drug of choice for chronic glucocorticoid replacement therapy. The dosage is normally 1 to 2 mg/kg/dose bolus, then 25 to 150 mg/day in divided doses for infants and young children and should be individualized. Older children receive a 1- to 2-mg/kg bolus, then 150 to 250 mg/day in divided doses (McGee, Howie, and Dice 1994). The treatment for mineralocorticoid deficiency is replacement therapy with oral fludrocortisone acetate (Florinef), 0.05 to 0.15 mg/day as a single dose. In infants receiving only formula, carefully regulated amounts of salt will be added to the formula. Weight gain, dizziness, and swelling of the hands or feet should be carefully observed and reported (McGee, Howie, and Dice, 1994).

Nursing Care Plans in the Home

Potential for Knowledge Deficit Related to Disease, Administration of Medication, Signs and Symptoms of Complications, and Prevention of Adrenal Crisis

The family and the child (when developmentally appropriate) must learn about the disease process, proper administration of the replacement medication, and adjustment of the hydrocortisone dose during times of physiologic stress. They also must recognize the signs and symptoms of adrenal insufficiency (undertreatment), hypercortisolism (overtreatment), and adrenal crisis.

The hydrocortisone preparation comes in a liquid form as Cortef and in pill form as Florinef.

If Cortef is used, parents should learn to shake the bottle vigorously before use to ensure that the preparation is thoroughly mixed. To ensure correct dosage, Cortef should be administered orally using a syringe for accurate measurement. Florinef can be crushed and dissolved in a small amount of formula or food. In children with congenital adrenal hyperplasia, the hydrocortisone is given three times daily, preferably every eight hours. Because the midafternoon dose is most frequently forgotten, the school nurse may be able to assist in giving it to the child to provide consistency.

Adrenal crisis occurs when the adrenal cortex cannot produce the additional levels of cortisol needed to prevent widespread vasodilation, shock, and death during times of physiologic stress. Physiologic stress includes trauma, surgery, and illness, especially when associated with high fever. The signs and symptoms of adrenal crisis are vomiting, dehydration, lethargy, hypotension, and shock. Signs and symptoms associated with adrenal dysfunction are listed in Table 9–2.

Parents must be instructed to double or triple the dose of hydrocortisone for several days during times of illness, especially when a high fever is present. They should contact the health care provider immediately for information about any signs or symptoms of adrenal crisis. Injectable hydrocortisone is available and can be used under the direction of the health care provider during significant illnesses, especially persistent vomiting. Children should wear Medic-Alert identification tags stating they have adrenal insufficiency.

Potential for Disturbance in Self-Concept Related to Appearance Changes Secondary to Early Onset of Pubic Hair, Enlargement of Clitoris or Penis, and Increased Height for Age

Children with precocious virilization are at risk of developing disturbances in self-concept. Precocious virilization can occur in poorly controlled 21-hydroxylase deficiency, the most

Table 9–2 Signs and Symptoms Associated with Adrenal Dysfunction

Hypercortisolism	Adrenal Insufficiency	Adrenal Crisis
Moon facies	Lethargy	Nausea
Increased body fat	Anorexia	Vomiting
Retarded growth	Weakness	Dehydration
Muscle weakness	Occasional vomiting	Lethargy
Hypertension	Weight loss	Hypotension
	Hyperpigmentation	Shock
	Virilization (in children with congenital adrenal hyperplasia)	

common form of congenital adrenal hyperplasia. In the school-age years, children begin to struggle with peer identity and the need for peer acceptance. Precocious development of pubic hair and enlargement of the penis or clitoris can enhance children's natural feelings of being different. These children can also, in turn, have difficulty with developing peer relationships and the development of a healthy self-concept.

Assessment of the child's feelings and understanding about body changes and differences is important. Explanations should be developmentally appropriate, positive, and supportive. Play therapy is useful for many children for them to explore and express feelings. Home care nurses can play a major role in assisting school personnel to developing programs that help students understand and accept individual differences.

Acceleration in growth may cause adults to have unrealistic expectations of the child. Parents and teachers may need assistance in developing appropriate expectations for the child based on age and not stature.

Potential for Alterations in Family Processes Related to Having a Child with Congenital Adrenal Hyperplasia or 21-Hydroxylase Deficiency

The diagnosis of congenital adrenal hyperplasia has an emotional impact on the family. It can be particularly stressful when the child has am-biguous genitalia or when the sex assigned to the child at birth is incorrect. Home care nurses are ideally positioned to support the family through the grieving process when parents struggle with acceptance of the child's illness. It is important to assess the family's level of understanding, coping style, feelings about the child's diagnosis, and support systems. Many parents are particularly interested in information concerning corrective surgery for ambiguous genitalia. Surgery, depending on the defect, occurs anywhere from three months to three years of age. Families may need reassurance that the child will look normal after surgery and help to explain the anomaly to other family members.

ALTERATION IN THYROID FUNCTION: HYPOTHYROIDISM

Thyroid hormones are important for normal growth, development, and metabolism in infancy and childhood. Hypothyroidism during childhood and adolescence can result from a variety of congenital or acquired defects. Thyroid function is regulated by circulating thyroid-stimulating hormone (TSH). Hypothyroidism may be congenital, resulting from a defect in or absence of the thyroid gland or deficiency in TSH or thyroid-releasing hormone (TRH). In North America, the majority of children with congenital primary hypothyroidism are detected through neonatal thyroid screening programs (Dallas and Foley 1996). The incidence of congenital hypothyroidism is 1 in 4,000 live births (Fisher 1994). Neonatal screening for hypothyroidism is part of the newborn screening tests in most states. Early identification and initiation of therapy have reduced the significant developmental delays previously associated with congenital hypothyroidism. The signs and symptoms of congenital hypothyroidism are listed in Table 9–3.

Hypothyroidism acquired in childhood and adolescence is caused most often by an autoimmune process known as Hashimoto's thyroiditis. Hypothalamic or pituitary disease may result in deficiencies of TRH or TSH with subsequent development of hypothyroidism. The signs and symptoms of acquired hypothyroidism are listed in Table 9–4.

The treatment for hypothyroidism is replacement therapy with L-thyroxine. The dose is 100 $\mu/m^2/day$ but must be individualized (Dallas and Foley 1996). The dose of L-thyroxine is adjusted for growth throughout childhood and adolescence.

Table 9–3 Symptoms and Signs of Congenital Hypothyroidism

Symptoms	Signs
Prolonged jaundice	Skin mottling
Lethargy	Umbilical hernia
Constipation	Jaundice
Feeding problems	Macroglossia
Cold to touch	Large fontanelles, wide sutures
	Distended abdomen
	Hoarse cry
	Hypotonia
	Dry skin
	Slow reflexes
	Goiter

Source: Reprinted from *Pediatric Clinics of North America*, Vol. 26, p. 46, with permission of W.B. Saunders Company, © 1979.

Nursing Care Plans in the Home

Potential for Knowledge Deficit Related to Disease, Administration of Medication, and Complications

Home care nursing of a child with hypothyroidism involves educating the family about the disease. Important points to include are the importance of giving the medication daily, signs and symptoms of hypothyroidism, and signs and symptoms of hyperthyroidism (overtreatment). Generic preparations of L-thyroxine may have variable potencies and therefore may provide inconsistent replacement therapy (Rees-Jones, Rolla, and Larsen 1980). L-Thyroxine is prescribed orally as a single daily dose and should be taken every day at the same time, preferably before breakfast, to maintain constant hormone level (Dallas and Foley 1996).

For infants, the pill is crushed in a small amount of formula or strained food and administered by a spoon. The medication should not be placed in a bottle of formula because the infant may not drink all the formula and not receive the full dose of L-thyroxine. For older children and adolescents, the nurse may need to assist the family in identifying methods of remembering the medication, such as a calendar or a weekly reminder pillbox.

Frequently, there are behavioral changes due to replacement therapy, which may occur in children with acquired hypothyroidism. Children may become more active but also may experience sleep disturbances and emotional lability. Parents and teachers need to be aware of anticipated behavioral changes. Symptoms of hyperthyroidism may be present for several weeks until the child's system adjusts to a normal thyroid state.

Potential for Self-Care Deficit Related to Developmental Delays Secondary to Low Thyroid Levels during First Two to Three Years of Life

Because of the increased incidence of developmental delay associated with congenital hy-

Table 9–4 Symptoms and Signs of Acquired Hypothyroidism

Symptoms	Signs
Slow growth	Decreased growth velocity
Puffiness	Increased upper to lower segment ratio
Decreased appetite	Delayed dentition
Constipation	Myxedema, mildly overweight
Swollen thyroid gland	Goiter
Lethargy	Delayed reflex return
Drop in school performance	Dull, placid expression
Cold intolerance	Pale, thick, carotenemia or cool skin
Galactorrhea	Muscle pseudohypertrophy
Menometrorrhagia	Delayed puberty Precocious puberty

Source: Reprinted from *Clinical Pediatric and Adolescent Endocrinology* by S.A. Kaplan (Ed.), p. 92, with permission of W.B. Saunders Company, © 1982.

pothyroidism, periodic assessment of the child's development is important. Development should be assessed by the Denver Development Screen Test (DDST) or other screening modes and definitively tested at three, five, and seven years (Fisher 1994). DDST is a standardized tool used to assess development in children from infancy through the preschool years. Children with suspected delays should be referred to the primary health care provider or a developmental center for further evaluation. Home care nurses can assist the family in the use of developmentally appropriate play activities for the child.

ALTERATION IN CARBOHYDRATE METABOLISM: DIABETES MELLITUS

Diabetes mellitus is a syndrome of altered carbohydrate metabolism resulting from an absolute or functional deficiency of insulin. Diabetes mellitus is a group of disorders characterized by high blood glucose levels and, in some in-

stances, poor glucose utilization. Noninsulin-dependent diabetes mellitus (NIDDM), or Type II diabetes, characterizes approximately 80 percent of all diabetes. However, NIDDM is not commonly found in children. Insulin-dependent diabetes mellitus (IDDM) is one of the most frequent chronic diseases in children in the United States. The frequency is, in fact, higher than all other chronic diseases of youth. Prevalence of IDDM in children is approximately 1.7 per 1,000 or roughly 1 in 580 children (LaPorte, Matsushima, and Chang 1995).

IDDM results from an absolute deficiency of insulin due to destruction of the beta cells. Insulin injections are necessary for life. Although IDDM can occur at any age, it is most common during youth and in younger adults. NIDDM occurs more frequently in obese adults older than 40 years and results from insulin resistance or decreased tissue sensitivity to insulin. Meal plans directed toward weight loss and oral hypoglycemic agents are primary treatments for NIDDM. Treatment may or may not include insulin.

The classic symptoms of diabetes in childhood are polyuria, polydipsia, polyphagia, and nocturia. Weight loss, lethargy, blurred vision, and candidal vaginitis may also be present. Enuresis may develop in a child who previously did not experience this condition at night. The plasma glucose concentration is elevated above 200 mg/dL (Drash 1986).

Insulin acts by binding to receptor sites located on the cell membrane and facilitating glucose uptake by the cells. When there is insufficient insulin or insulin resistance, the cells do not receive necessary amounts of glucose and starvation ensues. Deficiency of insulin leads to hyperglycemia with resultant glucosuria. Glucosuria occurs when the renal threshold of approximately 160 mg/dL is exceeded. Osmotic diuresis results in polyuria and accompanying losses of sodium and potassium. Relative or severe dehydration follows, which results in polydipsia. Other signs of dehydration may also be present such as sunken eyes, poor skin turgor, and/or dry mucous membranes. Intracellular glucose deficiency causes appetite increases. Weight loss occurs despite a normal or increased appetite.

Protein and fat stores are broken down to maintain energy supplies. Gluconeogenesis (glucose formed from protein) occurs, adding to the hyperglycemia, osmotic diuresis, and dehydration. Fat catabolism accelerates, with increased formation of ketone bodies. Accumulation of ketoacids leads to metabolic acidosis and compensatory rapid, deep (Kussmaul) breathing to "blow off" excess carbon dioxide. The characteristic fruity odor is due to these ketone bodies. Progressive dehydration, hyperosmolarity, and acidosis impair the level of consciousness and can result in coma. The effect of insulin deficiency is shown in Figure 9–1.

The diagnosis of IDDM is based on an elevated plasma glucose concentration, glucosuria, ketonuria, and history of polyuria and polydipsia. Oral glucose tolerance tests are rarely used in children. Because of increased public awareness, the diagnosis in children and adolescents occurs in many cases before the development of diabetic ketoacidosis (DKA).

DKA is one of the acute diabetic complications, and usually occurs in IDDM. After initial diagnosis, DKA most commonly occurs in children with intercurrent illness, who are under extraordinary familial or emotional stress or who miss insulin doses. DKA is clinically defined by absolute insulin deficiency with hyperglycemia

(usually with glucose levels above 200 mg/dL), glucosuria, ketonemia, ketonuria, and acidosis (pH below 7.30 and bicarbonate less than 15 mg/L) (Fishbein and Klein 1995). Treatment must be immediate, but done in the care of experienced pediatric endocrinologists, and consists of correction of the fluid and electrolyte imbalance, acidosis, and hyperglycemia. Rapid overcorrection can lead to fluid shifts and resulting cerebral edema. One of the best treatments of DKA is prevention through education of the child and family (Exhibits 9–2 and 9–3).

The goal of the treatment plan for children is to achieve normoglycemia while avoiding severe hypoglycemia, to maintain normal growth and development, and to maintain the emotional well-being of the child and the family. The goals for each child and family are individualized. For example, the primary goal for a child with recurrent episodes of DKA may be to keep the child out of the hospital. A goal for another child may be to prevent severe hypoglycemia.

The chronic complications associated with diabetes include retinopathy, cataracts, nephropathy, peripheral neuropathy, autonomic neuropathy, coronary artery disease, and peripheral vascular disease. Growth failure has also been documented in children with poorly controlled diabetes (Chase et al. 1985). The complications usually appear following 10 to 15 years of established diabetes.

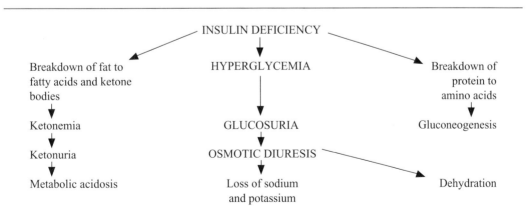

Figure 9–1 Effects of insulin deficiency.

Exhibit 9–2 Behavioral Objectives: Initial Education for Children with Type I Diabetes Mellitus and Their Families

Definition
- Define diabetes.
- Identify components of the treatment plan (meal plan, insulin therapy, and exercise).
- Explain the effect that a lack of insulin has on the body.
- Explain the difference between Type I and Type II diabetes.

Meal Plan
- Explain interrelationship among food, insulin, and exercise.
- State importance of good nutrition.
- Explain importance of meal plan in relationship to diabetes control.
- Identify types and amounts of food to be included in the meal plan.
- Explain modification of meal plan during sick days, party, travel, and eating out (especially dining in fast-food restaurants).

Exercise
- Explain benefit of exercise.
- Explain the influence of exercise on blood glucose levels.
- Explain when exercise is not recommended.
- Describe need to test blood glucose before, during, and after changes in exercise.
- Explain foods (amount and type) to be used to prevent hypoglycemia associated with exercise.
- Explain need to inform appropriate person concerning the possibility of hypoglycemia with exercise along with its recognition and treatment.

Insulin Therapy
- Explain effect insulin has on blood glucose level.
- Explain type, species, concentration, and amount of insulin to be taken.
- Demonstrate ability to draw up amount of insulin using proper technique, including two types of insulin.
- Demonstrate ability to inject insulin using proper technique.

- Explain importance of rotating insulin injection sites and use of rotation schedule.
- Explain daily administration of insulin and times of injection.
- Explain schedule for giving insulin.
- Explain peak action, onset, and duration of insulin used.
- Inform patient and family where to purchase insulin and syringes.

Monitoring
- Explain benefit of self-monitoring of blood glucose.
- Demonstrate ability to perform self-monitoring of blood glucose.
- Demonstrate ability to document results of self-monitoring of blood glucose in record book.
- State schedule for self-monitoring of blood glucose.
- Explain when to contact health care provider—when blood glucose levels are consistently above and below guidelines.
- Explain honeymoon period and its effect on blood glucose and insulin dosages.
- Explain rationale for monitoring urine ketone levels.
- Demonstrate ability to perform urine ketone testing.
- Demonstrate ability to record results of urine ketone testing.
- Explain when to perform urine ketone testing.
- Explain when to contact health care provider—when test is positive for ketones.
- Explain optimal blood glucose and urine ketone results in relationship to time of day and various situations.
- Explain rationale for urine glucose testing (if this method is used).
- Demonstrate ability to perform urine glucose testing (if this method is used).
- Demonstrate ability to record results of urine glucose testing (if this method is used).
- Explain when to contact health care provider: persistent glucosuria.

continues

Exhibit 9–2 continued

Acute Complications
- State possible symptoms of hypoglycemia and its treatment.
- Explain possible causes of hypoglycemia.
- Explain ways to prevent hypoglycemia.
- Explain how and when to use glucagon.
- Demonstrate ability to administer glucagon.
- Explain need to carry a form of simple sugar at all times.
- Describe possible symptoms of hyperglycemia.
- Explain causes of hyperglycemia and methods of prevention.
- Explain sick day rules and the need to continue insulin administration during illness.
- State when and how to contact health care provider in case of hypoglycemia, hyperglycemia, illness.
- Explain ketoacidosis, its causes and treatment.

Psychosocial Adjustment
- Parents verbalize that child has diabetes.
- Patient verbalizes that he or she has diabetes when developmentally appropriate.
- Patient verbalizes feelings about having diabetes and/or parents verbalize feelings about having a child with diabetes.

- Patient and family state that daily injections, meal planning, and exercise are the necessary treatment of diabetes.

Activities of Daily Living
- Explain how to fit routine into school setting and work.
- Explain importance of Medic-Alert tag for a form of diabetic identification.

Health Habits
- Explain need for good personal hygiene, daily foot care, and daily dental care.

Community Resources
- List resources in community for diabetes support and education.

Use of Health Care System
- Describe when and how to obtain emergency care.
- State follow-up plans.

Source: Goals for Diabetes Education by M. Franz et al., pp. 7–9, American Diabetes Association, Inc., © 1986; "Instruction Plan, Day 1—Day 7," Diabetic Home Care Program, Medical Personnel Pool, Inc., 1987.

Until recently, there was no general agreement on the best management for diabetes. However, in 1993, the Diabetes Control and Complications Trial (DCCT), a multimillion dollar 10-year study by the National Institutes of Health, was completed. The DCCT followed 1,400 people with IDDM, aged 13 to 39 years. Study participants were divided into two groups with one receiving standard or conventional treatment of the day (usually two injections of insulin daily) and the other group receiving four injections of insulin per day, an insulin pump, nutrition counseling, and behavioral support to maintain blood glucose levels at near-normal levels. This study found that the subjects who kept their blood glucose levels as close to normal as possible had a 60 percent reduction in their risks of development and progression of eye, kidney, and nervous system complications (American Diabetes Association 1996a). Because this study included only those who had insulin deficiency, not children, results cannot be generalized to all types of diabetes, although most practitioners think that the effects of hyperglycemia are common to all people with diabetes. It has become widely recognized that it is in the best interests of those with all types of diabetes to keep blood glucose levels as tightly controlled as possible without risking severe hypoglycemic episodes.

Exhibit 9–3 Behavioral Objectives: In-Depth Continuing Education and Counseling for Children with Type I Diabetes Mellitus and Their Families

Definitions
- Explain the cause of Type I diabetes mellitus.
- Explain the symptoms of poorly controlled diabetes.
- Explain how diabetes is diagnosed.
- Explain what is good diabetes control.
- Explain the benefit of good diabetes control.
- State behaviors necessary to achieve good diabetes control.
- Explain the effects of insulin deficiency.
- Explain the dawn phenomenon.
- Describe treatment of the dawn phenomenon.
- Explain the Somogyi effect.
- Describe how to prevent the Somogyi effect.
- Explain the effect of the counterregulatory hormones on blood glucose.
- Explain the honeymoon period and its effect on blood glucose.

Nutrition
- Plan appropriate meals from meal plan.
- Describe benefit of food in controlling blood glucose and lipids.
- Explain importance in maintaining consistency in caloric intake.
- State caloric level in percentage of fat, protein, and carbohydrates in meal plan.
- List nutrients in foods (carbohydrate [simple, complex, refined, fiber], fat, protein, vitamins, minerals, and water).
- Explain the function of these nutrients.
- Explain effects of these nutrients on blood glucose and lipid levels.
- List sources of fiber in meal plan.
- Explain differences between saturated and unsaturated fats.
- Explain benefit of reducing total fat, saturated fat, and cholesterol in meal plan.
- Explain benefit of reducing salt in meal plan.
- Explain how to modify meal plan in relation to changes in activity.
- Plan appropriate meals based on meal plan when eating out (especially with dining in fast-food restaurants).
- Explain how to incorporate "special treats" into the meal plan.

- Demonstrate ability to evaluate food products from information on food labels.
- Identify those dietetic and low-calorie foods that may be incorporated into meal plan.
- Explain how to incorporate dietetic and low-calorie foods into meal plan.
- Explain how to incorporate sweetening agents into meal plan.
- Describe effect that alcohol has on blood glucose.
- Explain how to modify meal plan during illness.
- Explain when to adjust (increase/decrease) caloric intake.

Exercise
- State benefits of exercise.
- Explain benefits of exercise on blood glucose and lipid levels.
- Identify types of exercise that could be incorporated into diabetes treatment plan.
- Explain the relationship among exercise, injection sites used, and blood glucose level.
- Explain the effect that timing of exercise has on blood glucose level.
- Explain the relationship among exercise, timing of meals, and blood glucose level.
- Explain how to choose injection sites to prevent hypoglycemia during and after periods of exercise.
- Explain effect that exercise has when hyperglycemia and/or ketosis is present.
- Explain how to adjust meal plan to prevent hypoglycemia during and after exercise.
- Explain benefit of monitoring blood glucose level before, during, and after exercise.
- Explain benefit of carrying concentrated carbohydrate source during periods of exercise.
- State that strenuous exercise can affect blood glucose levels for up to 12 to 24 hours.
- Explain the benefit of exercising with a companion and wearing appropriate identification outlining emergency care.

Medication
- Describe sources of insulin (beef/pork, pork, human).

continues

Exhibit 9–3 continued

- Identify the different types of insulin.
- State the time of onset, peak, and duration of insulins used.
- Explain benefit of site rotation.
- Explain plan for site rotation.
- Define lipohypertrophy.
- Define lipoatrophy.
- Explain how to prevent lipohypertrophy and lipoatrophy.
- Explain when insulin dose should be adjusted.
- Explain how to adjust insulin dosage based on guidelines.
- Explain effect other medications have on blood glucose levels.
- Explain care and storage of insulin during travel.
- Explain when insulin dosage should not be adjusted.
- Explain the proper way to reuse insulin syringes as well as the benefits and risks.

Monitoring
- Explain how to adjust treatment plan (exercise, meal plan, insulin dose) based on results of blood glucose monitoring to achieve desired blood glucose levels.
- Identify factors that cause fluctuations in blood glucose levels.
- Explain benefit of glycosylated hemoglobin in maintaining diabetes control.
- Explain how to relate results of glycosylated hemoglobin to treatment plan.
- State when to notify health care provider.

Acute Complications
- State causes of hypoglycemia.
- Explain how to prevent hypoglycemia.
- Explain mechanism of ketone production.
- Explain cause of ketosis.
- Explain treatment of ketosis.
- Define diabetic ketoacidosis.
- Explain how to prevent diabetic ketoacidosis.
- Explain signs and symptoms of diabetic ketoacidosis.
- Explain effect stress (emotional and physical) has on diabetes control.
- State sick day roles: adjustment in meal plan, monitoring, and insulin dose.

- State need to take insulin during illness.
- State when to notify health care provider.

Psychosocial Adjustment
- Patient states concerns about having diabetes.
- Parents state concerns about having child with diabetes.
- Patient explains the effect that diabetes has had on lifestyle.
- Patient and family state situations that cause stress.
- Patient and family state methods used to manage stress.

Health Habits
- Explain proper care of skin.
- Explain proper care of feet and nails.
- Explain proper dental care.
- Explain when to communicate with health care provider.
- Explain deleterious effect of smoking.
- Explain deleterious effect of drug abuse (alcohol and illicit drugs).

Long-Term Complications
- Explain benefit of good diabetes control.
- Explain complications that can be associated with diabetes.
- State need for annual ophthalmologic examination.
- State need for regular blood pressure monitoring.
- State when to notify health care provider.

Community Resources
- List community resources available to assist with special needs and concerns.
- Encourage visit to local American Diabetes Association chapter.

Use of the Health Care System
- State need for routine follow-up to health care provider.
- State need for periodic nutritional assessments.
- State need for continuous diabetic education.

Source: Goals for Diabetes Education by M. Franz et al., pp. 15–20, American Diabetes Association, Inc., © 1986.

Insulin Therapy

Insulin therapy for children and adolescents must be adequate for optimal growth and pubertal development. When insulin insufficiency occurs during childhood and adolescence, normal growth and development may be delayed.

Before the DCCT trials, most children and adolescents regularly took a standard split/mix of an intermediate-acting insulin and regular insulin, usually 30 minutes before breakfast and bedtime. However, with the DCCT experience, many centers have changed to using at least three and sometimes four injections of insulin. Types of insulin and injection times may vary according to the individual needs of the child (see Table 9–5). With newer, more comfortable 30-gauge syringes; cartridge pens for insulin administration; and the use of Humalog insulin (no need to wait 30 minutes after injecting), regimens have become more flexible and injections more comfortable. Most frequently, regular or Humalog insulin is given in combination with NPH or Lente. The intention of multiple daily dose regimens is to provide more flexibility in meal schedules and the opportunity to make adjustments for more or less food, exercise, or high blood glucose numbers. Most parents and older children are now taught to manipulate insulin doses based on blood glucose levels, food intake, and related exercise.

After the diagnosis of diabetes, many children move into a remission or "honeymoon" phase requiring decreased insulin doses. Otherwise, most children require approximately one unit of insulin per kg of body weight (Drash 1990). Individual variables that affect the total amount of insulin include level of exercise, eating patterns, and potential for insulin resistance.

Commercially prepared premixed insulins generally do not allow for the flexibility of daily dosage adjustment based on blood glucose values and exercise levels, which are especially variable in children. It is important to be able to adjust insulin to avoid hypoglycemia. Premixed insulins, however, may be useful in some adolescents who are unable or unwilling to alter their insulin doses.

Insulin is given subcutaneously using sites on the upper arms, thighs, upper outer quadrant of the buttocks, and abdomen. Abdominal injections in children with little subcutaneous abdominal fat, or in very young children, may not be advisable. Rotating sites in a consistent manner is advisable (for example, arms in the morning, legs in the evening). Injecting into the same area causes a buildup of fat, lipohypertrophy, which interferes with the absorption of insulin. If hypertrophied areas result from nonrotation of injections, insulin absorption will be poor in these areas and may take months to fade. However, when parents and children use a plan for site rotation, insulin absorption problems can be minimized. Plans for site rotation are variable, although consistency is important. Some children will use arms in the morning, legs at dinner, and hips at night. Figure 9–2 is a general guide for site rotation.

Insulin pump therapy provides a continuous basal infusion of regular insulin with bolus infusion before meals and snacks. A small, soft needle is placed subcutaneously and is replaced every 48 to 72 hours. Insulin infusion pumps have become more widely accepted for use in adolescents and adults. Some centers are now using pump therapy successfully in children, as well. Infusion pumps have not been widely used in children because of the added responsibility of pump care, which many children are unable or unwilling to do. The regimen for those using a pump involves testing blood glucose levels at least four times a day and a 3 AM test once a week to prevent nocturnal hypoglycemia. One detriment to pump therapy in the past related to contact sports, when children could not easily remove the pump. However, there are now catheters that disconnect at or above the needle site, which makes it possible for pumps to be removed for short periods for sports, swimming, bathing, etc.

Nutrition Therapy

Nutrition is an important component of the treatment regimen. The principles of nutrition

Table 9–5 Commercially Available Insulin

Product	Manufacturer	Onset (hrs)	Peak (hrs)	Duration	Species
Rapid Acting					
Humulin R	Lilly	0.75	2	6	Human
Novolin R	Novo Nordisk	1/2	1/2/2–5	8	Human
Velosulin BR (Buffered Regular for insulin pump therapy)	Novo Nordisk	1/2	1–3	8	Human
Iletin I Regular	Lilly	1/2/2–1	2–4	6–8	Beef/Pork
Iletin II Regular	Lilly	1/2/2–1	2–4	6–8	Pork
Purified Pork R	Novo Nordisk	1/2	1/2/2–5	8	Pork
Humalog	Lilly	0.25	1–2	3–4	Human Analog
Intermediate Acting					
Humulin N	Lilly	3	6–7	13	Human
Novolin N	Novo Nordisk	1 1/2	4–12	24	Human
Iletin I (NPH)	Lilly	1–3	6–12	24	Beef/Pork
Iletin II (NPH)	Lilly	1–3	6–12	18–24	Pork
Purified Pork R	Novo Nordisk	1 1/2	4–12	24	Pork
Humulin L	Lilly	1–3	6–12	12–28	Human
Novolin L	Novo Nordisk	2 1/2	7–15	22	Human
Iletin I (Lente)	Lilly	1–3	6–12	12–28	Beef/Pork
Iletin II (Lente)	Lilly	1–3	6–12	12–28	Pork
Purified Pork L	Novo Nordisk	2 1/2	7–15	22	Pork
Long Acting					
Humulin U	Lilly	4–6	14–24	36	Human
Mixtures					
Humulin 50/50	Lilly	1/2–1	6–12	24	Human
Humulin 70/30	Lilly	1/2–1	6–12	24	Human
Novolin 70/30	Novo Nordisk	1 1/2	4–12	24	Human

therapy for children and adolescents differ from those for adults. Children commonly do not require weight control but need calories for growth and development (Betschart 1993). The goals of nutrition therapy are appropriate blood glucose and blood fat levels, reasonable weight, and good nutrition (American Diabetes Association 1996b).

Nutritional goals involve eating well-balanced meals with foods from all the food groups, reducing foods high in simple sugars, maintaining consistency in the timing of the meals and snacks, and maintaining consistency in the amount of food eaten at each meal and snack. There is currently a variety of regimens that are useful in managing diabetes in children

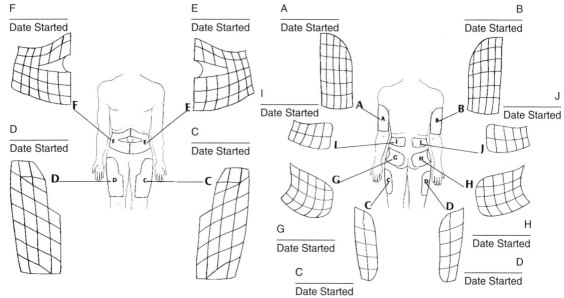

F _____ Date Started

E _____ Date Started

A _____ Date Started

B _____ Date Started

I _____ Date Started

J _____ Date Started

D _____ Date Started

C _____ Date Started

G _____ Date Started

H _____ Date Started

C _____ Date Started

D _____ Date Started

Injection Log

The BODY MAP is designed to help you record your insulin injections. Write down the date that you start an area. Place an X in the space on the map to show which site you used. One suggested pattern for using the map is to rotate your injections in one area for one week or until you have used each site in the area once. This system will help you rotate insulin injection sites over the 12 body areas and avoid using any one area or site too often.

Figure 9–2 Plan for site rotation. *Source:* Reprinted from the GETTING STARTED "Site Selection" brochure with permission of Becton Dickinson Consumer Products, Becton Dickinson and Company, Franklin Lakes, New Jersey, © 1985.

and adolescents. The traditional "exchange" diet (American Diabetes Association 1996b) continues to work well. In many instances, it is modified to account for carbohydrate intake and to make insulin adjustments accordingly. This is the principle behind the "carbohydrate counting" plan whereby the meals are planned according to the total carbohydrate content rather than by planning food groups. This method is useful in providing flexibility to meal planning and insulin therapy.

Most children older than six years require three meals a day plus snacks in midafternoon and at bedtime. Children younger than six years or who must go more than four or five hours between breakfast and lunch may require a morning snack. Meals and snacks are timed to correspond with the peak action of insulin. Therefore,

it is generally recommended that children and teens try not to deviate more than one hour from their normal schedules. The current recommendations from the American Diabetes Association (1996b) for adults are as follows:

1. Calories: Calories should be prescribed to achieve a desirable body weight.
2. Carbohydrates: The amount of carbohydrates should ideally be 55 to 60 percent of the total calories. The use of complex carbohydrates and foods high in fiber is recommended.
3. Protein: The recommended dietary allowance for protein is 0.08 gm/kg of body weight.
4. Total fat and cholesterol intake: The total fat and cholesterol intake should be re-

stricted, with the total fat intake less than 30 percent of the total calories and cholesterol intake less than 300 mg/day. Saturated fats should be replaced with unsaturated fats.

5. Alternative sweeteners: The use of sweeteners is acceptable.

6. Salt intake: The recommended sodium intake is 1,000 mg/100 kcal, not to exceed 3,000 mg/day.

7. Recent evidence shows that the use of sucrose as part of the meal plan does *not* impair blood glucose control in individuals with diabetes. Sucrose may be substituted for other carbohydrates and not simply added to the meal plan (American Diabetes Association 1996b). It has also been suggested that sweetened foods be added to a meal rather than eaten alone to prevent broad glycemic excursions.

Meal plans are individualized for the child and family. The meal plan provides a guide for food choices at meals and snacks. The types of meal planning used include the exchange meal plan; high-carbohydrate, high-fiber, low-fat meal plan; constant carbohydrate meal plan; and the glycemic index meal plan. It is important that parents or caregivers have a sound understanding of the meal plan. The child and/or adolescent with diabetes should see a dietitian at least annually to adjust calories and evaluate the meal plan.

Depending on the insulin regimen, children may require snacks throughout the day. Children younger than six years or those who experience a long time between breakfast and lunch usually require a morning snack (Betschart 1993). Most children also eat a midafternoon and bedtime snack to maintain appropriate blood glucose levels and prevent hyperglycemia. The timing of the snacks takes into account the peak action of the insulins and the periods of exercise.

Nutrition therapy is frequently the most difficult part of the diabetes regimen for parents. Trying to get young children to eat when they have taken insulin and are not hungry is a challenge and a worry. Fast foods, adolescent eating habits, and hectic schedules make food planning and preparation challenging for families. Home care nurses may be able to help parents plan, organize, and provide helpful hints to assist families in taking necessary steps. Supporting parents' efforts to make appropriate food adjustments around exercise, blood glucose numbers, and insulin regimens is an extremely important function.

Exercise

Exercise does not necessarily improve glycemic control, but it does have positive effects on cardiovascular fitness and long-term weight control, and enhances social interaction and esteem through team play. Adolescents with greater fitness have been shown to have greater insulin sensitivity (Arslanian et al. 1990).

In children with IDDM, the major glycemic concern of exercise is hypoglycemia. Preventing hypoglycemia is the goal of therapy for children who exercise. There can be an exercise effect on blood glucose that can last for many hours after the actual exercise. Additional carbohydrate with protein or fat may be eaten before activity. Sometimes it is preferred to use drinks such as Gatorade or fruit juice before, during, or after sports because of the difficulty of exercising with a full stomach. On specially active days, parents may be advised to test a blood glucose in the night to prevent nocturnal hypoglycemia. Parents may also be advised to supplement the bedtime snack with additional protein and fat on active days.

Injection of the pre-exercise insulin dose in a nonexercising area can be helpful to avoid hypoglycemia as insulin absorption is increased from exercising limbs. Adjustment of insulin dose and the use of supplemental carbohydrate-containing snacks may prevent exercise-induced hypoglycemia. Frequent monitoring of blood glucose levels should occur before, during, and after the exercise period to prevent hypoglycemia and to determine the efficiency of the insulin dose and the meal plan.

Monitoring

Self-Monitoring of Blood Glucose

Self-monitoring of blood glucose (SMBG) is essential to adequate management of diabetes. In 1986, the Consensus Development Conference on Self-Monitoring of Blood Glucose (American Diabetes Association 1987) recommended that blood glucose monitoring be used by all persons treated with insulin. In children, monitoring is especially necessary for the recognition and prevention of hypoglycemia in young children and/or those who cannot detect hypoglycemia themselves. Monitoring is also critical to decision making in the adjustments of food intake, insulin dosages, and exercise.

In general, it is recommended that blood glucose monitoring for children be done before each meal and bedtime snack, with additional tests if there are symptoms of hypoglycemia, hyperglycemia, ketosis, or illness (Betschart 1993). Occasional monitoring may also be recommended at 3 to 4 AM to detect a nocturnal drop in blood glucose or predawn increases in blood glucose due to the release of counterregulatory hormones (dawn phenomenon). It is especially important that parents test during the night if the child was hypoglycemic at bedtime or had an unusually active day.

Some children have difficulty monitoring before lunch for a variety of reasons, and therefore may sometimes not be required to do so. The decision to test regularly in school is based partially on the individual child's ability to cope with the monitoring situation, support from school personnel, perceived disruption to the classroom or schedule, and the child's willingness to do it.

The devices used for self-monitoring have become pocket-sized, portable, and easy to use. Lancets and lancing devices that are designed to give a blood sample have also become adjustable based on the child's or adult's skin thickness, finger size, and required sample size. Proper technique is required to achieve accurate results in blood glucose monitoring. It is essential to carefully follow manufacturer's instructions for performing SMBG to ensure accurate results. Inaccurate results can be due to insufficient blood sample size, expired strips, or wet fingers. Washing the hands with warm soapy water, milking the finger, and sticking the sides of the fingertips are techniques that result in increased blood flow. Adequate handwashing cleanses the finger of substances such as fruit juices that may lead to false high results.

Target ranges for blood glucose levels for children and adolescents must be individually determined. Generally speaking, however, target ranges might be 80 to 120 mg/dL at fasting and 80 to 180 mg/dL at other times of the day for children older than six years. For children youner than six years, goals may range from 90 to 200 mg/dL because of the concern that young children may have unrecognized hypoglycemia (Betschart 1993).

Periodic reassessment of monitoring technique is important. Problem areas frequently encountered include failure to obtain sufficient blood, not washing hands, wet fingers, and poor maintenance and care of the meter or strips. Children and adolescents will also at times fabricate results. One study showed that 40 percent of the children listed fabricated results and 18 percent failed to record some test results (Wilson and Endres 1986). It may be that the children's desire to please the parents and health care providers contributes to this problem. Results in the desired range frequently elicit praise whereas results in the hyperglycemia range far too often elicit accusations of "cheating" on the meal plan.

SMBG in and of itself will not affect diabetes control. The family and child must have knowledge of and guidelines for adjusting the treatment plan based on the results obtained. The guidelines for adjustment are individualized to reflect the insulin regimen, the specific meal plan, and the level of desired glycemic control.

Urine Testing

Although urine glucose testing does not accurately reflect the blood glucose level, it sometimes is a useful adjunct to blood glucose monitoring, especially when glycohemoglobin is high. Persistent glucosuria on first voided morning specimen can indicate nocturnal hyperglycemia, which may otherwise go undetected. Factors that influence the results include overall kidney function, volume of urine excreted, and medications such as ascorbic acid, penicillin, salicylates, cephalosporins, and chloral hydrate (Rotblatt and Koda-Kimble 1987). Hypoglycemia cannot be detected by urine glucose monitoring.

Urine ketone testing is an essential part of monitoring to detect ketosis and prevent diabetic ketoacidosis. Ketone testing should be done when blood glucose levels are above 240 and when the child is ill (Betschart 1993). Ketones may also be present in the urine after hypoglycemia. Detecting small amounts of ketones on initial voided specimens may help to detect nocturnal hypoglycemia.

Hypoglycemia Treatment

The risk of hypoglycemia can increase when near normoglycemia is achieved. Profound or prolonged hypoglycemia can result in neurologic impairment, seizures, or loss of consciousness. Early recognition of hypoglycemia and prompt treatment are important to prevent the progression of symptoms. Older children and adolescents most often recognize symptoms of hypoglycemia and take appropriate actions such as telling an available adult and eating something sweet.

Typical symptoms include shakiness, dizziness, hunger, drowsiness, fatigue, pallor, behavioral changes, headache, sweating, incoordination, and blurred vision. In young children, it is incumbent upon caregivers to recognize these symptoms. Infants and toddlers may show symptoms of extreme drowsiness, crying, irritability, and paleness.

If equipment is available, checking the blood glucose is important to confirm hypoglycemia before initiation of treatment. If equipment is unavailable, treatment should be initiated imme-

diately to prevent development of profound hypoglycemia.

The treatment includes the use of 10 to 15 g of a simple carbohydrate to cause a rapid increase in blood sugar followed by a protein or carbohydrate snack to prevent recurrent hypoglycemia. The goal is to increase the blood glucose level into the normal range. Generally, 10 to 15 g of carbohydrate are sufficient to treat hypoglycemia in children and young adolescents. A treatment plan for hypoglycemia in children is presented in Table 9–6. If symptoms of hypoglycemia do not improve in 10 to 15 minutes after treatment and blood glucose levels are not increasing, repeat the treatment (Siminerio and Betschart 1995).

The use of candy for treatment of hypoglycemia is not recommended in children because many children will eat it when it is not needed or a friend will eat it. In addition, some candy, such as chocolate, may not be effective in increasing blood glucose levels because of the proportional percentage of fat versus sugar. Candy can become a reward for being hypoglycemic. It is generally recommended that candy be fit into the diet in a more balanced way, such as at the end of a meal.

Glucagon is a hormone that, when injected, causes an increase in blood glucose by releasing glucose from glycogen stores in the liver. As the blood glucose level decreases to very low levels, the child may become combative, semiconscious, or have a seizure. A subcutaneous glucagon injection should be kept at a well-known place in the home or car to treat profound hypoglycemia. All parents and caregivers should learn to mix and inject glucagon and know to take it on vacations, long hikes, etc. It is generally recommended that children younger than six years receive 0.5 mg whereas children older than six years receive the full 1.0 mg. Nausea and vomiting may occur after administration of glucagon (Siminerio and Betschart 1995).

Prevention is the best treatment for hypoglycemia. A program of prevention includes eating meals and snacks on time, following the meal plan, and eating an extra snack when extra exer-

Table 9–6 Signs and Symptoms and Appropriate Treatment of Hypoglycemia

Signs and Symptoms	Treatment
Mild:	
Hunger	4–6 oz fruit juice
Dizziness	or
Shakiness	2–3 glucose tablets
Blurred vision	or
Drowsiness	½ can regular soda
Sweating	or
Headache	4–6 oz juice
Paleness	or
Irritability	2 teaspoons sugar
	or
	2 teaspoons honey
	Followed with a protein snack
Moderate:	
Behavioral changes such	15 g glucose gel by mouth
as lethargy, irritability	or
	icing or 4–6 oz juice or soda
	Follow with a protein snack/carbohydrate
	If symptoms persist and/or the child cannot or will not take by mouth, administer 0.5–1.0 mg glucagon
Severe:	
Seizure	0.5–1.0 mg glucagon intramuscularly or
Loss of consciousness	subcutaneously
Inability to eat, drink, or swallow	Followed with a protein/carbohydrate snack when child regains gag reflex

cise occurs. The rapid onset of hypoglycemia requires that parents, older children, and adolescents carry a readily available source of rapid-acting carbohydrate. Glucose tablets, gels, and juice boxes and crackers are convenient items. The wearing of a medical identification tag is also essential for emergency treatment.

Diabetic Ketoacidosis

The development of DKA in children with IDDM is a continual concern. Proper education and medical supervision can help avoid this complication. DKA can develop (1) if a child does not take insulin, (2) if a child does not take enough insulin, (3) if illness or infection is present, or (4) during periods of severe emotional stress. Signs of DKA include Kussmaul's breathing, sunken eyes, fruity/acetone breath, poor skin turgor, nausea, vomiting, and increasing sleepiness. As ketosis builds, ketones in the blood spill into the urine and are present on urine monitoring.

The following four guidelines should prevent the development of DKA with illness:

1. Never omit insulin. During illness, the dosage may need to be adjusted depending on the blood glucose level, the presence of ketones, and the ability to follow the meal plan.

2. Monitor the blood glucose and urine ketone levels every two to four hours.
3. Follow the meal plan if possible by substituting solid foods with equal amounts of carbohydrate liquids. If the child is vomiting or will not eat, provide foods high in carbohydrate, such as regular soda, Gatorade, regular Jell-O, and Popsicles.
4. Notify the physician when vomiting or ketones persist or when early signs of DKA are present (for example, abdominal pain, nausea, vomiting, Kussmaul's breathing, change in level of consciousness).

Nursing Care Plans in the Home

Potential for Knowledge Deficit Related to Initial and Continuing Education

Initial in-depth and ongoing education is crucial for children with diabetes, their families, and their caregivers. It is especially important for growing children to be followed carefully because, developmentally, different ages bring different diabetes-related concerns. Most children who are newly diagnosed have traditionally been hospitalized. However, in the current health care climate, there is increasingly a trend toward offering outpatient diabetes education. The setting for initial diabetes education can be the hospital, the outpatient area, or the home.

Assessment of the level of understanding, knowledge, and acceptance of diabetes is the initial step in the outpatient educational process. Initial education provides the child and family with basic information and skills needed for survival. Assessment of the health beliefs, cultural impact, social situation, lifestyle, and readiness to learn must be completed before an educational plan can be developed. The child's participation in diabetes education with age-appropriate material is essential and must be suitable for the child's developmental level. Individualization of the teaching plan based on the assessment is crucial for the success of diabetes education.

Ideally, the child should receive developmentally appropriate education and all family members and caregivers should also be educated. General behavioral objectives for the initial stage developed by the American Diabetes Association are listed in Exhibit 9–2 (Franz et al. 1986). Subsequently, continuing education provides the family with ongoing skills and knowledge needed to master self-sufficiency in daily management (see Table 9–7 and Exhibit 9–4).

The goal of the home health nurse should be to assist the child and family with understanding, flexibility, insight, motivation, and skills needed to make lifestyle changes. It is well known, however, in spite of best efforts, that it is difficult for many parents and children to learn well during acute illness and/or hospitalization. The shock of diagnosis and stress of the time can inhibit learning. The effectiveness of the education process may be diminished if sufficient time is not allowed for the child and family to work through the grief and turmoil experienced at diagnosis. Therefore, learning may actually be best in the home, in a more relaxed environment. Initial concepts can be reinforced at that time.

Play therapy using needle play is often helpful in assisting the child in adjusting to the treatment regimen. Children love to play with "safe" syringes, give shots to dolls or stuffed animals, or use figures to play out their concerns. Depending on the age of the child, a reinforcement system using stickers, hugs, and praise may be useful to help develop "sitting-still" behavior. For the older child, the stickers may be cashed in for special treats or special time with family members. The key is to reinforce appropriate sitting-still behavior while ignoring other behaviors. This system can also be used to encourage use of alternate injection sites.

The chronicity of diabetes and the ongoing nature of the education process make follow-up essential. Adjustments in the treatment regimen may be necessary as the child resumes a regular schedule of activities. Follow-up plans should

Table 9–7 Survival Skills Teaching Plan

Content Area	Specific Patient Objectives
Medication regimen	Able to prepare syringe for injection
	Able to inject self with insulin
	Able to state times for insulin or medication
Hyperglycemia/ketosis	Able to state signs and symptoms
	Knows when to call physician
	Knows reasons for hyperglycemia
Hypoglycemia	Able to state signs and symptoms
	Knows reasons for hypoglycemia
	Knows treatment for hypoglycemia
	Support person knows how to administer glucagon (IDDM)
Monitoring	Able to perform accurate self–blood glucose monitoring
	Able to test urine for ketones (IDDM)
	Can demonstrate how to record values in a daily log
Nutrition	Able to state correct meal plan
	Able to weigh or measure correct amounts of food
	Knows appropriate meal and snack times
Emergency information	Able to state how to reach physician or diabetes care team

Source: Reprinted from J. Betschart, Diabetes and Home Health Care: A Natural Combination, *Journal of Home Health Care Practice*, Vol. 4, No. 3, p. 5, © 1992, Aspen Publishers, Inc.

include return visits to the physician, dietitian, and nurse (see Tables 9–8 and 9–9).

School Issues

Because school-age children spend large portions of their days in school, it is reasonable to expect that school personnel become informed about diabetes care. Many children with diabetes feel different than their peers because of aspects of their treatment regimen. School personnel can help to minimize these differences and can be a valuable support to the family and diabetes regimen. Education of school personnel can decrease anxiety about diabetes and help to facilitate communication among parents, teachers, and the health care team.

The primary issue of importance for school personnel is an understanding of hypoglycemia recognition and treatment. The school nurse and teacher need information about the meal plan, the timing for the meals and snacks, how parties and special treats should be handled, the treat-

ment of hypoglycemia, and the monitoring of blood glucose and possibly urine ketone levels. The goal is to incorporate the diabetes treatment regimen into the school schedule so the child can participate in all activities. Under federal law, diabetes is considered a disability, and the school must evaluate and devise a plan of care for the child's special needs. The parents and school personnel should meet at the beginning of the school year to develop a plan that will fit diabetes care into the normal school schedule without much disruption and likewise meet the requirements of the diabetes regimen. Once this plan is established, there should be communication between the school and parents when there is a deviation from the plan, such as field trips or parties (see Chapter 19).

When possible, special treats can be incorporated into the child's regularly scheduled snacks or meal schedule. Parents may send alternative foods for special occasions such as diet soda, pretzels, plain cookies, or peanuts for days when

Exhibit 9–4 Essential Supplies

Medication Supplies

Enough stock of prescribed medications
Syringes (IDDM)
Magnifying glass (optional)

Monitoring Supplies

Monitoring device
Lancets
Strips appropriate to monitoring device
Urine test strips (IDDM)
Daily log

Hypoglycemia Treatment

Fruit juice or soda
Glucose tablets, sugar cubes, or cake icing
Crackers
Glucagon kit (1 mg)

Food Staples

Appropriate food groups
Sugar-free alternatives

Emergency Information

Physician or health care team telephone
   number
Support person telephone number

Source: Reprinted from J. Betschart, Diabetes and
Home Health Care: A Natural Combination, *Journal
of Home Health Care Practice,* Vol. 4, No. 3, p. 8,
© 1992, Aspen Publishers, Inc.

---

sweets or unplanned treats are served. Parents and children may also decide that it is acceptable to eat the usual treat. It is especially helpful if parties can be planned in advance because insulin doses may need to be adjusted on those days.

The administration of glucagon in school is variable according to state laws. However, upon physician's order, most schools designate a person to administer glucagon. In the absence of the school nurse, the designated person might be a secretary, another teacher, or willing volunteer.

Potential for Nonadherence as Related to Complexity of Treatment Plan

It is difficult for children and families to be consistent about their diabetes regimen. Some do well in some areas, such as taking medication and monitoring, yet struggle with food issues or recordkeeping. Patience, guidance, and promoting as much flexibility in the plan as possible will help to ensure that children and their families follow a specific treatment plan. The following factors have been associated with a lower adherence rate: a behavioral restriction or lifestyle change, a lengthy duration of treatment, no intermediate consequence from the nonadherence, and treatment behaviors required several times a day (Rapoff and Christophersen 1982). Some of the primary goals of home care are to assess, support, and promote adherence to the treatment plan. Chaotic home environments and chronic family stress can contribute to poorer metabolic control as a result of increased epinephrine responses or the frank omission of insulin (Betschart 1993).

The first step is to determine how fully the child and family are able to follow the treatment plan. Assessment tools include a self-report, observation of the child's and parents' behaviors as related to the treatment plan, and physical examination. To promote honesty in the self-report, health care providers should take a nonjudgmental approach. Interviewing the child and parent separately may also yield more accurate information because children may be more reluctant to share information in front of their parents. During the home visit, the nurse has an opportunity to observe the child's and parents' techniques in injections and monitoring. Education can be offered about the elements that need correction. Review of the child's record book can reveal information on the frequency of monitoring and the handling of problems. Today there are meters with memory to store day, date, time, and result, which make it much easier to retrieve and validate results.

Table 9–8 Long-term Management Teaching Plan

Content Area	Specific Patient Objectives
Medication regimen	Demonstrates how to rotate injection sites (IDDM)
	Knows properties of medications
	Knows how to adjust insulin based on blood glucose levels
Daily control	Knows how to balance medication, food, and exercise
Exercise	Can state reasons exercise is important
	Makes exercise part of routine management
	Knows how to prevent hypoglycemia during exercise
Complications	Sees ophthalmologist regularly
	Demonstrates how to examine feet
	Knows when to call physician for problems
	Knows potential complications such as impotency, neuropathy
Sickness	Knows to test urine for ketones (IDDM)
	Knows to take medication always, even when ill
	Knows to call physician for vomiting
	Knows diabetes control may go awry
Alcohol	Knows effects of drinking alcohol on blood glucose levels
	Knows to eat food when drinking
Medical identification	Wears some form of medical identification
Nutrition	Able to judge portion sizes
	Knows food groups
	Can make appropriate selections in restaurants

Source: Reprinted from J. Betschart, Diabetes and Home Health Care: A Natural Combination, *Journal of Home Health Care Practice,* Vol. 4, No. 3, p. 6, © 1992, Aspen Publishers, Inc.

Table 9–9 Teaching Plan for Nonessential Information

Content Area	Specific Patient Objectives
HbA$_{1c}$ (glycosylated hemoglobin)	Recognizes test as measuring average blood glucose control for preceding 2-month period
Travel	Knows to take extra supplies when traveling
	Knows to consult with health care team when traveling across time zones or out of the country
Etiology	States why diabetes may occur
Types	Identifies characteristics of NIDDM and IDDM
Pathophysiology	States the action of insulin in the body
	Understands effects of glucose levels on vessels
Stress	Understands the effect of physical and emotional stress on blood glucose levels
	Able to find and use a stress reduction method

Source: Reprinted from J. Betschart, Diabetes and Home Health Care: A Natural Combination, *Journal of Home Health Care Practice,* Vol. 4, No. 3, p. 6, © 1992, Aspen Publishers, Inc.

Several strategies can be used to promote adherence. One of the major causes of nonadherence is lack of understanding. Education should be selective, brief, and written. The child and parents should be involved in developing the treatment plan, and it should be tailored to the child's and family's characteristics. This includes developing a schedule for injections and meals, creating a meal plan around the family's food preferences, and choosing an exercise program that the child enjoys. Strategies for behavioral change should be based on goals that are specific and easily attainable. For example, if the child is not monitoring blood glucose levels four times daily, lowering the expectation to three times a day can promote more positive feelings about accomplishment. Meaningful rewards can be given after each improvement. The reward must be individually tailored and may include praise, material objects, money, or special time with a family member. It is important to reward the testing and not the blood glucose results. A behavioral contract is another technique that can be used. Contracting is a written agreement between the child and family and another person that clearly and specifically states the behavior to be changed and the reward to be provided for the specifically desired behavior. For example, Susan will check her blood glucose level before breakfast each day without being reminded to do so, and in return her mother will allow her to have a friend sleep over at the end of the week.

For children, adolescents, and families with complex emotional or behavioral problems, the primary health care provider should be notified. A referral may need to be made to a behaviorist, psychologist, psychiatrist, or therapist experienced in dealing with medical and behavioral problems.

Developmental Considerations

As in all chronic illness, there are developmental considerations of each age group that are impacted by the dynamics of diabetes. Children normally struggling with these normal developmental issues must also deal with the "overlay"

of diabetes issues. Sometimes this is when the child or teen "hits a sticking point." The challenge for parents is to fit diabetes care into the child's normal activities in a way that provides optimum diabetes control, emotional adjustment, and school performance. The difficult part is that many of the demands of diabetes care do not necessarily fit into normal developmental tasks for a child. For example, a child may not always feel like eating when it is time for meals and snacks. Learning to find a balance that makes the child content, does not create a family struggle, and takes care of diabetes concerns can become challenging.

It is common for parents and children to feel frustrated when they try hard to do all the right things, and diabetes control eludes them. Parents can feel frustrated trying to provide balanced and appropriate meals on time, making sure supplies are available, and feel trusting that caregivers know how to treat hypoglycemia.

Impact of Diabetes

Infant (Birth to Two Years)

An infant with diabetes should grow and develop normally. However, when an infant has diabetes, some of the normal developmental parts of infancy are affected by diabetes care. Infants may experience the following:

- need to sometimes eat or drink when they aren't hungry to keep blood glucose levels up
- require treatment for hypoglycemia with fast-acting glucose
- need to have blood glucose monitoring done frequently from a finger, toe, or heel stick
- need to have a feeding during the night
- occasionally need to be awakened to eat
- become dehydrated easily when blood glucose levels are high
- require responsible caregivers trained in diabetes management

Tips for Teaching.

- Because infants and young children cannot verbally communicate how they feel, one of the most important responsibilities of parents and caregivers is carefully observing their behavior and taking steps to protect them from extremes of high and low blood glucose levels.
- When an infant has low blood glucose and refuses food, sometimes sugar water, apple juice, or Kool-Aid is helpful. Sometimes cake decorator icing offered on the tip of the finger will help keep blood glucose levels up. Add cereal and, after six months, egg yolk, cottage cheese, plain yogurt, or meat to the late-night feeding to help keep blood glucose levels up at night.
- If the infant is breast fed, the mother can pump the breasts and store the milk so that the infant will not have calorie differences between formula and breast milk, and take milk easily.
- When choosing a meter, consider accuracy, ease of use for testing an infant, and blood sample size as factors in making your decision. Generally, for an infant, portability and amount of blood required are the most important considerations.
- Perform fingersticks with prickers or lancets that have adjustable depth penetration. You will need enough blood to accurately test, but use the least deep device possible. Acceptable sites are fingers, toes, earlobes, and the outer side of the heel.
- Inject insulin into the legs, arms, and upper-outer quadrant of the buttocks in an infant. Afterward, give the infant extra soothing or play for a few minutes.
- Use a disposable diaper liner to absorb urine to test urine for sugar and ketones. A urine test strip pressed into the diaper liner will work, or you can pull out the wet stuffing and put it inside a large syringe to "plunge" out a drop or two to test. The silica gel in regular disposable diapers is too absorbent to provide urine for testing.

- Call the physician or health care provider for help at the first signs of illness, vomiting, or diarrhea. Blood glucose and urine ketones will need to be monitored more frequently during an illness. Dehydration can easily occur and will need to be prevented. Signs of dehydration are little or no urine; dry, cracked lips and mucous membranes; sunken eyes; and poor skin turgor. Give the infant fluids with glucose such as juice, Pedialyte, or Jell-O water to prevent dehydration.

Toddler (Two to Three Years Old) and Preschool (Three to Five Years Old)

Many of the issues of infants with diabetes still apply to these age groups. Hypoglycemia remains the number one concern as children frequently become either poor or picky eaters and have unpredictable bursts of activity. Constant surveillance is essential for general safety and observation of signs of hypoglycemia. Parents and caregivers must be prepared to treat with juice, crackers, or whatever the child will take.

Minimizing the trauma of injections and fingersticks by doing them quickly and matter-of-factly can be helpful. Band-Aids are important for feelings of body intactness. Letting the child participate in the process will help him or her to feel that he or she has some control over it. Let the child know he or she was brave and/or did a great job holding still. Children do not understand why they must have these procedures done. Reinforcing the explanation that these procedures are important to keep them well is important.

Parents' sleep may be disrupted because they are either listening for their toddlers or treating their toddlers' hypoglycemia at night. The demands of toddlerhood are exhausting enough, then add the extra issues of the diabetes regimen, and parents can become weary. Sometimes it is also difficult to find a mature, reliable babysitter who is competent and comfortable in dealing with diabetes. However, it is extremely important for parents to find help so they can have a night out alone or time to themselves.

Tips for Teaching.

- Fingersticks and injections are "nonnegotiable." However, children do need reasonable time to prepare themselves. Suprising a child with procedures or performing them while the child is asleep can cause a child to be suspicious and afraid that he or she may be poked at any time. Hugs do wonders to console a child after a prick or injection. Invest in a supply of colored, "fun" Band-Aids.
- Keep as much to a regular schedule as possible. Try to maintain a cheerful, fun-loving, well-organized daily routine.
- Many children age three years and older can identify feelings of hypoglycemia. Talk with the child after an episode of hypoglycemia to help him or her pick up symptoms himself or herself. Ask if he or she was feeling hungry, shaky, sweaty, dizzy, tired, or had a headache.
- Working with a health care provider can help to match the insulin regimen to the way the child naturally eats. You may need to add or subtract snack foods, or change meal times somewhat. For example, if the child is a "poor breakfast eater" but will eat a hardy dinner, his or her insulin regimen can be adjusted accordingly.
- Parents who share caretaking tasks of diabetes prevent one parent from feeling overburdened from always being the "bad guy."
- Begin teaching children that if they feel signs of low blood glucose that they need to tell someone and to eat something sweet.
- When in preschool or day care, the staff will need to be educated about the signs, symptoms, and treatment for hypoglycemia and know how to treat it.
- If a young child becomes picky or refuses to eat or drink when hypoglycemic, sometimes getting the child to eat something small and "fun," such as a few M&M's, will increase blood glucose enough so that the child will cooperate and eat or drink juice, milk, or a cookie.
- If parents work, make certain that the babysitter, day care center, or preschool has adequate supplies, such as appropriate snacks, juice, and crackers, for hypoglycemia treatment and glucagon.
- Avoid battles involving the child saying "no" when possible. Provide acceptable choices. Do not ask, "Do you want your fingerstick now?" Instead, ask, "Shall we poke this finger or that one for your fingerstick?"
- Provide praise and reinforcement for "holding still," picking the injection spot, being brave, etc. Provide hugs and smiles for cooperative behavior. Hold child firmly in a bear hug, if necessary, restraining him or her for injections, discouraging temper tantrums or negative behavior until the child regains control. Loss of control is frightening for a child.
- Provide a quiet, gentle, consistent environment.
- Set limits; do not give in to unreasonable requests.

School-Age Children

Although concerns about hypoglycemia and hyperglycemia are still present, one of the primary issues of this age group is that of feeling "different" from peers. Parents and others try hard to balance blood glucose control with emotional aspects of the disease. Feeling or being different from everyone is of primary importance to many children with diabetes. For a child who must eat when everyone else is not, or shouldn't eat when everyone else is, or who eats crackers when others eat cupcakes, diabetes can be a problem. Other feelings of difference come into play with blood glucose monitoring and injections, especially during social gatherings such as "sleep-overs."

Parents, schoolteachers, and others who are sensitive to the issues can help to minimize the problem. Offering everyone a healthy snack food instead of cupcakes, or giving the child a private place to test blood and take an injection can help.

Frequently, friends and others will take on the attitude of the child himself or herself. Those who are open and matter-of-fact about their diabetes will usually have friends who respond in the same way. However, children who are embarrassed, sensitive, or desire privacy about their diabetes care should have their wishes for dealing with diabetes respected. They may eventually become more open as they are reassured that diabetes should not alter their friendships or activities.

Tips for Teaching.

- Help parents be organized and prepared. Keep plenty of snack foods that are portable to stock backpacks, school nurse office, gym teacher's supplies, etc. Juice boxes and crackers go everywhere!
- Ask to see the school lunch menu monthly. If the child buys lunch at school, discuss which foods are appropriate to eat and in what quantity, and arrange to replace inappropriate foods with others. Most schools will provide skim milk, fresh fruit, or juice when asked.
- Purchase an inexpensive extra glucose meter for the child to take to school or keep in the nurse's office. This avoids the child having to carry his or her only meter and the chance of breakage or loss of the only meter.
- Arrange a conference with all school staff involved. This may include the cafeteria worker, teacher, nurse, principal, playground aide, and bus driver. There should be a plan arranged for treating hypoglycemia, and everyone should know where supplies are kept. Decide who might be able to give a glucagon injection if necessary (see Chapter 19).
- Share the responsibility of diabetes care. Encourage the child to be independent in his or her care and to learn how to care for himself or herself. But, let the child know that you will be there to help, support, and supervise. Children are not developmentally able to take complete and responsible care of their diabetes. A parent or reliable caregiver should help the child oversee, write down numbers, supervise fingersticks, or double-check injections.
- When attending a party or special occasion, decide ahead of time how you will handle it. Sometimes your child may want to eat cake and ice cream with everyone else, and it may be "OK" for him or her to have only the ice cream, or something completely different. Make sure there are sugar-free beverages available.
- Work out a system of communication for blood glucose numbers and an arrangement for insulin injections if your child wants to sleep overnight at a friend's house. Inform other parents of your child's routine, any special needs, and how to treat a low blood glucose if it should occur.
- Consider diabetes camp as a way for your child to have fun, meet other children with diabetes, and have a safe camping experience. Many camps have educational programs that help children learn about their diabetes.

Adolescent Children

Children of this age can often manage their own diabetes regimen with guidance and supervision. They can accurately measure and inject insulin, do blood tests, and keep records. The issue is usually not one of capability, but taking the time and having the interest to care for diabetes. Children of this age will still look toward the power and protection of the parent, but not nearly to the degree as younger children. As children struggle for independence, they sometimes take two steps forward and one back. Sometimes they do well with managing things themselves; at other times they do not.

Many teens become busy in early adolescence with sports and activities. Even when they are not busy with structured activities they are still "busy." Diabetes tasks seldom fit easily into the child's schedule. It's not on their minds, even when they are reminded. The challenge can be getting the teen to do the things he or she needs to do to take care of himself or herself.

Managing diabetes around afternoon and evening sports or other activities can be challenging. The teen should be encouraged to do those activities he or she enjoys even if the scheduling does not necessarily fit into the diabetes plan. A diabetes nurse educator or dietitian can help devise a workable solution.

Diabetes also becomes a reminder that the teen is different from everyone else at a time when he or she is trying hard to be just like everyone else. "Blending in" becomes a priority. And the effect of diabetes on body image can be a concern to the teen who worries about arms and legs showing lumps or bumps, or black-and-blue marks.

Many teens, however, are capable and conscientious regarding their diabetes tasks. Others see diabetes as a nuisance and can be reluctant to partake in self-care activities if they cannot see an immediate benefit. They may intellectually know the advantages but have great trouble taking positive steps today because it will benefit them sometime later. This concept of delayed gratification is a mark of maturity and may improve over time.

Tips for Teaching.

- Help the teen to learn problem-solving skills regarding diabetes concerns. Sometimes teens can be creative with their solutions. For example, you might ask, "So, how do you suggest you work your insulin and dinner in with a 4 to 7 PM game?" You may need to say, "That solution of skipping dinner and insulin is unacceptable . . . try again." This gives the teen some control over the situation, but is still guided by the parent in his or her choices.

- Find medical identification that the teen will wear. These come in all shapes and sizes; in bracelets, necklaces, or ankle chains; and in stainless steel, gold, silver, or colorful stretch nylon.

- When possible, don't let diabetes issues be a focal point for an argument. Try to change the point of conflict to a nondiabetes issue such as makeup, homework, curfew, etc. The teen may then not use diabetes as an issue to test the system.

- Remain as firm and consistent as possible.

- Continue to provide hugs, praise, smiles, and pleasure for jobs well done.

- Give the teen the opportunity for some responsibility. Establish a trusting relationship.

- Consider diabetes camp as an excellent resource.

- Keeping surveillance and friendly interest in diabetes control helps teens focus on the tasks at hand. Knowing someone is watching, caring, and keeping them accountable can help them stay on target.

- Motivate teens with positive statements. Using threats or scare tactics to encourage teens to test or eat healthy foods rarely works and often backfires.

- Stressing the importance of diabetes control to athletic performance can help to motivate athletes to care for themselves.

- The privilege of driving should not be taken lightly. Teens who refuse to test or are irresponsible about their diabetes control should have driving privileges reconsidered.

- Encourage the teen to develop a good rapport with a health professional with whom he or she can openly discuss diabetes management, concerns, and questions.

REFERENCES

American Diabetes Association. 1987. Consensus statement on self-monitoring of blood glucose. *Diabetes Care.* 10:95–99.

American Diabetes Association. 1996a. Position statement on "Implications of the Diabetes Control and Complications Trial." *Diabetes Care* 19, suppl. 1:S50–02.

American Diabetes Association. 1996b. Nutritional recommendations and principles for individuals with diabetes mellitus. *Diabetes Care* 19, suppl. 1:S16–19.

Arslanian S., et al. 1990. Impact of physical fitness and glycemic control on in vivo insulin action in adolescents with IDDM. *Diabetes Care* 13:9–15.

Betschart, J. 1993. Childhood and adolescence. In *A core curriculum for diabetes education,* 2d ed., ed. V. Peragallo-Dittko, 447–75. Chicago: American Association of Diabetes Educators and the AADE Education and Research Foundation.

Blizzard, R., and A. Johanson. 1994. Disorders of growth. In *The diagnosis and treatment of endocrine disorders in childhood and adolescence,* ed. E. Wilkins, 404. Springfield, Ill.: Charles C Thomas.

Chase, H.P., et al. 1983–85. Techniques for improving glucose control in Type I diabetes. *Pediatrician.* 12: 229–35.

Dallas, J.S., and T.P. Foley. 1996. Hypothyroidism. In *Pediatric endocrinology*, 3d ed., ed., P. Lifshitz, 391–99. New York: Marcel Dekker.

Drash, A. 1990. Management of the child with diabetes mellitus: clinical course, therapeutic strategies, and monitoring techniques. In *Pediatric endocrinology: A clinical guide*, 2d ed., ed. F. Lifshitz, 681–700. New York: Marcel Dekker.

Drash, A.L. 1986. Diabetic mellitus in the child and adolescent: I. *Current Problems in Pediatrics.* 16:413–66.

Fishbein, H., and B.E. Klein. 1995. Acute metabolic complications in diabetes. In *Diabetes in America.* 2d ed., ed. M.I. Harris, et al, 283–92. Bethesda, Md: National Institutes of Health, National Institute of Diabetes and Digestive and Kidney Diseases.

Fisher, D.A. 1994. Hypothyroidism. *Pediatrics in Review* 15(6): 227–32.

Franz, M., et al. 1986. *Goals for diabetes education.* New York: American Diabetes Association.

LaPorte, R.E., M. Matsushima, and V.F. Chang. 1995. Prevalence and incidence of insulin-dependent diabetes. In *Diabetes in America,* 2d ed., ed. M.I. Harris, et al, 37–46. Bethesda, Md: National Institutes of Health, National Institute of Diabetes and Digestive and Kidney Diseases.

McGee, B., D. Howie, and J. Dice. 1994. *Pediatric drug therapy handbook & formulary 1995–6.* Hudson, Ohio: Lexi-comp, Inc.

Migeon, C.I., and R. Lanes. 1985. Adrenal cortex: Hypo- and hyper-function. In *Pediatric endocrinology,* ed. P. Lifshitz. New York: Marcel Dekker.

New, M.I., S. Pang, and L.S. Levine. 1985. An update of congenital adrenal hyperplasia. In *Pediatric endocrinology,* ed. P. Lifshitz. New York: Marcel Dekker.

Perheentupa, J., and P. Czernichow. 1994. Water regulation and its disorders. In *The diagnosis and treatment of endocrine disorders in childhood and adolescence,* ed. E. Wilkins, 1106–19. Springfield, Ill.: Charles C Thomas.

Rapoff, M.A., and E.R. Christophersen. 1982. Compliance of pediatric patients with medical regimens. In *Adherence, compliance and generalization in behavioral medicine,* ed. R.B. Stuart. New York: Brunner/Mazel, Inc.

Rees-Jones, R.W., A.R. Rolla, and P.R. Larsen. 1980. Hormone content of thyroid replacement preparations. *JAMA* 243:549.

Rotblatt, M.D., and M.A. Koda-Kimble. 1987. Review of drug interference with urine glucose. *Diabetes Care* 10:103–10.

Siminerio, L., and J. Betschart. 1995. *Raising a child with diabetes.* Alexandria, Va.: American Diabetes Associaton.

Wilson, D.P., and R.K. Endres. 1986. Compliance with blood glucose monitoring in children with Type I diabetes mellitus. *Journal of Pediatrics.* 108:1022–24.

BIBLIOGRAPHY

Koivosto, V.A., and P. Felig. 1980. Alterations in insulin absorption and in blood glucose control associated with varying insulin injection sites in diabetic patients. *Annals of Internal Medicine.* 92:59–61.

CHAPTER 10

Alterations in Renal Function

Janice C. Krueger

Before 1960, end-stage renal disease (ESRD) was uniformly fatal for both children and adults. Significant advances in technology, pharmacology, and immunology as well as the provision of Medicare coverage, regardless of the patient's age, have greatly improved life expectancy. Hundreds of thousands of patients, including children, have been able to receive renal replacement therapies (dialysis and transplantation) (National Institutes of Health 1993). However, these same advances in medical technology and the need for hospital cost containment have resulted in more complex care being done in the home. The burden of care for families of children with ESRD can be overwhelming, especially when it involves home dialysis, supplemental feeding, and the administration of recombinant human erythropoietin and/or recombinant human growth hormone. Referral for various home care services and other strategies to reduce stress and provide respite care are often necessary. This chapter focuses on the home care requirements and nursing considerations for children with chronic renal failure and ESRD.

ACUTE RENAL FAILURE

Acute renal failure is an abrupt reduction in renal function to a level insufficient to maintain homeostasis, resulting in the retention of nitrogenous wastes. The etiologies of acute renal failure are conventionally classified as prerenal, in-trinsic renal, and postrenal. Prerenal causes result from diminished renal perfusion, which may occur with severe dehydration, hemorrhage, septic shock, burns, and major trauma. Prompt correction of renal hypoperfusion by increasing the intravascular volume or cardiac output immediately returns function to normal (Feld, Springate, and Fildes 1986). Intrinsic renal causes include acute renal parenchymal disorders such as acute glomerulonephritis, hemolytic uremic syndrome, nephrotoxicity, and bilateral renal vein thrombosis. Repeated or prolonged ischemic insults may also lead to intrinsic renal failure and result in permanent damage. Postrenal causes result from the obstruction of urine flow by blood clots, stones, or tumor. To cause acute renal failure, the blockage must involve both kidneys.

Children with acute renal failure usually appear very ill. The kidneys abruptly cease to function, and the body does not have time to adapt. The manifestations of acute renal failure can be life-threatening and can affect every organ system. The child may present with decreased urinary output, hypertension, peripheral/pulmonary edema, anorexia and vomiting, cardiac arrhythmias, changes in mental status, and/or seizures. Laboratory studies may reveal marked azotemia, elevated serum creatinine, anemia, metabolic acidosis, hyperkalemia, hyperphosphatemia, and/or hypocalcemia.

In general, the management of acute renal failure is focused on supportive care and prevention. The goals of therapy are to support the child until the kidneys can recover from the acute insult and to prevent further kidney tissue damage. Depending on the cause and severity of the disease, the treatment regimen may include a variety of medications, nutritional support, blood products, and/or renal replacement therapy (acute dialysis or continuous hemofiltration).

The prognosis of acute renal failure varies with the cause and severity of the disease. As described by Feld, Springate, and Fildes (1986, 401), "renal failure is a potentially fatal, yet often reversible process demanding prompt and accurate diagnosis and meticulous attention to a wide variety of predictable and preventable complications." Most children with acute renal failure remain in the hospital until they no longer require dialysis. Although they may recover completely, they may be discharged to home with some degree of renal insufficiency, requiring medication, dietary restriction, and close follow-up. However, some children may not recover and may require long-term dialysis and transplantation.

CHRONIC RENAL FAILURE

The development of chronic renal failure is usually characterized as a relatively slow (over months to years) insidious process resulting in permanent and irreversible damage to both kidneys. It is usually defined as a reduction in kidney function to below 25 percent of normal (Foreman and Chan 1988). Recognition may be difficult because the early symptoms are often vague and nonspecific, such as lethargy, fatigue, headaches, anorexia, and nausea. However, chronic renal failure should be considered in any child who presents with anemia, hypertension, edema, or growth failure (Foreman and Chan 1988). The term chronic renal insufficiency is used to describe a reduction in kidney function from 50 to 25 percent of normal. These children may be completely asymptomatic except for mild azotemia and a slightly elevated serum creatinine. Chronic renal insufficiency almost always progresses to renal failure (Foreman and Chan 1988).

The incidence of chronic renal failure in children is not clearly known. Available data are based on the number of children accepted into dialysis/transplant programs (Harmon 1995; Gusmano and Perfumo 1993). These data do not address those children who receive only conservative management and those children who do not reach end stage until adulthood. According to Harmon (1995), the most recent data available from the United States Renal Data System (USRDS) and the North American Pediatric Renal Transplant Cooperative Study (NAPRTCS) suggest that approximately 2,500 children younger than 20 years begin treatment for chronic renal failure in the United States annually. Of these, approximately 100 children are younger than 2 years.

Based on data from USRDS and NAPRTCS, the diseases that cause ESRD in children differ significantly from those that cause ESRD in adults (Harmon 1995). Leading causes of chronic renal failure in young children include congenital abnormalities of the urinary tract (for example, posterior urethral valves, reflux nephropathy, dysplasia) and other inherited disorders (for example, cystic disease). Older children have a higher incidence of glomerular disease. In contrast to adults, virtually no children develop ESRD secondary to diabetes or hypertension (Harmon 1995).

Similar to acute renal failure, the manifestations of chronic renal failure can affect every organ system. Classic symptoms include fluid retention, hypertension, metabolic acidosis, anemia, and anorexia. Children with chronic renal insufficiency secondary to congenital obstructive uropathies and cystic diseases usually present with polyuria and may have severe salt wasting (Kohaut 1995). These children do not usually have difficulty with fluid retention or hyperkalemia until they approach end stage. In contrast, anemia is a predictable consequence of chronic renal failure, regardless of the underlying cause of the disease. The primary cause of anemia is decreased erythropoietin synthesis by the failing kidneys (Jabs and Harmon 1996). In addition, the life span of the red blood cell is reduced as a result of intestinal oozing and hemolysis (Jabs and Harmon 1996).

As their disease progresses, children with chronic renal insufficiency often develop renal osteodystrophy, a complex bone disease that features secondary hyperparathyroidism and a variety of bone deformities (Kohaut 1995). Renal osteodystrophy results from decreased excretion of phosphate by the kidney, bone demineralization due to the presence of parathyroid hormone, and the inability of the kidney to produce the active metabolite of vitamin D.

Growth retardation is a serious problem for children with chronic renal failure. Factors associated with growth failure in these children include anorexia and malnutrition, acidosis, renal osteodystrophy, anemia, sodium wasting, early onset of chronic renal insufficiency, and unresponsiveness to normal levels of growth hormone (Tönshoff and Fine 1996; Kohaut 1995; Wise and Case 1994). Issues related to growth retardation are increasingly emphasized because these children are now surviving to adulthood and because peritoneal dialysis and successful transplantation have not consistently been associated with significant catch-up growth (Kohaut 1995; Grimm and Ettenger 1992).

There is also evidence that chronic renal failure in children, particularly neonates, is associated with neurologic, cognitive, and psychosocial developmental delays. However, the prevalence and the factors associated with these delays are unclear. Future research should systematically study the relationships among a variety of developmental variables (for example, motor, language, social) and disease-related variables (for example, age of onset and duration of ESRD, treatment modality) (Frauman and Myers 1994).

Conservative Management

Conservative management is the first step in the treatment of chronic renal failure. In general,

it refers to the use of medications and dietary therapeutics to treat the manifestations of renal failure before the initiation of dialysis. The goals of conservative management are outlined in Exhibit 10–1. Even at this stage, the home care regimen can be extremely demanding and stressful for the child and the family. It may involve multiple oral medications, daily subcutaneous injections, dietary restrictions, and/or supplemental feeding. To achieve the optimal outcome for the child and family, it is important to use a multidisciplinary approach to care and to assist the family in developing appropriate support systems in the community (for example, local pediatrician, home health services, developmental evaluation clinic, school, support groups, mental health clinic).

Nutrition is the cornerstone in the management of chronic renal failure in children. The goal is to optimize growth and development while preventing or treating biochemical abnormalities (Harvey et al. 1996). However, adequate nutrition for growth may be difficult to achieve in the face of anorexia and difficult dietary restrictions. Dietary modifications are often used to prevent severe azotemia and hyperkalemia, to help control hypertension, and to prevent bone disease. Consequently, protein, potassium, sodium, fluid, and/or phosphorus may need to be restricted, while maintaining adequate protein and calorie intake for growth and development.

Exhibit 10–1 Goals of Conservative Management

- Encourage normal growth and development.
- Maintain normal electrolyte and water balance.
- Control anemia.
- Control metabolic acidosis.
- Control hypertension.
- Prevent bone disease.
- Prevent infection.
- Avoid nephrotoxins.

The dietary prescription must be tailored to the specific needs of the child. For example, some children may need a salt restriction to help control hypertension and edema, whereas others may require salt supplementation because of urinary salt wasting. Changes in nutritional status, progression of disease, and/or the initiation of dialysis may alter dietary requirements. Children who previously required a protein restriction may have significant protein losses in the dialysate after starting peritoneal dialysis, resulting in increased dietary protein requirements (Harvey et al. 1996).

Serial assessments of physical growth (weight, length/height, head circumference if three years old or younger), anthropometric measurements, dietary intake, gastrointestinal function, biochemical values, blood pressure, fluid status, and level of activity help determine nutritional status and dietary requirements (Harvey et al. 1996). Based on these assessments, the clinical dietitian can make recommendations for needed dietary changes. These recommendations should be communicated to the multidisciplinary team. The child, family, and team can then formulate a plan for achieving the requirements. The ability of the child and family to adhere to the plan and the palatability of the dietary prescription must be considered.

The plan should be communicated to all caregivers, including extended family members, teachers, day care workers, and other health care providers. Caregivers may require education related to appropriate food and fluid choices (for example, avoidance of high-potassium, high-sodium, or high-phosphorus foods and fluids). The child may be able to have certain foods and fluids in only limited amounts. Favorite foods, which are normally restricted, can often be allowed as treats (for example, one slice of pizza per week). Caregivers may also need guidance on how to maintain a fluid restriction (for example, measuring, dispensing, and recording fluid intake over 24 hours). It is important to teach caregivers that anything that is liquid at room temperature (for example, Jell-O, Popsicles, and ice) or that contains a lot of fluid

(for example, soup and melon) must be included in the fluid restriction. It is also important to use a familiar unit of measure (for example, ounces and cups). If the family has a scale, it can be taught to monitor fluid status based on changes in the child's weight. The family member who buys groceries and cooks may need education related to food preparation, evaluation and modification of recipes, and reading food labels.

Supplemental tube feedings (via nasogastric tube, gastrostomy tube, gastrostomy button, or duodenal tube) have been used successfully to improve growth and nutritional status. The formula selection and amount to be administered are dependent upon the specific needs of the child (see Chapter 8). There are several commercially available preparations, designed specifically for renal patients (with low protein, sodium, potassium, and phosphorus content). Although infants may require supplementation throughout the day, older children should be given continuous overnight feeding via a pump to allow for the development of an appetite during the day. It is often useful to involve a "feeding specialist" (for example, occupational therapist and/or psychologist) to help deal with oral sensitivity and food refusal.

Medications are also essential in the treatment of the manifestations of chronic renal failure in children. The types of medications and their indications are listed in Table 10–1. Optimal treatment often requires fine tuning of the dietary prescription and the medication regimen so that they complement each other. For example, the control of hypertension may require a combination of salt and fluid restriction, antihypertensives, and/or diuretics.

Similarly, the prevention and treatment of bone disease require dietary modification as well as medication. As the kidneys fail, they lose the ability to excrete phosphorus, leading to hyperphosphatemia and hypocalcemia. Hyperphosphatemia is treated with dietary phosphorus restriction and phosphate binders. The preferred binders are calcium carbonate, calcium citrate, and calcium acetate (Sanchez and Salusky 1996). They bind phosphorus in the intestine,

Table 10–1 Medications Used To Treat Chronic Renal Failure

Medications	Indications
Oral alkali preparations	Metabolic acidosis
Phosphate binders	Hyperphosphatemia, hypocalcemia, prevention and treatment of bone disease
Vitamin D preparations	Secondary hyper-parathyroidism, prevention and treatment of bone disease
Recombinant human growth hormone (rhGH)	Growth retardation
Recombinant human erythropoietin (rHuEPO)	Anemia
Iron supplements	Iron deficiency, rHuEPO therapy
Antihypertensives	Hypertension

which is excreted in the stool, and they provide supplemental calcium. For optimal effect, phosphate binders need to be taken with meals. Dosage varies from patient to patient and is adjusted according to serum phosphorus and calcium levels. Some patients and families can be taught to adjust the dosing so that the child takes more binder with big meals and less binder with small meals and snacks. It is also important that patients and families understand that other antacids cannot be substituted for these preparations. Many antacids contain magnesium or aluminum, which may be toxic for the child with chronic renal failure.

Vitamin D therapy is used to treat secondary hyperparathyroidism, as evidenced by persis-tently elevated parathyroid hormone (PTH) levels. Commonly used vitamin D preparations include calcitriol and dihydrotachysterol. The exact cause of secondary hyperparathyroidism is not clear. It may be related to a direct effect of hyperphosphatemia on PTH secretion, the accompanying hypocalcemia, or alterations in vitamin D synthesis (Sanchez and Salusky 1996). Poorly controlled secondary hyperparathyroidism results in parathyroid gland hyperplasia, which may necessitate surgical intervention.

As previously mentioned, growth retardation is a serious problem for children with chronic renal failure, and the pathogenesis is multifactorial. Despite the provision of adequate nutrition and the aggressive treatment of acidosis, renal osteodystrophy, and anemia, these children have continued to experience significant growth delays. There is now strong evidence that recombinant human growth hormone (rhGH) is a safe, efficacious, and well-tolerated treatment for growth retardation in this population (Tönshoff and Fine 1996; Kohaut 1995). Children with chronic renal failure are not growth hormone deficient, but they appear to need supraphysiologic doses of rhGH (0.05 mg/kg/day) to grow (Tönshoff and Fine 1996). The major side effect seems to be resistance to insulin. However, patients with chronic renal failure treated with rhGH have not developed overt diabetes (Tönshoff and Fine 1996). Recombinant human growth hormone is approved for use in patients with chronic renal failure (predialysis) and patients with ESRD (requiring dialysis). Although there is evidence that rhGH therapy may also improve growth velocity after transplantation, it may be associated with increased rejection and graft loss (Tönshoff and Fine 1996; Kohaut 1995).

Growth hormone therapy is intended for long-term (months to years) use in the home. The recommended length of therapy is controversial (Tönshoff and Fine 1996). Most children are treated with daily subcutaneous injections. Nursing responsibilities are focused on patient and family education, emotional support, and assistance with monitoring the response to therapy. Education should include aseptic technique, reconstitution procedures, storage of the reconstituted drug, injection techniques, and site rotation. Various teaching aids are available, including some from the manufacturer. Older children are often capable of performing self-injection. If a family member is taught to administer the injections, the child should be involved in the education process at an age-appropriate level and given an assigned task to help (Wise and Case 1994). Emotional support is important because waiting for a positive response to therapy can be frustrating (Wise and Case 1994). Children receiving growth hormone therapy require close follow-up to monitor for adverse effects and response to therapy.

Another important advance in the therapeutic regimen for children with chronic renal failure is the use of recombinant human erythropoietin (rHuEPO) for the treatment of anemia. Before the development of rHuEPO, children with chronic renal failure and ESRD were transfusion dependent. Complications of repeated transfusions included iron overload, transmission of infectious agents (for example, hepatitis viruses, cytomegalovirus, human immunodeficiency viruses) and sensitization to foreign human leukocyte antigens (HLAs) (Jabs and Harmon 1996). Repeated exposure to foreign HLA antigens is associated with longer waiting times for cadaveric kidneys and decreased graft survival after the transplant (Jabs and Harmon 1996). Recombinant human erythropoietin therapy consistently improves anemia, eliminates the need for blood transfusions, increases exercise tolerance and appetite, and decreases ventricular hypertrophy and uremic coagulopathy (Jabs and Harmon 1996). Iron deficiency limits the effectiveness of rHuEPO therapy; therefore, iron stores should be assessed before starting rHuEPO and monitored regularly throughout therapy. Hypertension that requires additional antihypertensive medication is the most significant side effect of rHuEPO (Jabs and Harmon 1996).

Recombinant human erythropoietin may be administered intravenously, subcutaneously, or intraperitoneally. The recommended starting dose is 50 to 100 u/kg three times a week. The maintenance dose must be individualized to maintain the hematocrit between 30 and 35 percent. The drug is supplied in single-dose, 1-mL vials containing either 2,000 u, 3,000 u, 4,000 u, or 10,000 u. Most children with chronic renal failure receive one to three 1-mL subcutaneous injections per week.

Similar to rhGH, nursing responsibilities for rHuEPO are focused on education, monitoring for side effects and response to therapy, and providing emotional support. In addition to injection techniques, site rotation, and drug storage, the family should be taught to monitor the child's blood pressure. It should be taught to keep a blood pressure record and be given specific guidelines for notifying the physician about variations in blood pressure. Unfortunately, subcutaneous epoetin alfa is painful for some patients, which may interfere with compliance and self-injection (Jabs and Harmon 1996). Topical anesthetics are not usually helpful. Mixing the drug with benzyl alcohol or lidocaine (Jabs and Harmon 1996) or numbing the injection site with ice may decrease the pain.

RENAL REPLACEMENT THERAPIES

When the signs, symptoms, and biochemical changes of chronic renal failure are no longer responsive to medication and dietary management alone, renal replacement therapy (dialysis or transplantation) is indicated. At this point, the patient is considered to have ESRD with a reduction in kidney function to approximately 8 to 10 percent of normal.

Dialysis (peritoneal and hemodialysis) removes metabolic waste products and excess fluid and helps maintain proper electrolyte and acid base balance (see Appendix 10–B for a nursing care plan). It does not correct alterations in erythropoietin or vitamin D synthesis. In fact, even the most effective dialysis regimen does not completely replace the normal kidney's ability to handle fluid and electrolytes. Therefore, the patient with ESRD usually requires dialysis in addition to the previously discussed conservative management regimen.

Transplantation is the treatment of choice for most children with ESRD (see Appendix 10–C for a nursing care plan). It is important, however, that patients and families realize that it is not a cure. Even though a well-functioning graft allows for a more normal lifestyle, the child is at risk for significant complications, such as rejection, infection, and malignancy. Although the child is free of dialysis, maintenance of a well-functioning graft requires medication, dietary modification, and close follow-up.

Education, assessment, and planning for end-stage care needs to start early, as soon as it is recognized that the child will require renal replacement therapy. The multidisciplinary team and the family should develop a plan of care based on medical considerations, patient and family preference, family dynamics, and home environment. The patient and family need adequate information about their options to make informed decisions. Some children may be suitable candidates for preemptive live donor transplantation before ever starting dialysis. Other children may require dialysis while waiting for a cadaveric kidney. If dialysis is necessary, the goal is to assist family members with fitting the dialysis regimen into their lives with as little disruption as possible. As stated by McDonald and Watkins (1996, 60), "Renal replacement therapy for the pediatric ESRD patient needs to be individualized, and one needs to view dialysis and transplantation as complementary parts of the lifelong treatment plan."

Peritoneal Dialysis

In general, peritoneal dialysis is the preferred dialysis modality for children. Advantages are listed in Exhibit 10–2. Absolute medical contraindications include omphalocele, gastroschisis, bladder extrophy, diaphragmatic hernia, and severe peritoneal membrane failure (Harvey et al. 1996).

Peritoneal dialysis is accomplished by repeated exchanges of dialysis fluid in the

Exhibit 10–2 Advantages of Peritoneal Dialysis

- Less traumatic
- Fewer dietary restrictions
- Better blood pressure control
- Better control of acidosis
- More suitable for home dialysis
- Less disruptive to school routine

patient's peritoneal cavity through a "permanent," surgically placed catheter. Each exchange (cycle) consists of the following consecutive steps:

1. outflow—drainage of dialysate as fast as possible by gravity (usually 15 to 20 minutes)
2. Inflow—instillation of fresh dialysis fluid as fast as possible by gravity, unless comfort is an issue (usually 5 to 10 minutes)
3. Dwell—period the dialysis fluid stays in peritoneal cavity (ordered by the nephrologist)

Dialysis occurs during the dwell phase. The peritoneal membrane is the dialyzer. It is a semipermeable membrane that allows free passage of small molecules (for example, water, electrolytes, and certain metabolites) between the blood supply in the peritoneal membrane and the dialysis fluid.

Dialysis works by diffusion and osmosis. Solute (for example, urea, creatinine, potassium, and uremic toxins) moves from an area of greater concentration to an area of lesser concentration until equilibration occurs. Because there is a high concentration of waste products (solute) in the bloodstream and none in the dialysis fluid, there is a net loss of waste products from the intravascular space into the dialysate in the peritoneal cavity. Water removal is governed by osmosis, which is largely dependent on the hypertonicity of the dialysis fluid. Dialysis fluid is available as 1.5 percent glucose (for minimal water removal), 2.5 percent glucose, and 4.25 percent glucose (for maximum water removal).

There are two types of peritoneal dialysis. Continuous ambulatory peritoneal dialysis (CAPD) involves doing four or five manual exchanges with warmed dialysis fluid per 24 hours, with an 8-hour overnight dwell. Each exchange takes 30 to 45 minutes. Although the procedure is simple, adherence to strict aseptic technique is critical. Many children and families prefer continuous cycler peritoneal dialysis (CCPD), which involves several shorter cycles (1 to 2 hours in length) overnight for 8 to 10 hours while the child and family sleep. The cycler facilitates the gravity exchange of preheated dialysate. The newer cyclers are "user friendly." They are compact, easy to set up and program, and have multiple safety features. CCPD alleviates the need for daytime exchanges and may decrease the risk of peritonitis because the dialysis catheter is opened only twice a day (for connect and disconnect procedures).

Ideally, the selection of the dialysis modality is based on patient and family preference. However, medical considerations may dictate a particular therapy. For example, some patients may require CCPD because of inadequate ultrafiltration (fluid removal) with the long dwell times of CAPD (Harvey et al. 1996). The nephrologist formulates an individualized dialysis prescription based on the child's residual renal function, peritoneal transport characteristics, and fluid status, as determined by intake and output, weight, and blood pressure. The prescription designates dwell volume (35 to 50 mL/kg with a maximum of 2 L), length of dwell, number of exchanges per day, glucose concentration, and the mechanics of delivery.

Peritonitis, which can be associated with significant morbidity, is the most common complication of chronic peritoneal dialysis. Other potential complications are listed in Exhibit 10–3. Peritonitis may be caused by bacteria, fungi, or mycobacteria. Gram-positive bacteria (for example, *Staphylococcus epidermidis* and *Staphylococcus aureus*) are the most common causative organisms (Tzamaloukas 1996). Persistent or recurrent bacterial peritonitis and fungal peritonitis can lead to catheter loss and/or peritoneal

Exhibit 10–3 Common Complications of Peritoneal Dialysis

- Peritonitis
  Bacterial
  Fungal

- Catheter site infection
  Exit site
  Tunnel

- Catheter malfunction
  Fibrin clots
  Dialysate leaks
  Omental wrapping
  Constipation
  Migration of the catheter out of the pelvis

- Hernias
  Inguinal
  Umbilical
  Incisional

membrane failure, necessitating temporary or permanent hemodialysis.

Common signs and symptoms of peritonitis include cloudy dialysate, diffuse abdominal pain, nausea, vomiting, and fever. The diagnosis is usually based on the presence of clinical manifestations, a positive dialysate cell count (100 or more leukocytes/mm^3 with more than 50 percent neutrophils), and a positive dialysate culture. Fourteen days of intraperitoneal antibiotics is recommended for the initial treatment of peritonitis (Tzamaloukas 1996). Persistent or recurrent infection may require an extended course of therapy, the addition of oral or parenteral antibiotics, and/or catheter removal.

It is generally accepted that (1) breaks in aseptic technique during connections or disconnections of the peritoneal dialysis system and/or (2) peritoneal catheter tunnel and exit-site infections can result in peritonitis. Other variables that may be associated with the development of peritonitis include host defense mechanisms, patient age, type and length of peritoneal dialysis therapy, catheter and equipment selection, and exit-site location. The prevention and treatment of peritonitis is the focus of many current research efforts.

Exit-site and tunnel infections deserve special mention because they may lead to persistent or recurrent peritonitis. Exit-site infection may be defined as erythema and/or purulent drainage at the site where the catheter exits the skin (Piraino 1996). A tunnel infection is usually defined as erythema, tenderness, or edema over the subcutaneous pathway of the catheter (Piraino 1996). Approaches to treatment vary widely and may involve antibiotics (systemic and/or topical), intensified local care, surgical debridement of the exit site, and catheter removal (Piraino 1996; Prowant 1996).

Protocols for routine exit-site care also vary widely among dialysis centers. Variations in routine care are related to the frequency of care, types of cleansing agents, and types of dressings. Some centers advocate keeping the exit site covered; others advocate that well-healed, noninfected exit sites may be left open to air. Various topical antibacterial preparations have been used as part of the routine care. No single protocol has proved to be superior in preventing infection (Piraino 1996).

Preventing trauma to the exit site and tunnel, especially with a new catheter, may be one of the most important measures in preventing infection. Trauma may result from tension or pressure on the catheter, excessively vigorous cleaning, or irritation from cleansing agents and adhesives (Prowant 1996). Gentle handling and immobilization of the catheter to minimize movement are particularly important (Prowant 1996). Good personal hygiene, handwashing before performing exit-site care, and aseptic technique for dressing changes on new catheters are also recommended (Prowant 1996).

Before beginning the formal education program for home peritoneal dialysis, the primary and backup caregivers must be identified. Occasionally, the home health nurse or aide may be able to attend at least some of the training. Caregivers may need to arrange for baby-sitting for siblings, anticipated absence from work, and

preparation of the home for dialysis supplies (Harvey et al. 1996).

There are wide variations among pediatric home training programs related to the length of the program (3 to 11 or more days) and to the setting (inpatient or outpatient) (Miller, Ruley, and Bock 1995). Although some standardization based on outcome studies is indicated, flexibility must be maintained to accommodate various learning styles and to ensure that caregivers are competent. There is also wide variation among centers related to the age at which the child is considered capable of assuming primary responsibility. Although even very young children should be encouraged to participate in their own care, the level of responsibility and the amount of supervision required must be individualized, regardless of age.

Suggested content for the home peritoneal dialysis training program is outlined in Exhibit 10–4. Many centers train each family in both CAPD and CCPD (Miller, Ruley, and Bock 1995). Various teaching tools (for example, videos, printed materials, and dolls with functional peritoneal catheters) and assistive devices are available.

Starting home dialysis can be frightening and overwhelming for the entire family. Coping and learning styles vary greatly. Personnel who provide home care training must be able to adapt to individual differences and to maintain open communication with the family to accomplish program objectives. With time, many families become sophisticated in their ability to make decisions and appropriately manage their children's dialysis. Other families require more guidance, including frequent reinforcement of basic principles. The multidisciplinary team and other health care providers should also be alert to changes in coping style, which may indicate increased stress and interfere with the caregiver's ability to care for the child.

Hemodialysis

Hemodialysis is accomplished by the flow of the patient's blood through the dialyzer. The

Exhibit 10–4 Content for Home Peritoneal Dialysis Training Program

- Complications of renal failure
- Role of medications, diet, and dialysis
- Physiology of peritoneal dialysis
- Importance of handwashing and good personal hygiene
- Basic principles of asepsis
  Connect and disconnect procedures
  Addition of medications to dialysate
- Mechanics of CAPD
  Exchange procedure
  Prescription
- Mechanics of CCPD
  Machine setup
  Programming prescription
  Responding to alarms
- Exit-site care
  Routine cleansing
  Prevention of trauma
  Assessment for and recognition of
  infection
- Monitoring of fluid status
  Weight
  Blood pressure
  Intake and output
  Relationship between ultrafiltration and
  dialysate glucose concentration
- Recognition of and appropriate response to
  complications
  Peritonitis
  Catheter malfunction
- Clinic routines
- Contact information

Note: CAPD, continuous ambulatory peritoneal dialysis; CCPD, continuous cycler peritoneal dialysis.

patient's blood is separated from the dialysate bath by a semipermeable membrane, which allows for the removal of fluid and solute across the membrane by differential diffusion. Although advances in technology have made it possible to safely dialyze infants and small children, the expertise required and the potential for complications usually preclude performing pediatric hemodialysis in the home.

Home care for pediatric hemodialysis patients is focused on adherence to diet and fluid restrictions, medication administration, and vascular access care. Most children undergo dialysis for three to four hours three times a week in a specialized facility. Waste products, excess fluid, and uremic toxins accumulate between treatments. Therefore, strict adherence to the prescribed dietary and medication regimen is imperative to prevent dangerous complications (for example, pulmonary edema, hyperkalemia, and hypertensive encephalopathy).

Maintenance of vascular access for hemodialysis may be a major problem for the pediatric patient. Adolescents may be candidates for primary arteriovenous fistulas or vascular synthetic grafts. Smaller children usually require central venous catheters. Potential complications include clotting and sepsis, both of which can lead to loss of the access. Patient education related to prevention of complications is outlined in Exhibit 10–5.

In general, children do not seem to tolerate chronic hemodialysis as well as peritoneal dialysis. Dialysis scheduling is relatively inflexible and may interfere significantly with school attendance and other age-appropriate activities. The dialysis procedure is potentially more frightening and more painful, especially if the child's access has to be cannulated for each treatment. In addition, older children often have to dialyze in adult units. Although the staff may be technically competent, they may be inexperienced and uncomfortable in caring for chronically ill children and their families.

Renal Transplantation

Successful renal transplantation continues to provide the best possible outcome for children with ESRD. Determining the optimal time for the transplant is a critical decision that requires careful consideration of multiple factors, including age of the patient, primary renal disease, source of the donor kidney, maximization of growth and development, and ability of the patient and family to follow through with care re-

Exhibit 10–5 Patient and Family Education for Prevention of Vascular Access Complications

---

Primary Fistula or Vascular Synthetic Graft

- Do not occlude blood flow to access (for example, no blood pressures, tourniquets, or other application of pressure).
- Do not allow venipunctures except by dialysis personnel.
- Palpate thrill or listen for bruit daily.
- Wash access with soap and water before needle cannulation.
- Recognize signs and symptoms of infection; report promptly.
- Know emergency procedures for bleeding.

Central Venous Catheter

- Reserve catheter for dialysis only (for example, no blood draws, parenteral therapy).
- Practice good personal hygiene.
- Keep dressing clean and dry.
- Secure the catheter to prevent trauma to the site.
- Recognize signs and symptoms of infection; report promptly.
- Check temperature routinely.
- Know emergency procedures for bleeding.

---

quirements after the transplant. Recipients younger than six years tend to do less well than older children and young adults (Grimm and Ettenger 1992; McDonald and Watkins 1996). Young children have decreased graft survival and increased mortality rates, which may be due to technical problems, heightened immune responsiveness, and/or altered cyclosporine metabolism (Grimm and Ettenger 1992). Age at the time of transplant and growth after the transplant appear to be related. Although younger children may have a worse long-term outcome, they appear to have more improvement in linear growth (Grimm and Ettenger 1992; McDonald and Watkins 1996). Adolescent recipients, however, experience a deceleration in growth (McDonald and Watkins 1996). Growth after transplant is also affected by the total steroid dose and graft function (Grimm and Ettenger 1992).

Consideration of the primary renal disease is important because some glomerular diseases are known to recur in the transplant. Recurrence may or may not result in graft failure. The primary disease, however, may influence the decision about whether to use a potential live donor.

Failure to adhere to the prescribed immunosuppressive regimen is a leading cause of rejection and subsequent graft loss, particularly among adolescents (Grimm and Ettenger 1992). Failure to adhere to the dialysis regimen may be an indicator of behavior after the transplant. Counseling for the child and family, introduction of behavior modification, or other psychological interventions may be indicated before performing the transplant. The multidisciplinary team and the family should carefully weigh all the factors related to the timing of the transplant and reach a joint decision to achieve the best possible outcome.

Selection of the appropriate immunosuppressive regimen is also a critical decision. There is wide variation in protocols among transplant centers. Most centers use a combination of oral glucocorticosteroids, cyclosporine, and azathioprine for prevention of rejection (maintenance therapy). Prednisone, the most commonly used corticosteroid, has broad anti-inflammatory effects on cell-mediated immunity (McDonald and Watkins 1996). Although prednisone continues to be the mainstay in most regimens, it has multiple adverse effects, including cushingoid appearance, poor growth, hypertension, increased susceptibility to infection, cataracts, and acne. Most centers attempt to minimize the total steroid dose to prevent these side effects (see Table 13–5 for immunosuppresive agents used in transplantation).

The use of cyclosporine, which inhibits T-cell response, represents an important advance in transplantation because it has improved graft survival rates and allowed for the minimization of steroid dosage (Grimm and Ettenger 1992). However, it, too, has multiple side effects and is difficult to use. The side effects include nephrotoxicity, hypertension, hyperkalemia, tremor, hirsutism, gingival hyperplasia, neurotoxicity, and increased risk of malignancy. Individual patient differences regarding absorption and metabolism, the potential for nephrotoxicity, and the existence of multiple drug interactions make appropriate dosing difficult. In addition, rejection is more difficult to diagnose because classic signs of acute rejection (for example, fever, graft tenderness, and oliguria) are often absent. There are now two cyclosporine preparations available, Sandimmune and Neoral. The newer preparation, Neoral, may have improved bioavailability. Interchanging the two preparations is not recommended by the manufacturer.

Azathioprine interferes directly with the growth and differentiation of immune cells and inhibits antibody production (McDonald and Watkins 1996). Common side effects include leukopenia, thrombocytopenia, hepatotoxicity, and increased risk of viral infection and malignancy.

There are several experimental immunosuppressive drugs currently under investigation. Two new agents, FK506 and mycophenolate mofetil, are commercially available and currently being used in some centers. FK506 is being used in place of cyclosporine, and mycophenolate mofetil is being used instead of azathioprine. Both drugs appear to be effective in reducing the incidence of rejection. Although the side effects are similar, advantages of FK506 over cyclosporine may include less hypertension, improved cosmetic appearance, and the potential for further reduction in steroid dosage (McDonald and Watkins 1996). However, FK506 may be associated with an increased incidence of post-transplant lymphoproliferative disease (McDonald and Watkins 1996). The major side effects of mycophenolate mofetil are leukopenia and gastrointestinal disorders, especially diarrhea (Sollinger 1995).

Although renal transplant recipients are at risk for surgical complications (vascular or urologic), the major long-term risks are rejection, infection, and malignancy. Rejection is usually classified as hyperacute, acute, or chronic. Hyperacute rejection occurs immediately post-transplant and is usually irreversible. Acute rejection occurs most often during the first year and is usually responsive to therapy. Chronic rejection is characterized by a slower, progressive increase in creatinine, which is usually not responsive to antirejection therapy. Patients and families must constantly deal with the threat of rejection. Data from NAPRTCS showed that 57 percent of live-related donor recipients and 73 percent of cadaveric recipients experienced at least one rejection episode during the first two years after transplantation (McDonald and Watkins 1996). NAPRTCS also found that only 52 percent of all acute rejection episodes are completely reversible (serum creatinine returns to baseline) and that the reversibility declines with each subsequent episode of rejection the patient experiences (McDonald and Watkins 1996).

The diagnosis of acute rejection may be difficult because the child may be essentially asymptomatic except for an elevated serum creatinine. Cyclosporine toxicity, partial obstruction, acute tubular necrosis (ATN), mild dehydration, and infection must also be considered as possible causes. In the absence of a surgically correctable problem or improvement with hydration, a kidney biopsy is usually performed. Acute rejection, chronic rejection, and ATN can be differentiated by biopsy. In addition, the biopsy may be helpful in diagnosing cyclosporine toxicity and infection. Before beginning antirejection therapy, which is associated with certain risks, the diagnosis of acute rejection should be confirmed by biopsy.

The initial treatment for acute rejection is usually high-dose glucocorticosteroid therapy. Intravenous methylprednisolone at a dosage of 5 to 30 mg/kg/day is usually given for a total of three to five doses (Grimm and Ettenger 1992). High-dose oral prednisone with a rapid taper over several days may also be used. Acute rejection episodes that are unresponsive to steroids are usually treated with antilymphocyte preparations (antithymocyte or antilymphocyte globulin, OKT3).

OKT3 has been shown to be effective in reversing steroid-resistant rejection in more than 90 percent of children treated (Grimm and Ettenger 1992). OKT3 is a mouse monoclonal antibody that blocks T-cell function and causes the early disappearance of circulating T cells. The dosage is 5 mg a day as an intravenous (IV) bolus for 10 to 14 days if the patient weighs 30 kg or more. The dosage is reduced to 2.5 mg for the patient who weighs less than 30 kg (Duffy and Nestor 1992). OKT3 must be filtered through a 0.22-micron low-protein binding filter before administration and then given as an IV bolus within one minute (without filter). Oral cyclosporine is usually discontinued at the initiation of OKT3 therapy and restarted three days before completing the course of OKT3 (Duffy and Nestor 1992). OKT3 has significant adverse side effects. The most serious and dramatic of these usually occur during the first two to three days of therapy. Adverse effects may include pulmonary edema, especially if the patient is fluid overloaded; high fever; chills; bronchospasm; headache; nausea; vomiting; diarrhea; and hypotension. Patients should be premedicated to decrease the severity of side effects. Because the side effects usually subside after the third or fourth day of therapy, it is often possible to give a number of doses on an outpatient basis (clinic or home) (Grimm and Ettenger 1992). Long-term side effects of OKT3 include an increased risk of infection and malignancy.

Infection is always a serious threat to the immunosuppressed patient. The use of powerful antilymphocyte preparations, either as prophylaxis or as antirejection therapy, increases the risk of infection. During the first few weeks post-transplant, serious infections are usually bacterial, related to central lines, catheters, the pulmonary toilet, or the wound. The most common causative organisms are *Staphylococcus aureus* and *Escherichia coli* (Grimm and Ettenger 1992). After the first month, the transplant recipient is at risk for opportunistic infection, which may be of bacterial, viral, fungal, or protozoan origin. Assessment for infection should include consideration of the time elapsed since transplant, the level of immune suppression, the patient's environment and travel history, and the prevalent hospital-acquired and community-acquired pathogens (Grimm and Ettenger 1992). Please see Table 13–7 for comparative infections observed post-transplant.

Cytomegalovirus (CMV), varicella, and Epstein-Barr virus (EBV) can be particularly problematic for the pediatric renal transplant patient because many young children are seronegative for these diseases at the time of transplant. Although reactivation of disease in seropositive patients can be a serious problem, there is increased morbidity and mortality for children who have a primary infection with CMV, varicella, or EBV in an immunosuppressed state (Grimm and Ettenger 1992; McDonald and Watkins 1996). Manifestations of CMV infection may include fever, neutropenia, thrombocytopenia, gastritis, hepatic dysfunction, pneumonitis, and renal transplant dysfunction. CMV may be associated with an increased risk of rejection and graft loss (Grimm and Ettenger 1992; McDonald and Watkins 1996). A primary varicella infection in a pediatric renal transplant patient can be overwhelming, resulting in encephalitis, pneumonitis, hepatic failure, pancreatitis, and disseminated intravascular coagulation (Grimm and Ettenger 1992). It is extremely important to instruct the parents of seronegative recipients to report any exposure to varicella. If given within 72 hours of exposure, varicella zoster immune globulin may prevent or attenuate primary infection. McDonald and Watkins (1996) recommend immunizing seronegative pediatric transplant candidates and their seronegative family members with varicella vaccine as long before transplant as possible. EBV is associated with the pathogenesis of the B-cell lymphoproliferative disease seen in transplant patients. Patients who are seronegative for EBV at the time of transplant and who receive antilymphocyte preparations (for example, antilymphocyte globulin (ALG), antithymocyte globulin (ATG), and OKT3) seem to be at greater risk for developing lymphoma (McDonald and Watkins 1996). The prognosis for post-transplantation lymphoproliferative disease seems to depend on cell type and the extent of the disease. Treatment may include withdrawal of immunosuppression, antiviral therapy, chemotherapy, immune therapy, and/or radiation therapy (McDonald and Watkins 1996).

Rehabilitation after transplant starts in the early postoperative period. Although there is wide variation among transplant centers, the length of the initial hospitalization is decreasing. Induction therapy with an antilymphocyte preparation, surgical complications, infection, delayed graft function, and/or severe hypertension may lead to an extended length of stay. Patients who have an uncomplicated course may be discharged in less than a week to a subacute facility, a nearby hotel or apartment, or their homes. The "uncomplicated" patient, however, still requires extremely close follow-up (for example, daily or every-other-day laboratory studies) and may have significant home care requirements. The child and family may need assistance with catheter care, wound care, and/or infusion therapy (for example, intravenous ganciclovir for CMV prophylaxis).

Appropriate patient and family education before and after discharge is critical to the success of the transplant. Suggested content for post-transplant education is outlined in Exhibit 10–6. The child should be included in the education process at an age-appropriate level. Because medications are so important, a detailed medication schedule is often helpful (see Appendix 10–A). Because the pharmacy may use either the generic or the brand name on the prescription, it is important to include both names of the medication on the patient's schedule. Prednisone tablets are available in several sizes (for example, 2.5, 5, 10, 20, and 50 mg). Prescribing only the 5-mg tablet decreases the risk of error. Although the child has to take more tablets initially, tapering the dose by either 5 mg (one tablet) or 2.5 mg (one-half tablet) is relatively easy for patients

Exhibit 10–6   Content for Patient and Family Education after Transplantation

- Definition of rejection (normal immune response to kidney)
- Importance of compliance with medications, clinic appointments, and laboratory studies (creatinine, cyclosporine level, white blood cell count)
- Medications
  Name
  Indication
  Dosage and administration
  Schedule
  Side effects
- Diet and fluid allotment
- Activity
  Lifting and driving restricted for four to six weeks
  Showers only, until wound completely healed
  Walking encouraged
  Sports limitations, if any
- Routine monitoring
  Temperature
  Blood pressure
  Weight
  Intake and output
- Recognition of and appropriate response to the following:
  Signs and symptoms of rejection
  Signs and symptoms of infection
- Early detection and prevention of complications
  Call for questions or concerns.
  Practice good personal hygiene.
  Avoid crowds and people with obvious infections.
  Call immediately for exposure to chickenpox.
  Check with transplant team *before* taking any other medication or receiving immunizations.
  Use sun protection (for example, sunscreen, hat, long-sleeved clothing).
  Obtain routine dental and eye examinations.
- Clinic routines and laboratory protocols
- Contact information

and families to understand. For some families, it may be necessary to tape the actual pills and capsules to the schedule.

In addition to learning the details about home care, the child and family need to understand that the first few months to one year after transplant may be stressful because of frequent clinic visits, multiple medication changes, and readmissions to the hospital. The greatest risk for acute rejection is during the first year after transplant, and treatment for rejection increases the risk for infection. After the first year, the child and family may need reeducation about the importance of health maintenance activities (for example, monthly serum creatinine determinations, eye examinations, and dental examinations) and the risk of noncompliance with the immunosuppressive regimen. Also please see Chapter 13 for further discussion of home care issues after transplantation.

IMPACT OF CHRONIC ILLNESS

The diagnosis of chronic renal failure in a child has a profound and lasting impact on the entire family. Chronic renal failure affects every aspect of the child's life, including physical appearance, energy level, diet, and socialization experiences (for example, peer and family relationships). Treatment is a long-term process, which may involve more than one kidney transplant with a return to dialysis after each graft loss. In addition, the family must deal with providing much of the direct care in the home and may be faced with choosing a family member as a donor for a kidney transplant. As stated by Frauman and Gilman (1990, 383), kidney failure "influences the family's lifestyle, residence, mobility, financial status, social life, and functioning as a unit."

Families cope with the stresses of chronic illness in many different ways, and coping styles may change over time. Some families appear self-reliant and handle the stress internally; others need a great deal of support from the health care team and other resources. It is not uncommon for the family of the newly diagnosed child to exhibit strong denial. Because the symptoms of chronic renal failure may be vague and nonspecific, it is often difficult for the child and family to accept the diagnosis, especially if the child is still making urine and does not have obvious physical signs of disease.

Some families become overprotective and child-centered, focusing all their attention and energy on the ill child (Frauman and Gilman 1990; Harvey et al. 1996). This pattern of functioning, which fosters helplessness and dependence in the child, is not healthy for the patient, the siblings, or the parents (Harvey et al. 1996). Parents often need assistance, support, and/or permission to engage in normal parenting behaviors (for example, discipline and toilet training) toward the chronically ill child. The child should be assisted to attain normal developmental milestones and to participate in age-appropriate activities (for example, school, day care, and social functions). This approach will help the child attain a normal self-image and help the family keep the chronic illness in perspective (Frauman and Gilman 1990).

Families with a child on home peritoneal dialysis grow tired of the daily dialysis schedule, medication regimen, and altered lifestyle (Watson 1995). As stress increases, the primary caregiver may appear depressed or anxious and may feel that other family members are not helping sufficiently with the child's care requirements. In addition, there may be other sources of stress in the family that demand attention (for example, work demands and marital relationship). Occasionally, resolving other family problems may take precedence over providing end-stage care. The more serious manifestations of increased stress may include missed clinic appointments, failure to perform dialysis or give medications, frequent episodes of infection, and the shift of too much responsibility for care to the ill child.

Families often need assistance with developing strategies to reduce stress and obtain respite. Early intervention is critical. Support groups are helpful because parents often derive a great deal of benefit from talking with others in a similar situation (Watson 1995). Family members, friends, church groups, and community volunteers may be able to provide occasional or regularly scheduled relief. Some families may be eligible for a home health aide through the social services department. Summer camps for children on dialysis are available in some areas of the country. Camps provide an excellent opportunity for children to develop peer relationships and to become more independent, while giving parents a break from the daily dialysis routine. It is important for parents to use strategies that allow them to support the normal development of their chronically ill child and to spend quality time with their other children and each other as well.

ROLE OF THE MULTIDISCIPLINARY TEAM

The multidisciplinary team approach to care is most appropriate for children with ESRD (Frauman and Gilman 1990; Harvey et al. 1996). The pediatric nephrologist directs the team and has overall responsibility for the treatment plan. Teams should include nurses, dietitians, and social workers. Involvement of other therapists (for example, physical and occupational therapists) may be required for specific children. Ideally, all team members should be experienced in dealing with the complexities of ESRD in the pediatric population. The team must meet frequently to formulate and refine the plan of care for each child. A well-functioning team is characterized by open communication and a mutual respect for the expertise of each member. It is critical to the child and family that all team members agree on and present a unified approach to care (Frauman and Gilman 1990; Harvey et al. 1996).

Although interventions and strategies are tailored to the specific needs of the child and family, the team should be focused on enhancing the family's ability to care for the child with ESRD. Team members should not foster overdepend-

ence or assume the care of the child (Frauman and Gilman 1990). Because the physicians may rotate call responsibilities, the dietitian, social worker, and nurse may have the most consistent communication with the family. The dietitian has expertise in assisting the family with meeting the child's nutritional needs. The social worker may provide several services, including counseling, referral to appropriate community resources (for example, social services and support groups), and assistance with the coordination of funding (for example, Medicare, private insurance, Children's Health Services, etc.). A nurse, such as a clinical nurse specialist (CNS), has the knowledge and expertise to provide education related to treatment options, medications, and other health care requirements. The CNS may be the primary liaison with the family and may be responsible for coordinating services among the various disciplines involved. Obviously, some responsibilities are shared across disciplines. For example, all team members are responsible for providing emotional support and appropriate, accurate information. In addition, each team member is responsible for supporting and reinforcing the teaching of other team members.

It is important that the ESRD team maintain effective communication about the plan of care with the health care providers in the community (for example, primary pediatrician, home health nurse, and school nurse). This communication allows local providers to support and reinforce the plan of care, and it increases the family's sense of security. In addition, the multidisciplinary team may gain valuable information about the child's and family's adaptation to ESRD.

ROLE OF THE HOME HEALTH NURSE

The home health nurse is a valuable resource for the child and family and for the multidisciplinary team. His or her role varies according to the needs of the child and family. Often, it involves providing direct care, such as home infusion therapy or teaching injection techniques for rHuEPO and rhGH. In addition, the home health nurse can assess the family's level of understanding about the disease and the plan of care, including the importance of medications, diet, and clinic appointments.

Even when the family has received extensive education at the hospital, caring for the child at home, without the dialysis or transplant staff, initially can be frightening. The role of the home health nurse may include providing emotional support, helping with procedures, and/or assisting with assessment and clinical decision making. Appropriate nursing intervention may be a significant factor in the prevention and/or early diagnosis of complications. As a consistent caregiver, the home health nurse may be the person who is able to help the child or adolescent assume more responsibility for self-care.

The home health nurse observes firsthand the family dynamics and the home environment. He or she may possess valuable knowledge and insight about the family's current sources of stress, acceptance of the diagnosis, and level of understanding of the treatment, all of which may impact the family's ability to follow through with the plan of care. It is extremely important that the home health nurse and the ESRD team communicate on a regular basis to share information and maintain a unified approach to care.

CONCLUSION

The outcome for children with ESRD has improved dramatically over the last three decades. However, the diagnosis of chronic renal failure is still overwhelming because the child and family must cope with some form of renal replacement therapy for the remainder of the child's life. Much of the care is provided in the home by the family, and the burden of care impacts every aspect of family life. A multidisciplinary team approach to care is appropriate to achieve the optimal outcome for the child and to assist the family in coping with the complexities of ESRD. In addition to formulating an individualized plan of care, the role of the team includes providing extensive education, emotional support, and assistance with developing appropriate coping strategies. It is important that the ESRD team develop relationships with health care providers in the child's community to maintain a unified approach to care. The home health nurse can be a particularly valuable link between the child and family and the ESRD team.

REFERENCES

Duffy, M.M., and A. Nestor. 1992. Nursing guidelines for muromonab-CD3 (OKT3). *ANNA Journal.* 19:493–95.

Feld, L.G., J.E. Springate, and R.D. Fildes. 1986. Acute renal failure: I. Pathophysiology and diagnosis. *Journal of Pediatrics.* 109:401–08.

Foreman, J.W., and J.C.M. Chan. 1988. Chronic renal failure in infants and children. *Journal of Pediatrics.* 113:793–99.

Frauman, A.C., and C.M. Gilman. 1990. Care of the family of the child with end-stage renal disease. *ANNA Journal.* 17:383–86.

Frauman, A.C., and J.T. Myers. 1994. Cognitive, psychosocial, and physical development in infants and children with end-stage renal disease. *Advances in Renal Replacement Therapy* 1:49–54.

Grimm, P.C., and R. Ettenger. 1992. Pediatric renal transplantation. *Advances in Pediatrics.* 39:441–93.

Gusmano, R., and F. Perfumo. 1993. Worldwide demographic aspects of chronic renal failure in children. *Kidney International* 43(suppl. 41):531–35.

Harmon, W.E. 1995. Treatment of children with chronic renal failure. *Kidney International* 47:951–61.

Harvey, E., et al. 1996. The team approach to the management of children on chronic peritoneal dialysis. *Advances in Renal Replacement Therapy.* 3:3–13.

Jabs, K., and W.E. Harmon. 1996. Recombinant human erythropoietin therapy in children on dialysis. *Advances in Renal Replacement Therapy* 3:24–36.

Kohaut, E.C. 1995. Chronic renal failure and growth in childhood. *Current Opinion in Pediatrics.* 7:171–75.

McDonald, R.A., and S.L. Watkins. 1996. Progress in renal transplantation for children. *Advances in Renal Replacement Therapy* 3:60–68.

Miller, D.H., J. Ruley, and G.H. Bock. 1995. Current status of pediatric home peritoneal dialysis training in the United States. *Advances in Peritoneal Dialysis* 11:274–80.

National Institutes of Health. 1993. *NIH consensus statement: Morbidity and mortality of dialysis* (Vol. 11, 2). Bethesda, Md.: National Institues of Health.

Piraino, B. 1996. Peritoneal catheter exit-site and tunnel infections. *Advances in Renal Replacement Therapy* 3:222–27.

Prowant, B.F. 1996. Nursing interventions related to peritoneal catheter exit-site infections. *Advances in Renal Replacement Therapy* 3:228–31.

Sanchez, C.P., and I.B. Salusky. 1996. The renal bone diseases in children treated with dialysis. *Advances in Renal Replacement Therapy* 3:14–23.

Sollinger, H.W. 1995. Mycophenolate mofetil for the prevention of acute rejection in primary cadaveric renal allograft recipients. *Transplantation* 60:225–32.

Tönshoff, B., and R.N. Fine. 1996. Recombinant human growth hormone for children with renal failure. *Advances in Renal Replacement Therapy* 3:37–47.

Tzamaloukas, A.H. 1996. Peritonitis in peritoneal dialysis patients: An overview. *Advances in Renal Replacement Therapy* 3:232–36.

Watson, A.R. 1995. Strategies to support families of children with end-stage renal failure. *Pediatric Nephrology* 9:628–31.

Wise, B., and B. Case. 1994. Recombinant human growth hormone. *ANNA Journal.* 21:87–89.

Medication Schedule

For _____
Date _____

Drug	Morning							Afternoon						Evening				
	6	7	8	9	10	11	12	12	1	2	3	4	5	6	7	8	9	10
Neoral (cyclosporine) 100-mg capsules			1 cap													1 cap		
Neoral (cyclosporine) 25-mg capsules			3 caps													3 caps		
Cellcept (mycophenolate mofetil) 250-mg capsules			3 caps													3 caps		
Deltasone (prednisone) 5-mg tablets			5½ tabs															

Prepared by _____

Nursing Care Plan for a Child on Dialysis

Nursing Diagnosis/ Patient Problem	Defining Characteristics	Nursing Interventions	Expected Outcome
High risk for injury related to biochemical changes	Azotemia Increased serum creatinine Hyperkalemia Metabolic acidosis Hyperphosphatemia Hypocalcemia Hyponatremia	*Provide prescribed diet. *Administer prescribed medications: oral alkali preparations, phosphate binders, vitamin D, salt supplements. *Assist with dialysis. Assess for signs and symptoms of electrolyte imbalance and uremia.	Child exhibits no uremic symptoms. Child maintains normal serum electrolytes. Child does not develop renal osteodystrophy.
Fluid volume excess related to failure of renal regulatory mechanisms	Rapid weight gain Hypertension Resting tachycardia Tachypnea, dyspnea Edema (peripheral/pulmonary) Congestive heart failure	Monitor vital signs, weight, and intake and output. *Maintain fluid and sodium restrictions as ordered. *Administer prescribed antihypertensive medications. *Assist with dialysis: monitor outflow and ultrafiltration. Monitor fluid status. Observe for side effects of antihypertensive medications.	Child exhibits no signs or symptoms of fluid overload.

*Denotes nursing intervention requiring a physician's order.

Nursing Diagnosis/ Patient Problem	Defining Characteristics	Nursing Interventions	Expected Outcome
Fatigue related to anemia	Decreased hemoglobin and hematocrit Lethargy Pallor Decreased activity tolerance Severe anemia • Tachycardia • Tachypnea • Shortness of breath • Dizziness and lightheadedness	*Administer rHuEPO and iron therapy as ordered. Provide emotional support and attempt to decrease pain from injections. Observe for bleeding tendencies. *Administer transfusion as ordered for severe anemia.	Child maintains hematocrit of 30% to 35%. Child participates in age-appropriate activities.
Nutrition alteration: less than body requirements related to anorexia, dietary restrictions, and protein losses in dialysate	Inadequate weight gain or weight loss Abnormal anthropometric measurements Decreased serum albumin Abnormally low blood urea nitrogen in comparison to serum creatinine	Monitor physical growth. *Provide adequate protein and calories for growth. Monitor dietary intake. Monitor gastrointestinal function. Consult with dietitian and "feeding specialist." *Provide supplemental tube feeding as ordered. *Assist with dialysis.	Child's intake contains adequate protein, calories, and essential nutrients.
Impaired growth and development: physical and psychosocial related to chronic renal failure	Inability to maintain steady growth curve Delay or difficulty in reaching appropriate developmental milestones (motor, language, cognitive, and psychosocial skills)	Monitor physical growth. *Provide adequate nutrition for growth. *Administer prescribed medications to control acidosis and anemia and to prevent bone disease. *Assist with dialysis. *Administer rhGH as ordered.	Child achieves maximum growth and developmental potential.

*Denotes nursing intervention requiring a physician's order.

Nursing Diagnosis/ Patient Problem	Defining Characteristics	Nursing Interventions	Expected Outcome
		Observe for side effects of rhGH and provide emotional support. Monitor developmental progress. Promote the use of existing skills and encourage activities that will help the child attain a higher skill level. Assist with referral to appropriate community resources (for example, developmental evalua- tion clinic and/or physical, occupational, and speech therapists).	
High risk for infection related to dialysis	Exit-site/tunnel infection: Erythema Edema Purulent drainage Tenderness Peritonitis Cloudy dialysate Abdominal pain Nausea and vomiting Fever Positive dialysate cell count and culture Hemodialysis access infection: Erythema Tenderness Purulent drainage Edema Sepsis Fever Chills	Minimize risk of infection: handwashing, aseptic technique, and prevention of trauma to access. Perform routine exit-site care per protocol. Monitor for signs and symptoms of infection. * Administer antibiotics as ordered. Refer to Exhibits 10–4 and 10–5 for patient and family education related to infection.	Child remains free of infection.

*Denotes nursing intervention requiring a physician's order.

Nursing Diagnosis/ Patient Problem	Defining Characteristics	Nursing Interventions	Expected Outcome
	Positive blood culture Lethargy and drowsiness Nausea and vomiting Hypotension Poor peripheral perfusion		
High risk for peritoneal catheter malfunction related to fibrin clots, dialysate leaks, omental wrapping, constipation, or migration of catheter	Fibrin present in dialysate Dialysate leaking at exit site Poor outflow Poor inflow Severe pain on inflow	*Add heparin to dialysate. Monitor for signs and symptoms of infection. *Administer stool softeners as ordered. Monitor bowel function. Consult dietitian for high-fiber diet. Notify physician for any signs of catheter malfunction.	Child experiences no catheter malfunction related to fibrin and constipation. Unavoidable catheter problems are detected early.
Knowledge deficit related to the disease process and the plan of care (diet, medications, and dialysis)	Verbalization of questions or problems Inability to articulate rationale for treatment Inability to perform care requirements	Assess readiness for learning. Select appropriate teaching strategies. Provide education for the child at an age-appropriate level. Provide accurate information at a rate that is appropriate for the individual. Assess level of understanding and ability to perform care requirements (for example, verbal feedback and return demonstration). Reinforce teaching as needed.	Child and family verbalize and demonstrate understanding of disease process and treatment regimen.

*Denotes nursing intervention requiring a physician's order.

Nursing Diagnosis/ Patient Problem	Defining Characteristics	Nursing Interventions	Expected Outcome
		Encourage child and family to keep a journal for questions or concerns. Continually assess for further knowledge deficit. Refer to section on Chronic Renal Failure and Exhibits 10–4 and 10–5 for content of education program.	
Body image disturbance related to chronic illness, growth retardation, and perception of being "different"	Poor growth Delayed pubescence Depression Irritability Helplessness, overdependence Social isolation (for example, school phobia) Lack of interest in age-appropriate activities "Hiding" dialysis access Noncompliance with diet, medications, and/or dialysis procedures	Provide age-appropriate education about the disease process and the treatment regimen. Encourage child to participate in all aspects of care. Allow child to participate in making decisions, if possible. Encourage participation in normal age-appropriate activities, especially school. Promote independence. Encourage verbalization of feelings and perceptions; acknowledge feelings and clarify misconceptions. Support positive coping mechanisms. Encourage parents to engage in normal parenting behaviors. *Assist with referral for professional counseling as needed.	Child participates in normal age-appropriate activities and peer relationships. Child actively involved in own care and management.

*Denotes nursing intervention requiring a physician's order.

Nursing Diagnosis/ Patient Problem	Defining Characteristics	Nursing Interventions	Expected Outcome
Coping, ineffective family, related to a child with chronic illness and multiple home care requirements	Verbalization of inability to cope Difficulty integrating treatment regimen into family life Primary caregiver exhibits signs of stress, anxiety, depression, or anger Inability to make appropriate decisions Noncompliance with medical regimen	Allow family to verbalize frustration, fatigue, stress, anger, and anxiety. Determine etiology of ineffective coping (for example, lack of knowledge or other current sources of stress). Support appropriate coping mechanisms. Assist with identifying alternative strategies for ineffective coping mechanisms. Encourage participation in a support group. Encourage utilization of respite care, if available. Assist with referral to other community resources as appropriate (for example, social services and counseling).	Family exhibits decreased stress and increased ability to care for child. Family uses appropriate coping mechanisms.

*Denotes nursing intervention requiring a physician's order.

Note: rHuEPO, recombinant human erythropoietin; rhGH, recombinant human growth hormone.

Nursing Care Plan for a Child with a Kidney Transplant

Nursing Diagnosis/ Patient Problem	Defining Characteristics	Nursing Interventions	Expected Outcome
High risk for injury related to recent kidney transplant surgery	Delayed graft function Infection: Central line Urinary tract Wound Respiratory Urinary obstruction or leak	Monitor vital signs, weight, and intake Observe for signs and symptoms of fluid excess or deficit. Assess for signs and symptoms of electrolyte imbalance and uremia. *Assist with dialysis, if indicated. *Provide prescribed diet, fluid allotment, and medications. Minimize risk of infection: handwashing; aseptic technique for care of central lines, urinary catheters, and wounds; aggressive pulmonary toilet. Encourage ambulation. Observe for signs and symptoms of infection. *Administer antibiotics as ordered. *Maintain patency of urinary catheter(s): irrigate as ordered. Encourage frequent voiding after removal of urinary catheter.	Child maintains normal fluid and electrolyte balance. Child experiences no evidence of complications.

*Denotes nursing intervention requiring a physician's order.

Nursing Diagnosis/ Patient Problem	Defining Characteristics	Nursing Interventions	Expected Outcome
High risk for injury related to rejection	Increased serum creatinine Decreased output Fever Graft tenderness Hypertension Flulike symptoms	*Administer prescribed immunosuppression (maintenance). Observe for signs and symptoms of fluid overload. *Administer antihypertensives, antipyretics, and diuretics as ordered. Monitor severity of pain, if present. Provide emotional support. *Administer antirejection therapy, including premedication, as ordered. *Administer viral prophylaxis therapy as ordered. Maintain IV access: monitor for signs and symptoms of infection and infiltration. Monitor for side effects of and response to therapy.	Child maintains normal fluid balance. Child responds to antirejection therapy. Child experiences no adverse effects from therapy.

High risk for injury related to side effects/adverse effects of immunosuppression	Increased serum creatinine
	Hypertension
	Hyperkalemia
	Leukopenia
	Gastrointestinal disorders
	CNS symptoms
	Infection/malignancy:
	  Fever
	  Fatigue/malaise
	  Transplant dysfunction
	CNS symptoms
	Respiratory symptoms
	Gastrointestinal symptoms
	Skin lesions
	Urinary tract symptoms
		Monitor vital signs, weight, and intake and output.
		*Obtain laboratory studies as ordered:
		  Serum creatinine
		  Serum electrolytes
		  Cyclosporine level (trough)
		  Blood cell count
		Minimize risk of infection and malignancy. (Refer to Exhibit 10–6 —Early detection and prevention of complications.)
		Report all new symptoms.
		*Administer prophylaxis or treatment for infection as ordered.
		Maintain IV access: monitor for signs and symptoms of infection and infiltration.
		Monitor for side effects of and response to therapy.
		Provide emotional support.
			Child experiences no serious adverse effects from immunosuppression.
			Unavoidable complications (for example, opportunistic infection, malignancy) are detected early.

*Denotes nursing intervention requiring a physician's order.

Nursing Diagnosis/ Patient Problem	Defining Characteristics	Nursing Interventions	Expected Outcome
Nutrition alteration: more than body requirements related to increased appetite and sodium retention from corticosteroids	Steady/excessive weight gain out of proportion to height Hypertension Edema	Monitor physical growth and blood pressure. *Maintain prescribed sodium restriction. Consult dietitian for assistance with weight control and salt restriction. Encourage walking and sports, as allowed. Encourage three well-balanced meals (no second helpings). Encourage limiting snacks: avoid concentrated sweets and high-carbohydrate, high-fat foods.	Child does not have excessive weight gain or symptoms of excessive sodium intake. Child's diet provides adequate nutrition for growth.
Fluid volume deficit related to inadequate oral intake and the kidneys' decreased concentrating ability	Failure to drink prescribed amount of fluid Decreased weight and blood pressure Laboratory values consistent with mild dehydration (increased creatinine, blood urea nitrogen, and hematocrit) Illness that causes excessive fluid losses (for example), fever, vomiting, diarrhea)	Monitor vital signs, weight, and intake and output. *Encourage oral fluids as prescribed. Assess for excessive fluid losses. *Administer intravenous fluids as ordered.	Child exhibits no signs or symptoms of fluid deficit.
Knowledge deficit related to potential complications and the importance of medications, diet, and continued medical care	Verbalization of questions or problems Inability to articulate rationale for treatment Inability to follow medication schedule Failure to seek appropriate follow-up	Refer to Appendix 10–B, Nursing Care Plan for a Child on Dialysis, for strategies. Refer to Exhibit 10–6 for content.	Child and family verbalize and demonstrate understanding of potential complications and treatment regimen.

*Denotes nursing intervention requiring a physician's order.

Nursing Diagnosis/ Patient Problem	Defining Characteristics	Nursing Interventions	Expected Outcome
Body image disturbance related to chronic illness, growth retardation, and side effects of immunosuppression	Cushingoid features Excessive weight gain Poor growth Acne Hirsutism Gingival hyperplasia Tremor Depression Social isolation Noncompliance with immunosuppressive regimen	Provide age-appropriate education about the disease process and the treatment plan. Explain that many side effects are dose dependent. Teach child how he or she can decrease severity of side effects (for example, weight control diet, exercise, care of acne). Encourage verbalization of feelings and perceptions; acknowledge feelings and clarify misconceptions. Support positive coping mechanisms. Encourage participation in normal age-appropriate activities, especially school. *Assist with referral for professional counseling as needed.	Child actively involved in normal age-appropriate activities and peer relationships. Child is compliant with immunosuppressive regimen.
Anxiety and fear related to success of transplant and long-term outcome for the child	Rejection episode(s) or other complications Frequent hospitalizations Child and parents verbalize fear and anxiety Child and parents exhibit signs of increased stress, anger, anxiety, frustration, or depression	Encourage verbalization of feelings and concerns. Provide emotional support. Provide accurate information and clarify misconceptions. Support positive coping mechanisms. Assist with identifying alternative strategies for ineffective coping mechanisms. Encourage normal parenting behaviors and normal family activities. *Assist with referral for professional counseling as needed.	Child and family exhibit decreased stress. Child and family use appropriate coping mechanisms.

*Denotes nursing intervention requiring a physician's order. Also see Table 13–9: Nursing Care Plan for the Child after Transplant.

Note: IV, intravenous; CNS, central nervous system.

CHAPTER 11

Impairment of the Musculoskeletal System

Kathleen Mauro

Musculoskeletal conditions for which home health care is needed can be categorized as either acute or chronic. Acute conditions require home health management for less than six months, whereas chronic conditions require management for longer periods and possibly a lifetime. The most frequently encountered acute conditions are developmental dysplasia of the hip (DDH) and osteomyelitis. Chronic conditions include Legg-Calvé-Perthes disease (LCP), limb abnormalities that require lengthening, cerebral palsy, and muscular dystrophy.

DEVELOPMENTAL DYSPLASIA OF THE HIP

The estimated incidence of DDH in the United States is one to two cases per 1,000 live births. The incidence is higher in populations that continue to tightly swaddle infants or use cradle boards. Females are affected six times more often than males, and in 20 percent of cases, both hips are involved (McCullough and Pellino 1994).

When DDH is diagnosed within the first six months of life, more conservative management such as a Pavlik harness (Figure 11–1) or casting may be used and potential outcomes are better (Speers and Speers 1992). However, if the diagnosis is made when the child is older than six months, treatment becomes more complex. In most of these older infants and children, the hip is actually dislocated and normal development of the hip socket has not occurred. In these cases, home traction can be used to stretch muscles and allow for hip reduction before surgical intervention and/or casting (Kramer, Schleberger, and Steffen 1990; McCullough and Pellino 1994).

If it is determined that the child is a candidate for home traction, the child is admitted for a brief hospitalization. A portable, modified Bryant's traction system such as the apparatus pictured in Figure 11–2 is obtained and applied (Hays 1995). In some treatment plans, a period of Russell's traction (Figure 11–3) precedes Bryant's traction (Kramer, Schleberger, and Steffen 1990). Bryant's traction is always applied to both legs. Parents and other potential caregivers are taught to apply the traction, maintain the equipment, adapt the procedure to activities of daily living (Figure 11–4), and observe for potential traction-related complications. Parents must demonstrate ability to care for their child in traction before discharge (Hays 1995). Inpatient teaching is reinforced by written handouts. The period of home traction is followed by surgery and casting or casting alone. See Exhibit 11–1 for general instructions for caring for a child in a cast at home and Appendix 11–A at the end of this chapter for a generic home care plan for a child with limited mobility secondary to a hip spica cast.

Because orthopedic plans are highly individualized, home health providers should carefully review any information that the parent received. The orthopedic management team should be

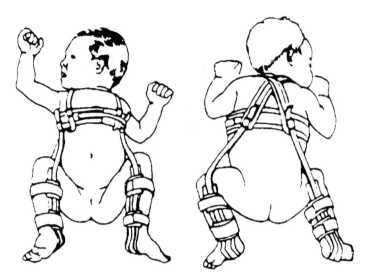

Figure 11–1 Application of the Pavlik harness. *Source:* Reprinted with permission from A. Speers & M. Speers, Care of the Child in a Pavlik Harness, *Pediatric Nursing,* Vol. 18, pp. 229–232, © Jannetti Publications, Inc.

contacted if further clarification of the orthopedic plan is needed. Home traction usually lasts two to three weeks. Children are allowed out of traction for a brief period each day, usually one to two hours. Special activities such as brief outings or car rides could be scheduled during this period (Hays 1995).

The generic care plan for use with a child experiencing an alteration in mobility secondary to

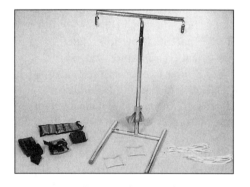

Figure 11–2 T-bar traction stand and weights. *Source:* Hays, M.A. (1995). Traction at home for infants with developmental dysplasia of the hip. *Orthopaedic Nursing,* *14*(1), pp. 33–4. Reprinted with permission of the publisher, the National Association of Orthopedic Nurses.

home traction is found in Appendix 11–B at the end of this chapter. Other generic pediatric home care nursing plans and care plans specific to many orthopedic conditions are available in the literature (Mourad 1995; Wong and Whaley 1996). These nursing plans can be modified for use with a specific child. It is recommended that a file of handouts, which are provided by the referring agency to the home health agency's clients, for parents and children be maintained to supplement or reinforce teaching.

It is essential that parents and caregivers are able to evaluate the child's skin integrity, assess circulation, conduct neurovascular checks, and implement appropriate interventions (Styrcula 1994a,b). One way to assess the caregiver's knowledge is to have the caregiver demonstrate procedures and assessments. Encourage the caregiver to use a flowsheet such as the one in Exhibit 11–2 to document time out of traction and the results of needed assessments. The flowsheet can be reviewed and modified as needed during future home care visits and shared with the orthopedic team at outpatient visits.

An alteration in mobility, even partial immobility, can result in appetite changes, constipation, sleep disturbances, irritability, discomfort,

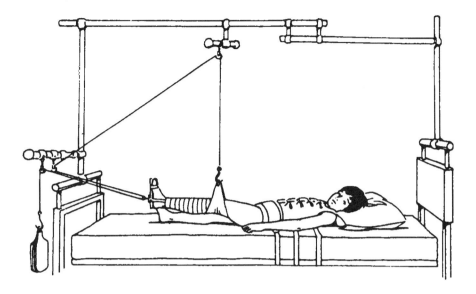

Figure 11–3 Russell traction. *Source:* Reprinted from D. Wong and L. Whaley, *Wong and Whaley's Clinical Manual of Pediatric Nursing,* p. 519, © 1996, Mosby-YearBook, Inc.

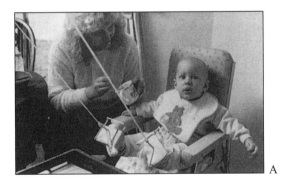
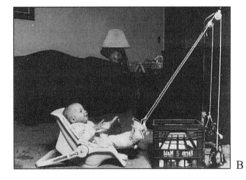

A   B

Figure 11–4 Child in traction demonstrating setup for high chair (A) and infant seat (B). *Source:* Hays, M.A., (1995). Traction at home for infants with developmental dysplasia of the hip. *Orthopaedic Nursing*, 14(1), pp. 33–4. Reprinted with permission of the National Association of Orthopedic Nurses.

and crying (Styrcula 1994b). Problems arising from the child's limited mobility are probably more challenging for parents and caregivers than monitoring traction equipment and making timely assessments. Anticipatory guidance may help prevent potential problems such as constipation, acknowledge the additional stress placed on the child's caregiver, and validate the need for diversional activities for both the child and caregiver.

LEGG-CALVÉ-PERTHES DISEASE

LCP is a self-limiting form of avascular necrosis of the femoral head. LCP occurs most commonly in children 2 to 12 years old with the

Exhibit 11–1 Caring for the Child in a Cast

- The cast and the skin above and below the cast need to be monitored frequently. A health professional should be notified if any of the following occur: burning sensation; numbness; odor; strange feelings; temperature changes; tingling; fluid coming from under or through the cast pain; or soft, broken, or cracked area on cast.
- Swelling can be prevented or decreased by raising the arm or leg in a cast above the level of the child's heart.
- Joints and muscles not casted need to be exercised. Remember movement can be fun when incorporated into a game.
- Petal the cast by using soft adhesive tape to cover the rough edges. Use three-inch strips. Begin by adhering the tape to the inside border of the cast. Bring the strip over the cast edge and adhere it to the outside of the cast.
- Do not put anything inside the cast in an attempt to scratch the skin. Sometimes blowing cool air into the cast with a hairdryer or scratching the opposite extremity will help relieve itching. If any object falls inside the cast and cannot be removed, notify a health professional.
- Children in body casts and full leg casts should receive a sponge bath. Smaller casts can be wrapped and sealed in plastic and kept out of the water while a child bathes or showers. Plaster casts should remain dry.
- Young children in a cast must be safely restrained in a safety seat when traveling in a car. Older children must still be restrained with a seat belt.
- See Appendix 11–A for nursing care plan for a child with a hip spica cast.

Source: Data from D. Wong and L. Whaley, *Wong and Whaley's Clinical Manual of Pediatric Nursing,* 4th edition, © 1996, Mosby Year Book, Inc.

highest incidence occurring in children 4 to 8 years old. Males are affected four times as often as females. The exact etiology is unknown, but LCP has been associated with transient synovitis, trauma, infection, and metabolic bone disease (McCullough and Pellino 1994; Serlo, Heikkinen, and Puranen 1987).

The disease progresses through four stages. Many children are asymptomatic during the initial avascular stage when necrotic bone develops. During the second, or fragmentation stage, symptoms increase. The child develops a limp, the hip becomes painful, or pain may be referred to the knee. Hip infusion occurs and hip range of motion may decrease. Immature cells begin to replace necrotic bone, and the redeveloping femoral head becomes susceptible to molding defects. During the third stage, lasting one to three years, reossification and remodeling occur as the necrotic bone is reabsorbed. During the next one to three years the final healing stage occurs and normal bone cells replace immature cells (McCullough and Pellino 1994).

Early initiation of treatment for LPD is essential for the prevention of deformity, and younger children tend to have a better prognosis. Most orthopedic treatment plans involve a period of limited mobility, limited weight bearing, and containment. The treatment goal of containment is to facilitate the development of a normal femoral head contour by "containing" or maintaining the femoral head within the acetabulum. Casting, orthotics, traction, surgery, or a combination of treatment modalities can be used. Surgery is usually reserved for more complicated cases or for children and/or families who are unable to comply with less invasive treatment plans. Another major treatment goal is to regain and/or maintain full range of motion in the hip joint (McCullough and Pellino 1994).

Home health providers must become familiar with the child's orthopedic treatment plan. Although some children can be followed radiographically, children requiring home health follow-up require more complex treatment interventions such as traction. A soft boot is applied to the foot, and Russell's traction (refer to Figure 11–3) is applied (Styrcula 1994b). Traction serves to facilitate circulation with the hip joint, prevent venous stasis, and allow the femoral head to develop normally (Serlo, Heikkinen, and Puranen 1987). Length of time in traction within

Exhibit 11–2 Sample Flowsheet for Assessment of Child in Cast or Traction

DATE:					
TIME:					
TOES					
Skin					
Vascular					
Color					
Temp					
Cap refill					
Sensation					
Range of motion (ROM)					
FOOT					
Skin					
Vascular					
Color					
Temp					
Pulses					
Sensation					
ROM					
LEG					
Skin					
Vascular					
Color					
Temp					
Pulses					
Sensation					
ROM					
EQUIPMENT					
Traction					
Cast					
BODY ALIGNMENT					
FLUIDS					
BOWEL MOVEMENT					
OUT OF TRACTION					
ACTIVITIES					
INTERVENTIONS					
CAREGIVER					

a 24-hour period varies and some children require traction only at night.

Children with LPC often experience periods of acute pain. Refer to Appendix 11–C at the end of this chapter for a nursing plan for a child with an alteration in comfort level. For additional information on pain including pain assessment scales, please see Chapter 14. The pain associated with LPD is due to inflammation, synovitis, and spasm. Discomfort, which is a primary concern of both the child and parent, can be managed with bed rest, salicylates, and traction with abduction. Additional pain medication should be used as needed to provide pain relief. Complementary pain management therapies, such as music, massage, video programs, and relaxation, should also be considered.

LIMB LENGTHENING

Uneven limb length and structural bone deformity may be the result of metabolic bone disease, growth retardation, infection, trauma, radiation therapy, congenital defects, or neuromuscular conditions such as polio or cerebral palsy. Technology acquired from the former Soviet Union now makes it possible to correct many structural bone deformities using external fixators (Dunwoody 1994; Newschwander and Dunst 1989). The population of children with external fixator devices requiring home health care has been increasing rapidly. Therefore, knowledge related to the management of such children in the home has become more essential.

Limb lengthening and limb modification procedures are accomplished by surgery in combination with the application of an Ilizarov external fixator or similar device. The surgical procedure includes a corticotomy, accomplished through a small incision, in which two-thirds to three-fourths of the circumference of the bone cortex is cut. The remaining one-third to onefourth of the circumference of the bone cortex is fractured. Because the medullary cortex is not cut, the surgical result is the creation of a potential growth area. New "lengthening" bone forms in the created growth area (Figure 11–5).

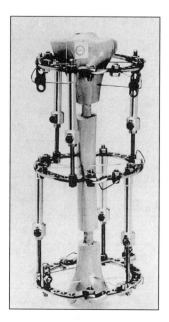

Figure 11–5 Bifocal corticotomy with Ilizarov fixator. *Source:* Reprinted from Newschwander, G.E. and Dunst, R. (1989). Limb lengthening with the Iliazrov external fixator. *Orthopaedic Nursing*, 8(3), pp. 17. Reprinted with permission of the publisher, National Association of Orthopedic Nurses.

The Ilizarov external fixator, a combination of metal rings, rods, and wires, is used to manipulate the growth pattern. Growth takes place through controlled distraction. As healing begins to occur in the created gap, distraction or further separation within the gap is created by moving the metal rings further apart and/or by applying greater tension to the wires (Newschwander and Dunst 1989). The Ilizarov external fixator can be used to immobilize fractures, lengthen and widen bones, and correct rotational deformities (Dunwoody 1994). Children with Ilizarov external fixators must be followed closely and are usually scheduled for weekly outpatient visits.

In addition to being monitored for pain or potential complications due to impaired mobility and potentially impaired neurovascular status, children with external fixators must be closely monitored for complications due to impaired skin integrity (Appendix 11–D). Caregivers must closely observe for signs and symptoms of infection at pin and wire insertion sites. Pin care, as prescribed by the orthopedic surgeon, must be routinely carried out. Early signs or symptoms of skin infection such as crusting or tenting around pin sites must be immediately reported to the surgeon. Early intervention is essential because wound infection can compromise treatment or progress to osteomyelitis.

OSTEOMYELITIS

Osteomyelitis, infection of the bone, most commonly occurs in children younger than 12 years. Osteomyelitis can occur from hematogenous spread, infected soft tissue, or direct wounds. Thus, osteomyelitis may occur secondary to the spread of bacteria from ear, skin, and respiratory infections or as the result of open fractures or surgical procedures. *Staphylococcus aureus* and *Haemophilus influenzae* are the most common causative organisms isolated in children (Morse et al. 1994).

As bacteria proliferate within the bone, inflammation occurs. As the inflammation process continues, pus, vascular congestion, and edema occur as the result of normal immunologic responses. Soon, vascular pressure within the bone reaches arterial pressure. Inadequate arterial circulation results in further ischemic injury and necrosis within the rigid bone (Morse et al. 1994).

Because osteomyelitis is potentially a difficult infection to treat, early diagnosis and initiation of appropriate antibiotic therapy are critical. Once treatment is initiated, impaired circulation may prevent adequate levels of antibiotics from reaching the infection site. Potential complications of acute osteomyelitis include soft tissue abscesses, cutaneous sinus tracts, a shortened limb, and a chronic form of the disease.

Home management of osteomyelitis focuses on continuing antibiotic therapy and monitoring for signs and symptoms of increased infection. Intravenous (IV) antibiotic therapy usually lasts four to six weeks. IV antibiotic therapy may be delivered through a peripheral intermittent infusion or a central venous catheter such as a Broviac or Hickman. (See Chapter 8 for care of central lines.) Therefore, parents and caregivers must be taught to maintain and monitor the IV site, administer antibiotics, and observe for potential side effects. IV antibiotic therapy is usually followed by approximately four to eight weeks of oral antibiotic therapy.

CEREBRAL PALSY

The estimated incidence of cerebral palsy varies from 1.5 to 5.0 cases per 1,000 live births. Cerebral palsy refers to a collection of neuromotor disorders of central origin (motor cortex, basal ganglia, or cerebellum), with the essential clinical finding being neuromotor impairment. Prenatal, perinatal, and postnatal factors that contribute to the development of cerebral palsy include asphyxia and infection. Intraventricular bleeding with resultant necrosis of white brain matter is strongly associated with cerebral palsy morbidity (Hill and Volpe 1995). Studies indicate, however, that a large proportion of the cases of cerebral palsy remain unexplained (Rosen and Dickenson 1992; Nelson, Swaiman, and Russman 1995). This fact may be especially disconcerting to the parents who ask, "Why was my child affected?" Despite earlier optimism that cerebral palsy was likely to disappear with improvements in obstetric and neonatal care, there has reportedly been no decrease in its frequency in the past two decades and cerebral palsy continues to be the most frequent childhood disability (Molnar 1992).

During the neonatal period, an infant who has sustained a severe insult to the brain may display a weak suck and uncoordinated swallow. Parents may describe a "floppy" or hypotonic infant. There are often abnormalities of the grasp, Moro, and stepping reflexes (see Chapter 16). Abnormal posturing and muscle tone may be present. Seizures occur in about one-half of the children but less frequently in children with diplegia and dyskinetic cerebral palsy (Molnar 1992).

Exhibit 11–3 Impaired Physical Mobility

Goals:

- Maintain independent movement within the environment to the fullest extent possible.
- Recognize complications of immobility and prevent or treat.
- Minimize potential for injury.

Interventions:

- Assess the degree of neuromuscular impairment and assess functional abilities, including activity tolerance, coordination, strength, endurance, level of discomfort or pain, joint range of motion. Document using scale indicating "independent," "independent with equipment," assistance necessary from another person, assistance necessary from another person and equipment, and "dependent."
- Assess the effects of perceptual and cognitive impairment.
- Discuss purposes of mobility, prevention of disuse phenomena, stimulation and motivation, and ability to complete activities of daily living.

- Meet child's safety needs and minimize potential for injury by supervised ambulation, helmets, seat belts, correct-fitting wheelchairs with appropriate safety features, and restrainers to assist with positioning. Assess for presence of risk factors for injury.
- Use assistive devices (orthotics, splints, and braces) to facilitate protection and stimulation of weak muscles, relaxation of tight muscles, joint support, functional positioning, prevention of contractures, and delay in progression of abnormal postures.
- Establish home recreation and exercise program.
- Teach proper positioning to prevent complications and encourage compliance with treatment program to delay or prevent complications.
- Assess for complications of immobility and note effects in the following areas: integumentary (skin breakdown), respiratory (infection and decreased vital capacity), neuromuscular (circulation, weakness, and contractures), gastrointestinal (appetite, digestion, and elimination), genitourinary (infection and continence), and psychosocial (attitude, self-concept, and socialization). Discuss, teach, and reinforce with caregivers.

Cerebral control of movement develops as the infant matures. Failure to attain motor milestones and a change in muscle tone from hypotonic to hypertonic may become evident. Evaluation of delayed or abnormal motor development must take into account the wide range in variability and quality of performance in achievement of milestones. Thus, establishing an early definitive diagnosis of cerebral palsy is difficult in some children because specific manifestations indicating neuromotor impairment may not be present.

Variations of clinical manifestations in the continuum of this disorder result from differing degrees of involvement. Children with spastic hemiplegia (one side of body) or spastic quadriplegia (all four extremities) make up the largest group. Clinical manifestations include increased muscle tone, increased stretch reflexes, and muscle weakness. Contractures of the affected joints occur because of spasticity, which may be mild to severe. In hemiparetic cerebral palsy, which is the most frequent clinical type, fine motor function of the hand is the most severe impairment. Sensory deficits, cortical neglect, and unawareness of the paretic side may also be present. Despite the limited function of the hemiparetic hand, these children are expected to become independent in daily activities unless perceptual or cognitive deficits interfere with self-care skills (Molnar 1992). Greater involvement of the lower extremities is more common in the child with quadriparetic cerebral palsy. A "scissoring" gait results as bilateral contractures rotate the hips inward. The usual motor pattern also includes plantar flexion of the feet, poor trunk control, and flexion contractures of the wrist and fingers. Oromotor involvement, manifested by tongue protrusion, impaired swallowing, and dysarthric speech may be present to varying degrees (see Exhibit 11–3).

Spastic diplegia is the common term applied to a variation of spastic quadriparesis in which the upper extremities are only mildly affected. Athetoid cerebral palsy, the second most common type of neuromotor dysfunction, manifests as writhing, uncontrolled muscular activity that appears when the child is 18 months of age or older. These abnormal involuntary movements include facial grimacing, tongue and mouth dystonic movements, and rotary or twisting movements of the hands and feet. Muscle tone fluctuates, and abnormal movements may disappear during sleep. If the child is anxious or physically stimulated, the abnormality of the movements may intensify. A mixed pattern of cerebral motor deficit may occur with elements of spasticity and athetosis.

Cerebellar impairment of balance and coordination characterizes ataxic cerebral palsy, which is the least frequent clinical type. Clinical manifestations include a wide-based, unsteady gait and uncoordinated upper extremity function. "Overshooting" when reaching for a toy is characteristic. Speech may be monotonous and drawling.

Management of spasticity includes specialized treatment techniques aimed at inhibition of the patterns of abnormal reflex activity and facilitation of normal motor patterns. Orthopedic management includes the use of positioning devices and, in selected cases, surgery (Sprague 1992).

Injection of phenol or alcohol solution into the peripheral nerve or motor points of a spastic muscle results in a decrease in tone due to chemical neurolysis. Although the effects are transient, good results and no significant side effects have been reported (Molnar 1992). Occasionally, children undergoing tibial nerve block will experience painful paresthesias, which may last from three to four weeks and can almost always be managed with mild analgesics. Hydrotherapy can have a soothing effect. The relative benefits and goals of each treatment regimen

must be communicated effectively to the family to avoid unrealistic expectations because the underlying motor dysfunction is not corrected. Use of medications for the control of spasticity requires careful monitoring for adverse side effects. Adjunctive medication may be required for control of seizures and other associated conditions. See Chapter 6 for medications commonly used to treat seizures.

Auditory and visual deficits are reportedly more common in children with cerebral palsy when compared with children without disabilities. Early recognition and correction of these deficits will minimize interference with the child's functioning to the extent possible. One should remember, however, that the child with cerebral palsy may have normal intellect capabilities.

A comprehensive care plan and follow-up must be developed for infants identified as "high risk" in addition to those infants with a known neurologic dysfunction. Infant research studies support the concept of early intervention during infancy and the first three years of life (Molnar 1992). An infant's responsiveness to a wide variety of stimuli and enjoyment of social contacts have also been found to correlate highly with the capacity to cope with frustrations and challenges presented by the environment. Notable achievements in this area include the use of specially adapted electromechanical toys. As a result, more children with severe disabilities (developmental level, six months to eight years) can experience increased opportunities for interaction and exploration, enhancing their motor and perceptual development. Through the use of specially designed switches, children can control some part of the environment, often for the first time. In addition, the concept of cause and effect, a foundation for future learning, is within their realm of experience. Similarly designed switches can eventually be used to drive an electric wheelchair or operate an environmental control device. The toys also serve as an introduction to the use of augmentative communication devices. See Chapter 18 for physical and occupational therapy interventions.

It is critical for professionals to advocate for children with cerebral palsy and to educate families about potential resources for their children. An excellent reference for parents is *Cerebral Palsy: A Complete Guide for Caregiving* by Miller and Bachrach (1995).

In summary, goals for children with cerebral palsy and their families include the following:

- Maximize the child's potential for achieving independence in movement and mobility, communication, and self-care.
- Minimize the deleterious effects of associated conditions (for example, seizures, auditory and visual deficits, cognitive impairments).
- Assist the family in dealing with the special demands in caring for their child through education, emotional support, and communication and coordination of the necessary resources.

Treatment includes adaptive devices to facilitate movement and self-care abilities; augmentative communication devices; therapeutic handling and positioning; and modification of spasticity with medications, such as dantrolene (Dantrium), diazepam (Valium), baclofen (Lioresal), benztropine (Cogentin), and clonazepam (Clonopin), peripheral nerve blocks, and orthopedic surgery.

Additional nursing goals are included in Exhibits 11–4 through 11–13.

MUSCULAR DYSTROPHY

The muscular dystrophies are the largest group of muscle diseases that occur during childhood. Duchenne's dystrophy, the most common and most extensively studied type, occurs in approximately 0.14 per 1,000 children. Progressive muscle weakness and increasing disability characterize the four types of muscular dystrophy. All four have a genetic origin; however, the most common form, Duchenne's, is found only in males and is transferred as a recessive, sex-linked trait. Elevated enzyme levels in

Exhibit 11–4 Potential Impairment of Skin Integrity

Goals
- Minimize risk for skin breakdown.
- Prevent, recognize, and treat complications.

Interventions
- Plan with the family and child an effective skin-care regimen to prevent breakdown and to recognize and treat problems. Some children may be able to use and position a mirror to inspect less accessible parts of their bodies.
- Discuss use of methods to increase circulation and alter or eliminate pressure: exercise including active and passive range of motion, position change, positioning devices, lotions or ointments, skin barriers, alternate pressure mattresses or waterbeds, and flotation pads or gel cushions for wheelchairs.
- Observe pressure areas, institute effective care, and begin treatment when problems arise.

this type have led to speculation that a biochemical deficit in the muscle tissue may be a causative factor. Additionally, early recognition of this exceptionally high enzyme activity level will facilitate genetic counseling.

Onset of symptoms of Duchenne's dystrophy start during the preschool phase when weakness in the legs, stumbling, and flat feet are noted. (For other types of dystrophies, the onset of symptoms may not occur until late childhood, adolescence, or early adult life.) Wasting of the muscles occurs, but the muscles actually seem to grow larger, especially in the calves, because of increased fat and fibrous tissue. The weakness progresses to the pelvic area, leading to a waddling gait, difficulty in getting up from the floor (Gowers's sign), toe walking, and difficulty in climbing stairs. Lordosis and scoliosis develop. As more areas become involved, ambulation becomes difficult and confinement to a wheelchair is necessary. The disease continues on a steady, downhill course until almost all voluntary muscles are affected and the child is bedridden.

Most children do not survive past age 21 years, with death resulting from respiratory or cardiac complications. Goals in nursing care of these children include the following:

- Maintain safe ambulation.
- Maintain function and independence through range of motion, surgery to release contracture deformities, bracing, and performance of activities of daily living. Reduce preventable complications by early recognition and intervention.
- Help child and family understand and cope with the nature of the condition and to deal with the restrictions imposed on their lives.

Exhibit 11–5   Ineffective Airway Clearance/ Breathing Pattern

Goals
- Minimize risk for occluded airway or respiratory distress.
- Prevent or recognize and treat complications.
- Effectively clear secretions within level of ability.

Interventions
- Assess for signs and symptoms of increased respiratory effort and respiratory distress, including secretions audible or visible in airway that cannot be independently cleared, change in breath sounds, retractions, use of accessory muscles, asymmetrical chest wall movement, tachypnea, tachycardia, diaphoresis, pallor, and cyanosis.
- Discuss and review with caregivers the indications for calling the physician and/or rescue squad. Assess plans for emergency intervention and assist in their development.
- Use adaptive seating and positioning to improve pulmonary function.
- Use aggressive pulmonary toilet, assisted coughing, and postural drainage when required.
- Instruct in use and side effects of prescribed antibiotics.

Treatment includes supportive measures, supervision, special braces, aids, and equipment. A lightweight body brace, individually constructed, may help to delay deterioration and abnormality. Physical therapy and orthopedic procedures can minimize deformities (see Chapter

---

Exhibit 11–6   Alteration in Nutrition

Goals
- Maintain body weight in relation to metabolic need while maintaining optimal health.
- Attain desirable body weight with optimal health.

Interventions
- Assess for consumption of adequate fluids and calories, including the use of assistive devices. Encourage self-feeding using long-handled utensils, drinking tubes, and other devices as recommended.
- Assess effectiveness of swallowing facilitation techniques, including use of verbal cueing, modification of food type or consistency, positioning.
- Observe caregivers' ability to tube feed, including preparation of equipment, placement of tube, position check, safety, and administration of feeding. Assess knowledge of common tube feeding problems such as constipation, diarrhea, abdominal cramping, vomiting, plugged tube, and aspiration. See Chapter 8 for alterations in metabolic functions.
- Note behavior, response, and tolerance of dietary regimen. Provide adequate diet teaching emphasizing the need for food with high fiber content to facilitate normal elimination.
- Assess hydration status by reviewing pattern of weight gain, intake versus output, skin turgor, and condition of mucous membranes.
- Note condition of teeth and compliance and ability to provide effective oral hygiene program to include flossing and brushing, as well as avoidance of cariogenic foods.

18). Exercise, rest, and diet needs are normal. Assistance in activities of daily living is required, along with reduction of architectural barriers and modification of clothing. Relationships with staff should be supportive, with assistance provided in decision making as care needs increase. Long-term support is necessary in dealing with fears of death and grieving. The parents should be given genetic counseling.

The therapy program should be tailored to the child's needs and abilities. Active participation of the family in a home program of activities and exercises and school, social, and recreational activities is encouraged. The child should be helped to develop and enhance self-help skills for maximum independence. The home care nurse can provide supportive interactions for the family and child.

The child with muscular dystrophy and cerebral palsy requires the combined services and involvement of an interdisciplinary health care team. The home care nurse can assist the family to clarify roles and responsibilities and to coordinate various services. The use of nursing diagnoses provides a focus for discharge and home care planning. Nursing diagnoses facilitates communication with nurses in community agencies and other resources for continuing care (Gordon 1994).

Nursing goals and interventions for children with cerebral palsy and muscular dystrophy are presented in Exhibits 11–3 through 11–12 and should be viewed in relation to the specifics of the disease condition and the assessed needs and problems of the child and family (Doenges and Moorhouse 1996).

Exhibit 11–7 Alteration in Bowel Elimination

Goals

- Establish regular pattern in bowel functioning.
- Resume elective bowel function pattern.

Interventions

- Assess usual and current pattern of bowel function.
- Evaluate dietary intake.
- Determine need for use of medications, enemas, or natural laxatives.
- Promote normalization of bowel function with use of bowel program including diet high in fiber and bulk, adequate amount and type of fluid intake (using some type of incentive or reward program may be helpful for some children), activity exercise as tolerated, stool softeners, laxatives as prescribed, privacy and scheduled times for defecation, and normal and comfortable position (see Chapter 8).

Exhibit 11–8 Self-Care Deficit: Feeding, Bathing, Hygiene, Dressing, Grooming, and Toileting

Goals
- Achieve self-care to the fullest possible extent.
- Achieve activities of daily living within limits of situation.

Interventions
- Continually assess and evaluate potential for self-care capabilities and activities.
- Change daily routines as indicated.
- Identify barriers and assist in the provision of necessary adaptations and assistive devices to facilitate self-care activities. Help with the selection and modification of clothing.
- Review and reinforce instructions from the interdisciplinary team; continually evaluate care plan with child and family to identify progress and needed modifications.
- Assess child and family response to level of and/or changes in functioning. Provide support and referral to appropriate resources as needed.

Exhibit 11–9 Anticipatory Grieving

Goals

- Feelings are appropriately expressed.
- Difficulties in the process of grieving are identified and resolved.

Interventions

- Assess current needs and behaviors involving child and family. Note family interaction patterns and alterations imposed by disease. See Chapter 20 for parents' perspective on pediatric home care.
- Provide assistance to child in expressing feelings and dealing with changes in familiar patterns. Incorporate family and significant others in support structure.
- Give information, identify strengths, and refer to other resources as appropriate (counseling, support groups, spiritual resources).

Exhibit 11–10 Sensory-Perceptual Alteration (Visual, Auditory)

Goal

- Improve ability to interact with the environment and respond to it adaptively.

Interventions

- Assess level of functioning through periodic ophthalmologic and auditory screening.
- Provide opportunities for self-initiated activities such as specially adapted toys. General concepts for provision of stimuli include the following: must be individually tailored for infant or child, be variable over time and in intensity, and capture the child's attention to elicit a response. Placement of such stimuli should present a challenge, however, within the scope of the child's ability.
- Review environmental safety aspects and use of assistive devices, including hearing aids, communication devices to promote acquisition of language skills, and/or effective communication patterns.

Exhibit 11–11 Diversional Activity Deficit/ Powerlessness

Goals

- Engage in meaningful activities appropriate for tolerance and abilities.
- Initiate coping actions appropriate for identified problems.
- Maintain appropriate level of social interaction.

Interventions

- Determine ability to participate, mobility requirements, and interest in leisure activities that are available.
- Identify child's locus of control.
- Motivate or stimulate child's involvement in needs identification and activity planning; acknowledge reality of situation and child's perceptions and concerns and provide for physical and mental activities.
- Explore options for activities given child's strengths and abilities.
- Show respect and concern for the child and family and assist in dealing with feelings of hopelessness and anger.
- Continue school as long as possible and encourage socialization and diversional activities.

Exhibit 11–12   Impaired Home Maintenance Management

Goals
- Function in home environment with use of available resources and appropriate modifications.
- Environment is clean and safe and facilitates optimal growth and development.

Interventions
- Assess level of physical functioning as well as cognitive and emotional functioning.
- Reduce architectural barriers in as many areas as possible.
- Identify learning needs, available support systems, and financial resources.
- Support child and family in their ability to maintain a safe environment that promotes and encourages independence. This includes establishment of a realistic home care plan, identification and acquisition of necessary equipment, structural modifications to facilitate care, as well as discussion and planning with family opportunities to have respite from care of child. Modify plans as disease state changes or progresses.

Exhibit 11–13   Disturbance in Body Image/ Self-Concept

Goals
- Verbalize understanding of body differences and acceptance of self.
- Recognize and incorporate changes into self-concept in an accurate manner with preservation of self-esteem.

Interventions
- Assess level of knowledge about present condition or diagnosis and child and family responses to changes in function.
- Assess adaptation to grief response related to changes in function and/or prognosis; modify as disease progresses.
- Acknowledge and accept adaptation and grief response while setting limits on maladaptive behavior.
- Provide information, reinforce explanations, and refer to support groups or counseling as appropriate.
- Encourage positive attitudes and effective communication patterns.

REFERENCES

Doenges, M., and M.F. Moorhouse. 1996. *Nurse's pocket guide: Nursing diagnoses with interventions.* 5th ed. Philadelphia: F.A. Davis.

Dunwoody, C.J. 1994. Modalities for immobilization. In *Orthopedic nursing,* ed. A.B. Maher, S.W. Salmond, and T.A. Pellino, 277–310. Philadelphia: W.B. Saunders Company.

Gordon, M. 1994. *Nursing diagnosis process and application.* 3d ed. St. Louis: C.V. Mosby.

Hays, M. A. 1995. Traction at home for infants with developmental dysplasia of the hip. *Orthopaedic Nursing* 14: 33–40.

Hill, A., and J.J. Volpe. 1995. Hypoxic-ischemic cerebral injury in the newborn. In *Pediatric neurology principles and practice: Vol 1,* ed. K.F. Swaiman, 489–507. St. Louis: C.V. Mosby.

Kramer, J., R. Schleberger, and R. Steffen. 1990. Closed reduction by two-phase skin traction and functional splinting in mitigated abduction for treatment of congenital dislocation of the hip. *Clinical Orthopaedics and Related Research* 258:27–32.

McCullough, L., and T.A. Pellino. 1994. Congenital and developmental disorders. In *Orthopedic nursing,* ed. A.B. Maher, S.W. Salmond, and T.A. Pellino, 617–700. Philadelphia: W. B. Saunders Company.

Miller, F., and S.J. Bachrach. 1995. *Cerebral palsy: A complete guide for caregiving.* Baltimore: Johns Hopkins University Press.

Molnar, G.E. 1992. Cerebral palsy. In *Pediatric rehabilitation,* ed. G.E. Molnar, 481–533. Baltimore: Williams & Wilkins.

Morse, C.O., et al. 1994. Infections of the musculoskeletal system. In *Orthopedic nursing,* ed. A.B. Maher, S.W. Salmond, and T.A. Pellino, 843–81. Philadelphia: W.B. Saunders Company.

Mourad, L. 1995. *Plans of care for specialty practice: Orthopedic nursing.* Milwaukee: Delmar Publishers.

Nelson, K.B., K.F. Swaiman, and B.S. Russman. 1995. Cerebral palsy. In *Pediatric neurology principles and practice: vol 1,* 2d ed., ed. K.F. Swaiman, 471–88. St. Louis: C.V. Mosby.

Newschwander, G.E., and R.M. Dunst. 1989. Limb lengthening with the Ilizarov external fixator. *Orthopaedic Nursing* 8, no. 3:15–21.

Rosen, M.G., and J.C. Dickenson. 1992. The incidence of cerebral palsy. *American Journal of Obstetrics and Gynecology* 167, no. 2:417–32.

Serlo, W., E. Heikkinen, and J. Puranen. 1987. Preoperative Russell traction in Legg-Calvé-Perthes disease. *Journal of Pediatric Orthopedics* 7:288–90.

Speers, A.T., and M. Speers. 1992. Care of the infant in a Pavlik harness. *Pediatric Nursing* 18:229–232, 252.

Sprague, J.B. 1992. Surgical management of cerebral palsy. *Orthopaedic Nursing.* 11, no. 4:11–18.

Styrcula, L. 1994a. Traction basics: Part III types of traction. *Orthopaedic Nursing* 13, no. 4:34–44.

Styrcula, L. 1994b. Traction basics: Part IV traction for lower extremities. *Orthopaedic Nursing* 13, no. 5: 59–68.

Wong, D., and L. Whaley. 1996. *Wong and Whaley's clinical manual of pediatric nursing.* 4th ed. St. Louis: C.V. Mosby.

BIBLIOGRAPHY

Corbett, D. 1988. Information needs of parents of a child in a Pavlik harness. *Orthopaedic Nursing* 7, no. 2:20–23.

Mubarak, S., et al. 1981. Pitfalls in the use of the Pavlik harness in congenital dysplasia, subluxation and dislocation of the hip. *Journal of Bone and Joint Surgery American.* 63:1239–48.

Home Care Plan for Child with Alteration in Mobility Secondary to Hip Spica Cast

Nursing Diagnosis	Child Goals	Interventions	Rationale	Home Caregiver Teaching
Alteration in mobility secondary to hip spica cast	Child will maintain normal peripheral neurovascular status.	Monitor skin color and temperature, capillary refill in foot, foot and lower leg pulses, and cast fit. Determine how lower leg and area under the cast "feels" to the child. Monitor sensation in foot and lower leg.	Normal color, temperature, capillary refill, and pulses are indicators of adequate tissue perfusion. A tight cast can constrict extremity and impede circulation. Discomfort, tingling, or unusual sensations can indicate skin irritation or excessive pressure. Prolonged pressure can result in tissue or nerve damage and compartmental syndrome.	Briefly discuss neurovascular status. Demonstrate indicators of adequate status and follow with return demonstration. Discuss potential alterations in status and recommended interventions. Review how to contact appropriate health care provider if caregiver has questions or problems develop. Encourage questions.

Nursing Diagnosis	Child Goals	Interventions	Rationale	Home Caregiver Teaching
	Child will be free of skin irritation from cast.	Observe skin in close proximity to cast. Check cast fit daily. Observe for unusual cast odors. Maintain adequate perianal hygiene.	Skin areas in close proximity to cast are prone to irritation due to friction between cast and skin. Young children grow rapidly and can require frequent cast changes. Loose casts produce unnecessary friction, which can result in tissue damage. Odor may indicate skin breakdown or foreign body under cast. Inadequate hygiene and soiling can promote bacterial growth, which results in skin breakdown. Excessive moisture will cause cast to deteriorate.	Discuss effect of excess pressure on skin and tissue. Point out potential pressure areas. Discuss early indicators of tissue break-down such as swelling, redness, and tenderness. Discuss need for keeping cast clean and dry, increased risk for skin breakdown, and importance of frequent diaper changes or toileting modifications for older children.
	Child will participate in diver-sional activities.	Develop a variety of potential activities based on child's developmental level and attention span and vary setting.	Small children who are confined and/or bored may be more difficult to comfort. Early initiation of and frequent changes in activity level	Discuss child's and family's normal routine and areas of potential modification. Provide anticipatory guidance on child demands,

Nursing Diagnosis	Child Goals	Interventions	Rationale	Home Caregiver Teaching
			can prevent or relieve boredom or discomfort and decrease caregiver burden over the long term.	stress, and diversional activities for child and caregiver. Encourage expression of concerns.
	Child will maintain full range of motion (ROM) in foot.	Supervise ROM.	Limited mobility, even for short periods, can result in loss of full ROM and delay recovery.	Demonstrate active and passive foot and knee ROM. Encourage questions.

Home Care Plan for Child with Alteration in Mobility Secondary to Traction

Nursing Diagnosis	Child Goals	Interventions	Rationale	Home Caregiver Teaching
Alteration in mobility secondary to home traction	Child will maintain normal peripheral neurovascular status.	Monitor skin color and temperature, capillary refill in toes, and pulses in foot on affected side. Monitor sensation in affected extremity. Document findings on flowsheet.	Normal color, temperature, capillary refill, and pulses are indicators of adequate tissue perfusion. Redness indicates tissue irritation. Impaired sensation can indicate increased pressure on nerve and progress to nerve damage. Documentation facilitates communication among caregivers and early intervention.	Briefly discuss neurovascular status. Demonstrate indicators of adequate status and follow with return demonstration. Discuss potential complications and interventions to restore status. Provide flowsheet or encourage caregiver to develop a flowsheet. Demonstrate recording findings on flowsheet. Encourage questions.
	Child will be free of skin breakdown.	Observe potential pressure points and skin in close	Dependent body areas are prone to venous stasis which increases	Discuss effect of excess pressure on skin and tissue. Point out

271

Nursing Diagnosis	Child Goals	Interventions	Rationale	Home Caregiver Teaching
		proximity with external equipment. Observe for edema.	risk for skin breakdown. Friction from sheets and loose wraps can cause skin break-down.	potential pressure areas. Discuss early indicators of tissue break-down such as swelling, redness, and tenderness. Review traction application. Encourage questions.
		Ensure that foam boot and/or Ace wraps and straps are not too loose or tight. Maintain adequate hygiene especially in perianal area.	Edema can indicate venous stasis and tissue injury. Tight wraps can impair circula-tion. Loose Ace wraps may result in inadequate traction pull. Prolonged skin contact with waste products in combination with immobility will result in faster skin breakdown.	Discuss increased risk for skin breakdown and importance of frequent diaper changes for young children or toileting modifications for older children.
	Child will maintain normal bowel function.	Monitor and document intake and bowel elimina-tion. Provide increased fluids and dietary fiber as appropriate for age.	Decreased activity can result in appetite changes and decreased peristalsis and increases risk for constipation. Documentation facilitates	Discuss relation-ships among diet, appetite, bowel function, and immobility. Stress preven-tion of constipa-tion and importance of dietary fiber.

Nursing Diagnosis	Child Goals	Interventions	Rationale	Home Caregiver Teaching
			communication among caregivers and early intervention.	Discuss potential dietary modifications for this child.
	Child will participate in diversional activities.	Develop a variety of potential activities based on child's developmental level and attention span. Incorporate fine and gross motor activities and vary setting.	Small children who are confined and/or bored may be more difficult to comfort. Early initiation of and frequent changes in activity level can prevent or relieve boredom or discomfort and decrease caregiver burden over the long term.	Discuss child's and family's normal routine and areas of potential modifications. Provide anticipatory guidance on child demands, stress (see Chapter 19), and diversional activities for child and caregiver. Encourage expression of concerns.
	Child will maintain full range of motion (ROM) in knee and foot distal to affected hip.	Supervise and document range of motion exercise.	Limited mobility, even for short periods, can result in loss of full ROM and delay recovery. Documentation of activity will facilitate adherence to routine.	Discuss and demonstrate active and passive ROM (see Appendix 16–A) taking into consideration the clinically indicated restrictions for this child. Encourage questions.

Home Care Plan for Child with an Alteration in Comfort Level

Nursing Diagnosis	Child Goals	Interventions	Rationale	Home Caregiver Teaching
Alteration in comfort	Child will be physically comfortable.	Maintain proper body alignment. Use pillows and rolled towels. Modify child's position frequently. Use diversional activities as needed.	Improper alignment places abnormal stress on muscles and joints and increases risk for contracture and deformity. Muscle stress can cause spasms and pain. Diversional activities can reduce the discomfort caused by boredom and time can seem to pass more quickly.	Demonstrate proper body alignment using pillows and rolled towels as needed. If possible, use child for demonstration. Discuss how to modify areas within the home to accommodate child and traction equipment. Discuss and demonstrate common improper alignment positions that child may assume. Provide anticipatory guidance on child's comfort needs and diversional activities. Encourage expression of concerns and ask questions.

Nursing Diagnosis	Child Goals	Interventions	Rationale	Home Caregiver Teaching
	Child will be psychologically comfortable.	Discuss child's concerns about condition and treatment. Provide appropriate reassurance. Provide the opportunity for child to make some autonomous decisions regarding routines, diversional activities, and self-care.	Children need an opportunity to discuss their fears and concerns and have their questions answered. Clarification of the issues can decrease stress. Developmentally appropriate reassurance meets child's emotional needs. Individuals need to feel some control over their environment.	Discuss child's stage of cognitive (see Chapter 13) and psychological development, and needs related to stages. Mention that children may have unrealistic fears based on their incorrect interpretations of what they may have heard or seen. Assist parents in determining which types of decisions child can make.
	Child will be free of pain.	Use a valid, reliable, and age-appropriate method to assess the child's level of pain such as the FACES scale (Wong and Whaley 1996). Incorporate nontraditional therapies such as touch, massage, applications of heat or cold, music, aroma-therapeutics,	A consistent reliable method of assessing pain is essential for adequate pain management especially when multiple caregivers are involved in care. Nontraditional therapies have been documented to increase relaxation and decrease pain sensation. An inadequate dose	Briefly discuss pain and instruments available for assessment. Instruct in use of assessment method selected. Discuss and provide reading materials on alternative pain-management therapies. Encourage questions. Discuss appropriate dose and potential

Nursing Diagnosis	Child Goals	Interventions	Rationale	Home Caregiver Teaching
		and relaxation techniques into pain manage-ment. Provide an adequate dose of pain medication when needed. Document pain level and pain intervention on a flowsheet.	or schedule will not provide appropriate relief. Docu-mentation is essential for eliciting patterns over time and success of selected interventions.	side effects. Provide pain documentation flowsheet (see Appendix 14–B). Demonstrate how to use flowsheet.

Alteration in Skin/Bone Integrity Secondary to External Fixator

Nursing Diagnosis	Child Goals	Interventions	Rationale	Home Caregiver Teaching
Alteration in skin/bone integrity secondary to external fixator	Child's pin and wire sites will remain clean and free of exudate.	Observe skin at pin and wire insertion sites. Provide pin-site care as ordered by surgeon.	Close observation of sites required for assessment and early intervention. For example, redness may indicate early infection. Pin-site care will decrease risk for infection by removing bacteria and drainage from the skin. Bacterial growth and/or prolonged skin contact with drainage can result in skin breakdown and wound infection.	Discuss normal wound appearance and expected drainage. Reinforce pin- and wire-site care as ordered by physician. Review potential sources of pathogens. Review method for obtaining and paying for needed supplies. Encourage questions.
	Child will not demonstrate signs of	Observe pin and wires sites for skin color changes,	Skin redness may indicate early infection. Presence and	Discuss early indicators of infection such as swelling,

Nursing Diagnosis	Child Goals	Interventions	Rationale	Home Caregiver Teaching
infection at pin and wire sites. Child remains free of exudate.	tenting, or drainage. Note absence or characteristics (color, consistency, amount) of drainage.	characteristics of drainage may indicate a need for intervention. For example, clear watery drainage may indicate venous stasis because the extremity has been in a dependent position for an extended period. Purulent drainage may indicate wound infection.	redness, tenting, tenderness, and increased or purulent drainage. Discuss potential interventions and when to contact health care providers. Encourage questions.
	Child will maintain proper distraction.	Review procedure for increasing distraction. Examine fixator device.	Procedure as ordered by physician for increasing distraction must be followed for optimal thera-peutic results. Fixator device must be intact for proper distraction to occur.	Review physician's orders with caregiver with special attention to when and how much screws will be turned to maintain ad-equate distrac-tion. Discuss scheduled outpatient follow-up.
	Child will maintain normal peripheral neurovascular status of extremity.	Monitor skin color and temperature, capillary refill, and pulses in extremity being treated. Monitor sensa-tion in affected extremity.	Normal color, temperature, capillary refill, and pulses are indicators of adequate tissue perfusion. Redness indicates tissue irritation.	Briefly discuss neurovascular status. Demon-strate indicators of adequate status and follow with return demonstra-tion. Discuss potential compli-cations and

Nursing Diagnosis	Child Goals	Interventions	Rationale	Home Caregiver Teaching
		Document findings on flowsheet.	Impaired sensation can indicate increased pressure on nerve, excessive distraction, and progress to nerve damage. Documentation facilitates communication among caregivers and early intervention.	interventions to restore status. Provide flowsheet or encourage caregiver to develop a flowsheet. Demonstrate recording findings on flowsheet. Encourage questions.

CHAPTER 12

Impairment of the Hematopoietic System

Sharon Frierdich and Anne Armstrong Griffin

Hematologic disorders manifested in children and adolescents encompass a wide spectrum of clinical pathologies. Causation of the illnesses is related to functional abnormalities, production failure, or depletion of specific cellular components of the blood. The symptoms, illness course, and management strategies will vary with each clinical problem. Many of these disorders have an undetermined outcome or response to treatment. Subsequently, the home care needs of the children with these various disorders require an individualized approach.

In developing a care plan for a child with a hematologic disorder, the nurse should have knowledge of the normal variances in cellular production of blood component levels that occur throughout childhood. An understanding of the pathophysiology and the treatment of the specific disease is also required. Finally, it is important to assess the impact of the illness on the child and family.

CHILDHOOD HEMATOPOIETIC DISORDERS

Hyperbilirubinemia

Hyperbilirubinemia is an elevated bilirubin level that produces jaundice. Clinical jaundice is visible at serum bilirubin levels of 5 to 7 mg/dL. Approximately 50 percent of all newborns, and

a higher percentage of premature infants, develop physiologic jaundice (Gourley and Odell 1989).

There are several factors that contribute to a physiologic increase in bilirubin levels. First, in extrauterine life, there is an increase in red blood cell breakdown due to the decreased oxygen requirements in the extrauterine environment. Also, erythrocyte production ceases for a few days after birth. There is a large pool of erythrocyte precursors in the bone marrow, liver, and spleen and because they are not used, the rapid death of these cells contributes to increased bilirubin production.

Second, there is an impaired ability in the first few days of life to excrete bilirubin. The increased breakdown load cannot be handled by the liver because of an intermittent deficiency of glucuronyl transferase. Last, intestinal bacteria, which break down indirect bilirubin, is not present at birth, so unconjugated bilirubin formed is free to be absorbed (Goodman 1987). Physiologic jaundice usually does not exceed safe bilirubin levels greater than 12 mg/dL and is corrected after four days.

Breast-fed infants can also develop increased bilirubin levels. Substances in breast milk (for example, pregnanediol and free fatty acid) inhibit glucuronyl transferase in the liver (Alonso et al. 1990). Discontinuation of breast-feeding usually reduces the bilirubin level to normal, although mothers can continue to breastfeed their infants if bilirubin remains at safe levels.

Serum bilirubin concentrations above 12 mg/dL in a full-term infant should be investigated beyond routine screening. Also, conjugated hyperbilirubinemia, rather than unconjugated hyperbilirubinemia, is always a sign of pathology (Whitington and Gartner 1993). In severe cases of jaundice, usually due to serious blood incompatibility, or a rapid increase in serum bilirubin, an exchange transfusion may be indicated. Donor red blood cells are administered, while the infant's blood is slowly removed through the umbilical vein.

Phototherapy is used to treat physiologic jaundice and some cases of pathologic jaundice. Phototherapy is used in the majority of full-term infants who have jaundice when their serum bilirubin concentrations reach or exceed 20 mg/dL. Phototherapy reduces serum bilirubin concentration mainly by the mechanism of photoisomerization of bilirubin. Photoisomerization is defined as a change in the configuration of the bilirubin molecule as a consequence of the absorption of light energy (Ennever 1986). A blue-range light source is known to decompose bilirubin from unconjugated to water-soluble bilirubin. Much of the bilirubin is in the intestine and contributes to an enhanced enterohepatic circulation of bilirubin during phototherapy. Only tissue bilirubin is subject to the photodynamic reaction, and the light penetrates only approximately 2 mm of the skin. Therefore, it is imperative that as much skin as possible is exposed to the light energy source.

Modern treatment involves placing fluorescent or special "superblue" lights over the crib or incubator. The infant is undressed so that much of the body surface is exposed to the light. The child's eyes and gonadal cells are protected at all times. Warmth is carefully monitored and ensured by the use of an incubator or plastic shield over the crib. More recently, a filtered fiberoptic light source eliminating ultraviolet (UV) and infrared radiation has been used in the form of a blanket. The advantage to the biliblanket is that the infant's eyes do not need to be covered as long as the biliblanket is shielded and continuous phototherapy is provided even when holding or feeding the infant.

Home care agencies are presently making phototherapy a viable treatment option in the home. Infants who have uncomplicated, nonprogressive hyperbilirubinemia are eligible for phototherapy using overhead phototherapy lights or a biliblanket.

Discharge Teaching Issues

The appearance of jaundice in the newborn may be anxiety producing to the parents, especially if this is their firstborn. Parents of children with jaundice need information concerning the cause and potential treatment. Parents of children with pathologic jaundice who will receive an exchange transfusion need to be instructed about the risks and benefits of this procedure. Often, infants with pathologic jaundice remain hospitalized after their mothers have been discharged after giving birth. Parents should be encouraged to visit often. Parents of children with physiologic jaundice need assurance regarding the benign nature of the condition and that the golden yellow color will eventually disappear. Mothers who are breastfeeding their infants need to know that jaundice may last longer in their infants than in bottle-fed infants.

Home phototherapy is an option for children who have nonprogressive hyperbilirubinemia and require only a few days of treatment. The nurse needs to assess the ability as well as the desire of the parents to perform this treatment in the home. The benefit of home phototherapy is that it allows the child to be discharged with the mother, fostering parent-infant bonding. In addition, it allows the mother to continue breastfeeding and there are less interruptions in the family unit.

Parents will require instruction on equipment use, schedule of treatments, and the special care of the infants receiving phototherapy. A nursing care plan for home phototherapy is found in Appendix 12–A.

All infants who develop jaundice should be followed frequently with an initial visit one week after discharge. They should be checked for signs of anemia. If kernicterus occurred, the child will require periodic evaluations for observation of developmental delays and auditory and neuromuscular abnormalities. If problems exist, parents will require rehabilitative counseling to maximize the abilities of the child.

Anemias in Childhood

Anemias are the most common hematologic disorders seen in infancy and early childhood. Anemia is defined as a reduction in the number of red blood cells or blood hemoglobin concentration. This results in a decrease in the oxygen-carrying capacity of the blood; therefore, the signs and symptoms are reflective of decreased oxygenation to the tissues.

Signs and symptoms are also dependent on the rapidity in the development of the anemia. Most chronic disorders have an insidious onset and therefore the body is allowed time to compensate for the decrease in the number of red blood cells.

The most prevalent signs and symptoms noted with all anemias include pallor of skin and mucous membranes and an increased cardiac output and heart rate to meet the demand for oxygen. When anemia progresses, the child may show signs of weakness, shortness of breath, anorexia, irritability, dizziness, headaches, and fatigability with exertion. In severe anemia, signs of cardiac failure, dyspnea, edema, increasing weakness, and weight gain may occur.

Diagnosis of the spcific cause of the anemia is assisted by the history of occurrence of symptoms and laboratory data. A complete blood cell count is usually the first test to be performed. Evaluation of these results can determine the extent of the anemia, decrease of other cellular components, and morphology of erythrocytes (size, shape, and amount of hemoglobin). Other tests that may be essential in determination of the cause of anemia include bone marrow aspira-

tion, hemoglobin electrophoresis, reticulocyte count, bilirubin, and iron values.

Iron-Deficiency Anemia

Iron-deficiency anemia remains the most common type of anemia that occurs during infancy and childhood. It is most frequently reported when the child is between six months and three years of age and again when the child is in adolescence. The factors that most often lead to iron deficiency in children are rapid growth, insufficient absorption, and blood loss (Pearson 1990).

The healthy newborn usually has sufficient iron derived from breakdown of maternal red blood cells for up to three to four months. After this time, because of the rapid growth of the infant, the iron stores need to be replenished. Therefore, iron-deficiency anemia is most frequently observed in premature infants and infants who, after four months of age, consume a diet of non–iron-containing cow's milk with little solid food. Adolescents, especially females, experiencing rapid growth with the onset of puberty are also at risk for development of iron-deficiency anemia. Approximately as many as 25 percent of adolescent girls and 40 percent of infants have some degree of iron-deficiency anemia (Lanzkowsky 1985).

Iron deficiency can occur as a result of loss of blood through the intestines due to intolerance or hypersensitivity to milk. Ingestion of drugs that cause gastrointestinal bleeding, such as salicylates, and parasitic infections can also lead to intestinal blood loss. Malabsorption syndrome or prolonged diarrhea can prevent absorption of iron even with sufficient intake (Dallman, Yip, and Oski 1993).

Children with iron-deficiency anemia usually present with symptoms of anemia and may also have tarry stools in the case of gastrointestinal blood loss. A history of dietary intake and elimination patterns is essential in making the diagnosis. The complete blood cell count will show hypochromic (pale) and smaller (low mean corpuscular hemoglobin [MCH]) erythrocytes with decreased hemoglobin value. Ferritin levels are usually low: the total iron binding capacity may be elevated with low iron levels. Free erythrocyte protoporphyrin (FEP), a precursor to heme, may be elevated (Oski 1993).

Children who are diagnosed with severe anemia and show signs of cardiac failure should initially receive packed red blood cell transfusions when correction is promptly required. The transfusion therapy should be administered at a slow rate to elevate hemoglobin to 4 to 5 g/dL to correct the immediate anoxia.

The goals of treatment of iron-deficiency anemia are to replace the iron deficiency and correct the underlying cause of the anemia (Penrod et al. 1990). The treatment of choice is oral supplementation of iron for five to six weeks. A therapeutic trial of oral iron supplementation should result in an increase in hemoglobin between the 5th and 10th days, as well as an increase in the reticulocyte percent. Instructions should be provided to correct practices that contributed to the development of the anemia (for example, inadequate fortified diet, use of salicylates, and other drugs that cause gastrointestinal bleeding). Malabsorption syndromes and milk hypersensitivity often require discontinuation of milk products or a trial with an alternative milk or nonmilk formula.

Sickle Cell Anemia

Sickle cell disease is the most common inherited hemoglobinopathy in the United States, affecting predominately individuals of African, Mediterranean, Middle Eastern, and Indian ancestry (Lane 1996). Sickle cell trait is present in 8 percent of the population, and the disease affects 1 in 200 to 500 newborns in the United States (Weathers, Pearson, and Gaston 1989). Children with sickle cell trait are usually asymptomatic except at times of prolonged hypoxic episodes, whereas sickle cell anemia is associated with multiple acute and chronic problems.

Sickle cell disease is transmitted as an autosomal-dominant disorder in which adult hemoglobin (HbA) is partly or completely replaced by sickle hemoglobin (HbS). The gene is partially expressed in the heterozygous state, or sickle cell trait, as part normal hemoglobin and part sickle hemoglobin (HbSA).

Sickle cell anemia is the complete expression of sickle hemoglobin (HbSS), with variant combinations with sickle cell–hemoglobin C (HbSC) or sickle cell–thalassemia B disease.

Hemoglobin S arose as a spontaneous mutation and deletion of the beta hemoglobin gene on chromosome 11, believed to selectively protect carriers from falciparum malaria. This abnormality results in the replacement of an amino acid on the hemoglobin chain from glutamine in hemoglobin A to valine in sickle hemoglobin. This abnormal amino acid will affect the shape (crescent or sickle shape) and solubility of the hemoglobin molecule, especially under the conditions of low oxygen and pH.

The transformation or polymerization of deoxygenated red blood cells to rigid rodlike tactoids causes them to become lodged in blood vessels. Hyperviscosity, cellular adherence, and possibly hypercoagulopathy also contribute to the vascular effects (Francis and Johnson 1991). Vascular flow impairment results in decreased blood flow, vessel infarction, thrombosis formation, and ischemia to the surrounding tissue. This is known as sickle cell crisis. A crisis may be precipitated by infection, fever, cold exposure, hypoxia, strenuous physical activity, dehydration, stress, and extreme fatigue. During periods of adequate oxygenation and hydration, the red blood cells retain their normal shape. Repeated cycles of transformation from a sickled (deoxygenated) to an unsickled (oxygenated) red blood cell destroys the membrane integrity, thus decreasing the life span of the cell from the usual normal 120 days to approximately 12 days.

Newborn hemoglobinopathy screening, now required in many states, allows for early identification of children with sickle cell disease. The diagnosis of sickle cell disease is determined by evidence of normocytic, normochromic anemia and sickle cells on the blood cell count. Elevations in the reticulocyte count and the bilirubin level are also noted. Hemoglobin electrophoresis can help make a definitive diagnosis by detection of hemoglobin abnormality, thus differentiating the sickle cell trait versus the disease and its hemoglobin variants.

There are several types of sickle cell crises. Vaso-occlusive crisis is the most common type of crisis experienced, resulting in veno-occlusion and ischemia. The symptoms manifested are related to the specific site of occlusion and areas of ischemic tissues. In children between the ages of three months and four years, the most common site of crisis is the painful swelling of the metacarpals and metatarsals of the fingers and toes, known as hand-foot syndrome. Episodes of bone pain, especially in the extremities, often begin after the age of three years. Abdominal pain crisis, or girdle crisis, is due to the infarction of the mesenteric vessels, or infarction of liver or spleen. Pulmonary infarctions may lead to "acute chest syndrome," marked by rapidly progressive dyspnea and pleuric pain. Acute chest syndrome is often primarily or secondarily associated with an infection. Central nervous system crisis, which may occur at the mean age of seven years, resembles the symptoms of a cerebrovascular accident and may result in minor to severe neurologic impairment. Priapism, or painful erection of the penis, may result in partial or complete impotence if not corrected within 24 hours (Reid 1995).

Splenic sequestration crisis is uncommon but may be rapidly fatal. It occurs most often in children younger than 1 year, but it also may occur later in childhood. It results from the pooling of a large amount of blood in the spleen, causing a dramatic drop in blood volume. This can lead to hypovolemic shock and cardiovascular collapse. The initial symptoms include abdominal girth enlargement with pain, nausea and vomiting, paleness, and marked fatigue and lethargy.

Erythroblastopenic or aplastic crisis is a decrease in the production of red blood cells as noted by low reticulocyte or nucleated red blood cell count. There is a decrease in production of red blood cells in the bone marrow, along with a shorter life span and destruction of the circulating red blood cells. Therefore, there is a profound drop in hemoglobin. The most common causes of aplastic crisis are infections, primarily viral infections. The symptoms are directly related to the percentage drop in hemoglobin.

Short- and long-term complications occur in the body organs as a result of multiple episodes of crises. The spleen initially becomes enlarged because of congestion of sickle cells. Over time, the splenic sinuses will become compressed and fibrinotic until they become a shrunken fibrotic mass. Consequently, the spleen is unable to filter bacteria and children become more susceptible to infections.

Cirrhosis of the liver can be the sequela of the impaired hepatic blood flow and capillary obstruction. The liver becomes enlarged and tender. Hepatitis infections and hemosiderosis may also damage the liver function. By the age of 18 years, 42 percent of individuals with sickle cell disease have cholelithiasis. Gallstones occur as frequently as one in four patients by the age of 25 years because of accretion of calcium bilirubinate in the gallbladder. Surgical removal of the gallbladder may be indicated (Lanzkowsky 1995).

The glomerular capillaries of the kidney may become congested with sickle cells, leading to fibrosis and eventually to nephrotic syndrome. The initial symptoms of ischemia are hematuria, proteinuria, enuresis, dysuria, and inability to concentrate urine.

Orthopedic complications, which occur because of hyperplasia of the bone marrow and hypoxia, include osteoporosis, osteomyelitis, and aseptic necrosis of the epiphyses of long bones in arms and legs. Children with sickle cell anemia are usually of shorter stature than those children without sickle cell disease.

Cardiomegaly and myocardial dysfunction are caused by ischemic fibrosis and hemosiderosis. Electrocardiogram (ECG), radiologic, and echocardiogram findings can be diagnostic of increase in heart size, decrease in heart function, and arrhythmias. Congestive heart failure and myocardial infarction are consequences of heart damage.

Lung infarctions resulting from pneumonias and acute chest syndrome may initially decrease oxygen saturation. After repeated damage, chronic obstructive lung disease may develop, resulting in dependency on oxygen administration.

Thrombosis and ischemic episodes of the central nervous system (CNS) are estimated to affect 6 to 10 percent of children with sickle cell anemia, with a recurrence rate as high as 67 percent (Pegelow et al. 1995). Symptoms such as headaches, convulsions, aphasia, and decrease in motor strength and movement may be manifested. Major deficits in motor control, learning ability, or other neurologic impairments may be permanent.

Cutaneous ulcers of the legs occur as a result of decrease of sluggish blood flow to the lower extremities and tissue ischemia. There is also reduced healing of these lesions because of the causative factors.

There is a decrease in sexual maturation development in both girls and boys. Tanner stage V is usually not achieved until the mean age of 17 years in boys and girls with sickle cell anemia (Lanzkowsky 1995).

Sickled cells are rapidly destroyed, causing hemolysis. Increased erythropoiesis to compensate for anemia results in production of extramedullary sites. Prominence of the face and skull are due to this fact. Increased hemolysis results in jaundice and hemosiderosis. Often, children with sickle cell anemia will also have deficits in folic acid and vitamin B_{12}. Evaluation of these deficiencies is essential to avoid progressive anemia.

Retinal vein dilation, neovascularization, hemorrhages, and choroid and retinal atrophy may lead to proliferative sickle cell retinopathy as early as the age of 10 years. Early intervention with laser or cryotherapy may prevent loss of sight.

Sensorineural hearing loss can also occur over time because of infarctions. Ocular screening and audiograms should be performed on a yearly basis for children older than 10 years (Vichinsky 1991).

The overall prognosis for any one child with sickle cell anemia is unpredictable, but the majority of individuals do live into the third decade of life. The severity of the disease and the number of complications appear to be major factors. Active management strategies provided by comprehensive medical staff, family, school staff, and home care providers have improved survival time and quality of life.

Management of sickle cell anemia should emphasize prevention of complications. Prophylactic antibiotic therapy, usually with penicillin, is advocated starting at three to four months of age and 24-valent pneumococcal vaccine at 2 years of age, with revaccination occurring at 4 years of age. *Haemophilus influenzae* and hepatitis and all other vaccinations should be administered at routine health care checks. Prompt reporting of fever and workup is essential for all children with sickle cell anemia. Parents should be instructed on how to feel the spleen in an infant and report an increase in abdominal girth size.

Crisis episodes may not require hospitalization, especially if the child is afebrile, is able to achieve good pain control with oral analgesics, is drinking adequately, and does not suffer from complications. Hospitalization is often required when the child is febrile and requires intravenous antibiotics, hydration, analgesics, and blood transfusions or exchange transfusions. Oxygen therapy may also be required.

Hypertransfusions are recommended for children who have suffered from a major complication related to sickle cell disease, such as acute chest syndrome or cerebrovascular accident. This therapy requires transfusing the child every three to four weeks to maintain an HbS level less than 30 percent and a total hemoglobin at 12 g/dL. This will suppress the bone marrow production of HbS red blood cells. Unfortunately, hypertransfusion therapy may result in an increase in iron stores in the body and may require chelation therapy when the ferritin level is greater than 2,000 and marked saturation of iron stores or significant organ damage occurs because of hemosiderosis (Wayne 1993).

Most recently, there have been attempts to increase the level of fetal hemoglobin through the use of certain chemotherapy agents, such as Hydroxyurea and 5-Azacytidine. It is thought that fetal hemoglobin-stimulating agents may decrease the incidence of severe complications if fetal hemoglobin (HbF) is greater than 10 percent and decrease the number of painful crises if greater than 20 percent. These agents may also increase the hemoglobin content within the cell and alter the properties of the red cell membrane to make it less formidable and adherent to vessels (Charache et al. 1995). The safety of these agents used over a long period has not been determined.

Bone marrow transplantation is a curative approach for children with sickle cell anemia. This procedure is performed only when a child has suffered from a severe complication of sickle cell anemia and has a matched histocompatible sibling without disease (Johnson et al. 1994). Allogenic bone marrow transplantation is not without its own potential complications (see section on bone marrow and peripheral stem cell transplantation).

Future investigations of the role of gene therapy may have practical application if a technique to correct the abnormality in the red blood cell of the child with sickle cell anemia can be achieved.

Thalassemia

Thalassemia refers to a variety of anemias associated with a decreased production of one or more of the normal polypeptide chains (beta or alpha) of the adult hemoglobin (HbA). Thalassemia occurs most frequently in children of Mediterranean ancestry, although it can occur in children of African or Asian decent as well. In many populations, alpha- and beta-thalassemia and structural hemoglobin variants exist together, resulting in a wide variety of anemias with various severity of symptoms.

Thalassemia major (homozygous beta-thalassemia) is the most severe variety. It is also known as Cooley's anemia. Beta-hemoglobin chain defects become evident at approximately six months of age when the infant's stores of fetal hemoglobin are reduced. Like other severe hemolytic anemias, the abnormal erythrocytes are not effective and have a shortened life span. The red blood cells will be hypochromic (pale) and microcytic (small) and have a low mean corpuscular volume (MCV) of hemoglobin. Hemoglobin levels can be as low as 5 g/dL. The serum iron level is high because iron cannot be incorporated into synthesis of hemoglobin. Iron saturation is usually 100 percent and fetal hemoglobin is usually high, whereas adult hemoglobin remains normal. Osmotic fragility is decreased, serum ferritin is high, and the bone marrow aspirate reveals a megaloblastic bone marrow.

Usually, thalassemia major is detected in children by symptoms of failure to thrive and pallor; these children are unable to produce normal beta-hemoglobin. Examination may reveal hepatosplenomegaly and jaundice. As the child begins to use extramedullary sites for the production of hematopoiesis, he or she develops abnormal facies, such as frontal bossing, prominence of malar eminences, depression of the bridge of the nose, and exposure of central upper teeth. Over time, there may be generalized osteoporosis, pathologic fractures, and spinal cord compression (Johanson 1990).

Endocrine disorders such as delayed growth and puberty, diabetes mellitus, adrenal insufficiency, hypothyroidism, and hypoparathyroidism are not uncommon. Cardiac abnormalities from chronic anemia, increased plasma volume, and myocardial iron overload can often lead to fatal cardiac failure. Hemosiderosis of the liver results in cirrhosis and the hypersplenism results in sequestration of not only red blood cells, but leukocytes and platelets as well (Festa 1985).

Supportive care is primarily to provide hypertransfusion therapy every three to four weeks to maintain a hemoglobin between 10.5 and 11 g/dL. The goal of hypertransfusion therapy is to suppress erythropoiesis, thereby decreasing sites of extramedullary production. This will decrease the characteristic cosmetic changes and skeletal weakness. It may also decrease the need for a splenectomy and decrease cardiac complications (Pearson 1987). Aggressive chelation therapy should be initiated at the time transfusion therapy is begun. The purpose of chelation therapy is to remove excess intracellular iron and to bind to free extracellular iron for excretion in the urine (Cohen 1989).

A splenectomy may be therapeutic when the spleen becomes so enlarged that it is significantly uncomfortable to the patient and may suffer a traumatic rupture. Removal of the spleen is also indicated when there are increased requirements for blood transfusions, and there is severe leukopenia and thrombocytopenia. Before surgical removal of the spleen, the child should receive a pneumococcal vaccination and also follow a treatment regimen that includes taking penicillin daily.

Because these patients will be more at risk for infections, all fevers should be reported to the physician.

It is recommended that children with thalassemia take supplemental vitamin C to aid in iron excretion and vitamin E to protect erythrocyte membrane with its antioxidant effects (Festa 1985). Other supportive care includes the untransfused patient taking folic acid daily, hepatitis B vaccine for those receiving hypertransfusion therapy, and close monitoring for potential cardiac and endocrine problems. Children who develop congestive heart failure may need to take digitalis and diuretics. Endocrine interventions may include L-thyroxine growth hormone, estrogen or testosterone replacement, and insulin for diabetes mellitus. A cholecystectomy may be indicated for gallstone formation. Leg ulcers are not an uncommon development in the older child, and elevation of lower extremities periodically throughout the day is recommended. Evidence of ulcer develop-

ment should be brought immediately to the attention of the child's physician.

There are several recent new directions in the management of children with thalassemia major. Oral chelation, although not approved for use in the United States, is being used in other countries with some success (Nathan 1990). Fetal hemoglobin synthesis agents, such as hydroxyurea, and 5-azacitidine, whose use was previously described for sickle cell anemia, is being advocated for trial with thalassemia. These agents ameliorate the symptoms by increasing the hemoglobinization of the thalassemic red cell and result in more effective erythropoiesis.

Bone marrow transplantation with an HLA-identical sibling is a curative mode of treatment and results are promising especially with young individuals who received few transfusions and are without serious organ damage (Lucarelli et al. 1990). Heart transplants have been carried out for severe hemochromatic myocardiopathy in the absence of cirrhosis of the liver (Albertini 1990).

Gene therapy, in which the normal globin genes could be inserted into marrow stem cell, may ultimately be utilized in the future.

Aplastic Anemia

Aplastic anemia is a serious disorder caused by a production failure of red blood cells, white blood cells, and platelets. Aplastic anemia can be acquired, or it can be a congenital defect. Congenital aplastic anemias comprise approximately 25 percent of childhood aplastic disorders. Fanconi's anemia is the most common congenital aplastic anemia. This condition is genetically transmitted as an autosomal recessive trait. In addition to pancytopenia, symptoms include microcephaly, defects in the radii and thumb, cardiac and renal abnormalities, deafness, dwarfism, and hyperpigmented rash. Disorders such as dyskeratosis, congenital Schwachman's syndrome, and WT syndrome are other congenital disorders associated with bone marrow failure that occur less frequently (Shahidi 1987).

Acquired aplastic anemia can occur as a result of exposure to chemicals and toxins such as benzene, hydrocarbons, petroleum solvents, and pesticides. In addition, bone marrow depression can also be related to certain drugs, such as chemotherapy, certain antibiotics, and anticonvulsants. Large doses of radiation may also be a causative factor. In some cases, aplastic anemia can be the sequela of contracting viral infections, such as hepatitis and measles. In 70 percent of the cases, acquired aplastic anemia is idiopathic or no etiology is identified (Lanzkowsky 1995).

The complete blood count will show a decrease in circulating erythrocytes with a low reticulocyte percent as well as low platelets and white blood cells. Confirmation of aplastic anemia is made through a bone marrow aspirate demonstrating a hypocellular marrow.

The exhibiting signs and symptoms are related to the degree of severity of anemia, thrombocytopenia, and neutropenia.

Severe aplastic anemia was classified by Camitta and colleagues in 1976 as having at least two of the following: a neutrophil count less than 500/mm^3, a platelet count less than 20,000/mm^3, and a reticulocyte count below 1 percent after correction for hematocrit. In addition, the bone marrow smear must be hypocellular. Mild to moderate aplastic anemia is distinguished from severe by increased bone marrow cellularity.

The treatment of choice for moderate to severe aplastic anemia in children who have a histocompatible locus antigen (HLA)–matched sibling is an allogenic bone marrow transplant. This option has a 70 percent cure rate. The odds are increased to 85 percent if the child has not received prior transfusions that would cause sensitization to histocompatible antigens. Another source of stem cells can be umbilical cord blood from an HLA-matched newborn sibling. Only approximately 25 to 30 percent of affected children have an HLA-matched sibling (Lanzkowsky 1995).

Patients who have minor symptomatology or who do not have a compatible bone marrow donor may have cellular production stimulated by various therapies. Antithymocyte globulin (ATG) and antilymphocyte globulin (ALG) are serums produced by immunization of horses or rabbits with human peripheral blood and are cytotoxic reagents with activity against marrow cells. ATG or ALG is usually administered over four to six hours intravenously for approximately eight consecutive days concurrently with steroid therapy. This therapy alone has a 50 percent partial or complete response rate. When this treatment is combined with the administration of cyclosporin-A, the response rate increases to 65 percent (Gluckman 1992). ATG and ALG can have several adverse effects, such as allergic reactions and serum sickness; therefore, children are hospitalized for this therapy. They may be discharged with instructions to follow a regimen including steroids and cyclosporin-A as oral medications. Long-term use of steroids is not without potential complications, and the levels of cyclosporin-A need to be monitored closely to prevent untoward effects.

The role of colony-stimulating growth factors, such as granulocyte colony-stimulating factor (G-CSF) , granulocyte-macrophage colony-stimulating factor (GM-CSF), and other newer factors are being explored for their potential benefits as therapy for aplastic anemia (Kojima et al. 1991). Immunoglobulin infusions have also been used with occasional success.

Children with aplastic anemia require supportive therapy of red blood cells and platelet transfusions. Unfortunately, many patients develop antiplatelet antibodies and become refractory to platelet transfusions. More conservative limits are set as criteria for transfusions. Aminocaproic acid (Amicar) is usually prescribed to decrease use of platelet transfusions and prevent bleeding. Chelation therapy may be necessary for iron overload due to multiple blood transfusions. Blood products should be irradiated to deactivate lymphocytes that can cause graft-versus host disease (GVHD) from repeated transfusions.

Infections are a major problem in children who remain neutropenic. These children must take all the usual precautions of immunosuppressed individuals (see Appendix 12–H). They are placed on prophylactic trimethoprim-sulfamethoxazole to prevent pneumocystis infections and oral antifungal therapy. Intravenous administration of broad-spectrum antibiotics is required for febrile episodes. Granulocyte infusion for severe life-threatening sepsis remains a controversial therapy.

Children who have severe anemia, thrombocytopenia, and neutropenia and who are not responsive to therapy have an extremely poor prognosis. Life expectancy ranges from several months to years.

Discharge Teaching Issues

Anemias caused by nutritional deficiencies have a short course if the proper nutrients are replaced. Inherited hemolytic disorders such as sickle cell disease and thalassemia are chronic disorders and require lifetime management. The course of other anemias, such as aplastic anemia, is uncertain and dependent on the success of the treatment. The major issues for discharge teaching for a family of a child with anemia include the following: (1) disease and treatment plan; (2) nutritional counseling; (3) conservation of physical energy; (4) avoidance of infection; (5) pain relief and comfort measures; (6) genetic counseling, if applicable to disease transmission; and (7) coping with the impact of the disease on the child and family.

Disease and Treatment. Because there are specific variables related to the source of the anemia, family members require an explanation of the disease, causative factors, prognosis, and potential complications. They also need instruction on interpretation of laboratory values and frequency of medical follow-up visits. The specific treatment plan should be outlined, and the route of administration and dosage of medications should be explained. Expected side effects of therapy should be reviewed as well.

Written information on the disease and treatment should be provided. Many of the support organizations for the various anemia groups have prepared instructional material that is useful in the teaching process.

Parents should receive information on contacting health care personnel who will assist in the management of their child's care, especially when problems arise. They need guidelines on when they should contact their local health care providers versus their specialty physician.

Nutritional Counseling. Nutritional counseling should focus on the dietary sources to replenish nutrients causing the anemia, such as iron, vitamin B_{12}, and folic acid. All children may benefit from learning to eat a well-balanced diet, especially a diet high in folic acid and vitamin B_{12}, which is required for the regeneration of red blood cells. In the case of children who already have an excess of iron supplies in their bodies (for example, those suffering from sickle cell anemia and thalassemia), foods containing a high source of iron should be avoided. The nurse needs to assist the parents in assessing the special dietary needs of their child. Parents should receive assistance in planning meals based on the developmental and cultural food preferences. Resources should be provided to assist families with budget restraints that impact on proper nutrition. Methods to increase dietary intake, such as small frequent meals, should be offered when the child has chronic fatigue.

Conservation of Physical Energy. Parents require information on methods to conserve the child's energy and promote adequate tissue oxygenation. Young children, when allowed, will self-regulate their activities and not overextend their tolerance capacity. Older children may become exhausted when trying to maintain the same level of activity as their peers. Parents and children require information to maximize the child's energetic periods to meet the child's developmental needs. Most children with chronically low hemoglobin levels are able to adapt to lower than normal oxygen concentrations. The effects are most noted during periods of strenuous exercise or periods of stress.

Therefore, children should participate in activities that are interesting and challenging yet require minimal energy expenditure. Gym teachers and coaches should also be made aware of the fact that children with anemia may need frequent rest periods and should not be pushed to compete beyond their capability.

Adolescents require additional information regarding their condition and sexual activity. Pregnancy may place additional demands on a female. In addition, adolescents may be taking certain medications that may be harmful to a fetus. Therefore, specialized counseling is required as the boy or girl enters puberty and before sexual activity is initiated.

Additional oxygenation may be efficacious in certain situations. If home oxygen is to be used, family members require instruction on the proper use and safety measures.

Red blood cell transfusions (and other blood products) infused in the home has become a growing practice for patients requiring frequent transfusion therapy. The nurse must receive specific physician orders on the type and amount of blood product to be infused and the length of time of infusion. The product should be checked for correct typing, expiration date, and other significant data (for example, irradiated, filtered, volume-reduced, etc.) before initiation of transfusion. Many children also require pre-medications, such as acetaminophen or diphenhydramine to prevent chills and fevers that may accompany transfusions.

The child should be closely monitored for potential complications associated with transfusion therapy. Any symptoms indicative of a transfusion reaction should prompt the nurse to discontinue the transfusion and report the incident immediately to a physician.

Protocols for administration of emergency medications should be developed to expedite interventions when transfusion reactions occur. Parents should be instructed to report symptoms of advancing anemia, especially severe headaches, fatigue, weight gain and edema, and shortness of breath. These manifestations may be indicative of congestive heart failure.

Avoidance of Infection. Avoidance of infection should be stressed because of the increase in oxygen demand during infectious periods. These precautions are especially important for children with sickle cell disease to prevent the initiation of a crisis and for children with aplastic anemia who are immunosuppressed.

Maintenance of good health practices, such as good hygiene, regular dental care, and updating immunizations, should be encouraged. Children with aplastic anemia require special instructions, especially in the area of immunizations, due again to their immunosuppressed state.

Children with anemias are prone to the development of skin breakdown and poor healing due to decreased tissue oxygenation. Methods to prevent skin breakdown, such as using good protective equipment while participating in sports, should be initiated. Any source of skin breakdown should be reported immediately, and proper care of the area should be taught.

The importance of pneumococcal prophylaxis and twice a day dosing of penicillin should be stressed when the child has a nonfunctional spleen or has had a splenectomy. Compliance with daily antibiotic therapy should be assessed especially in the older school-age child and adolescent.

Parents should be alerted to report signs and symptoms of infection immediately, especially when their child becomes febrile. They should be taught how to take a temperature accurately and have a thermometer available.

Pain Relief and Comfort Measure. Pain is a symptom primarily related to sickle cell anemia during crisis episodes or dealing with chronic pain, such as aseptic necrosis. Other children with anemia may experience headaches and also abdominal pain due to enlargement of liver and spleen. The prevention of vasoconstriction through limited exercise, good hydration, warmth, and decreased stress should be emphasized. Adolescents should also be counseled on avoidance of cigarette and alcohol use.

All pain should be carefully assessed. Whenever possible, a developmentally appropriate pain scale should be utilized by the the child to describe the intensity of their pain. Because most of the pain the children experience is overt, it is important to trust the child's subjective interpretation of its location and intensity. In the case of sickle crisis pain, it is important to note it can change in its intensity and location throughout the crisis episode. For chronic pain, a regimen of oral analgesics provided round-the-clock is advocated. Narcotic use may be necessary for moderate to severe pain. Parents and older children need reassurance that their child will not become addicted to narcotic use if medications are taken for pain alone (see Chapter 14 for additional information on pain control). Table 12–1 lists medications used to treat anemias.

Children with concurrent platelet disorders should not receive aspirin or nonsteroidal pain products, because they can inactivate platelet function.

Comfort measures, especially during sickle cell disease crisis, should be used. Keeping the child warm, and providing rest and support to the areas of discomfort are helpful. Packs should be used only when ordered by a physician. Parents should check for warm temperature before applying warm packs on a child. Cold packs should be avoided because they cause vasoconstriction.

Children with chronic pain should also be instructed on the use of behavioral methods to control pain, such as biofeedback, relaxation training, self-hypnosis, distraction techniques, and massage therapy. Health care providers specializing in pain control can assist the family in incorporating these techniques into their pain management programs.

Genetic Counseling. When a child is diagnosed with a genetic anemia, all family members should be tested. The results of the testing should be provided in a clear, honest manner while being sensitive to the impact this may have on the parents. Parents and older children should be encouraged to express their concerns and feelings regarding the transmission of the disease to their offspring. If family planning options are requested, information should be provided.

Coping with Impact of Anemia. Children with chronic anemia have to cope with physical restraints on their activities, body alterations, decreased growth, sexual immaturity, and often decreased life expectancy. These impairments and stressors will present different issues as the child grows. These children need the opportunity to express their concerns, feelings, and attitudes.

They require an evolving explanation of the tests for the disease and purpose of treatment. Because of frequent hospitalizations, outpatient checkups, and home illnesses, school personnel need to be alerted to the special needs of the student. Anemia may also result in a decreased level of attention or learning deficits (for example, the child with sickle cell disease who has a cerebral vascular accident (CVA)). Tutorial programs should be implemented when necessary to sustain academic performance.

The family must learn to adjust when a child has a chronic or life-threatening disorder. Parents may feel guilt over the transmission of the disease, which may create an additional coping burden. Parents may be expected to perform technically advanced procedures, such as caring for a central venous catheter or administering desferoxamine infusions or monthly B_{12} injections in the home. The nurse can help the family maintain a sense of normalcy, set realistic expectations for the child, and encourage the expression of family members' concerns, especially the well siblings who may observe special attention given to the child with anemia.

The family should be made aware of support organizations and resources. Many organizations specific to certain anemias have been established and offer excellent resources to the families affected by the disorder. Often, there are local support groups or camps for children with anemia or their family members to attend.

Table 12–1 Medications Used To Treat Anemias

Medication	Purpose	Dosage	Side Effects
Antilymphocyte globulin (ALG)	Suppression of immune system	10 mg/kg/day IV over 6 hours × 8 days + prednisone 40 mg/m²/day × 5 days + cyclosporin-A 40 mg/kg/day over 12 hours + 1 mg/kg methyl-prednisolone × 4 days	Chills, fever, pruritus, anaphylaxis, hypotension, "serum sickness," phlebitis
Corticosteroids	Stimulation of bone marrow production	Dosage dependent upon specific disorder	Mood swings, shortened stature, masks signs of infection, hypertension, water retention, "moon face," truncal obesity, acne, decreased glucose tolerance
Cyclosporine	Suppression of immune system	8 mg/kg/day over 14 days, then 15 mg/kg/day (monitor cyclosporine-A (CSA) levels closely to achieve trough 200–500 mg/L)	Nausea, vomiting, diarrhea, hypertension, electrolyte wasting, headaches, seizures, anxiety, depression, tremors, nephrotoxic, hepatotoxic, ototoxic, gingival hyperplasia, flushing
Desferoxamine	Chelation of excess iron	20–40 mg/kg/day slow IV or subcutaneous infusion over approximately 10–12 hours	Allergy, tinnitus, tubular neuropathy, hypotension with rapid infusion, dysesthesia, cataracts, optic neuritis, visual disturbances
Ferrous sulfate	Increase serum iron	Therapeutic replacement: 5–6 mg/kg/day	Nausea, vomiting, diarrhea (5%), constipation (10%), dental stains, false stool guiac, dark stools
Folic acid	Replacement of folic acid	1–5 mg/day for 7 days	Allergic sensitization

continues

Table 12–1 continued

Medication	Purpose	Dosage	Side Effects
Penicillin	Antibiotic after splenectomy	125 mg PO bid (<5 years) 250 mg PO bid (>5 years)	Abdominal discomfort, rash, allergic reactions, anaphylaxis
Vitamin B$_{12}$	Replacement of vitamin B$_{12}$	Initial: 100 mcg intramuscularly (IM) 1–2 weeks Maintenance: 30–50 mcg IM monthly	Pulmonary edema, congestive heart failure, anaphylaxis, transient diarrhea, itching, exanthema, pain after injection

Note: IV, intravenous; IM, intramuscular; PO, by mouth.

Because the life expectancy may vary with the chronic anemias, the family needs to be kept abreast of new therapies and recommendations. Family members should be aware that anticipatory grief is a normal emotion, especially when a serious acute episode occurs in the course of the illness. Open and honest communication should be fostered in the family, and family members should be encouraged to share feelings, especially when dealing with such topics as death.

Home care plans for children with anemia are presented in Appendixes 12–B through 12–E.

BLEEDING DISORDERS IN CHILDHOOD

Bleeding disorders in children can be caused by abnormal structure or function of blood vessels; decreased production, destruction, or sequestration of platelets or abnormal platelet function; and congenital or acquired coagulation deficiencies (Lusher 1993). A complete child and family history, a physical examination, and a laboratory evaluation are essential in the diagnosis of the specific cause of the disorder.

The signs and symptoms of increased bleeding may be localized or generalized. The skin and mucous membranes are frequent sites of bleeding. Bruising and/or petechiae (flat, nontender, red spots) may be evident on the skin,

especially on dependent areas, bony prominences, and areas of trauma. Frequent or prolonged epistaxis and oral mucosal bleeding are common. Patients with more severe disorders may show signs of conjunctival or retinal hemorrhage, melena, hematuria, gastrointestinal bleeding, menorrhagia, and hemarthrosis (bleeding into joints). Intracranial hemorrhage, a life-threatening consequence, may occur spontaneously.

Idiopathic Thrombocytopenic Purpura

Thrombocytopenia, a decrease in circulating platelets, may result from known etiology such as platelet loss, hemolysis, infection, and specific autoimmune disorders. Certain drugs such as aspirin, indomethacin, nonsteroidal anti-inflammatories, sulfonamide derivatives, and chemotherapeutic agents can depress platelet production or interfere with platelet function. The origin of idiopathic thrombocytopenic purpura (ITP) is related to elevated IgG and IgM levels, although the exact relationship between a preceding viral illness and immune destruction of platelets has yet to be determined (Goebel 1993).

There are two forms of ITP—acute and chronic. Acute ITP is characterized by a rapid onset of severe thrombocytopenia, a history of recent viral infection, and a spontaneous recovery in a few weeks to two months (Goebel 1993). ITP lasting longer than six months usually results in a chronic, long-term course.

Presenting symptoms of ITP are dependent on the degree of thrombocytopenia. The complete blood cell count reveals a reduced number of platelets, although a bone marrow examination, if performed, reveals a normal to slight increase in megakaryocytes. Results of coagulation studies are normal. Management of acute ITP involves supportive measures to prevent bleeding (for example, avoidance of aspirin and aspirin-containing products, intramuscular injections, shaving with razor blade, and risky and traumatic activities). Table 12–2 lists medications used in the treatment of thrombocytopemia.

Usually, acute ITP does not require medications because of spontaneous remission. Corticosteroid therapy is started in severe cases and tapered slowly after response. Chronic ITP may require long-term use of corticosteroids. Intravenous gamma globulin has been shown to be beneficial in patients refractory to other therapy. Splenectomy is reserved for children who experienced clinically significant bleeding and in whom ITP persisted for more than one year (George et al. 1996). Platelets are transfused only for active, emergent bleeding. Many patients with chronic ITP are advised to take aminocaproic acid (Amicar) to prevent fibrinolysis (clot breakdown).

Hemophilia

Hemophilia A (factor VIII deficiency) and hemophilia B (factor IX deficiency) are genetically transmitted disorders inherited as X-linked recessive traits, although spontaneous mutations do occur. Males are affected and females are carriers. Hemophilia affects all races equally.

The severity of the disorder is dependent on the plasma level of factor (VIII or IX). Hemophilia is characterized by prolonged bleeding after injury and spontaneous hemarthrosis (bleeding into joints).

Hemophilia A is the most common form of hemophilia, occurring in 1:10,000 males; it is four times more common than hemophilia B (Pfaff and Geninatti 1993). Hemophilia A is characterized by the absence of the anti-hemophilia factor (factor VIII) that is required in the formation of thromboplastin. The defect in hemophilia B (or Christmas disease) results from a deficiency of factor IX, the plasma thromboplastin component.

The factor levels required to maintain normal hemostasis range from 60 percent to 120 percent. When factor levels are less than 1 percent, the child has severe hemophilia and a bleeding tendency may be noted during the newborn period with cephalohematoma occurring after vaginal delivery or prolonged bleeding occurring after circumcision. Bruising with handling or palpable hematomas after immunizations may occur. Bleeding episodes become more common once the toddler begins to crawl, pulls to stand, and starts to walk. The resultant bumps and falls result in more frequent bruising and mouth lacerations that may be difficult to control.

As children grow older and activity becomes more strenuous, they begin to develop hemarthrosis. This condition produces a swollen, hot, painful joint and restricted mobility. Repeated hemarthroses causes degeneration of the synovial membrane, with resultant muscle weakness and loss of joint stability. This joint then becomes a "target joint." Further bleeding over time may lead to erosion of the joint cartilage and resultant arthritic and crippling deformities (Bell, Candy, and Audet 1995). Recent research suggests that a prophylactic regimen of factor infusions (for example, on Monday, Wednesday, and Friday) may maintain a factor level sufficient to prevent spontaneous joint bleeds and subsequent permanent joint damage (Nilsson et al. 1992).

Other sites of frequent bleeding are the muscles of the extremities, which may be managed with local measures. Massive soft-tissue bleeds, particularly into the iliopsoas or retro-

Table 12–2 Medications Used in the Treatment of Thrombocytopenia

Medication	Purpose	Dosage	Side Effects
Corticosteroids	Increase platelet production	Dependent upon specific disorder	Mood swings, shortness of stature, masks signs of infection, hypertension, water retention, acne, "moon face," truncal obesity, decreased glucose tolerance
Gamma globulins (IVIG)	Increase platelet production	100 mg/kg/month (0.6 mL/kg) IV or IM	Nausea, vomiting, chills, flushing, loss of consciousness, anaphylactic reaction, facial swelling, abdominal pain
Penicillin	Antibiotic: prophylactic after splenectomy	125 mg PO bid (< 5 years) 250 mg PO bid (> 5 years)	Abdominal discomfort, rash, allergic reactions, anaphylaxis
Anti-D immunoglobulin (WinRho® Solvent Detergent)	Increase platelet production	Acute ITP: 250 IU/kg on days 1 and 2 (125 IU/kg if hemoglobin <10) Chronic ITP: 250 IU/kg	Nausea, vomiting, chills, flushing, loss of consciousness, anaphylactic reaction, facial swelling, abdominal pain, destruction of red blood cells (use with caution in children with anemia)

Note: IV, intravenous; IM, intramuscular; PO, by mouth; ITP, idiopathic thrombocytopenic purpura.

peritoneal space, can lead to anemia or vascular compromise. These bleeds may require factor replacement for up to one week to prevent rebleeding and allow for reabsorption of the hematoma (Furie et al. 1994).

Head, neck, or spinal hemorrhage is the major cause of death in children with hemophilia. Factor replacement in children with a history of CNS insult should not be delayed.

Children who have moderate hemophilia (1 to 5 percent factor levels) tend to experience varying degrees of bleeding with less frequent joint involvement. Those with mild hemophilia (5 to 25 percent) may not show symptoms until they experience a severe injury, surgery, or tooth extraction.

In most children with hemophilia, small cuts and abrasions will stop bleeding in a few minutes after application of firm pressure. Treatment for deeper lacerations, trauma, and joint bleeding requires replacement of the deficit plasma factors to control bleeding. These products are administered intravenously. The treatment of choice is purified, virally inactivated factor VIII or factor IX concentrates of which there are several products on the market.

Factor concentrates are made from human pooled plasma from as many as 20,000 to 30,000 donors. Improvement in donor screening, purification and viral inactivation processes, and the inclusion of recombinant technology have created factor concentrates that will most likely never transmit human immunodeficiency virus (HIV) to a patient and that significantly decrease the risk of transmission of hepatitis and other viruses (Bell, Candy, and Audet 1995).

The half-life of factor VIII is 8 to 12 hours and that of factor IX is 18 to 24 hours; therefore, prolonged or extensive bleeding usually requires more than one infusion. The amount of factor to be infused depends on the severity of the bleeding and the weight of the child. Life-threatening situations require an initial 100 percent factor replacement level (50 units/kg of body weight for factor VIII, or 100 units/kg of body weight for factor IX) followed by repeated dosages or a continuous infusion (Pfaff and Geninatti 1993).

Other bleeding episodes may require only a 25 to 50 percent replacement. Evaluation of the success of replacement therapy should be monitored by appropriate laboratory tests.

Desmopressin acetate (DDAVP) is the treatment of choice for children with mild hemophilia A who respond to this synthetic form of antidiuretic hormone. This can be administered intravenously, subcutaneously, or intranasally (Stimate), which is more convenient for home use. DDAVP is not effective in all children, so a trial must be performed to determine an adequate increase in factor VIII levels. It also is limited by its potential to cause tachyphylaxis, so it is not useful when frequent treatments are necessary. DDAVP is not useful in the management of hemophilia B (Bell, Candy, and Audet 1995).

Approximately 15 to 30 percent of children with severe hemophilia A develop antibodies or inhibitors to factor VIII that destroy the factor replacement when infused. The incidence of inhibitors is less frequent in those with mild to moderate disease and in those with hemophilia B.

When a child does not respond after replacement therapy, it should be determined whether an inhibitor is present. Inhibitor levels should also be measured at the annual visit and before surgical procedures. Management of bleeding in the presence of an inhibitor is more challenging, but alternative products or treatment protocols have proven to be successful.

Children should undergo an orthopedic and physical therapy evaluation annually. As they grow they may require orthopedic surgery for joint aspiration, arthroscopy, or synovectomy. Such procedures should be thoroughly discussed before the surgery. Rehabilitation after the surgery should be done in collaboration with a physical therapist experienced in the care of hemophilia and related complications.

von Willebrand Disease

The most common inherited bleeding disorder, von Willebrand disease, occurs equally in males and females and is characterized by excessive bruising, bleeding from mucous membranes, epistaxis, and menorrhagia. The von Willebrand factor protein plays a key role in hemostasis by initiating platelet adhesion at sites of injury. It is also the carrier protein for factor VIII, which is integral to the creation of the fibrin clot (Scott and Montgomery, 1993). Symptoms and severity of bleeding may vary even among family members.

There are several different types of von Willebrand disease and identification of the type through laboratory studies is critical to selecting an appropriate therapy (Montgomery 1993). The most common form of VWD is Type I and for most children with this mild form of VWD their bleeding symptoms respond to treatment with DDAVP.

Children with types IIA and IIB and severe von Willebrand disease (Type III) require infusions of exogenous von Willebrand protein such as that found in the intermediate purity factor VIII concentrates such as Humate-P, Alphanate, and Koāte to manage bleeding (Logan 1992). These children often experience bleeding symptoms similar to those of a child with hemophilia.

Discharge Teaching Issues

The child and family require instruction on the etiology of the bleeding disorder. Genetic counseling should be made available to interested family members when the disorder is inherited.

The major goals of discharge planning for a child with a defect in hemostasis are instructions on (1) prevention of bleeding; (2) management of bleeding episodes; (3) rehabilitation after significant bleeding episodes such as hemarthroses, intramuscular bleeds, or surgeries; and (4) the future implications of the bleeding disorder on the child and family.

Prevention of Bleeding

Parents need to learn to maintain a balance for their child by providing a safe environment while fostering normal development and a sense of independence to help promote self-esteem. Parents usually benefit from specific suggestions on the types of activities to promote at various stages of their child's growth.

Young children are most vulnerable to bleeding as they become increasingly mobile and learn to walk. Extra padding can be added to pants to protect the sensitive knees of children who are still crawling. Gates should be placed to prevent access to stairs. Carpeting on floors, pads on edges and corners of fireplaces, and padded cribs and side rails will cushion falls. Throw rugs are often a hazard and should be avoided. Children learning to walk have better traction with bare feet than socks or booties. Toys should be selected that are soft, especially those that may be chewed. Big Wheels are preferable to tricycles because they are less likely to tip, and the healthy habit of wearing a bicycle helmet, a must for safe cycling at any age, should be initiated with the first tricycle.

Older children should be involved in making wise choices regarding sports participation, hobbies, and careers that will not increase their risk of bleeding. Regular physical activity is encouraged to build strong musculature and maintain normal weight, which will help prevent bleeding

into muscles and joints. Involvement in specific sports activities should be discussed with a physician. School personnel should be informed if there are any limitations regarding physical activities.

Oral care should be performed with a soft toothbrush and flossing is discouraged when bleeding results. Taking rectal temperatures and the use of enemas and suppositories should be avoided. Tight, constricting clothing should not be worn. Older children should be taught to handle sharp objects with caution. Adolescents should be instructed to shave with an electric shaver. Females should refrain from tampon use and report increased or prolonged menstrual flow.

Children with bleeding disorders should not receive products that contain aspirin. Instruct families to read the list of ingredients for over-the-counter cold preparations. Nonsteroidal anti-inflammatories should be used only with the consent of a physician. Table 12–3 lists factor concentrates and medications used in coagulation disorders. The child should wear a Medic-Alert emblem to alert others to the child's increased risk of bleeding. Immunizations should be given subcutaneously rather than intramuscularly to avoid painful muscle hematomas.

Parents must be advised to consult their health care provider before a child's dental work or surgery. Special precautions may be necessary at these times even if the child has had no prior major hemorrhage.

Treatment and Care during Bleeding Episodes

Action should be initiated immediately when bleeding occurs. Superficial cuts and abrasions usually respond to firm pressure applied for 10 to 15 minutes. When epistaxis occurs, the child should lean forward to avoid swallowing blood and apply pressure to the nose for 15 minutes. Hemarthroses in the child with hemophilia should be immediately managed by *R*est, *I*nfusion of factor concentrate, application of *C*old packs, and *E*levation of the limb (RICE). A sup-

Table 12–3 Factor Concentrates and Medications Used in Coagulation Disorders

Medication	Purpose	Dosage	Side Effects
Aminocaproic acid (Amicar)	Antifibrinolytic: Stabilizes clots, prevents clot lysis: used for oral and nosebleeds	100 mg/kg every 6 hours	Nausea, diarrhea, malaise, headache, abdominal discomfort. Do not give in presence of hematuria.
Cryoprecipitate	Used in life-threatening circumstances *only* when factor VIII concentrate unavailable	60–100 units factor VIII in each bag: Dosage same as for Factor VIII below.	Cannot be virally inactivated: risk of hepatitis and HIV
Desmopressin (DDAVP)	Promotes release of factor VIII and von Willebrand factor stores in mild hemophilia A and mild type I von Willebrand disease	0.3 mcg/kg/dose IV in normal saline run over 20 minutes	Facial flushing, blood pressure, headache, fluid retention, hyponatremia, water intoxication
Monoclonally purified factor VIII (Monoclate, Hemofil M, AHF-M)	Virally inactivated factor replacement for hemophilia A, derived from human plasma	Body weight in kg × % factor level desired ÷ 2 = dosage in units *or* 20–30 units/kg for minor bleeds 40–50 units/kg for significant or life-threatening bleed	*For all factor replacement products: allergic reactions rare
Recombinant factor VIII (Bioclate, Kogenate, Helixate, Recombinate)	Genetically engineered factor replacement for hemophilia A, not derived from human plasma	Dosage same as for monoclonally purified Factor VIII	*For all factor replacement products: allergic reactions rare
Intermediate purity factor VIII (Koāte, Humate-P, Alphanate)	Derived from human plasma rich in von Willebrand factor: used in severe or type III von Willebrand disease	Dosage same as for monoclonally purified Factor VIII	*For all factor replacement products, allergic reactions rare
Ultrapure coagulation factor IX concentrate (AlphaNine SD, Mononine)	Virally inactivated. Derived from human plasma; contains factor IX solely	30-40 units/kg for minor bleeds 60-80 units/kg for significant or life-threatening bleeds	*For all factor replacement products: allergic reactions rare

continues

Table 12–3 continued

Medication	Purpose	Dosage	Side Effects
Recombinant factor IX	Gentically engineered factor replacement for hemophilia B. Not derived from human plasma	Dosage same as for ultrapure coagulation Factor IX concentrate	
Stimate (intranasal DDAVP)	High concentration of desmopressin for intranasal use, for treatment of minor bleeding in mild hemophilia A and mild type I von Willebrand disease	Delivers 150 mcg/ spray. Give children who weigh less than 50 kg one spray in one nostril or 150 mcg. Give children who weigh more than 50 kg one spray in each nostril or 300 mcg.	Side effects same as for desmopression (DDAVP)

Note: IV, intravenous; HIV, human immunodeficiency virus.

ply of cold packs should be kept readily accessible. Oral bleeds including those from dental procedures may be managed with aminocaproic acid (Amicar) alone.

Symptoms that indicate a potential intracranial bleed, such as headaches, loss of consciousness, slurred speech, unexplained vomiting, and loss of sensation or movement, should be reported to the health care provider as soon as possible. Children with hemophilia should be infused immediately. Black tarry stools, hematemesis, and hematuria should also be reported, as should hip pain, throat or neck swelling, chest or abdominal pain or injury, and any injuries to the eye.

Children who have chronic thrombocytopenia will require platelet transfusion when signs and symptoms of bleeding are evident. Platelet transfusions are usually administered in the health care setting.

Parents of children with hemophilia or von Willebrand disease can be taught to manage certain minor or common hemorrhages at home through the administration of the appropriate factor product or the intranasal form of DDAVP (Stimate). Parents need to demonstrate knowledge of the type of product their child uses as well as the correct procedure for mixing, dose calculation, venipuncture technique (as warranted), and administration. Parents should be taught to avoid delay in administering therapy or seeking treatment. A properly functioning refrigerator is necessary to maintain efficacy of the products.

Usually, the first few bleeding episodes prove traumatic and stressful for the family. Parents should be counseled to remain calm and supportive to decrease their child's anxiety. They also need to recognize their critical role as advocates for their child within the health care setting. Telephone numbers of contact personnel should be kept near the telephone. Day care providers, extended family, and school personnel should receive instruction on proper steps to take in the event of bleeding. Parents will feel more comfortable in taking respite leave when they know their child will be well supervised and cared for appropriately.

Rehabilitation after Bleeding Occurs

Children with chronic coagulation disorders benefit from a comprehensive interdisciplinary approach to care as is often seen at hemophilia treatment centers. An essential component of the program is incorporation of physical therapy. Such a program should be initiated when the diagnosis is made, and intervention should occur throughout childhood into adult life.

Hemarthrosis is a common bleeding manifestation in patients with hemophilia. Repeated bleeding into joint spaces can result in chronic synovitis and cartilage destruction. Osteoporosis, subchondral bone cysts, malalignment of bones, and limb asymmetry are often late sequelae. Repeated muscle hemorrhage may cause fibrotic tissue and shortened muscles, leading to joint contractures. After bleeding into the joints and muscles occurs, a physical therapist should be consulted to suggest appropriate splinting and a progressive exercise and strengthening program. Pain relief measures such as infusion of factor before therapy and administration of analgesia as needed should be administered because pain often interferes with mobility and participation in exercise and physical therapy programs. Factor infusion before therapy also decreases the risk of rebleeding with active and passive motion.

Children who survive a significant intracranial hemorrhage may have multiple temporary or permanent physical and/or sensory defects. They require a complete assessment by speech, occupational, and physical therapists to determine their specialized needs (see Chapters 18 and 19).

The Impact of the Disease on Child and Family

Living with a disorder that places restriction on participation in activities can be stressful for the child and family. Steroidal therapy for children with thrombocytopenia may alter the appearance of these children. Counseling should be made available to encourage the development of strategies for successful interactions with peers and the promotion of a positive self-esteem.

Parents may require guidance in setting limits with their child and providing age-appropriate discipline. Overprotection of their child should be discouraged. Occasionally, parents are suspected of child abuse by persons who observe a child's bruises and are unaware of the bleeding tendency. Parents may also feel guilty if the bleeding disorder is inherited. Fathers frequently express difficulties coping with a son who is unable to engage in stereotypically male activities because of a risk of bleeding. Anticipatory guidance regarding these concerns should be addressed soon after the diagnosis is made and as needed when concerns arise.

For any child receiving factor concentrates or blood products, the risk of acquiring hepatitis and HIV should be discussed. Because of advances in donor screening, blood testing, and viral inactivation processes and the incorporation of recombinant DNA technology into the development of factor concentrates, families may be assured that from what is known at this time the risk of contracting a virus from therapies currently available is extremely low. Nonetheless, annual testing of a child's HIV and hepatitis status and appropriate counseling should be offered. The hepatitis B series, which is currently recommended by the American Academy of Pediatrics for all children, and the hepatitis A vaccination should be administered. For those children who may have acquired the AIDS virus or hepatitis before the recent advances in technology, the services of specialists in these diseases should be sought.

Information on local and national resource organizations and support services should be made available. Many hemophilia treatment centers sponsor summer camps for children with coagulation disorders as well as support groups for family members.

Home care plans for children with thrombocytopenia and coagulation disorders are presented in Appendices 12–F and 12–G, respectively. Tables 12–2 and 12–3 provide specific information on medication and factor administration for bleeding disorders.

IMMUNODEFICIENCY IN CHILDREN

Altered immune function in children can result from an absence or malfunction of components required for either cellular immunity (T lymphocytes), humoral immunity (B lymphocytes), or both. An immunodeficiency disorder may be an inherited genetic trait (primary) or result from an unrelated illness or treatment (secondary) (Shearer 1996).

Combined Immunodeficiency

Several syndromes have combined deficiencies in cellular and humoral immunity that result in recurrent life-threatening infections and failure to thrive. Severe combined immunodeficiency syndrome (SCIDS) is one such congenital disorder that occurs as an X-linked recessive disorder or occasionally an autosomal recessive disorder. Lymphocyte analysis reveals an absence of mature T cell–bearing lymphocytes and only a few B cells with mature antigens, although most infants with SCIDS do not produce immunoglobulins (Shearer 1996).

Children with SCIDS usually manifest illness within the first few months of life. Intractable diarrhea, thrush, increasingly severe respiratory infections, and frequent bouts with bacterial, viral, and fungal organisms of low pathogenicity are common. Bone marrow transplantation from a histocompatible sibling donor is the most promising treatment of this otherwise fatal disease.

Success has been demonstrated as well with engraftment of parental haplotype-mismatched bone marrow transplantation. Although finding an appropriate donor requires an exhaustive search, matched unrelated bone marrow transplantation has proven successful in some cases (Hong et al. 1996).

Ataxia-telangiectasia is an autosomal recessive disorder characterized by telangiectases (initially in the conjunctiva of the eye), cerebellar ataxia usually noted as the child begins to walk, and recurrent sinopulmonary infections leading to bronchiectasis. The immunologic findings indicate deficiencies of IgG, IgA, and IgE and an abnormality in T cell immunity. No treatment currently exists that interferes with the ongoing CNS degeneration, and, although supportive treatment may prolong the survival rate of children with this disorder, it is uniformly fatal (Hong et al. 1996).

Wiskott-Aldrich syndrome, an X-linked recessive disorder, is characterized by thrombocytopenia, eczema, and recurrent infections. The immunodeficiency occurs as a result of progressive dysfunction of the thymus gland leading to defective T cells with a deficiency of IgM (Hong et al. 1996). Children with Wiskott-Aldrich syndrome experience bleeding that increases in severity with concurrent bacterial or viral infection. They are also prone to lymphoreticular malignancies mostly of the brain. Infections may be treated with the antibiotics or antivirals of choice, and monthly gamma globulin may prove to be successful. Transfusions with fresh platelets are appropriate for acute bleeding episodes. Although splenectomy may improve the platelet count, the increased risk for sepsis after a splenectomy must be considered. The treatment of this disorder with matched-donor bone marrow transplantation has proven to be successful.

Gene therapy may be a viable option for the treatment of these primary immunodeficiencies. Home care plans for the immunosuppressed child and for the child after bone marrow transplantation are presented in Appendixes 12–H and 12–J, respectively. Supportive care agents for the immunosuppressed child may be found in Table 12–4.

Human Immunodeficiency Virus/Acquired Immunodeficiency Syndrome

Among infants and children, the HIV epidemic is growing and, in 1994, was the seventh leading cause of death in children one to four years old (Bertolli et al. 1995). Despite the initial concentration of pediatric HIV cases in urban metropolitan areas of the northeastern and western regions of the United States, the identification of HIV in children is now being made across the nation. HIV, the retrovirus causing acquired immunodeficiency syndrome (AIDS), contains the reverse transcriptase enzyme which upon attachment to and infection of the helper-inducer

Table 12–4 Supportive Care Agents for Immunosuppressed Children

Medication	Purpose	Dosage	Side Effects
Acyclovir	Herpes simplex prophylaxis and varicella-zoster	5 mg/kg/dose bid increase to 10–20 mg/kg/dose tid or qid if breakthrough occurs	Nausea, vomiting, diarrhea, anorexia, neurotoxicity, headache, dizziness, encephalopathic changes, hypotension, nephrotoxicity, increased LFTs
Amoxicillin	Dental prophylaxis	50 mg/kg (max 3 g) PO 60 min before procedure then 25 mg/kg (max 1.5 g) PO q 6 hours after one dose	Allergic reaction, nausea
Amphotericin B	Antifungal	1.0 mg/kg/day (give test dose of 1 mg before starting)	Fever, chills, hypotension, dyspnea, renal toxicity, flushing, anaphylaxis, pain, (monitor electrolytes)
Azithromycin	Prophylaxis against *Mycobacterium avium* complex (MAC)	5–12 mg/kg/dose q day	Diarrhea, nausea, vomiting, palpitation, chest pain, dizziness, ototoxicity, fatigue, rash, photophobia
Chlorhexadine	Antifungal and antibacterial	10–15 cc bid swish and spit (do not swallow)	Staining of teeth
Clarithromycin	Prophylaxis against MAC	7.5 mg/kg/dose bid	Diarrhea, nausea, headache, abdominal discomfort
Clotrimazole	Antifungal	10 mg troche prn daily	Increased LFTs, nausea, vomiting
Filgrastim (G-CSF)	Stimulates neutrophil production	5 mcg/kg/dose subcutaneously (IV over 2 hours—dilute only in D5W). If concentration <15 mcg/mL, albumin 1 mg/mL should be added.	Bone pain, rash, fever, malaise, mild splenomegaly, headache, hyperuricemia, ARDS

continues

Table 12–4 continued

Medication	Purpose	Dosage	Side Effects
Fluconazole	Antifungal	3–6 mg/kg IV or PO q day	Nausea, increased LFTs, skin rash (rare)
Ganciclovir	CMV prophylaxis	5 mg/kg q 12 hours IV (adjust based on renal function)	Anaphylactic reaction, hypotension
Immunoglobulin	Passive immunity	250 mg/kg IV (maximum 20 g)	Anaphylactic reaction, hypotension
Itraconazole	Antifungal	100 mg q day (age 3–16)	Nausea, vomiting, headache, fatigue, rash, anorexia, dizziness, hypokalemia
Nystatin	Antifungal	200,000–500,000 units tid to qid (swish and swallow)	Nausea, diarrhea
Pentamidine	Prophylaxis against *Pneumocystis carinii* pneumonia	300 mg nebulized once per month (two puffs of albuterol before administration of drug)	Hypoglycemia, nephrotoxicity, hypotension
Rifabutin	Prophylaxis against MAC	5 mg/kg q day	Rash, neutropenia, gastrointestinal intolerance
Sargramostim (GM-CSF)	Stimulates neutrophil-monocyte production	250 mcg/m²/day subq (IV over 2 to 6 hours—dilute in NS)	Bone pain, rash, fever, malaise, mild splenomegaly, headache, hyperuricemia, ARDS
Trimethoprim-sulfamethoxazole	Prophylaxis against *Pneumocystis carinii* pneumonia	150 mg/m²/day in two divided doses; Monday, Tuesday, Wednesday only	Pancytopenia, allergic reaction, nausea, vomiting, diarrhea

Note: LFTs, liver function tests; ARDS, adult respiratory distress symdrome; D_5W, dextrose5 water; CMV, cytomegalovirus; NS, normal saline; PO, by mouth; IV, intravenous; max, maximum; q, every.

T cells (CD4 cells) assemble deoxyribonucleic acid (DNA) from the viral ribonucleic acid (RNA). The CD4 cell is responsible for helping to coordinate the immune system's defense against infectious agents. The resultant destruction of the host cell by the viral RNA releases a new HIV virus, which circulates and attaches to other target CD4 cells (Falloon et al. 1989;

Casey 1995). The clinical manifestations of pediatric AIDS are the result of this attack on the immune system as well as the spread of the virus to the CNS. Frequent and recurrent bacterial infections, behavioral and mental deterioration, the fact that developmental milestones are not experienced or are lost and neoplasms are characteristic of HIV in children (Rodriquez and Hard 1995).

Mode of Transmission

The risk factors for HIV infection in children have changed over the last 10 years. Those children who acquired HIV through contaminated blood products or factor concentrates did so before the availability of serologic testing in 1985 (Wilfert 1994). With the institution of blood donor screening and viral inactivation of factor concentrates, HIV transmission through blood products has almost been eliminated (Bertolli et al. 1995). Sexually active adolescents, those involved in intravenous drug use, or those children who are sexually abused are at risk for contracting the virus. Sexual contact with an HIV-infected partner has become the primary mode of transmission of the disease to women of child-bearing age (15 to 44 years old), and perinatally acquired disease accounts for virtually all new cases of HIV infection in children younger than 13 years (Bertolli et al. 1995). The risk of transmission of HIV infection from an infected mother to her unborn or newborn child ranges from 15 to 40 percent (Wilfert 1994); in 1993, more than 6,600 infants were born to HIV-infected women (Bertolli et al. 1995). Maternal transmission of HIV may occur in utero, during labor and delivery, or to a lesser extent through breastfeeding.

A recent study has shown that the administration of the antiretroviral agent zidovudine (AZT) to pregnant women starting at week 14 of gestation through labor and delivery and subsequently to the newborn for the first six weeks of life can decrease the rate of perinatally acquired HIV to 8 percent (Conner et al. 1994). Women should be offered HIV counseling and testing in the early stages of pregnancy. Those who test positive for HIV should receive further counseling and be offered AZT to decrease the risk of transmission of the virus to their children. The risks and benefits of other antiretrovirals regarding pregnant women are currently being investigated.

Diagnosis in Newborns and Infants

Several laboratory tests assist in the diagnosis of HIV. The enzyme-linked immunosorbent assay (ELISA) can detect antibodies to HIV. The Western Blot differentiates antibodies according to molecular size (Centers for Disease Control 1989) and is used to "rule out" any false-positive results from the ELISA test. The diagnosis of HIV in children younger than 18 months who have infected mothers is complicated because a positive HIV antibody test result reflects passively acquired maternal antibodies. Therefore, the polymerase chain reaction for HIV DNA (HIV DNA PCR) or HIV culture is used to diagnose HIV in children younger than 18 months who have infected mothers (Centers for Disease Control 1995).

Disease Progression

HIV infection is broadly manifested in children, from those who are asymptomatic to those who rapidly progress to severe immune disease and early death. The Centers for Disease Control and Prevention has published standardized criteria and guidelines for the classification of HIV in children based on infectious processes, immune status, and clinical condition (Centers for Disease Control 1994). The more common AIDS-defining conditions include *Pneumocystis carinii* pneumonia (PCP), lymphoid interstitial pneumonia, recurrent serious bacterial infections, wasting syndrome, recurrent herpes, mycobacterium avium complex, HIV encephalopathy, cytomegalovirus (CMV) disease, lymphomas, and invasive candidal infections.

Children tend to develop AIDS more rapidly than adults, with three to five years as the median age of perinatally infected children to develop AIDS-defining characteristics (Bertolli et al. 1995). Factors that appear to indicate rapid disease progression in perinatally infected children include the presence of AIDS-defining conditions in a child younger than one year (for example, PCP, a detectable virus in the serum of a newborn, and the severity of the mother's disease at the time of delivery (Bertolli et al. 1995). HIV encephalopathy is also associated with a shorter survival rate (Wilfert 1994). There is a subset of HIV-infected children with slowly progressing disease 10 years or more beyond infection who have not been diagnosed with AIDS. Conditions that influence this slow disease progression are not yet identified.

PCP occurs in HIV-infected infants most frequently between three and six months of age and is often associated with a poor outcome. All infants born to HIV-infected women should begin PCP prophylaxis therapy (trimethoprim-sulfamethoxazole [Bactrim]) at four to six weeks of age regardless of their HIV status. Once it has been determined that HIV infection does not exist, the PCP prophylaxis treatment may be discontinued (Centers for Disease Control 1995).

Children with HIV infection and their families benefit from a supportive, trusting relationship with an easily accessible primary care provider, as do all children. Because of the rapid advances being made in the understanding and management of HIV infection in children, the primary care provider will find consultation and ongoing dialogue with a specialist in pediatric HIV care beneficial. For the infant or child with indeterminate or asymptomatic HIV, the emphasis of care is on the prevention of frequent or opportunistic infections while ensuring that the child's physical, developmental, emotional, and social needs are met. Regular visits to the clinic to monitor growth and development and to conduct laboratory monitoring are important.

Antiretroviral Therapy

Although there is no cure for HIV presently, treatment strategies are constantly evolving. The use of antiretroviral therapy that prevents replication of the virus through inhibition of reverse transcriptase has proven to be effective in delaying disease progression in both adults and children. Routine monitoring of clinical status as well as laboratory studies of CD4 cell counts as a reflection of immune status and viral burden (RNA PCR or P24 antigen) are critical to determine the point at which to initiate antiretroviral therapy. The most widely accepted clinical symptoms of HIV disease progression in children are neurodevelopmental delay or deterioration and growth failure (Tudor-Williams and Pizzo 1996). Therapy is not routinely started in HIV-infected children who do not experience any symptoms and have a healthy immune status. Clinical trials have indicated that more than one antiretroviral given in combination is more effective than monotherapy in preventing HIV disease progression (Hammer et al. 1996). Several of these reverse transcriptase inhibitors are available now for use in children (several years after their availability for use in adults) and are listed in Table 12–5. Once antiretroviral therapy has been initiated, periodic clinical and laboratory monitoring is critical to identify disease progression and to monitor drug toxicity. Parents should be made aware of the importance of regular follow-up and blood testing. Local providers and laboratories should be provided with the necessary information to accurately monitor progress. Protease inhibitors, currently in use in adults, are starting to be used to treat children.

Teaching Issues

Family members of a child with an immune deficiency will benefit from an understanding of the normal function of the immune system and the implications the specific defect will have on the health of their child and their family. The family's or caregiver's ability to provide for the child's physical, nutritional, and general health care needs should be assessed. Instruction on appropriate home and personal hygiene measures to prevent infection as well as early signs and symptoms of infectious processes should be made available. A common concern for the family living with HIV is prevention of trans-

Table 12–5 Medications Used in the Treatment of HIV/AIDS

Medication	Purpose	Dosage	Side Effects
AZT/zidovudine	Antiretroviral: Reverse transcriptase inhibitor	0–6 weeks: 2 mg/kg/ dose qid PO 4 weeks–13 years: 90– 180 mg/m$_2$/dose qid PO ≥13 years: 100 mg/dose five times daily PO or 200 mg/dose tid	Anemia, neutropenia, liver function tests
DDI/Didanosine	Antiretroviral	90–135 mg/m^2/dose/bid PO	Pancreatitis, peripheral neuropathy, retinitis
DDC/Zalcitabine	Antiretroviral	0.01 mg/kg/dose tid PO ≥ 13 years: 0.75 mg t.i.d.	Peripheral neuropathy, mouth sores, pancreatitis
D$_4$T/Stavudine	Antiretroviral	1 mg/kg/dose bid PO ≥ 13 years: 30–40 mg bid PO	Peripheral neuropathy, nausea, vomiting, diarrhea, pancreatitis
3TC/Lamivudine	Antiretroviral	3 months–12 years: 4 mg/kg/dose bid PO ≥ 12 years: 150 mg/ dose bid PO	Anemia, neutropenia, headache, nausea, diarrhea, fatigue
Nevirapine	Antiretroviral	Dosage under investi- gation for children	Rash: can be severe
Saquinavir/SQV	Protease inhibitor	Dosage under investi- gation for children	Gastrointestinal, hemolytic anemia, ALT, CPK
Ritonavir/RTV	Protease inhibitor	Dosage under investi- gation for children	Gastrointestinal common, ALT, GGT, CPK, multiple drug interactions
Indinavir/IDV	Protease inhibitor	Dosage under investi- gation for children	Nausea, vomiting, headache, must take with lots of fluids to prevent kidney stone

Note: PO, by mouth; CPK, creatinine phosphokinase.

mission of the virus to other family members, friends, or caregivers. Universal precautions should be explained underscoring that HIV is not casually transmitted. Parent or caregiver re- lations with the child can and should be affec- tionate and loving. The home care plan for the child with HIV or AIDS may be found in Appen- dix 12–I.

Prevent or Minimize Infections

Total prevention of infection may not be a practical expectation because the majority of infections are opportunistic or have an endogenous source. Therefore, social isolation of the child is not recommended. The home environment should be evaluated for proper heat, electricity, running water, and toileting facilities, as well as appropriate garbage disposal. Pets in the home should have had appropriate immunizations and the child should not come into contact with the pet's excreta. Vaporizers or home humidifiers, if used, should be cleaned weekly following manufacturer's guidelines to prevent dispersion of fungus.

Teaching the child good physical hygiene is recommended. Handwashing after play, contact with animals, and toileting should be taught. Routine oral care after meals and at bedtime and visits to the dentist twice a year are necessary. The mouth should be assessed for evidence of oral candidiasis, ulcerations, or dental caries. Nystatin suspension or clotrimazole troches may be prescribed prophylactically to prevent oral yeast infections. Children with recurrent herpes lesions may be placed on prophylactic acyclovir.

Children with a primary immunodeficiency may be immunized using an inactivated vaccine but may not be able to mount an immune response. Because of the potential susceptibility of the child with HIV to illness, the American Academy of Pediatrics guidelines for childhood immunizations should be followed, although the child must receive inactivated (Salk) polio vaccine rather than the live (Sabin) oral vaccine. Siblings and children whose parents are HIV infected should also receive the inactivated polio vaccine because the live virus, which inhabits the gastrointestinal tract of the recipient for approximately three weeks, may be passively transmitted to the immunosuppressed person. Because of the high fatality rate from measles in children with HIV, they should receive measles-mumps-rubella (MMR) despite its being a live vaccine. Children with HIV have an increased risk of *Streptococcus pneumoniae* and those

older than two years should receive the pneumococcus vaccine.

Precautions against contracting chickenpox should be discussed. The new varicella (chickenpox) vaccine is also a live vaccine and should be avoided. Parents need to be reminded to immediately report if their child is exposed to another child with chickenpox lesions or who has broken out with lesions within 48 hours of contact. These precautions also apply to any exposures to persons with active shingles (herpes zoster). After such an exposure, children with HIV or other immunodeficient disorders should receive varicella-zoster immune globulin (VZIG) (Boland and Czarniecki 1995). This intramuscular injection given within 96 hours of exposure will prevent or attenuate the course of chickenpox. School personnel should be informed to contact parents if there is an outbreak of chickenpox in the classroom. If chickenpox develops, the child usually requires five to seven days of intravenous acyclovir.

Growth-related problems are common in children with immunodeficiencies and frequently they may present with failure to thrive and an increased caloric demand despite a loss of appetite. The vicious cycle of undernutrition, which can impair the immune status and subsequently result in an infectious process, should be avoided. Culturally sensitive nutritional counseling, which considers the child's preferences and family's financial ability to provide supplemental nutrition, is a routine part of care. Close monitoring of growth parameters and a complete diet history help to detect nutritional changes early. Food should be properly cleaned and stored, and meats adequately cooked to avoid introduction of food contaminants. Normal cleaning of dishware and eating utensils with hot water and soap is sufficient to disinfect surfaces.

Children with oral lesions or chronic diarrhea will require special attention to maintain proper nutrition and fluid and electrolyte balance. Weight loss should be reported and etiology determined. Supplemental nutrition via nasogastric or gastrostomy tubes, or total parenteral nutrition via a venous access device, is often required as the disease progresses, and parents will need to learn proper technique for home administration (see Chapter 8).

Recurrent pulmonary infection or lymphoid interstitial pneumonitis (LIP) leading to bronchiectasis is common in children with an immunodeficiency. Parents need to be alert to alterations in respiratory status and taught pulmonary percussion and drainage to assist in secretion removal during infections. Percussion is avoided in the child with thrombocytopenia. Prophylactic use of trimethoprim-sulfamethoxazole (TMP/sulfa) (Bactrim) is prescribed for those whose immune status puts them at risk for PCP. Baseline and annual chest radiographs are a routine part of care. Yearly tuberculosis screening is indicated for children older than one year (see Chapter 5 for information on pulmonary percussion and drainage).

Encephalitis is a major concern when considering HIV-infected children, the primary cause of developmental delay, and the fact that developmental milestones may be achieved and sebsequently lost. This CNS insult results from HIV or other CMV, herpes, or varicella-zoster viruses and is an AIDS-defining illness. Specialists in physical, occupational, and speech therapy may be needed in the home to assist the child and family living with motor abnormalities and cognitive impairment. Neurologic and developmental evaluations are a routine part of care (see Chapter 18).

Promote Early Reporting of Symptoms and Treatment

Children who are immunosuppressed may be unable to elicit the usual symptoms of infection, or initiation of symptoms may indicate the infection is already progressive. It is, therefore, essential that infectious episodes are identified early and treatment initiated immediately.

Parents should be instructed to report fever, vomiting, diarrhea, excessive fatigue, any unusual rash, or other symptoms of infection that are of concern. A fever may be the initial sign and parents should be taught to use and read a thermometer. The child should be immediately evaluated by a physician and appropriate cultures and tests performed to establish the source of infection. Children may be hospitalized initially to begin therapy and be observed for response. Home administration of intravenous antibiotics or antifungal medications can then be used once an organism has been identified and the child is noted to be responsive. Parents will require specialized instruction or administration guidelines. They also need to report breakthrough fevers because infections not responsive to therapy may occur during the treatment regimen.

Foster Healthy Adaptation of Child and Family

There is a tendency for parents of a child who is immunosuppressed to isolate their child from "normal" social interactions. Parents need guidance to promote independence and provide as normal as possible a lifestyle for their child. Regular school attendance and participation in peer activities should be encouraged. Remember that a child's HIV status is confidential information protected under the law and unauthorized disclosure without a parent's written permission carries legal ramifications (see Chapter 19 for information on working with the school system).

Parents and children benefit from meeting other families in similar situations. Parents should also receive information on agencies and organizations that can provide information, resources, and support.

Families of children with HIV and AIDS often require additional support. Frequently, at least one other family member, if not all, are infected. Ensuring adequate health care for adult family members is critical. Respite care and potentially foster care for children should be sought.

Resources within the extended family need to be identified and used. Families usually benefit from the advocacy, support, and legal services made available through local AIDS service organizations (ASOs).

Parents should be informed of the experimental treatments and the risks and benefits to their child. Treatments, such as bone marrow transplantation, may require that family members be treated far away from home. This may cause disruption of the home or family unit. Counseling should be provided to decrease emotional and financial stress.

Most immunodeficiency disorders are fatal and the family should be encouraged and allowed to express their feelings and concerns. Guilt is a common emotion expressed by parents who transmit a disorder genetically or through an acquired route. Anticipatory grief, especially when the child has a serious infection, is often expressed. Family members should be encouraged to express their feelings regarding the death of a child in the family. A hospice care referral may be helpful if the terminally ill child is cared for in the home (please see Chapter 14 for further information on hospice care).

THE CHILD WITH CANCER

Approximately 8,000 children are diagnosed with cancer each year in the United States, reflecting an increase of about 0.7 percent per year. Despite the rarity of cancer in children, it remains the leading cause of death due to disease under the age of 15 years. It is important to emphasize that the long-term survival rate for all sites of childhood cancer is now over 70 percent (American Cancer Society 1996). Therefore, the goal to successful management of the child with cancer and the family is to develop a support network among the medical center, home, and community to promote the individual's growth and development throughout the treatment phase and beyond.

The epidemiology of the majority of childhood cancers remains unknown. Ecogenetic epidemiology studies are being performed to try to identify certain genetic and environmental risk factors that contribute to the development of childhood cancer. These studies have shown that the majority of children who contract cancer are not associated with known risk factors and that a complex interaction of ecogenetic factors is probably related to the cause (Mooney 1993). Unlike adult cancers, the importance of routine screening for early detection has minimal significance because of the rarity of the cancer types and the often rapid onset of the disease. Many of the presenting symptoms mimic common childhood maladies, which are often ruled out before the diagnosis of cancer. These factors are important to stress to parents who may be feeling guilty about causing the cancer or not seeking more specialized medical care earlier.

Childhood cancer encompasses a variety of diseases (Figure 12–1), each unique in treatment approach and overall prognosis.

Discharge Planning Issues

The agenda for discharge teaching is established by the specific cancer type, prognosis, forms of therapy, and the short- and long-term effects of the disease and treatment. The psychosocial and financial impact of the cancer diagnosis on the child and family necessitates anticipatory counseling and referral to support services.

Childhood Cancers

Acute Leukemia

Acute leukemia is the most frequently occurring cancer in children, accounting for approximately 2,500 new cases in the United States each year. The two major types of leukemia are acute lymphocytic leukemia (ALL) and acute myeloid leukemia (AML).

Leukemia involves a malignant transformation of a blood cell with duplication in the bone marrow and infiltration through the peripheral blood system. Initial symptoms are due to this process and include bone marrow suppression (bleeding and easy bruising, fatigue and pallor, and infections); involvement of the liver, spleen, and lymph nodes with potential increase in size of structure; and arthralgia related to leukemia infiltration in bones and joint spaces. Neurologic symptoms may be present in children with CNS leukemia. The absolute diagnosis is made by microscopic evaluation of the bone marrow contents.

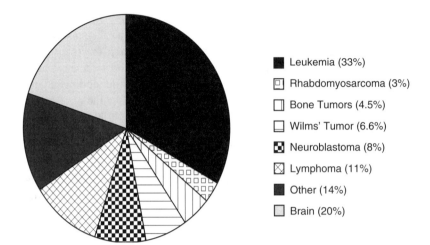

Leukemia (33%)
Rhabdomyosarcoma (3%)
Bone Tumors (4.5%)
Wilms' Tumor (6.6%)
Neuroblastoma (8%)
Lymphoma (11%)
Other (14%)
Brain (20%)

Figure 12–1 Incidence of cancer that occurs during childhood in the United States. *Source:* Data from W.A. Bleyer, The Impact of Childhood Cancer on the United States and the World, *Cancer,* Vol. 40, p. 366, 1990.

Acute lymphocytic leukemia comprises 75 percent of all leukemias in children. The disease-free survival rate is now 70 to 80 percent at five years (American Cancer Society 1996). The two most important good prognostic factors are an initial white blood count less than 50,000/mm^3 and the child's age being 1 to 10 years. Children who present with symptoms that are associated with higher risks require more aggressive therapy, whereas children who present with symptoms that are associated with lower risks will require less therapy, thus minimizing short- and long-term effects of treatment.

The phases of treatment usually include a one-month induction of chemotherapy to achieve a remission of the leukemia.

Remission is achieved in approximately 95 percent of all children by the end of this phase, but it is not a cure. The consolidation phase occurs in the following month and treatment includes weekly intrathecal chemotherapy. Children who have CNS blasts, evidenced by blasts in the spinal fluid at the time of diagnosis, will receive cranial radiation at this time. Maintenance therapy will usually last two to three years and consists of low-toxicity drugs, many of which are administered orally and at home,

therefore requiring fewer visits to the medical center. Even when remission has been achieved, undetectable blasts remain. Recent studies have shown that incorporation of one or two intensification phases of therapy during maintenance can reduce minimal residual disease, destroy resistant clones, and decrease disease in sanctuary sites, such as the CNS and testes. The intensification phase does add to the treatment morbidity but has increased survival for children with ALL (Tubergen et al. 1993).

Also, more recently, children who present with such high-risk symptoms as poor cytogenetics and failure to obtain remission by induction day 28 and have an HLA-matched sibling may proceed to receiving a bone marrow transplant when remission is obtained (Pinkel 1993).

Presently under investigation is the utilization of leukemic cell-targeted monoclonal antibodies with adherent toxins (immunotoxins) that adhere to antigens on the surface of the blast cell, incorporate the toxin into the cytoplasm, and cause cell death. Using biologic therapy during periods of low tumor burden may be an evolving therapy adjunct (Uckun et al. 1992).

Children who have a relapse of ALL while on chemotherapy, or within six months of discontinuation of therapy, have poor long-term survival. However, more aggressive treatment regimens or a matched allogeneic bone marrow transplant from a sibling donor or matched-unrelated donor has improved the disease-free survival rate to approximately 30 percent (Torres et al. 1989).

AML encompasses 20 percent of childhood leukemias. AML can occur at any age in childhood. Treatment results are not as optimistic as with ALL, with the five-year disease-free survival rates being 45 to 50 percent in children younger than 18 years (Steuber et al. 1989). Prognostic factors in AML are less clearly defined because of the heterogeneous group of this leukemia. Chemotherapy is aggressive and myelosuppressive. The initial treatment support is required for such complications as coagulopathies and tumor lysis syndrome, followed by intervention for long periods of marrow suppression. The course of therapy usually lasts 9 to 12 months. Children in remission who have an HLA-matched sibling and have a bone marrow transplant have a 60 percent long-term survival rate (Amadori et al. 1993).

A rare type of AML, acute promyelocytic leukemia, can be treated with ALL-trans retinoic acid and chemotherapy. ALL-trans retinoic acid is a differentiating agent that promotes maturation of promyelocyte blast into mature granulocytes. This drug, which is administered orally, can decrease the coagulopathy complications noted in induction, yet can lead to leukocytosis. The effect of ALL-trans retinoic acid is also temporary and the patients will require further therapy (Fenaux et al. 1993).

Children with acute nonlymphocytic leukemia (ANLL) and who are refractory to chemotherapy and who do not have an HLA-compatible sibling may seek transplantation through a matched-unrelated donor if a search for a candidate is successful.

Chronic Leukemias

Chronic myelogenous leukemia (CML) is the most common myeloproliferative disease in childhood and comprises 2 to 5 percent of the leukemias. There are two types of CML—adult CML (with positive Philadelphia chromosome) and juvenile CML. In the course of CML, there is a clonal evolution from a slow proliferative phase into an accelerated expansion of blasts and eventually to an acute crisis. This transformation may take several years. Early therapy with such chemotherapy drugs as hydroxyurea or busulfan can be used for symptomatic patients and for leukocytosis (Griffin 1986). Alpha-interferon daily injection therapy and 13-cis-retinoic acid have also provided temporary improvement and decreased acceleration of CML (Dow et al. 1991).

It has been well documented that a transplant from an HLA-matched sibling or matched-unrelated donor can be the only cure for this disease. It is recommended that a bone marrow transplant be performed during the early chronic phase of the disease process for optimal results (Synder and McGlave 1990; Gamis et al. 1993).

Lymphomas

Cancer of the lymphoid system includes Hodgkin's disease and non-Hodgkin's lymphoma. Hodgkin's disease occurs primarily in adolescents, whereas non-Hodgkin's lymphoma commonly occurs between the ages of 5 and 15 years (Parkin et al. 1988).

Hodgkin's disease usually presents as painless lymphadenopathy. Systemic symptoms such as malaise, anorexia, fever, night sweats, and pruritus (known as "B" symptoms) occur during the advanced stages of the disease.

It is important to know the full extent of the disease and histologic type to determine staging, prognosis, and treatment plan. Laboratory data, such as a complete blood count; sedimentation rate; ferritin, copper, and transferrin levels; and alkaline phosphatase may be serum markers for the extent of the disease.

A chest radiograph is essential to rule out a mediastinal mass. Computed tomography (CT) scans of the chest, abdominal, and pelvic areas are common noninvasive methods to evaluate pulmonary and retroperitoneal involvement. Gallium scanning is advantageous in children with pulmonary involvement. Bone marrow aspiration should be performed to assess infiltration. The use of lymphangiogram and exploratory laparotomy and splenectomy remain controversial. A staging laparotomy is usually not performed if the child has advanced disease or if the choice of treatment will not be altered by the findings (Lister et al. 1989).

The treatment of children with Hodgkin's disease depends on the age of the child, stage of the disease, and tumor burden. Localized disease may involve only the use of radiation.

Children who have more extensive tumor involvement or who exhibit "B" symptomatology, such as weight loss, fever, and night sweats, over a six-month period will require chemotherapy and possibly radiation to sites of involvement (Donaldson and Link 1991).

Long-term survival rate for Hodgkin's disease is between 80 and 90 percent (Kennedy et al. 1992). Children who relapse after the initial treatment may be able to achieve a remission with salvage chemotherapy. An autologous bone marrow transplant may be recommended when relapse occurs after utilization of only chemotherapy and within one year of completion of initial treatment or for children who are refractory to their treatment (Seeger and Reynold 1991).

Non-Hodgkin's lymphoma (NHL) results from proliferation of malignant cells of lymphocytic or histiocytic lineage that have spread throughout the lymphoid system, usually resulting in generalized disease at diagnosis (Magrath 1993). The malignant cells appear undifferentiated, with rapid turnover, and usually rapidly respond to treatment. The initial symptoms are dependent on pressure to tissues caused by a space-occupying tumor. NHL may also infiltrate into the bone marrow and CNS.

There are three major types of NHL—diffuse lymphoblastic, diffuse undifferentiated (Burkitt's and non-Burkitt's), and diffuse histiocytic or large cell lymphoma (Burke 1990). Because of the rapid progression of this disease, diagnostic and staging tests need to be performed expeditiously. A biopsy sample from lymph node,

bone marrow, or effusion fluid may contribute to making the diagnosis. Chest, abdomen, and pelvic CTs; bone scan; gallium scan; and lumbar puncture are a few of the tests used to determine the extent of the disease.

Chemotherapy is the mainstay of therapy for NHL. During the induction phase, the child will need close monitoring and support for complications caused by rapid destruction of the malignant cells that have invaded organ structures. It is not uncommon to develop tumor lysis syndrome during this phase.

Remission is achieved in 85 to 90 percent of children within a six-week period of treatment. The majority of regimens, especially for lymphoblastic-type lymphomas and those that involve the head and neck, incorporate some type of intrathecal therapy. Multidrug aggressive chemotherapy regimens for approximately six months usually result in five-year disease-free survival from 90 percent for localized disease to 65 to 80 percent for more disseminated disease (Link 1990; Anderson 1993).

Children with NHL who experience a relapse and are able to achieve a remission with another chemotherapy regimen may be candidates for an autologous bone marrow transplant (if no bone marrow is involved) or an HLA-matched or matched-unrelated donor bone marrow transplant.

Brain Tumors

Brain tumors are the most common form of solid tumor in children, predominately occurring between the ages of 5 and 10 years (Albright 1993). Infratentorial brain tumors are the most frequent tumors occurring in the pediatric population. These tumors include cerebellar astrocytomas, medulloblastomas, brain stem gliomas, and ependymomas. Less common supratentorial tumors include craniopharyngiomas, optic nerve gliomas, and pineal tumors (Finlay et al. 1987b). Signs and symptoms of a brain tumor are influenced by tumor size, rate of growth, and location. The most common presenting signs and symptoms of an intracranial neoplasm are increased intracranial pressure and focal neurologic deficits. Symptoms of increased intracranial pressure in very young children may include irritability, listlessness, vomiting, failure to thrive, and macrocephaly (Albright 1985). Older children may experience headaches, vomiting (usually on awakening) impaired vision, seizures (usually focal), disturbances in gait and balance, mental somnolence, and personality changes. Children who have a primary spinal tumor or intramedullary seeding of intracranial tumor may have symptoms of compression of the spinal cord. Back pain, especially when in supine or with Valsalva maneuver, muscle weakness, gait disturbances, and other neurologic and sensory changes below the level of the tumor are often manifested (Gomez et al. 1982).

Neurologic examination and imaging studies (CT and magnetic resonance imaging [MRI]) are usually the most effective methods of diagnosis (Barnes 1990). Positron emission tomography (PET) scanning may be a helpful tool in differentiating tumor from necrotic tissue. Children often need to be sedated to obtain quality studies. CT or MRI with contrast should include spinal films, if there is a potential of seeding down the spine. Cerebral spinal fluid (CSF) may be required for testing for CSF spread. Bone marrow aspirates, bone scan, and abdominal CT are recommended for medulloblastoma and ependymoma workups, because these may be sites of metastatic spread.

Surgery is usually indicated to biopsy, debulk, or completely remove the tumor if possible. Surgery is also required for placement of ventricular shunts or reservoirs when CSF flow becomes obstructed. New surgical techniques with microinstrumentation, lasers, ultrasonic aspirators, etc. now allow for new possibilities in the area of neurosurgery (Finlay et al. 1987a). Every attempt should be made to remove those tumors that are curative by surgery alone, such as cerebral low-grade astrocytomas or germ cell tumors.

There have been advances in radiation therapy that decrease toxicity and provide a more exact field. Brachytherapy and hyper-

fractionated dosing of radiation are two examples (Finlay et al. 1987a). Children need to be fitted into molds and many require sedation to prevent movement out of the field.

Chemotherapy is playing an increasing role in the treatment of brain tumors. Chemotherapy is used to treat residual disease in children younger than one year to prevent the use of radiation at a time when radiation can have marked impact on intellect and physical development (Duffner et al. 1993). Chemotherapy has been shown to be adjunct therapy to conventional radiation and surgery for several pediatric brain tumors (Packer et al. 1991; Sposto et al. 1989). Certain chemotherapy drugs can also act as radiosensitizer agents to increase the sensitivity of cells to radiation (Kovnar et al. 1990). Finlay (1992) has noted some success in using high-dose chemotherapy followed by autologous hematopoietic rescue with bone marrow or peripheral stem cells for children with recurrent brain tumors.

Survival rates have improved over the years but vary greatly, from 90 percent for cerebellar astrocytoma to less than 10 percent for a brain stem tumor. Prognosis is dependent on tumor histology, resectability, degree of dissemination, and response to treatment.

Many of these children develop serious long-term effects from the tumor and its treatment. The management of these children must include periodic evaluations of the effects on learning, rehabilitation needs, and endocrinopathies because their condition may change over the years (Radcliffe et al. 1992; Livesey et al. 1990).

Wilms' Tumor

Most children are diagnosed with Wilms' tumor or nephroblastoma between one and five years of age. Most children are diagnosed because of a large abdominal mass, with other infrequent symptoms of malaise, anorexia, fever, hematuria, and hypertension also appearing (Crist and Kun 1991). Usually, one kidney is involved, although there are rare bilateral presentations.

Most Wilms' tumors are due to a sporadic mutation, but 1 percent of cases may be familial. Other rare congenital anomalies have been reported in 12 to 15 percent of cases, with the most common being aniridia, hemihypertrophy, Beckwith-Wiedemann syndrome, and genitourinary tract anomalies (Green et al. 1993).

Abdominal and chest CTs are essential diagnostic tools. Metastatic disease to the lungs and abdomen should be ruled out before surgical intervention. Surgical removal of the tumor with nephrectomy of the involved kidney is the major method of diagnosis and staging. If possible, the tumor should be removed without any spillage. Excision of involved nodes and other areas of spread should also be attempted. When two kidneys are involved, every effort to salvage the least affected kidney should be attempted. The extent of tumor involvement and histologic type will determine adjuvant therapy.

Chemotherapy is required in all cases, although a present study is exploring the option of no chemotherapy for stage 1 Wilms' tumor of good histology. The length of treatment and the type of drugs are dependent on the stage of disease. Abdominal radiation therapy is not required for children who have grossly resected tumors and with favorable histologic features. The prognosis for children with Wilms' tumor is approximately 90 percent for five-year survival, with the best out-come in those who present with local involvement and favorable histology (D'Angio et al. 1989).

Initial follow-up involves checking for evidence of metastatic disease in the abdomen and lungs, whereas long-term follow-up includes evaluation of the function of the remaining kidney.

Neuroblastoma

Neuroblastomas are tumors that most often arise along the sympathetic neural pathway or from the neural crest cells of the adrenal gland. This tumor is most often seen in children younger than five years. Signs and symptoms are dependent on the size of the tumor and its location. The most common presenting feature is a large abdominal mass, with metastases occurring at time of onset in 75 percent of the cases (Hayes and Smith 1989). The head and neck are the second most frequent presenting sites.

Radiologic studies, such as body scanning with iodine B_1 (131 I) metaiodobenzylguanidine (MIBG), can assist in tumor detection. Urinary catecholamines, if present, can be used as a tumor marker. The oncogene, N-myc, when amplified in the tumor cell, correlates highly with rapid tumor progression and poor prognosis (Oppedal 1989).

Children with localized but unresectable disease have a good prognosis with chemotherapy (Hayes and Smith 1989). The goals of treatment for children with advanced disease are the following: (1) to attain significant reduction of tumor size so that a complete or subtotal resection can be achieved; (2) to eliminate residual disease with use of chemotherapy and radiation therapy; and (3) to pursue a purged autologous bone marrow transplant to eliminate occult metastatic disease. Even with aggressive surgery, chemotherapy, radiation therapy, and bone marrow transplantation, the survival rate for the majority of children with advanced neuroblastoma is less than 20 percent (Berthold 1990).

Investigational therapies are being attempted to increase the survival rate in children who do not respond to initial therapy. Some of these approaches include radiolabeled MIBG, monoclonal antibody therapy, and differentiating agents such as retinoic acid (Cheung 1990; Castleberry 1990).

Rhabdomyosarcoma

Rhabdomyosarcoma is a tumor that arises from striated muscle tissue. This tumor can occur anywhere there is striated muscle and presents as a soft tissue mass of primitive rhabdoblasts or more undifferentiated mesenchymal cells. Rhabdomyosarcoma occurs most frequently in the period from early childhood to adolescence (Raney and Tefft 1993).

Signs and symptoms of rhabdomyosarcoma are dependent on the size of the tumor and location. The most common sites are the head and neck (40 percent), genitourinary tract (20 percent), and extremities (20 percent). Three histologic subtypes account for the majority of the cases—the embryonal and botryoid type (63 percent), which most often is involved in the head and neck disease; the alveolar type (19 percent), which usually involves the extremities and trunk; and the undifferentiated type (10 percent) (Lawrence et al. 1997). Embryonal tumors in general have a more favorable outcome than the alveolar type of rhabdomyosarcoma (Shapiro et al. 1991).

Diagnostic evaluation to determine the extent of the disease and clinical staging includes radiologic scans, histologic findings from biopsy, and bone marrow biopsy. CSF examination is required for tumors located in the head and neck region.

Complete surgical removal is attempted whenever possible. Radiation therapy to the primary and metastatic sites and aggressive chemotherapy regimens are also used. Patients with CNS disease receive intrathecal chemotherapy (Raney and Tefft 1993). The three-year survival rate, overall, is presently 73 percent. Children with parameningeal primary site have a three-year survival rate of 57 percent. Children who have widespread disease at diagnosis, including bone marrow involvement, usually have a poor prognosis (Maurer et al. 1989).

Bone Tumors

The two most common bone tumors are osteogenic sarcoma and Ewing's sarcoma. Bone tumors most often occur during the adolescent period of maximum growth velocity. Boys are more affected than girls (Link and Eiber 1989).

Osteogenic sarcoma is a cancer arising from the bone-producing mesenchymal cells most often occurring in the shafts of the long bones such as the distal femur, proximal tibia, and proximal humerus. Patients usually complain of a painful mass and a radiograph of the bone will often show the bone changes and the mass. A CT of the lungs and bone scan are essential to rule out metastatic spread. A surgical biopsy of the mass will confirm the diagnosis.

Surgical removal of the tumor through amputation or excision with limb salvage is essential for survival. Chemotherapy before surgery can reduce tumor size in the majority of cases so that a limb-salvage procedure can be attempted. A limb-salvage procedure is not recommended if good normal tissue margins cannot be achieved during the excision, or when further limb growth would result in marked leg length discrepancy. Surgical removal of metastatic lung disease is also indicated to maximize the chance for cure (Meyer and Malawer 1991).

Aggressive chemotherapy regimens following complete excision for approximately eight months to one year have resulted in a three-year disease-free 66 percent survival rate. Utilization of newer chemotherapy drugs may increase the survival statistics (Rosen et al. 1987).

Ewing's sarcoma is a small-cell malignancy probably derived from primitive neural tissue (Cavazzana et al. 1987). In contrast to osteosarcoma, Ewing's sarcoma most commonly involves the axial skeleton (40 percent) but can also arise at extraosseous sites. The initial symptoms are similar to osteogenic sarcoma, and the diagnosis involves tumor biopsy and radiologic test for metastatic workup. Complete surgical excision of the tumor is always attempted (Meyers 1987).

Unlike osteogenic sarcoma, Ewing's sarcoma is responsive to high-dose radiotherapy delivered to residual disease. Aggressive adjuvant chemotherapy is also essential (Horowitz 1993). Approximately 73 percent of children diagnosed without metastatic disease have been cured, except for those with pelvic primaries, whose five-year survival rate is approximately 50 percent. Children who have metastatic disease at diagnosis or experience a relapse have a dismal prognosis (Meyers 1987).

Children with localized disease and who receive multimodal therapy have a 70 percent disease-free survival rate (O'Conner and Pritchard 1991). Those individuals with disseminated disease and relapse who underwent an autologous bone marrow transplant continue to do poorly (Link and Eiber 1989).

Retinoblastoma

Retinoblastoma is an embryonic tumor of the retina. Most children are diagnosed before five years of age. Retinoblastoma may be bilateral in 30 percent of the cases. The unique significance of this tumor is its genetic transmission and susceptibility in children to secondary malignancies regardless of treatment in 10 to 15 percent of the cases (Donaldson, Eghert, and Lee 1993).

Retinoblastoma can extend beyond the retina into the vitreous fluid, choroid, optic nerve, and subarachnoid space. Metastases can occur to the CNS, bone marrow, lymph nodes, and liver (Grabowski et al. 1987).

Leukokoria ("cat's eye reflex") and strabismus are common presenting signs of retinoblastoma. Other signs and symptoms include a red, inflamed eye and visual impairments. Clinical evaluation by ophthalmologic examination and CT and MRI scans can help determine the degree of ocular involvement. Radiographic tests and bone marrow aspiration can determine the extent of metastatic disease (Green 1985).

Enucleation is curative and indicated in advanced disease when there is little chance of preserving the child's vision, extension of the tumor into the anterior chamber, or unresponsiveness to other forms of therapy (Shields, Shields, and Sivalingarm 1989).

Recent newer approaches in radiation therapy may provide tumor control in approximately 60 percent of the cases, while retaining some vision. Cryotherapy or focal radiation using radioactive plaques may be successful in treating localized disease (Abramson, Jereb, and Ellsworth 1981; Abramson, Ellsworth, and Rozakis 1982). Hematoporphyrin photodynamic therapy is the combination of an argon laser photocoagulator with a hematoporphyrin derivative that is concentrated 10 times greater in tumor cells than in normal retinal cells (Ohniski 1986). Chemotherapy is used to reduce the treatment field.

Chemotherapy improves the survival rate in children with extraocular disease but is of no advantage in intraocular disease with metastatic spread (White 1991). Intrameningeal spread should be treated with cranial radiation and intrathecal chemotherapy.

The overall survival rate is excellent with approximately 95 percent of children with localized disease free of tumor 5 to 10 years after diagnosis. Even children with extraorbital disease have a greater than 35 percent survival rate (Donaldson, Eghert, and Lee 1993). With increasing survival rates, there is evidence of an increasing incidence of secondary cancers as the patients reach their third decade, including osteosarcoma, small-cell lung sarcoma, and cancer of the bladder, prostate, and breast (Derkinderen et al. 1987). Most of these individuals have the bilateral form of retinoblastoma. It is postulated that these individuals have a genetic predisposition to develop cancer.

Cancer Treatment and Associated Side Effects

The use of a combination of treatment modalities has played a major role in increasing the survival rates in children with cancer. Specific treatment is based on the disease, stage of disease, age of the child, and prognosis.

Surgery

Surgery is the oldest form of cancer therapy, although dramatic advances have occurred in surgical techniques throughout the years. The role of surgery may be diagnostic, curative, or palliative. Most often, surgery is performed to biopsy the tumor for diagnosis and clinical staging. When appropriate, partial and complete removal of solid tumors is important to facilitate the action of radiation therapy and chemotherapy against a smaller tumor mass. Surgery has a role in palliative care to reduce patient discomfort (for example, tumor removal or nerve blocks). Surgical procedures are often indicated to diagnose infectious complications, such as lung infections, or to insert therapeutic devices (for example, central line catheters, ventricular reservoirs, and shunts). The goals of postoperative care are to prevent complications, such as infection and hemorrhage, and provide adequate pain relief. Most surgical procedures require short-term physical rehabilitation, whereas other surgeries (for example, enucleation, amputation, and colostomy) have a permanent impact on the physical and psychological adjustment of the child.

Radiation Therapy

Advances in radiation technology include computerized simulation strategies for more exact targeting of the field. In addition, innovative approaches, such as hyperfractionation, intraoperative radiation, and brachytherapy assist directing radiation to the field, while helping to spare damage to normal tissue. Chemicals concurrently administered with radiotherapy can increase the radiation effectiveness (radiation sensitizers) or shield normal cells from radiation damage (radiation protectors) (Noll 1990).

Selection of radiation therapy as a primary treatment modality is dependent on the radiosensitivity of the tumor and the age of the child. The potential gains of radiation therapy must be weighed against the late effects on the child and availability of alternative therapy.

The type of radiation used, the field to be irradiated, the maximal dose, and the fractionation of total dose need to be determined to maximize effectiveness while limiting complications. Young children will often require sedation and molds to decrease movement and exposure outside the field to be irradiated. Parents should be instructed on the importance of maintaining skin markings if they are not permanent.

Side effects of radiation therapy are dependent on the site irradiated and the dose of radiation. Cranial irradiation may result in partial or complete alopecia. The hair loss could be permanent in that area if high doses are used. Children may also experience somnolence syndrome, beginning several weeks after cranial radiation, characterized by headaches, nausea, and marked fatigue. Learning disabilities may be

late sequelae of cranial irradiation, especially in the young child (Duffner et al. 1991).

Irradiation to the head and neck region may result in irritation and dryness of the eyes, dryness and stomatitis of the oral mucosa, dental problems, taste alterations, and esophagitis. Radiation to the lung may result in pneumonitis. Abdominal irradiation can cause nausea, vomiting, and diarrhea. Skin irritation may become intensified in patients receiving anthracycline chemotherapy (doxorubicin, Daunomycin, or dactinomycin) or through prolonged sun exposure (O'Rourke 1987).

Immunosuppression can occur when large areas of marrow are included in the field. Other late effects of radiation may include skeletal defects, decrease in muscle mass, endocrine abnormalities, sterility, and secondary cancer (Maher 1996).

Chemotherapy

Chemotherapy has a primary role in the treatment of most cancers that occur during childhood. Treatment protocols often use repeated doses of a combination of antineoplastic agents to produce a greater antitumor effect, prevent development of tumor resistance, and minimize toxic effects on normal tissues.

The choice of antineoplastic drugs, dose, route of administration, and schedule are dependent on the specific disease protocol. Each drug will have unique side effects, which are summarized in Table 12–6.

Biologic Therapies

There have been significant advances in biologic therapies over the past few years. Scientific advances in recombinant DNA technology and hybridization have provided mechanisms to synthesize immune components that when administered can have direct antitumor effects, have passive antitumor mechanisms, or provide hematopoietic support and protection (Sondel 1993).

Interleukin 2 (IL-2), also known as T-cell growth factor, is a cytokine that stimulates the

Table 12–6 Common Pediatric Antineoplastic Drugs

Drug Name (AKA)	Nadir	N/V	Oto	Alopecia	Heart	Liver	Renal
5-Fluorouracil (*5-FU*)	9–21 days	X		X			
6-Mercaptopurine (*6MP*)	11–23 days					X	
6-Thioguanine (*6TG*)						X	
Bleomycin				X			
Busulfan	10–30 days					X	
Carboplatinum (*Paraplatin*)	21 days	X				X	X
Carmustine (*BCNU*)	3–5 wks	X		X	↓BP	X	X
Cisplatin (*CDDP*)	7–10 days	X	X				X
Cyclophosphamide (*Cytoxan*)	7–14 days	X		X			X
Cytarabine Ara-C, Cytosine arabinoside	7–14 days	X		X			
Dacarbazine (DTIC)	2–4 wks	X		X			
Dactinomycin (*Actinomycin D*)	10–14 days	X		X			X
Daunomycin (*Daunorubicin*)	10–14 days	X		X	X		
Doxorubicin (*Adriamycin*)	14 days	X		X	X		
Docetaxel (*Taxotere*)	8–14 days	X		X			X
Etoposide (*VP-16*)	7–14 days	mild			↓BP		
Fludarabine	8–15 days	X					X
Idarubicin	7–14 days	X		X	X	X	
Ifosfamide (*Ifex*)	7–14 days	X		X			X
L-Asparaginase							
Lomustine (*CCNU*)	3–6 wks	X		X		X	
Melphalan	14–21 days	X		X			
Methotrexate (*Mtx*)	7–14 days	X-high doses					X
Paclitaxel (*Taxol*)	10 days	X		X	↓BP, AP		X
Peg-Asparaginase (*Oncaspar*)							
Prednisone					↑BP		
Procarbazine	4 wks	X		X			
Thiotepa	7–28 days	X		X			
Topotecan (*Hycamtin*)	15 days	X		X			X
Vinblastine (*Velban*)							
Vincristine (*Vcr, Oncovin*)							

Protectors: MESNA, urinary protection: hypotension, headache, fatigue, limb pain, N, D., + urine ketones
Leucovorin, marrow salvage with Mtx: *must* administer at stated time intervals, rash

Stomatitis	Pulm	Neuro	Vesicant	Derm	Anaphylaxis	Comments
X		X		X		eye irritation
				X		PO on empty stomach
				X		PO on empty stomach
	X			X	X	PFTs, flulike syndrome
	X				X	PFTs
					X	audiometry
	X	X	irritant			
		X			X	audiometry
						check urine s.g. and heme; SIADH
				X		conjunctive irritation at high doses; steroid eyedrops
			irritant			flulike syndrome
			X	acne		yellow color; radiation recall
X			X			red color; MUGA; EKG; ECHO; anthracycline; pink tinged urine; radiation recall
X			X			red color; MUGA; EKG; ECHO; anthracycline; pink tinged urine; radiation recall
X		X		X		joint pain, conjuctivitis, third spacing, fever
		X			X	monitor BP 5 days
X	X	X				mental status deterioration, pancreatits
X			X			red color; MUGA; EKG; ECHO; anthracycline 4x
		X				Mesna
				X	X	IM; check urine glucose; check fibrinogen. If anaphylaxis, may use Erwinia or PEG asparaginase.
		X				
X	X			X		
X	X	X		X		yellow color; high doses, must rescue; sun sensitivity; check urine pH high doses, hold TMP-Sulfa high dose
X		X				joint pain 2–3 post administration
				X	X	IM; check urine glucose; check fibrogin; half-life 5x longer than L-Asparaginase
				acne		mood swings; check urine glucose; check BP; cushingoid; taper off after long-term use
X		X		X		AVOID alcohol, high tyramine foods, barbiturates, hypotensive agents, antihistamines, narcotics
X		X				
X				X		fatigue, headaches
		X	X			assess for constipation, jaw pain, toe walking, ptosis; SAIDH
		X	X			assess for constipation, jaw pain, toe walking, ptosis; SAIDH

production of T lymphocytes and natural killer cells and enhances natural killer cell and lymphokine-activated killer cell activity (Chang and Rosenberg 1989). Treatment with IL-2 depends on its passive augmentation or mobilization of cells capable of destroying neoplasms (Bordon and Sondel 1990). Investigational therapy using IL-2 primarily after aggressive therapy, and therefore directed at residual disease or minimal tumor burden, is presently the focus of research studies. IL-2 is being delivered after therapy for AML, neuroblastoma, and after bone marrow transplantation (Nasr et al. 1989).

Interferons (IFNs), members of the cytokine network, have a number of immune effects. IFNs have antiviral (inhibit viral replication), antiproliferative (inhibit the division of tumor cells), and immunomodulatory (stimulate production of immune cellular components) properties (Dutcher 1993). IFNs have shown promise in treatment of such malignancies in children as chronic myelogenous leukemia and non-Hodgkin's lymphoma (Dutcher 1993).

Tumor necrosis factor (TNF) is a cytokine that has been noted to exhibit direct cytotoxicity to tumor cells and stimulates the production of other cytokines and immune cells (Old 1985). Studies to date have shown synergistic activity with TNF with chemotherapy agents, such as doxorubicin and actinomycin D and with IL-2 and interferon (Watanabe et al. 1988; Semenzato 1990). Its future as a biologic agent is uncertain in pediatric oncology.

Monoclonal antibodies (MoAbs) are a fusion of antibody-producing cells with myeloma cells to produce antibodies specific to adhere to antigens, usually a glycoprotein, on the surface of cancer cells. Unfortunately, few cancer-specific antigens have been identified or the antigens are also shared with their nonmalignant normal cells (Moldawer and Murray 1985). Murine MoAbs developed from mouse B lymphocytes (antibody-producing cells) were first used. They were noted to cause severe allergic reactions in the recipients and produce human antimouse antibodies (HAMA) that decreased efficacy

(Dillman, Beauregard, and Halpern 1986). Newer chimeric (part mouse and human) and human MoAbs have decreased these reactions.

The effectiveness of MoAbs as a single agent has not been impressive. When the MoAb attaches to the surface of the cancer cell, it makes it more recognizable to the components of the immune system for destruction, such as macrophages and neutrophils, and activates the complement system. This is known as antibody-dependent cellular cytotoxicity (ADCC). Minimal tumor burden is needed to respond to this type of therapy (Quesada 1986). MoAbs attached to conjugates have had greater utilization in cancer detection and treatment. MoAbs attached to various radionucleotides are being used in scanning techniques for detection of disease (Miraldi, Nelson, and Karly 1986).

MoAbs can be attached to a toxic substance, such as ricin or pokeweed, and can be directed against specific tumor cell lines, be internalized into the cell, and cause cell death. MoAbs can also be conjugated with chemotherapy agents, radiation, and biologic agents to internalize these substances into cancer cells (Fitzgerald and Pastan 1989). Immunoconjugates potentially target the toxin or antineoplastic agent directly to the cancer cell, thereby sparing normal tissue of toxicity. There are several promising investigations using immunotoxins in the treatment of leukemia and other childhood cancers (Hertler and Frankel 1989).

Hematopoietic growth factors or colony-stimulating factors are glycoprotein hormones that regulate the proliferation and differentiation of hematopoietic progenitor cells and the function of the mature blood cell (Metcalf and Morstyn 1991). With the biosynthesis of these growth factors, we can influence the process of hematopoiesis. The growth factors predominately have been named for the major target-cell lineage they affect.

Erythropoietin stimulates the production of erythrocytes; granulocyte colony-stimulating factor targets only the granulocytes; macrophage colony-stimulating factor (M-CSF) stimulates macrophage production; and granulo-cyte-macrophage colony-stimulating factor targets both the granulocyte and macrophage lineages. Growth factors with more pleuripoient or early cell line stimulation are under investigation, as well as thrombopoietin, which can target platelet production (Clark and Kamen 1987).

The American Society of Clinical Oncology Expert Panel (1994) has made specific recommendations for the utilization of hematopoietic growth factors, mainly G-CSF and GM-CSF, in clinical practice. Preventive use after chemotherapy may be initiated if the probability of febrile neutropenia is 40 percent or greater and with subsequent cycles of chemotherapy when febrile neutropenia occurred in that individual. Colony-stimulating factors may also be used if prolonged neutropenia (even without febrile episode) delayed further therapy. In the area of bone marrow or peripheral stem cell transplantation, colony-stimulating factors can be used to mobilize stem cells for harvesting and after transplantation to hasten myeloid recovery. The panel also recommended starting treatment 24 to 72 hours after completion of chemotherapy and continuing until the absolute neutrophil count reached 10,000/mm³. Although the panel stated that there were fewer side effects with G-CSF, it made no comment regarding which product to use.

The major side effects of biologic therapies are the flulike symptoms of fever, chills, arthralgias, and excessive fatigue. Rarely, the child may also demonstrate symptoms of capillary leak syndrome and third-spacing of fluids resulting in cardiopulmonary effusions and symptoms of renal failure. There may also be electrolyte changes and, therefore, these levels should be closely monitored. As previously stated, use of monoclonal antibodies may result in allergic reactions, demonstrated by a mild rash to anaphylactic reaction. The hematopoietic growth factors usually are associated with more minor symptoms, primarily minor bone pain and flulike symptoms.

Bone Marrow and Peripheral Stem Cell Transplantation

The utilization of bone marrow transplantation (BMT) and peripheral stem cell transplantation (PSCT) as a treatment modality to rescue or replace healthy hemopoietic stem cells is increasing. Exhibit 12–1 lists the variety of hematologic, immunologic, metabolic, and malignant disorders for which BMT and PSCT are being used in children.

There are several differences between harvesting bone marrow cells and harvesting peripheral stem cells. The bone marrow donor has numerous aspirations of bone marrow drawn out from the iliac bone. This usually is a painful procedure and requires anesthesia and surgical setup. After harvest, the donor may experience pain and is at risk for infection at the donation site. Harvesting peripheral stem cells requires the donor to have several sessions on a phoresis machine (usually three sessions) to obtain the required stem cells for transplantation. This is an outpatient procedure and has limited risks. To prime the PSCT donor for the egress of stem cells into the peripheral circulation, the donor undergoes chemotherapy and/or is given growth factors several days before the harvest. As blood counts begin to escalate, the phoresis is begun and the number of CD34 cells (stem cells) being donated are counted until the required amount is collected (Bensinger et al. 1993). Because PSCT is less costly and poses fewer risks to the donor, this method of obtaining hematopoietic stem cells is growing in popularity. Another source for PSCT is utilization of infant umbilical cord blood harvested at the time of birth (Broxmeyer et al. 1991).

Donor selection is a second consideration in the transplant process. An autologous donation involves the patient being the recipient of his or her own bone marrow or peripheral stem cells. The bone marrow or peripheral stem cells are healthy and without disease or purged of malignant disease before infusion back into the patient. An allogenic bone marrow or peripheral

- Hematologic Malignancies
    Acute Lymphocytic Leukemia
    Acute Myelogenous Leukemia
    Progressive Myelodysplasia (Monosome 7)
    Chronic Myelogenous Leukemia
- Lymphomas
    Hodgkin's Disease
    Non-Hodgkin's Lymphoma
- Solid Tumors
    Neuroblastoma
    Brain Tumors
    Ewing's Sarcoma
    Rhabdomyosarcoma
    Wilms' Tumor
    Retinoblastoma
- Bone Marrow Failure
    Fanconi's Anemia
    Diamond Blackfan
    Severe Acquired Aplastic Anemia
    Kostmann's Syndrome (congenital
        neutropenia)
- Red Blood Cell Dysfunction
    Thalassemia
    Sickle Cell Anemia
- Immunodeficiencies
    Wiskott-Aldrich Syndrome
    Severe Combined Immunodeficiency
        Disease (SCID)
    Chronic Granulomatous Disease
    Chédiak-Higashi Syndrome
    Adenosine Deaminase Deficiency
- Metabolic Disorders
    Mucopolysaccharidosis
    Hunter's Syndrome
    Hurler's Syndrome
    Maroteaux-Lamy Syndrome
    Metachromatic Leukodystrophy
    Adrenoleukodystrophy
    Lesch-Nyhan Syndrome
    Type IIA Glycogen Storage Disease
- Other
    Osteopetrosis

Source: Data from H.M. Lazarus, (1992). Pharmacologic Advances in Bone Marrow Transplantation: Improvement in Supportive Care, *Mediguide to Oncology,* Vol. 2, No. 2, 1992.

stem cell donor is used when healthy stem cells from a recipient are required to replace malignant, absent, or abnormally functioning bone marrow cells in the patient. An allogenic donor is selected based on the criteria of having suitably histocompatible HLA and mixed leukocyte culture (MLC) matched to the patient. Ideally, six of the HLA loci are identical (Anasetti et al. 1989). A sibling has a 25 percent chance of being a perfect match. When an identical sibling cannot be found, an unrelated phenotypically identical donor may be identified using the National Marrow Donor Program (Beatty et al. 1985).

After collecting the source of stem cells (bone marrow or peripheral stem cells), red blood cells are removed and the source is filtered. If the stem cells are to be used at a later time, the cells are preserved in dimethyl sulfoxide (DMSO) and frozen.

The patient then needs to follow a preparative regimen of chemotherapy and, at times, undergo radiation therapy. The goal of the preparative regimen prior to bone marrow transplantation is to eliminate the malignancy or dysfunctional bone marrow cells and to sufficiently immunosuppress the patient to prevent engraftment rejection.

The choice of the preparative regimen is determined by the disease, age of patient, prior therapy and effects on the patient's health, and the source of the marrow (Applebaum 1996).

After the preparative regimen, the bone marrow or peripheral stem cells are transfused into the patient. The bone marrow or peripheral stem cells are transfused through a central line catheter similar to that used in a blood transfusion. Complications may include volume overload, shortness of breath, chills, fever, and urticaria. These symptoms are usually treated with antihistamines, antipyretics, or slowing the rate of infusion. Cryopreserved bone marrow or stem cells are removed from a liquid nitrogen tank and thawed in a warm water bath before infusion. The DMSO preservative is metabolized and excreted via the lungs and emits a strong garliclike odor, which may cause nausea for the patient. An antiemetic may be administered to control this symptom. Institutions usually have policies for close monitoring of patients throughout the infusion process.

The time after infusion is spent awaiting engraftment of the stem cells in the recipient bone marrow. It is thought that another advantage of PSCT versus BMT is that peripheral stem cells have a faster engraftment rate (Bensinger et al. 1994). Also, the use of growth factors, such as G-CSF or GM-CSF, after the infusion of stem cells has accelerated bone marrow engraftment (Nemunaitis et al. 1991).

There are several acute complications that can develop as a result of the toxicities of the preparative chemotherapy and radiation therapy. Total alopecia usually occurs, and, for children who have not experienced this effect before, it may be difficult emotionally. Nausea and vomiting can be minimized by the serotonin-inhibitor antiemetics provided "around-the-clock." Skin erythema can be reduced with use of water-based moisturizer. If the patient receives a conditioning chemotherapy agent that can cause hemorrhagic cystitis, such as cyclophosphamide, prophylactic use of mesna, and vigorous hydration may reduce the incidence of this side effect. Mucositis of the gastrointestinal tract usually occurs five to seven days after transplant. An aggressive oral hygiene regimen needs to be established and use of patient-initiated dose analgesia or continuous infusion of narcotics can assist in providing comfort to patients until healing occurs (Hill et al. 1990).

Because children usually do not wish to eat or eat very little during the time they are experiencing mucositis, they need to be nutritionally supported with intravenous nutrition and electrolyte supplementation. Most of their medications during this stage are delivered by the intravenous route.

Veno-occlusive disease may develop as a result of chemotherapy-radiation damage to the hepatic cells and the venous endothelium, obstructing blood flow leaving the liver. This condition is characterized by ascites, tender hepatomegaly, and jaundice, with elevations in liver enzymes. The goal of therapy is mainly to maintain intravascular volume and good renal perfusion through supportive measures (McDonald et al. 1993).

For approximately two to three weeks after the transplant, the patient will be severely pancytopenic. Red blood cell and platelet transfusion support will be necessary to treat anemia and thrombocytopenia. Because of the child's high risk of developing infection, many institutions place the child in a room that is heptafiltered and require good handwashing. All visitors should be screened for illnesses. The child usually should follow a neutropenic diet and needs to wear a high-filtration mask when leaving his or her room. Routine administration of an antifungal agent such as fluconazole and antiviral agents such as acyclovir and immunoglobulin infusions and administration of CMV-negative blood products (if CMV is negative at time of transplant) are prophylactic measures for neutropenia. Patients who are positive for excretion of CMV should receive ganciclovir prophylaxis at the time of engraftment (Goodrich et al. 1993). Trimethoprim-sulfamethoxazole is usually started twice daily, two days per week once engraftment occurs to prevent *Pneumocystis carinii*. Febrile patients with neutropenia should be cultured and broad-spectrum antibiotic therapy should be started to prevent septicemia. These antibiotics and antifungal agents may be modified based on culture results and the patient's clinical status.

Complications involving other organs, such as cardiac, pulmonary and renal insufficiency, should be monitored closely with appropriate tests and scans performed throughout the transplant process.

Graft-versus-host disease is a complication that can occur when the allogeneic T lymphocytes transferred with the graft mount an immune-mediated response against the patient's cells. GVHD of the skin is manifested as an erythematous maculopapular rash, which often involves the palms and soles, and may progress in intensity. GVHD of the liver is characterized by an increase in bilirubin, transaminase, and alkaline phosphatase. Gastrointestinal GVHD usually results in anorexia and diarrhea (Sullivan 1994). A biopsy of the skin, liver, or gastrointestinal mucosa may help make this diagnosis. The two most common agents used to prevent GVHD are methotrexate and cyclosporine and have a greater effect when used together (Storb et al. 1989). Once acute GVHD develops, other agents such as steroids, antithymocyte globulin, and monoclonal antibodies against T lymphocytes are often used (Martin et al. 1991).

Discharge criteria after BMT or PSCT will vary with each institution. Most institutions will expect the child to be afebrile and no longer taking antibiotics. The patient should be blood-product independent or require minimal support that could be transfused in the outpatient setting. The patient should also have begun to have an oral intake of greater than 50 percent of baseline nutrient requirements. Supplemental nutrition and hydration may be administered in the home. The child should be able to tolerate oral medications that he or she will need to take at home such as prophylactic antimicrobials, anti-GVHD medications, antiemetics, or antihypertensives.

The child is usually followed closely at the transplant facility for the first one hundred days after the transplant. There are usually restrictions regarding being out in crowds, wearing a high-filtration mask, and participation in occupational and physical rehabilitation exercises. Complete physical examinations are required to check for sites of infection, GVHD, or developing late effects of the transplant. Blood counts and blood chemistries are monitored closely for continued engraftment and potential complications. Children with malignant disorders may require procedures such as bone marrow aspirations or spinal taps to evaluate disease status. The decision when the child can resume his or her usual activities and return home is usually based on the child's immune status recovery based on quantitative immunoglobulin tests. Some institutions will also test titers for prior vaccinations and revaccinate with attenuated vaccines for low levels.

The transplant process may not be completely finished after the child is allowed to go home from the medical center. Several late complications can develop because of the transplant. Parents and home care providers need to obtain knowledge of potential problems that can occur and when to seek assistance from their local medical staff or the transplant staff (see Appendix 12–J, The Child after Bone Marrow Transplantation).

Teaching Issues before Discharge

Discharge teaching for a child with cancer and the family should incorporate content specific to the disease, treatment, anticipated short- and long-term effects of treatment, related home care, and precautions. In addition, counseling is directed toward decreasing family stress, maintenance of a normal lifestyle as much as possible, and access to support and financial resources.

A family conference is usually planned once the diagnosis of cancer is made. The goals of this conference are to provide initial information and address specific concerns and questions. Significant others, such as grandparents, are encouraged to attend. Adolescents and parents can be instructed together. Younger children will need a modified teaching approach geared to their developmental ages. Parents are encouraged to audiotape the sessions for future reinforcement. Written instructions should be provided for reference.

Disease and Prognosis

Parents are provided information regarding the child's specific cancer, potential etiology, concept of metastasis, and prognosis. The treatment modalities and side effects are explained. A treatment schedule or timetable should be provided. If the child is eligible for a research study, parents require protocol information, such as the purpose of the study, the risks and benefits in participating, and alternative therapy if they do not choose to participate. They should also receive the schedule of planned tests and procedures.

Side Effects of Therapy

Teaching issues related to the acute side effects of therapy should emphasize preventive measures when applicable and care of the child when the symptoms occur. Parents should receive information on "when" and "who" to contact when problems arise at home.

Hair Loss. Alopecia, or hair loss, may involve not only scalp hair but also eyelashes, eyebrows, and axillary and pubic hair. Instructions should include the anticipated degree, duration, and time hair loss will begin. Hair regrowth may occur in some cases while children are still receiving therapy. The child and family need to know that the color and texture may vary from that before treatment. Parents and child should be encouraged to express their fears and concerns regarding this change in appearance. Suggestions for protective and cosmetic coverings, such as wigs, scarves, or hats, should be provided.

The scalp should be covered when in bright sunlight to prevent sunburn and covered in cold conditions.

Skin Changes. Care for potential skin problems, such as rashes, acne, irritated skin, hyperpigmentation, and photosensitivity should be discussed. Rashes and skin erythema are usually transient but should be reported. The causative agent may or may not be the cancer therapy. Other sources, such as tape sensitivity, other drugs, or infections should be investigated.

Acne is usually the result of corticosteroid therapy or a side effect of dactinomycin. The skin should be kept clean. The use of benzoin peroxide topical cream is usually advised. Oral or topical antibiotics are prescribed when there is widespread folliculitis.

Hyperpigmentation is the result of increased levels of melanin-stimulating hormone. The areas most often affected are nailbeds, teeth, gingiva, and along veins used for chemotherapy. Skin may also be hyperpigmented in areas of irradiation. This discoloration may take many months to fade after discontinuation of therapy. Many chemotherapy drugs will make the skin more sensitive to ultraviolet rays. Sites of prior irradiation will also be more sensitive. Even short exposure in direct sunlight may result in sunburning. Parents should be instructed to apply a waterproof sunblock of sun protection factor (SPF) 15 on their child before the child goes outdoors. Protective clothing and hats are also recommended. Teens should be discouraged against tanning in sun and using tanning lamps and beds.

Dry, irritated skin may be a result of certain drugs and radiation. Frequent application of a nonalcohol-base moisturizing cream such as Eucerin may be helpful. No harsh soaps, creams, powder, or cosmetics should be used on irritated areas. Avoiding direct contact with heat and cold is essential. Tight-fitting clothes and harsh fabrics can exacerbate the condition. Antipyretic medications may be necessary if the child scratches the area. A moisturizing lip balm should be applied frequently to prevent dryness of lips. Children often prefer flavored lip balm.

Gastrointestinal Effects. Gastrointestinal side effects most commonly reported are stomatitis, anorexia, nausea and vomiting, diarrhea, and constipation. These symptoms are usually temporary but can be the source of discomfort for children undergoing cancer therapy.

Before the start of therapy, the child should have a panorex of jaw and be examined by a dentist, if possible. Braces and other orthodontic appliances should be removed before therapy and any emergency dental work should be performed to prevent future source of infection. Any child with a central line catheter will require prophylactic antibiotics before any dental work is performed. Routine oral care is encouraged. The recommended procedure is brushing teeth after meals with a soft toothbrush and fluoride toothpaste. Flossing is discouraged when platelet count is below 20,000/mm^3 and the absolute neutrophil count is below 500/mm^3. The oral cavity should be rinsed with chlorhexidine oral rinse. Chlorhexidine has antibacterial and antifungal ability, but it does stain the teeth. Because chlorhexidine must not be swallowed, it should be swabbed in the mouths of younger children with a sponge stick. A fluoride rinse may be recommended once a day. Parents and older children should inspect the mouth for signs of yeast infection or ulcerations. Many children are taking prophylactic antifungal medication, such as oral nystatin, clotrimazole troche, or systemic fluconazole.

Chewing sugarless gum can assist in stimulating saliva production, a natural infection control measure. Artificial saliva is available for use when production is diminished due to therapy. Children are also encouraged to drink frequently if the mouth is dry.

Stomatitis is the result of damage to the epithelial cells of the mucosa by therapy and results in painful ulcerations, hemorrhage, and often secondary infections. This condition may interfere with adequate oral intake. With minor ulcerations, parents are instructed to apply a topical anesthetic (benzocaine, lidocaine, or dyclonine product) to the area, especially before eating. A mixture of dyclonine, Maalox, and diphenhydramine is often effective. Children should be encouraged to eat cool, bland foods during this time and avoid spicy, acidic, or irritating foods and liquids. Medications may be needed for pain control. Parents should be advised to check their child's temperature before administration of acetaminophen to determine if their child has an infection. If the child is unable to eat or drink sufficient amounts or is experiencing severe pain, hospitalization may be indicated for parenteral pain control and nutrition.

Esophagitis, or ulceration of the esophagus, is less easily managed than oral stomatitis. Swallowing topical anesthetics is not recommended in small children because of the potential for aspiration from loss of gag reflex. Children with esophagitis usually require temporary hospitalization for pain control and hydration and to receive their medications intravenously.

Nausea and vomiting are symptoms frequently observed as a consequence of chemotherapy and abdominal radiation. Recent development of serotonin antagonist antiemetics (granisetron, ondansetron) has dramatically decreased the incidence of nausea, especially when used with dexamethasone. Antinausea medication should be administered before the start of chemotherapy and given "around the clock" during the therapy and until nausea ceases. The serotonin antagonist antiemetics are not effective against delayed nausea, which occurs several days after the completion of chemotherapy. Other effective antiemetics, such as Compazine and metaclopramide, should be combined with low-dose diphenhydramine because of their potential for extrapyramidal reactions, and diphenhydramine should continue for 24 hours after discontinuation of the antiemetic. Other drugs that may be used are lorazepam, haloperidol, chlorpromazine, and promethazine. Older school-age children and adolescents may try dronabinol (cannabinoid) for antiemetic effect.

Older children and adolescents who develop anticipatory nausea and vomiting may benefit from oral lorazepam before coming to the clinic or hospital.

Children should not be forced to eat or drink when nausea or vomiting is expected to be of short duration. Small frequent feedings or a clear-liquid diet is better tolerated. Minimizing sights and sounds and adverse smells, while providing enjoyable, relaxing distractions, is recommended. Young children should be positioned in a semiupright position after feedings to prevent aspiration if vomiting should occur.

Anorexia can occur for multiple reasons. These include taste alterations, nausea and vomiting, stomatitis, oral infections, dryness of oral mucosa, or as a direct effect of cancer.

Children often request different foods once treatment is started, because their taste sensation may be altered. They may experience a decrease in the acuity of their taste sensations. Common taste changes are aversions to bitter foods, such as beef, pork, and chocolate. Poultry and fish are often preferred as well as salty foods. Sweet foods do not often taste good. Parents should experiment with various food types and elicit suggestions on what foods the child likes to eat.

Taking older children grocery shopping allows them to have choices regarding food selection. Mealtime should be a pleasant experience, and food should not be used as a control issue.

Children on high-dose corticosteroid therapy will have an increase in appetite and sodium retention. The parents and child should be prepared to expect the child to gain weight, especially facial and truncal obesity. They should receive nutritional guidance on limiting the child's intake of salty foods and keep cheese and milk intake at a moderate level.

The weight and growth of the child should be monitored closely. A nutritional consultation may be necessary if the child is consistently losing weight. Nutritional supplementation is usually not tolerated well in younger children. Many children on aggressive therapy may suffer from anorexia and weight loss and will require total parenteral nutrition at home. This usually requires hospitalization for a few days to educate the caregivers and to make sure the child is tolerating the mixture. Close monitoring of electrolytes and liver function is required with parenteral nutrition use. Nasogastric feedings are also used, although many children often perceive the passage of the tube as traumatic.

Diarrhea may occur as a side effect of therapy and can be a sign of a gastrointestinal infection or malabsorption syndrome. Parents are instructed to report when their child suffers from persistent diarrhea. Suggestions should be provided for a low-residue diet and avoidance of high-bulk foods, caffeine beverages, and milk and milk products. The child is encouraged to drink plenty of liquids, such as Pedialyte, to replace lost electrolytes. Severe diarrhea may require more aggressive monitoring and interventions.

During periods of diarrhea, the rectal area should be kept clean and dry. At the start of diarrhea, an agent to prevent skin irritation should be applied to the rectal area. Such products as Vaseline Constant Care or A&D antibacterial ointments are often recommended. Antidiarrheal medications such as Kaopectate may be needed but should be prescribed by the oncologist.

Constipation may result from *Vinca*-alkaloid chemotherapy (vincristine, vinblastine) but may also be related to decreased activity, stress, narcotic use, or decreased roughage in diet. Parents are encouraged to provide more bulk in their child's diet and increase the child's intake of liquids. Encouraging mobility and exercise is also recommended. Stool softeners such as Colace, PeriColace, Naturcil, or Lactolose are prescribed for routine use when constipation is an expected symptom to prevent impaction. Parents are advised to avoid use of strong laxatives, suppositories, or enemas without the permission of the oncologist.

Hematologic Changes. Bone marrow suppression may result from tumor invasion of bone marrow, irradiation of bone marrow sites, and chemotherapy. The result is a decreased number of circulating blood cells. Parents should be instructed in the interpretation of a complete blood count, platelet count, and differential of the percentage of white blood cells and in the resulting care based on the values. A decrease in red blood cell production, bleeding, or hemolysis can cause symptoms of anemia. Hemoglobin or hematocrit levels are indicative of the degree of anemia. Parents are instructed to report symptoms such as paleness, fatigue, poor appetite, irritability, headaches, dizziness, and shortness of breath, which may be symptoms of anemia in their child. Most children will receive a transfusion with packed red blood cells when the hemoglobin value is less than 8 g/dL.

A decrease in the number of platelets can predispose the child to bleeding. Platelet counts lower than 5,000 to 20,000/mm^3 usually indicate the potential for bleeding and the need for platelet transfusion. Parents are instructed to report any signs of spontaneous bleeding such as epistaxis, bleeding gums, blood in urine or stool, bleeding around central line exit sites, or prolonged menstrual periods. Multiple bruises or petechiae are usually symptoms of thrombocytopenia and should be reported.

Preventive measures against bleeding should be recommended. Children should avoid rough contact sports, wear appropriate protective sports gear with activity, wear loose-fitting clothes, and avoid diving head first when swimming. Adolescents should avoid a straight-blade razor and use an electric razor for shaving. Children should not receive aspirin or ibuprofen products, which may alter platelet function. During bleeding episodes, firm pressure should be applied. If bleeding persists longer than 10 to 15 minutes, the parents should notify the physician. If the child suffers a head injury, parents should notify the physician immediately because of the potential for a CNS hemorrhage.

Infectious Complications. Infection is a frequent complication in children with cancer and is one of the major causes of morbidity and mortality in this population. Children are predisposed to infections due to immunosuppression caused by the disease and its treatment. Bone marrow suppression by chemotherapy results in neutropenia, beginning approximately one week after initiation of treatment and lasting 10 to14 days or longer. The use of growth factors (G-CSF or GM-CSF) after chemotherapy can influence the length and degree of neutropenia. Parents are taught how to administer growth factors usually subcutaneously, although they can be administered intravenously and started 24 to 72 hours after the completion of therapy. Growth factors are discontinued when the neutrophil count is 10,000/mm³.

Parents are initially fearful of exposing their child to potential sources of infection (for example, school, shopping malls, and church). They need to be reassured that most of the infections children contract are from their own bodies (that is, endogenous infections). Therefore, placing them in a "protective bubble" would not prevent the occurrence of infection.

Parents are instructed on the importance of the absolute neutrophil (granulocyte) count. The count is calculated by multiplying the percentage of neutrophils (segs, bands) by the total white blood cell count. When the result is less than 500/mm³, the child is at increased risk for bacterial infections. Parents are also informed that the child may not demonstrate the usual

signs and symptoms of infection in a neutropenic state. Parents should have a thermometer in the home and be instructed in reading the thermometer correctly. They should immediately notify the physician if the child develops a temperature greater than 101°F (38.3°C). They should not give acetaminophen to a child who has a low-grade temperature because it will delay the identification of the fever. In addition, they should report frequent cough or shortness of breath. Any sign of skin breakdown, pain, rash, erythema, or drainage on any area of the body should be reported. The physician should be notified when stomatitis or oral candidiasis occurs. Pain on defecation or rectal area skin breakdown may indicate a rectal abscess that requires immediate attention.

Good handwashing is the best preventive measure against infection. Children should be taught to wash hands after using the toilet, after playing outside or with other children's toys, after playing with pets, and before eating. Other members of the family should also take the same precautions.

Children should not be responsible for cleaning up pets' excreta, bird cages, fishbowls, or litter boxes. Household pets should have their vaccinations up to date.

Bedside humidifiers and vaporizers are usually not recommended because they are often difficult to clean and, therefore, often grow mold and fungus. Room-size humidifiers usually come with instructions on how to add special cleaning solution periodically to keep the solution clean.

Fresh fruits and vegetables should be washed well. Some institutions recommend cooking all unpared fruit and raw vegetables. Meats should be cooked well. Raw fish should be avoided. Children should not drink unpasteurized milk or milk products.

Children should not receive live immunizations (for example, immunizations for measles, mumps, rubella, and oral polio) because of the risk of immunocompromised patients contracting the illness. It is often recommended that siblings not receive the oral live polio (Sabin) vaccine but instead receive the inactivated polio (Salk) vaccine because the live virus is excreted in the stool. Diphtheria-pertussis-tetanus (DPT) and influenza vaccines may be given to a child, as well as hepatitis B series and varicella vaccine, but these vaccines may produce an ineffective therapeutic defense response due to the child's poor humoral immunity. "Catch up" on immunizations is recommended one year after completion of therapy when the immune system has recovered.

Children exposed to measles who have not had prior immunization should immediately receive pooled serum immune globulin in an attempt to prevent getting this illness.

Parents are instructed to notify the physician if there is a measles outbreak in the child's school or neighborhood.

Varicella-zoster exposure (chickenpox, shingles) may result in serious illness if contracted by a child with cancer. Parents are instructed to immediately report their child's exposure to chickenpox or shingles. An exposure is defined as one hour in direct contact with a person who has chickenpox lesions or shingles or develops chickenpox within two days after the contact.

Varicella-zoster immunoglobulin can be administered within 72 hours after exposure to eliminate the risk of developing chickenpox or to attenuate the course of the disease. The half life of VZIG is short, and the immunoglobulin must be readministered if the child is subsequently exposed after three weeks.

Children receiving aggressive therapy should receive prophylactic trimethoprim-sulfamethoxazole twice a day, two or three days per week, to prevent the development of *Pneumocystis carinii* pneumonia, a common infection acquired by immunosuppressed patients. Also, systemic antifungal coverage with fluconazole once a day is recommended to prevent fungal infections.

Neurologic Effects. Neurologic changes, such as peripheral neuropathy, are common in children receiving *Vinca* alkaloids. Early signs of this side effect include jaw pain, tingling of the fingers and toes, decreased reflexes, tremors, and weakness of extremities. Parents are encouraged to report problems with coordination such as stumbling or toe walking. Modifications in therapy and physical therapy exercises or bracing may be required if symptoms become severe. Leukoencephaly is a temporary neurologic condition that may occur after cranial radiation or after intrathecal chemotherapy. It occurs from inflammation of meninges and results in headaches, nausea, somnolence, and, at times, mental confusion and depression. A short course of steroids can decrease inflammation and resolve symptoms.

Cardiopulmonary Effects. Cardiopulmonary complications may occur as a consequence of cancer, infection, or direct toxicity of therapy. Parents are instructed to report symptoms in their child, such as shortness of breath, frequent cough, and progressive fatigue, that may indicate a problem. Periodic evaluation of cardiac function, with a stress/rest ejection fraction or echocardiographic scan, should be performed when the child is receiving drugs that have been known to cause cardiotoxicity. Pulmonary function tests are recommended to evaluate lung function before administration of drugs that may cause fibrosis. Inflammation of the lungs, or pneumonitis, may occur after lung radiation. Steroids can decrease the inflammation and decrease symptoms, such as chronic cough and shortness of breath.

Renal Effects. Renal effects by tumor involvement, cancer therapy, other nephrotoxic drugs, or infection may adversely affect the child's excretory function. Parents are instructed to promptly report oliguria, dysuria, or blood in the urine.

Some chemotherapy agents will temporarily discolor the urine. Parents and child should be informed so that they are not alarmed about the color of the urine, especially if a reddish hue, which may resemble blood. Kidney function determined by urine samples for urinalysis or creatinine clearance collection, or serum analysis for blood urea nitrogen and creatinine are often evaluated before administration of potentially nephrotoxic chemotherapy. Irritation of the bladder due to the metabolite of cyclophosphamide and ifosfamide chemotherapy may result in bleeding or hemorrhagic cystitis. Children should be encouraged to drink during and after administration of these drugs, even though they are receiving large amounts of intravenous fluids during administration and several hours after drug infusion. A new drug called mesna prevents the chemotherapy drug from forming the harmful metabolite. Therefore, mesna is usually administered during cyclophosphamide and ifosfamide therapy.

Many of the nephrotoxic chemotherapy drugs cause destruction of the tubules of the kidneys. The result is that often there is electrolyte wasting and inability to reabsorb electrolytes. Many children require supplemental electrolytes, such as magnesium, phosphate, or potassium, on a temporary basis.

Hepatic Effects. Many of the drugs are associated with hepatotoxicity because they are metabolized in the liver. Children are monitored for this effect by caregivers periodically checking serum liver function test results. Parents are instructed to report jaundice.

Endocrine Effects. Endocrine abnormalities may occur with certain drugs. Abnormality in pancreatic function may result in usually transient diabetes, especially with high doses of corticosteroids or use of asparaginase, which may require insulin therapy.

Reproductive Effects. Adolescents should receive counseling regarding sexuality issues. It is important to assess the knowledge of sexuality and sexual behavior of the patient. All adolescents who are sexually active should be informed of birth control measures while receiving therapy. It should be remembered that certain antibiotics impede the efficacy of birth control pills.

Postpubescent females should be prepared for potential amenorrhea while receiving therapy and that this condition does not ensure they will not be able to conceive during this period. Some females may experience heavy menses, especially during periods of thrombocytopenia. These individuals may take birth control pills continuously to temporarily cease menses during treatment. Vaginal candidal infections are not uncommon; therefore, vaginal pain, itching, or discharge should be reported.

Postpubescent males who may become sterile from the treatment should be given the option to cryopreserve their sperm before the start of therapy, if time allows. Males should be informed of potential transient impotence with the use of certain drugs, such as the *Vinca* alkaloids. Both males and females should be instructed to avoid sex practices that may potentially cause infections, specifically anal sex.

Safety Issues

Family members should also receive information about safe handling of chemotherapy agents in the home to decrease their exposure to these potentially harmful agents (Exhibit 12–2).

Late Effects of Therapy

Over the past decade, there has been awareness of the need for long-term follow-up of survivors of cancer experienced in childhood. Late complications have developed as a consequence of the disease, specific therapies, or complications of therapy. Screening for potential problems and early management may prevent or minimize the impact on the physical functioning of the child. The psychological sequelae to the child and family members should also be assessed.

Alterations in growth, musculoskeletal abnormalities, and hormone deficiencies have been observed as a result of specific therapies. Organ damage (for example, liver, heart, and lung damage) from therapy may become more evident later in life when these organs are stressed (for example, during pregnancy); therefore, function of these organs should be evaluated periodically. CNS effects should be considered in children with CNS tumor, with infection or hemorrhage

Exhibit 12–2 Chemotherapy Safety In The Home

Chemotherapy drugs are given to destroy cancer cells. They can affect normal cells as well, which accounts for the side effects some people experience. There is some concern that direct exposure to these drugs by people who do not have cancer may be harmful. Therefore, unnecessary exposure should be avoided. This handout is to provide you with practical guidelines when caring for someone receiving chemotherapy or handling chemotherapy.

1. How can I get exposed to chemotherapy?

Direct exposure can occur from actual contact on skin or through inhalation. Exposure can occur with skin contact by urine, vomit, and stool from a person receiving chemotherapy and for 48 hours after the chemotherapy has stopped.

2. How can I best protect myself from exposure to chemotherapy?

Here are some general safety guidelines to follow:
- You should wear latex gloves when handling any linens or utensils contaminated by chemotherapy or body waste.
- After removing the latex gloves, you should always wash your hands with soap and water. (If allergic to latex, you may wear vinyl gloves.)
- Contaminated disposable items, such as gloves, paper towels, diapers, etc., may be disposed of in a plastic bag and thrown in routine garbage.
- Contaminated washable items, such as linens, towels, cloth diapers, etc. should be washed separately using routine detergent.
- When cleaning up spilled chemotherapy or body waste, wear latex gloves, wash area with soap and water, then rinse area well.
- Dispose of body waste, such as urine, vomit, or stool, in toilet. Close lid before flushing. Flush toilet twice.
- If any contaminated body waste or chemotherapy comes into contact with your skin, immediately wash skin with soap and water, then rinse and pat dry.
- If any contaminated body waste or chemotherapy splashes in eye, immediately rinse out eye(s) with fast-running lukewarm water for five minutes. Keep affected eye(s) open while rinsing. Then call regional Poison Control Center for your area.
- Do not put chemotherapy to be taken orally into your hands. Pour the prescribed amount into a medicine cup or the cover of the medicine container.
- If crushing chemotherapy pill(s), place pill(s) in small plastic bag and secure. Then crush with spoon. Dispose of bag after pouring chemotherapy into a medicine cup.
- Keep chemotherapy out of reach of children or pets.
- Return any unused chemotherapy to your pharmacy for proper disposal.

3. Who should I ask if I have more questions about chemotherapy exposure?

If you have further concerns or questions, please talk to the oncology doctor, nurse, or pharmacist.

to the brain, or who have received radiation to the head or intrathecal chemotherapy. Periodical neuropsychological testing is recommended to evaluate CNS impairments in the child, such as memory retention or learning disabilities. These problems may become evident as the child progresses to more complex educational challenges.

Gonadal function and sexual ability may be impaired. Some females may experience early menopause due to therapy. Genetic predisposition to cancer has been observed in rare cases, specifically regarding retinoblastoma. When appropriate, genetic and fertility counseling should be provided to the parents, adolescents, and young adults.

It has been documented that persons who have been treated for childhood malignancies have an increased risk for the development of a second neoplasm. This has been observed most often in children who have received high doses of radiation and alkylating chemotherapy agents. There is considerable concern over the increasing incidence of females who receive high-dose radiation to the lungs and later develop breast cancer. Instructions about the early signs and symptoms of cancers experienced during adulthood should be given as the child enters adulthood.

The psychological impact on the patient and family members also needs to be assessed, even after the "cure." Parents and siblings may have suffered adverse psychological effects due to the experience of cancer in the family. As children grow into adulthood, they may have evolving concerns related to their cancer experiences. Adolescents have reported difficulty in obtaining jobs and health insurance. They may require guidance and advocacy regarding social discrimination and their legal rights.

As children with cancer enter adolescence, they should receive information about the potential late consequences of cancer and the treatment they received. They should be encouraged to continue to seek routine health care and receive a summary of their disease and treatment history, especially if they move to another geographic area. Anticipatory counseling, periodic physical examinations, and testing are ideally directed by a multidisciplinary health care team familiar with the late effects of cancer occurring during childhood.

Psychosocial and Financial Issues

The diagnosis of cancer in a child, regardless of prognosis, represents an extremely stressful experience for every member of the family. Although cancer that occurs during childhood is now termed a chronic illness because of the high survival rates, the course of treatment is intertwined with numerous acute episodes. Coping styles, additional stressors, areas of strengths, and the quantity and quality of the family's support network will vary. If parents are divorced or separated, the impact of the illness may affect two family units.

The following coping tasks for parents identified by Hoffman and Futterman (1971) continue to be valid:

- anticipatory mourning for the loss of the "well" child
- maintaining a sense of mastery over their grief to be able to continue to respond to day-to-day responsibilities
- helping their child cope and adapt to the illness, while encouraging normal development
- maintaining the integrity of the family and responding to each of the needs of the individuals

Fawzy and colleagues (1995) state the four major therapeutic interventions most effective in cancer care—education regarding disease, treatment and self-care, behavioral training, and individual psychotherapy and group therapy. In pediatric oncology, these interventions need to be applied to every member of the family at his or her level of acceptance and development.

Parents often require guidance in communicating with their children about the disease and the treatment. Role modeling communication techniques and providing informational material are helpful. Children often require information about how to respond to the reactions and comments of well-meaning friends and relatives. Other family members and friends may be pessimistic regarding their outlook of the child's health or offer suggestions that may weaken the parents' ability to cope with the reality of the situation. Other persons, unable to cope themselves, may withdraw from relationships with the family. Methods to redirect these reactions into constructive assistance by providing information and suggestions of support are helpful.

Parents should also receive anticipatory counseling on common issues that result in marital stress. Continued open communication between couples is essential. There is no room for blaming the partner for the illness or for the additional burdens as a result of the illness. Respect for the roles that the mother and the father assume in maintaining the income, insurance coverage, and meeting the needs of the family should be addressed. Parents should try to find private time to share feelings and strengthen their union. Often, parents find association with other parents of children with cancer beneficial for recognition of the normalcy of their feelings and responses, as well as additional support and information. Self-help parent groups, such as the Candlelighters, should be identified as a potential aid to parents (see resources in Appendix A at the end of this book).

It is not unusual for the family to have additional financial concerns related to the child's illness. Financial counselors should be consulted to help the family. Agencies that can provide support should be identified. Parents should identify an insurance case manager who can assist them in knowing what interventions will be covered and where they should obtain home care supplies and medications (refer to Chapter 3).

Parents should receive counseling in fostering the normal development in their child with cancer. The child with cancer should not be treated as "special," because this may influence the expectations of the child later in adult life. The child may also fantasize that special treatment means he or she is really more ill than he or she is being told. Parents should continue to provide consistent limits and appropriate discipline. They should foster the child's independence rather than promote overprotectiveness.

Children who receive information about the disease and treatment at an age-appropriate level are able to respond amazingly well. Their questions should be answered as honestly and calmly as possible. They should be encouraged to express their fears and concerns. Often, a child psychologist or child life specialist can help the child express these feelings that he or she would suppress around the parents. Whenever possible, the child should be allowed choices to assist him or her in maintaining control.

The major issue in coping for young children is fear of separation from parents. Parents should be allowed to accompany their child for tests and procedures and "room-in" during hospitalizations. Although the majority of children with cancer are sedated for intrusive procedures, such as bone marrow aspirates and lumbar punctures, parents should be encouraged to be present to provide support. Parents should be aware that often young children may perceive the procedures performed on them as a result of their bad deeds. They need reassurance that these events are not a consequence of wrongdoings.

School-age children and adolescents often fear the reactions of their peers to their change in appearance, predominately hair loss. Many pediatric oncology institutions have a school re-entry program to assist in the integration of the child into the classroom.

Information related to the following should be shared with school personnel:

- disease, treatment, and expected absences
- expected side effects of therapy and changes in appearance
- limitations in physical and academic performance due to the disease or treatment
- psychological adaptation of the child and family members
- importance of notification of parents of chickenpox or measles exposure of the child, and avoidance of live viral vaccinations
- the possibility of designing a tutorial program in the home, if necessary
- preparation of classmates for the child's return to school
- continued communication with parents and health care providers to assess the child's changing needs

The teacher, school nurse, home care nurse, or a member of the pediatric oncology team should share information with the classmates before the child's return to the school. These visits are beneficial in reducing the fears the friends and fellow students may express about the cancer, such as "cancer is contagious" or "that everyone with cancer dies." With simplistic explanations, students can understand cancer, its treatment, and reasons for side effects of therapy. Students are encouraged to be empathetic (for example, by asking them, "How would you want to be treated if you had to get medicine that made your hair fall out?"). Preparation of the classmates helps reduce the embarrassment and social isolation often felt by the child with cancer that may lead to school phobia. Teachers should also receive guidance in setting appropriate academic performance expectations for the child with cancer. They should not just pass the child because they feel sorry for the individual, but at the same time they should modify the amount of work required of the child to prove understanding of the learning concept (see Chapter 19).

Older children and adolescents often benefit from participation in support groups, camps, and other activities designed to acquaint them with other children sharing the cancer experience. Camps for children with cancer are designed to encourage independence and stress normalcy, rather than the role of being sick.

Siblings are also affected by the diagnosis of cancer in a brother or sister. They may feel they may have caused the disease or that they can contract it. They may be angry and jealous over the parental attention and gifts the sick child is receiving. They may be embarrassed by the child's change in appearance. Often, siblings are affected by the change in the family routine and their usual participation in activities. They may perceive the child with cancer as not having the same expectations or receiving discipline for wrongdoings. Siblings are often burdened with providing progress reports on the sick child's condition to friends and relatives, instead of engaging in conversations focused on them. Parents require counseling on supporting their children who are not sick. The well children also require age-appropriate information and the assurance that nothing they did or did not do caused the cancer. They should receive special time to reaffirm they are also loved and receive attention and praise for their accomplishments. Parents should encourage the children to express their feelings in acceptable ways. Changes in

siblings' roles and responsibilities should be minimized, and maintenance of their usual routine and activities encouraged. Allowing the sibling to offer suggestions on how he or she could be helpful during this difficult time allows the sibling to feel a sense of pride in contributing without being forced. Parents should receive information on special programs that assist siblings in coping with a brother or sister with cancer. Siblings are often encouraged to visit during hospitalization or clinic visits to have a realistic idea of what their brother or sister is experiencing.

Nursing Care Plan in the Home

Discharge from the security of the hospital after the diagnosis of cancer is often perceived by most families as stressful. They often receive a lot of information while under the stress of being told the diagnosis, in a limited period, and on multiple facets of home care (for example, symptoms to report, care of central lines, administration of medications, etc.). Parents are frequently unsure of their capability to meet the demands that cancer in the family entails. The home care nurse can assist the family in the psychological transition to the home, as well as offer support and reinforcement in providing care to the child with cancer.

A method of communication should be established between the pediatric oncology nurse and the home care nurse. The initial referral should relate information about the cancer, treatment plan, discharge teaching, and home care needs. Periodic updates should follow, especially after acute episodes or change in treatment plan.

The following are the primary goals in caring for a child with cancer in the home: (1) reinforcement of discharge teaching; (2) prevention and early identification of complications; (3) rehabilitation to optimal physical ability; (4) access to community resources; and (5) promotion of family cohesion, communication, and positive adaptation of each individual to the chronic illness.

Reinforcement of Discharge Teaching

Family members may have retained little information after the diagnosis was made. The home care nurse needs to assess the knowledge of the family and identify areas for reinforcement of teaching. Specific areas of reinforcement include the following:

- information regarding the cancer and treatment plan
- various therapies and schedule
- purpose, dosage, and schedule for medications to be taken in the home
- expected side effects of current therapy
- home care and precautions related to side effects of therapy
- schedule for blood tests, scans, and follow-up appointments
- telephone contacts if problems arise
- additional care needs of child (for example, administration of colony-stimulating factor, total parenteral nutrition, antibiotics, central line care, etc.)

Often, parents need assistance in differentiating among normal deviations in health, side effects of therapy, and recurrence of cancer. For example, the parents of a two-year-old girl were concerned by her irritability and low-grade temperature. They thought her symptoms were related to her leukemia or treatment, when careful examination revealed the child was breaking in her molars and "teething," and this was her usual response to this normal physical milestone.

It cannot be assumed that parents and children will be compliant in taking chemotherapy and other supportive-care medications. Parents should be encouraged to develop a system to remind them what medications their child is to take (for example, calendar, weekly pillbox, etc.). Children should be watched to make sure they are taking their medicine, especially if it has a noxious taste. Adolescents may not take their medications because they are so involved in their daily activities or are seeking to gain control over the cancer. This high-risk group requires special attention in determining compliance without inferring guilt.

Prevention and Early Identification of Complications

Minor problems may quickly become oncologic emergencies in a child receiving therapy for cancer. Any concerns about the child's health status should be immediately reported to the pediatric oncologist or nurse. The home care nurse can validate that a problem should be reported. The home care nurse is in a unique position to observe the environment of the child and make suggestions that could decrease infections, provide safety measures in the home, and identify any potential problems in providing home-based care.

Rehabilitation to Optimal Physical Ability

Cancer may result in temporary or permanent physical disabilities in some children. Children may experience impairment due to amputation or neurologic sequelae. There may be a loss of sensory function due to blindness or decreased hearing. Each child will require assessment of his or her special needs. Additional home care or school services may be required, such as occupational or physical therapy. Special supplies and appliances may be necessary to provide care in the home. The home care nurse is in a position to assist the family in acquiring these special care services.

Provision of Access to Community Resources

The home care nurse may be more aware than the family of local resources and agencies that may benefit the families of children with cancer. In addition, the nurse can act as patient advocate in the community to assist in acquisition of the required resources.

The nurse may be aware of parent support groups, and other organizations in the geographic area may be identified that provide educational materials, as well as psychological support (see the resource section in Appendix A found at the end of this book).

The nurse or local social worker may be familiar with local agencies or organizations that provide financial support, assistance with transportation, respite care, or baby-sitting services. The nurse can also assist parents with the completion of numerous and often complicated agency forms.

Promotion of Family Cohesion, Communication, and Positive Adaptation to the Chronic Illness

The home care nurse is in a unique position to evaluate potential problems in the emotional adjustment of family members. A visit planned immediately after discharge can establish a relationship with the family and address its initial questions, concerns, and feelings related to the cancer.

The ongoing role of the nurse is to foster a sense of control and independence for the family and encourage family members to take it "one day at a time." If adjustment problems are identi-

fied, the nurse can provide counseling or make referrals for psychological support.

Unfortunately, not all children will remain in remission of their disease or respond favorably to treatment. Recurrences of the disease add stress on the family system with the threat of death of the child. At this time, many parents may seek unproven methods of cancer treatment (Johnson, Rudalph, and Hartman 1979), and health care professionals need to share realistic optimism on treatment options and assist family members in making decisions.

When all therapy options are exhausted and the child's condition is terminal, the parents may require assistance in discussing this fact with their children. They may require guidance in making choices surrounding their preference in care of the child who is dying. If they want their child to die in the home, the home care nurse and/or hospice nurse will have a pivotal role in providing comfort measures for the child and emotional support for the family, relatives, and friends. Discussion on the care of the terminally ill child is located in Chapter 14.

REFERENCES

Abramson, D.H., B. Jereb, and R.M. Ellsworth. 1981. External beam radiation for retinoblastoma. *Bulletin of the New York Academy of Medicine.* 57:787.

Abramson, D.H., R.M. Ellsworth, and G. Rozakis. 1982. Cryotherapy for retinoblastoma. *Archives of Ophthalmology.* 100:1253.

Albertini, F. 1990. Bone marrow transplantation inpatients with thalassemia. *New England Journal of Medicine* 322:419.

Albright, A.L. 1993. Pediatric brain tumors. *CA: A Cancer Journal for Clinicians.* 43:272.

Albright, A.L. 1985. Brain tumors in neonates, infants and toddlers. *Contemporary Neurosurgery* 7:1.

Alonso, E.M., et al. 1990. Unconjugated bilirubin absorption in breast-milk jaundice. *Pediatric Research.* 27:100A.

Amadori, S., et al. 1993. Prospective comparative study of bone marrow transplantation and post-remission chemotherapy for childhood acute myclogenous leukemia. *Journal of Clinical Oncology.* 11:1046.

American Cancer Society. 1996. Cancer Statistics 1996. *A Cancer Journal of Clinicians,* 46:25.

American Society of Clinical Oncology Expert Panel. 1994. Indications for using colony stimulating factors. *Journal of Clinical Oncology* 12:2471.

Anasetti, C., Amos, D., Beatty, P.G., et al. 1989. Effect of HLA compatibility on engraftment of bone marrow transplants in patients with leukemia and lymphomia. *New England Journal of Medicine* 320:197.

Anderson, J., et al. 1993. Long-term follow-up of patients treated with COMP or LSA2-L2 therapy for childhood non-Hodgkin's lymphoma—A Report of CCG-551 from The Children's Cancer Group. *Journal of Clinical Oncology* 11:1024.

Applebaum, F. 1996. The use of bone marrow and peripheral blood stem cell transplantation in treatment of cancer. *CA: A Cancer Journal for Clinicians.* 46:1424.

Barnes, P.D. 1990. Magnetic resonance in pediatric and adolescent neuro-imaging. *Neurologic Clinics.* 8:741.

Beatty, P.G., et al. 1985. Marrow transplantation from related donors other than HLA-identical siblings. *New England Journal of Medicine.* 313:765.

Bell, B., D. Candy, and M. Audet. 1995. Hemophilia: An updated review. *Pediatrics in Review* 16, no. 8:290.

Bensinger, W., et al. 1993. Autologous transplantation with peripheral blood mononuclear cells collected after administration of recombinant granulocyte-colony stimulating factor. *Blood* 81:3158.

Bensinger, W.I., et al. 1994. Peripheral stem cells (PBSCs) collected after recombinant granulocyte colony stimulating factor (rh G-CSF): An analysis of factors correlating with the tempo of engraftment after transplantation. *Journal of Hematology* 87:825.

Berthold, F. 1990. Overview: Biology of neuroblastoma. In *Neuroblastoma: Tumor biology and therapy,* ed. C. Pochedly, 1–27. Boca Raton, FL: CRC Press.

Bertolli, J., et al. 1995. Epidemiology of HIV disease in children. *Immunology and Allergy Clinics of North America* 15, no. 2:193.

Boland, M., and L. Czarniecki. 1995. Nursing care of the child. In *HIV/AIDS—A guide to nursing care,* ed. J. Flaskerud and P. Ungvarski, 185–219. Philadelphia: W.B. Saunders Company.

Bordon, E.C., and P.M. Sondel. 1990. Lymphokines and cytokines as cancer treatment: Immunotherapy realized. *Cancer* 65:800.

Broxmeyer, H.E., et al. 1991. Umbilical cord blood hematopoietic stem of repopulating cells in human clinical transplantation. *Blood Cells* 17:313.

Burke, J. 1990. The histopathologic classification of non-Hodgkin's lymphomas: Ambiguities in the working formulation and two newly reported categories. *Seminars in Oncology.* 17:3.

Camitta, B.M., et al. 1976. Severe aplastic anemia: A prospective study of effect of early marrow transplantation on acute mortality. *Blood* 48:63.

Casey, K. 1995. Pathophysiology of HIV-1, clinical course, and treatment. In *HIV/AIDS—A guide to nursing care,* ed. J. Flaskerud and P. Ungvarski, 64–80. Philadelphia: W.B. Saunders Company.

Castleberry, R.P. 1990. Chemotherapy for neuroblastoma. In *Neuroblastoma: Tumor biology and therapy,* ed. C. Pochedley, 305. Boca Raton, FL: CRC Press.

Cavazzana, A.O., et al. 1987. Experimental evidence for a neural organ of Ewing's sarcoma of bone. *American Journal of Pathology.* 127:507.

Centers for Disease Control and Prevention. 1989. Interpretation and use of western blot assay for serodiagnosis of human immunodeficiency virus type 1. *Morbidity and Mortality Weekly Report* 38:(S-7).

Centers for Disease Control and Prevention. 1994. Revised classification system for human immunodeficiency virus infection in children under 13 years of age. *Morbidity and Mortality Weekly Report* 43:(RR-12).

Centers for Disease Control and Prevention. 1995. Revised guidelines for prophylaxis against *Pneumocystis carinii*

pneumonia for children infected with or perinatally exposed to human immunodeficiency virus. *Morbidity and Mortality Weekly Report* 44:(RR-4).

Chang, A.E., and S.A. Rosenberg. 1989. Overview of interleukin 2 as an immunotherapeutic agent. *Seminars in Surgical Oncology.* 5:385.

Charache, S., et al. 1995. Effect of hydroxyurea on the frequency of painful crisis in sickle cell anemia. *New England Journal of Medicine.* 330:1317.

Cheung, N.K. 1990. Immunology and targeted immunotherapy of neuroblastoma. In *Neuroblastoma: Tumor biology and therapy,* ed. C. Pochedly, 51. Boca Raton, FL: CRC Press.

Clark, S.C., and R. Kamen. 1987. The human hematopoietic colony-stimulating factors. *Science* 236:1229.

Cohen, A., J. Mizazin, and E. Schwartz. 1989. Rapid removal of excessive iron with daily high-dose intravenous chelation therapy. *Journal of Pediatrics* 2, no. 5:151.

Connor, E., et al. 1994. Reduction of maternal-infant transmission of human immunodeficiency virus type I with zidovudine treatment. *New England Journal of Medicine* 331:1173.

Crist, W.M., and L.E. Kun. 1991. Common solid tumors of childhood. *New England Journal of Medicine.* 324:461.

Dallman, P., R. Yip, and F. Oski. 1993. Iron deficiency and related nutritional anemias. In *Hematology of infancy and childhood,* ed. D.D. Nathan and F.A. Oski. Philadelphia: W.B. Saunders, Company.

D'Angio, G.J., et al. 1989. Treatment of Wilms' tumor: Results of the Third National Wilms' Tumor Study. *Cancer* 64:349.

Derkinderen, D.J.U., et al. 1987. Non-ocular cancer in hereditary retinoblastoma survivors and relatives. *Ophthalmic Pediatric Genetics* 8:23.

Dillman, R.O., J.C. Beauregard, and S.E. Halpern. 1986. Toxicities and side effects associated with intravenous infusion of murine monoclonal antibodies. *Journal of Biological Response Modifiers* 5:73.

Donaldson, S., and M. Link. 1991. Hodgkin's disease: Treatment in young children. *Pediatric Clinics of North America* 38:457.

Donaldson, S.S., P.R. Eghert, W-H Lee. 1993. Retinoblastoma. In *Principles and practices of pediatric oncology,* 2d ed., ed. P.A. Pizzo and D.G. Poplack. Philadelphia: J.B. Lippincott Co.

Dow, L., et al. 1991. Response to alpha-interferon in children with Philadelphia chromosomic-positive chronic myelocytic leukemia. *Cancer* 68:1678.

Duffner, P., and M.E. Cohen. 1991. The long-term effects of central nervous system therapy on children with brain tumors. *Neurologic Clinics.* 9:479.

Dutcher, J.P. 1993. Interferons and interleukins in cancer therapy. *Mediaguide to Oncology* 12:1.

Ennever J.F. 1986. Phototherapy in a new light. *Pediatric Clinics of North America* 33:603.

Falloon, J., et al. 1989. Human immunodeficiency virus infection in children. *Journal of Pediatrics.* 114, no. l:1.

Fawzy, F.L., et al. 1995. Critical review of psychosocial interventions in cancer care. *Archives of General Psychiatry* 52:100.

Fenaux, P., et al. 1993. Effect of all-transretinoic acid in newly diagnosed acute promyelocytic leukemia: Results of multicenter randomized trial. *Blood* 82:3241.

Festa, R. 1985. Modern management of thalassemia. *Pediatric Annals* 14:9.

Finlay, J.L. 1992. High-dose chemotherapy followed by bone marrow "rescue" for recurrent brain tumors. In *Pediatric neuro-oncology: New trends in clinical research,* ed. R.J. Packer, W.A. Bleyer, and C. Pochedly, 278. Chur, Switzerland: Harwood Academics.

Finlay, J.L., et al. 1987b. Progress in childhood brain tumors. *Hematology Oncology Clinics of North America* 1:753.

Finlay, J.L., R. Uteg, and W.L. Geise. 1987. Brain tumors in children: Advances in neurosurgery and radiation oncology. *American Journal of Pediatric Hematology/Oncology* 9:256.

Fitzgerald, D., and I. Pastan. 1989. Targeted toxin therapy for the treatment of cancer. *Journal of the National Cancer Institute* 81:1455.

Francis, R., and C. Johnson. 1991. Vascular occlusions in sickle cell disease: Current concepts and unanswered questions. *Blood* 77:1405.

Furie, B., S. Limentani, and C. Rosenfield. 1994. A practical guide to the evaluation and treatment of hemophilia. *Blood* 84(1):3–9.

Gamis A.S., et al. 1993. Unrelated-donor bone marrow transplantation for Philadelphia chromosome-positive chronic myelogenous leukemia in children. *Journal of Clinical Oncology* 11:834.

George, J., et al. 1996. Idiopathic thrombocytopenia purpura: A practice guideline developed by explicit methods for the American Society of Hematology. *Blood* 88:3.

Gluckman, E., et al. 1992. Multi-center standardized study comparing cyclospoin alone, and antithymocyte globulin with prednisone in the treatment of sever aplastic anemia. *Blood* 79:2540.

Goebel, R. 1993. Thrombocytopenia. *Emergency Medicine Clinics of North America* 11, no. 2:445.

Gomez, M.R., R.V. Grover, and S.F. Mellinger. 1982. Tumors of the brain and spinal cord. In *The practice of pediatric neurology,* Vol. 2, 2d ed., ed. K.F. Swaimnan, and F.S. Wright, 823. St Louis: C.V. Mosby.

Goodman, J. 1987. Nursing care of the high risk infant. In *Child and family: Concepts of nursing practice,* ed. M. Smith, J. Goodman, N. Ramsey. New York: McGraw-Hill Book co.

Goodrich, J.W., et al. 1993. Ganciclovir prophylaxis to prevent cytomegalovirus disease after allogeneic bone marrow transplant. *Annals of Internal Medicine.* 118:173.

Gourley, G.R., and G.B. Odell. 1989. Bilirubin metabolism in the fetus and neonate. In *Human gastrointestinal development,* ed. E. Lebenthal, 581. New York: Raven Press.

Grabowski, E.F., et al. 1987. Extraocular retinoblastoma: Sustained remission in 10 to 12 children treated with irradiation and combination chemotherapy. *Pediatric Research* 21:2999.

Green, D.M. 1985. Retinoblastoma. In *Diagnosis and management of malignant solid tumors in infants and children,* ed. D.M. Green, 90. Boston: Martinez Nijhoff.

Green, D.M., et al. 1993. Wilms' tumor (nephroblastoma, renal embryoma). In *Principles and practices of pediatric oncology,* 2d ed. ed. P.A. Pizzo and D.G. Poplack, 713. Philadelphia: J.B. Lippincott Co.

Griffin, J. 1986. Management of chronic myelogenous leukemia. *Seminars in Hematology* 23:20.

Hammer, S., et al. 1996. A trial comparing nucleoside monotherapy with combination therapy in HIV-infected adults with CD4 cell counts from 200 to 500 per cubic millimeter. *New England Journal of Medicine* 335:1081.

Hayes, F.A., and E.I. Smith. 1989. Neuroblastoma. In *Principles and practices of pediatric oncology,* ed. P.A. Pizzo and D.G. Poplack, 607. Philadelphia: J.B. Lippincott Co.

Hertler, A.A., and A.E. Frankel. 1989. Immunotoxins: A clinical review of their use in the treatment of malignancies. *Journal of Clinical Oncology.* 7:1932.

Hill, H.F., et al. 1990. Self-administration of morphine in bone marrow transplant patients reduces drug requirements. *Pain* 41:121.

Hoffman, E., and E.M. Futterman. 1971. Coping with waiting: Psychiatric intervention and study in the waiting room of pediatric oncology clinic. *Comprehensive Psychiatry* 12:67.

Hong, R., et al. 1996. Disorder of T-cell system. In *Immunologic disorders in infants and children,* 4th ed. ed. E.R. Stiehm. Philadelphia: W.B. Saunders Company.

Horowitz, M.E., T.F. Delaney, M.M. Malawer, and M.G. Tsokos. 1993. Ewing's sarcoma family of tumors: Ewing's sarcoma of bone and soft tissue and the peripheral primative neuroectodermal tumors. In *Principles and practice of pediatric oncology,* 2d ed. ed. P.A. Pizzo and D.G. Poplock. Philadelphia: Lippincott.

Johanson, N. 1990. Musculoskeletal problems in hemoglobinopathy. *Orthopedic Clinics of North America* 21:191.

Johnson, F., et al. 1994. Bone marrow transplantation for sickle cell disease: the United States experience. *American Journal of Pediatric Hematology/Oncology* 16:22

Johnson, L., L. Rudalph, and J. Hartman. 1979. Helping the family cope with childhood cancer. *Psychosomatics* 4:241.

Kennedy B., et al. 1992. Survival of Hodgkin's disease by stage and age. *Medical and Pediatric Oncology.* 20:100.

Kojima, S., et al. 1991. Treatment of aplastic anemia in children with recombinant human granulocyte colony-stimulating factor. *Blood* 77:937.

Kovnar, E.H., et al. 1990. Preirradiation cisplatin and etoposide in treatment of high-risk medulloblastoma and other malignant embryonal tumors of the central nervous system: A phase II study. *Journal of Clinical Oncology* 8:330.

Lane, P. 1996. Sickle cell disease. *Pediatric Clinics of North America* 43:639.

Lanzkowsky, P. 1985. Problems in diagnosing iron deficiency anemia. *Pediatric Annals* 14:621.

Lanzkowsky, P. 1995. *Manual of pediatric hematology and oncology.* New York: Churchill Livingstone.

Lawrence W., et al. 1997. Prognostic significance of staging factors of the UICC staging system in childhood rhabdomyosarcoma: A report from intergroup rhabdomyosarcoma study (IRS). *Journal of Clinical Oncology.* 5:46.

Link, M.P., and F. Eiber. 1989. Osteosarcoma. In *Principles and practices of pediatric oncology,* ed. P.A. Pizzo and D.G. Poplack, 689–711. Philadelphia: J.B. Lippincott Co.

Lister, T.A., et al. 1989. Report of committee convened to discuss evaluation and staging of patients with Hodgkin's disease: Cotswolds meetings. *Journal of Clinical Oncology* 7:1630.

Livesey, E.A., et al. 1990. Endocrine disorders following treatment of childhood brain tumors. *British Journal of Cancer* 61:622.

Logan, L. 1992. Treatment of von Willebrand disease. *Hematology/Oncology Clinics of North America* 6:1079.

Lusher, J. 1993. Disease of coagulation: The fluid phase. In *Hematology of infancy and childhood,* ed. D. Nathan and F.A. Oski. Philadelphia: W.B. Saunders Company.

Magrath I.T. 1993. Malignant non-Hodgkin's lymphomas, in children. In *Principles and practices of pediatric oncology,* 2d ed., ed. P.A. Pizzo and D.G. Poplack, 537. Philadelphia: J.B. Lippincott Co.

Maher, K.E. 1996. Late effects of radiation therapy: Quality of life. *Cope,* September/October 4.

Martin, P.J., et al. 1991. A retrospective analysis of therapy for acute graft-versus-host disease: Secondary treatment. *Blood* 77:1821.

Maurer, H.M., et al. 1989. Intergroup Rhabdomyosarcoma Study III: A preliminary report of overall outcome. *Proceedings of American Society of Clinical Oncology* 8:296.

McDonald, G.B., 1993. Venocclusive disease of the liver and multi-organ failure after bone marrow transplantation: A cohort study of 355 patients. *Annals of Internal Medicine* 118:255.

Metcalf, D., and G. Morstyn. 1991. Colony-stimulating factors: General biology. In *Biologic therapy of cancer,* ed. V.T. Devita, S. Hellman, and S.A. Rosenberg, 417. Philadelphia: J.B. Lippincott Co.

Meyer, W.H., and M.M. Malawer. 1991. Osteosarcoma clinical features and evolving surgical and chemotherapeutic strategies. *Pediatric Clinics of North America* 38:317.

Meyers, P. 1987. Malignant bone tumors of children: Ewing's sarcoma. *Hematology/Oncology Clinics of North America* 1:667.

Miraldi, F.D., A.D. Nelson, and C. Karly. 1986. Diagnostic imaging of neuroblastoma with radio-labeled antibody. *Radiology* 161:413.

Moldawer, N.P., and J.L. Murray. 1985. The clinical use of monoclonal antibodies in cancer research. *Cancer Nursing* 8:207.

Mooney, K.H. 1993. Biologic basis of childhood cancer. In *Nursing care of the child with cancer,* ed. G. Foley, D. Footchman, and K. Mooney, 25. Philadelphia: W.B. Saunders Company.

Nasr, S., et al. 1989. A phase I study of interleukin-2 in children with cancer and evaluation of clinical and immunologic status during therapy. *Cancer* 64:783.

Nathan, D. 1990. Oral iron chelators. *Seminars in Hematology* 27:83.

Nemunaitis, J., et al. 1991. Recombinant granulocyte macrophage colony stimulating factor after autologous bone marrow transplantation for lymphoid cancer. *New England Journal of Medicine* 324:1773.

Nilsson, I., et al. 1992. Twenty-five years experience of prophylactic treatment in severe hemophilia A and B. *Journal of Internal Medicine* 232:25.

Noll, L. 1990. Chemical modifiers of radiosensitivity—theory and reality: A review. *International Journal of Radiation Oncology, Biology, Physics* 11: 665.

O'Conner, M.I., and D.J. Pritchard. 1991. Ewing's sarcoma: Prognostic factors, disease control, and the reemerging role of surgical treatment. *Clinical Orthopaedics and Related Research* 262:78.

Ohniski, Y., Y. Yamana, and M. Minei. 1986. Photo radiation therapy using argon laser and hematoporphyrin derivative for retinoblastoma. *Japanese Journal of Ophthalmology* 30:409.

Old, L. 1985. Tumor necrosis factor (rTNF). *Science* 2300: 630.

Oppedal, B.R., et al. 1989. N-myc amplification in neuroblastoma: Histopathological, DNA ploidy, and clinical variables. *Journal of Clinical Pathology* 49:1148–1152.

O'Rourke, M.E. 1987. Enhanced cutaneous effects in combined modality therapy. *Oncology Nursing Forum* 14:31.

Oski, F. 1993. Iron deficiency in infancy and childhood. *New England Journal of Medicine* 329:190.

Packer, R.J., et al. 1991. Improved survival with use of adjuvant chemotherapy in treatment of medulloblastoma. *Journal of Neurosurgery* 74:433.

Parkin, D.M., et al. 1988. The international incidence of childhood cancer. *International Journal of Cancer* 42:511.

Pearson, H. 1987. Diseases of the blood. In *Nelson's textbook of pediatrics,* 13th ed., ed. R.E. Behrman and V.C. Vaghan. 13th ed. Philadelphia: W.B. Saunders Company.

Pearson, H. 1990. The nutritional anemias. In *Pediatrics: Principles and Practice,* ed. F.A. Oski et al. Philadelphia: J.B. Lippincott Co.

Pegelow, C., et al. 1995. Risk of recurrent stroke in patients with sickle cell disease treated with erythrocyte transfusions. *Journal of Pediatrics* 126:896.

Penrod, J., et al. 1990. Impact of iron status of introducing cow's milk in second month of life. *Journal of Pediatrics Gastroenterology and Nutrition* 10:462.

Pfaff, J., and M. Geninatti. 1993. *Hemophilia. Emergency Medicine Clinics of North America* 11(2):337.

Pinkel, D. 1993. Bone marrow transplantation in children. *Journal of Pediatrics* 122:331.

Quesada, J.R. 1986. Biological response modifiers in cancer therapy: A review. *Texas Medicine* 85:42.

Radcliffe, J., et al. 1992 Three and four-year cognitive outcome in children with non-cortical brain tumors treated with whole-brain radiotherapy. *Annals of Neurology* 32:551.

Raney, R.B., and M. Tefft. 1993. Rhabdomyosarcoma and the undifferentiated sarcomas. In *Principles and practice of pediatric oncology,* 2d ed., ed. P.A. Pizzo, D.G. Poplack. Philadelphia: J.B. Lippincott Co.

Reid, C., ed. 1995. *Management and therapy of sickle cell disease* (NIH Publication No. 95-21 1T). Washington, DC: U.S. Department of Health and Human Resources, Public Health Services.

Rodriguez, G., and R. Hard. 1995. Immunopathogenesis of AIDS. *Immunology and Allergy Clinics of North America* 15:225.

Rosen, G., et al. 1987. Pre-operative therapy for osteosarcoma: Selection of post-operative adjuvant chemotherapy based on response of the primary tumor to pre-operative therapy. *Cancer* 49:1221.

Scott, J.P., and R. Montgomery. 1993. Therapy of von Willebrand disease. *Seminars in Thrombosis and Hemostosis* 19:37.

Seeger, R.C., and C.P. Reynold. 1991. Treatment of high risk solid tumors of childhood with intensive therapy and autologous bone marrow transplantation. *Pediatrics Clinics of North America* 38:393.

Semenzato, G. 1990. Tumor necrosis factor: A cytokine with multiple biological activities. *British Journal of Cancer* 61:354.

Shahidi, N. 1987. Fanconi anemia, dyskeratosis congenita, and WT syndrome. *American Journal of American Genetics,* suppl. 3:263.

Shapiro, D.N., et al. 1991. Relationship of tumor cell ploidy to histologic subtype and treatment outcome in children and adolescents with unresectable rhabdomyosarcoma. *Journal of Clinical Oncology* 9:159.

Shearer, W. 1996. How to recognize and evaluate immunodeficiency. Presentation at the Wisconsin Allergy Society Meeting, Spring Green, WI. October.

Shields, J.A., C.L. Shields, and V. Sivalingarn. 1989. Decreasing frequency of enucleation inpatients with retinoblastoma. *American Journal of Ophthalmology* 108:185.

Sondel, P. 1993. Biological and immunological approaches to comprehensive therapy for pediatric malignant conditions. *Cancer* 71 (suppl.):3429.

Sposto, R., et al. 1989. The effectiveness of chemotherapy for treatment of high grade astrocytoma in children: Results of randomized trial: A report of Children's Cancer Study Group. *Journal of Neuro-Oncology* 7:165.

Steuber, C.P., et al. 1989. Prognostic factors and treatment outcome in childhood acute myeloid leukemia (AML): The POG experience. In *Acute myelogenous leukemia: Progress and controversies,* ed. R.P. Gale, 193. New York: Wiley-Liss.

Storb, R., et al. 1989. Methotrexate and cyclosporine alone for prophylaxis of graft-versus host disease in patients given HLA-identical marrow grafts for leukemia: Long-term follow up of a controlled trial. *Blood* 73:1729.

Sullivan, K.M. 1994. Graft-versus-host disease. In *Bone marrow transplantation,* ed. S.J. Forman, K.G. Blume, and E.D. Thomas, 339. Boston: Blackwell Scientific Publications.

Synder, D.S., and P. McGlave. 1990. Treatment of chronic myelogenous leukemia with bone marrow transplantation. *Hematology/Oncology Clinics of North America* 4:535.

Torres, A., et al. 1989. Allogenic bone marrow transplantation versus chemotherapy in treatment of childhood lymphoblastic leukemia in second complete remission. *Bone Marrow Transplantation* 4:609.

Tubergen, D., et al. 1993. Improved outcome with delayed intensification for children with acute lymphomacytic leukemia and intermediate presenting features: A

Children's Cancer Group phase trial. *Journal of Clinical Oncology* 11:527.

Tudor-Williams, G., and P. Pizzo. 1996. Pediatric human immunodeficiency virus infection. In *Immunodeficiency disorders in infants and children,* 4th ed. ed. E.R. Stielun, eds. Philadelphia: W.B. Saunders Company.

Uckun, F., et al. 1992. Immunotoxin therapy of relapsed B-linage ALL: A clinical phase I dose escalation study of B43 (anti-CD-19) pokeweed antiviral protein (PAP) immunotoxin. *Blood* 80(suppl.):205.

Vichinsky, E. 1991. Comprehensive care of sickle cell disease: Its impact on morbidity and mortality. *Seminars in Hematology* 28:220.

Watanabe, N., et al. 1988. Synergistic cytotoxicity of recombinant tumor necrosis factor and various anti-cancer drugs. *Immunopharmacology and Immunotoxicology* 10:117.

Wayne, A., S. Kevy, and D. Nathan. 1993. Transfusion management of sickle cell disease. *Blood* 5:1109.

Weathers, D., H. Pearson, and M. Gaston. 1989. Newborn screening for sickle cell disease and other hemoglobinophies. *Pediatrics* 83:813.

White, L. 1991. Chemotherapy in retinoblastoma: Current status and future directions. American Journal of Pediatric Hematology. *American Journal of Pediatric Hematology-Oncology,* 13:189.

Whitington, P.F., and L.M. Gartner. 1993. Disorders of bilirubin metabolism. In *Hematology of infancy and childhood,* ed. D.D. Nathan and F.A. Oski, 84. Philadelphia: W.B. Saunders Company.

Wilfert, C. 1994. Pediatric HIV infection: Epidemiology and natural history. *Opportunistic Complications of HIV.* 3:50.

BIBLIOGRAPHY

Appedal, B.R., et al. 1989. N-myc amplification in neuroblastoma: Histopathological, DNA ploidy, and clinical variables. *Journal of Clinical Pathology.* 49:1148.

Derthold, F. 1990. Overview: Biology of neuroblastoma. In *Neuroblastoma: Tumor biology and therapy,* edited by C. Pochedly. p. 1, Boca Raton, Fla: CRC Press.

Lucarelli, G., et al. 1990. Bone marrow transplantation in the patient with thalassemia. *New England Journal of Medicine.* 322:417.

Rivera, G., et al. 1993. Treatment of acute lymphoblastic leukemia: 30 years experience at St. Jude Children's Research Hospital. *New England Journal of Medicine.* 329:1289.

Segel, G. 1988. Anemia. *Pediatrics in Review.* 10(3):77.

The Child with Hyperbilirubinemia Receiving Phototherapy

Nursing Diagnosis	Expected Outcomes	Nursing Interventions
1. Knowledge deficit related to hyperbilirubinemia and purpose and procedure of phototherapy	Parents verbalize knowledge of disease and purpose and procedure of phototherapy. Parents communicate their concerns and feelings about home phototherapy. Parents demonstrate ability to assemble and use phototherapy unit. Child does not develop any harmful effects due to phototherapy. Bilirubin level returns to normal.	Assess prior knowledge, ability, and desire to learn. Assess support in home for respite (someone will need to be with child at all times). Assess instructional needs of other significant caregivers. Instruct parents in the following: • Cause of hyperbilirubinemia • Normal breakdown mechanism of hemoglobin and excretion (urobilinogen in urine—dark urine); sterobilingen in stool—brown stool • Purpose of phototherapy—Instruct parents to document in log every four hours during phototherapy. • Child's temperature • Hours of treatment • Oral intake • Output • Specific gravity • Position change • Eye patches (overhead unit only) • Diaper coverage (protect gonadal areas) Instruct on use of phototherapy unit. *Overhead Unit* • Use correct light for type of infant bed. • Reading temperature probe • Light source remains 30 inches from bed.

Nursing Diagnosis	*Expected Outcomes*	*Nursing Interventions*
		• Measure output of light by placing bilimeter probe next to top center of infant's trunk. If the reading is less than 8, reposition the infant centrally and repeat reading. If still <8, obtain new light
		• Plexiglass shield intact over light to prevent ultraviolet rays and to protect child from bulb breakage
		• Unit placement should be away from drafts, heat vents, and heavy traffic areas
		• Caretaker should avoid prolonged exposure under light and wear sunglasses near light source
		Instruct in preparation of child including the following:
		• Application of eye patches over closed eyes of child and checked hourly
		• Mouth and nose are not obstructed
		• Methylcellulose eye drops application (if prescribed)
		• Report eye drainage to physician
		• Turn every 2 hours to maximize skin exposure
		• Child is placed on abdomen and sides propped with blankets to prevent aspiration
		• Child is without clothes except disposable diaper
		• Child is never fed in unit
		• Diaper covers gonads
		Biliblanket
		• Cover white "paddle" of biliblanket with disposable cover.
		• Place "paddle" on infant's back or chest with cord towards infant. White side next to infant's skin. Place infant shirt over the biliblanket and secure shirt as usual. Wrap baby snugly in blanket.
		• Turn on machine to highest setting (rearrange clothing to prevent light scatter up to face).

Nursing Diagnosis	Expected Outcomes	Nursing Interventions
		• Do not remove blanket for feedings.
		• Registered nurse should determine daily bilirubin levels by drawing blood by a heel stick (as prescribed by physician) with bililight turned off.
		• Laboratory should call physician with results.
		• Home care nurse should communicate with physician for further orders.
2. Potential for impairment of skin integrity related to phototherapy	Child has normal skin reactions to phototherapy.	Instruct parents about the following: • Avoidance of skin lotion • Appearance of maculopapular rash is common and disappears spontaneously • Appearance of a severe gray-brown discoloration ("bronze baby syndrome") that clears three weeks after therapy is discontinued • Reporting extreme skin erythema, dryness, and blistering to physician

3. Potential for altered body temperature related to hypothermia or hyperthermia	Child does not develop hypothermia or hyperthermia.	Instruct parents to do the following:
		• Maintain temperature in room at 72°F.
		• Check child's temperature every hour (physician to specify expected temperature)
		  –If too warm, reduce temperature in room.
		  –If too cold, wrap child in three blankets and increase room temperature.
		  –Recheck temperature in 30 minutes: if normal return to unit; if still abnormal, call physician.

4. Potential for fluid volume deficit related to insensible loss due to heat and frequent loose stools	Child does not become dehydrated.	Instruct parents to do the following: • Offer frequent feeding • Child should take four or more extra ounces of liquid. • If breastfeeding, encourage at least 8 feedings daily plus additional water.

Nursing Diagnosis	*Expected Outcomes*	*Nursing Interventions*
		• Record number and color of stools. • Weigh infant every four to eight hours • Call physician if decreased intake of fluids or urine output or projectile vomiting.
5. Potential for alteration in parental role related to overhead photo-therapy and fatigue of caregiver.	There is a period of infant bonding. The child is not affected by sensory deprivation.	Child is removed from unit every two hours, and eye patches are removed for feedings and interaction with parents. Parents are provided with suggestions for stimulation of infant when eye patches are applied (music, voice, and touch) and when out of unit (visual stimula-tion).

The Anemias in Childhood (General)

Nursing Diagnosis	Expected Outcomes	Nursing Interventions
1. Health maintenance: risk factors for anemia	Appropriate referrals are made for children who are suspected to have anemia.	Assess for signs and symptoms of anemia, such as the following: • pallor • irritability • poor feeding and weight loss • decreased attentiveness • weakness • fatigability with exertion Assess for inadequate diet. Assess for other contributing causes such as chronic diarrhea or intestinal blood loss. Assess decreased financial resources or cultural preferences that may influence proper nutrition.
2. Knowledge deficit related to cause and treatment plan for anemia	The parents verbalize knowledge regarding cause of anemia and home therapy. Child takes medications.	Instruct in cause of anemia. Instruct in expected signs and symptoms. Instruct in meaning of laboratory results and frequency of tests. Instruct in treatment plan. Instruct on schedule and dose of medications (for example, folic acid). Instruct in importance of follow-up medical checkups.
3. Potential for infection related to increased risk due to tissue hypoxia	Child exhibits no sign of infection or skin breakdown.	Instruct in good hygiene measures. Report elevated temperature and other signs of infection to physician.

Nursing Diagnosis	Expected Outcomes	Nursing Interventions
4. Alteration in tissue perfusion related to anemia	Child remains active and alert appropriate for age and capability. Parents demonstrate safe and proper use of oxygen in home environment (if required). Administer transfusions in the home safely (if required).	Assess level of child's activity tolerance. Counsel parents concerning maximizing child's energy. • Assist child with activities of daily living. • Support activities during peak energy time that stimulate development and independence. • Provide sedentary projects when child is most exhausted but prevent boredom and withdrawal. • Alert significant others (baby-sitter, teacher, tutor) to child's physical tolerance. • Plan rest periods between activities. Report progressive signs of anemia, especially cardiac failure: • shortness of breath • extreme weakness and fatigue • edema and weight gain Provide oxygen for use if ordered by physician (see Chapter 5 for oxygen therapy). Obtain order for premedications and emergency care from physician. Check compatibility of blood product with ABO and Rh factor of patient. Administer premedications if ordered. Check if product was irradiated if ordered. Check expiration date, time, and filter product if ordered. Infuse product as ordered by physician. Check vital signs according to protocol. Document according to protocol. Notify physician of any adverse reaction.
5. Alterations in nutrition related to fatigue and anorexia	Child maintains or gains weight as appropriate. Child consumes foods required to correct anemia.	Obtain a 24-hour diet history. Instruct parents to provide frequent small meals to conserve child's energy. Counsel parents on deficiency in child's diet. Counsel parents on importance of mealtime as a pleasant experience. Check child's weight periodically.

Nursing Diagnosis	Expected Outcomes	Nursing Interventions
6. Potential for ineffective child coping related to decreased physical ability and multiple intrusive procedures	Child is less anxious and adjusts to altered abilities. Child demonstrates less fear with procedures.	Counsel child, at age-appropriate level, regarding the following: • cause of symptoms • purpose of test and procedures • reasons for certain home precautions Observe parent's ability to meet the needs of the child. Encourage child to assist in planning activities appropriate to capability.
7. Potential for ineffective coping related to additional stressors to family members	Family members communicate their fears and concerns.	Encourage expression of feelings and concerns of parents, siblings, and significant others. Discuss feelings of parental guilt about potentially causing anemia in the child. Inform family members of signs of progress. Anticipate stressful periods and need for respite care for child. Counsel parents regarding special needs of other children for attention and maintenance of as normal routine as possible. Assist in providing resources for family.

The Child with Sickle Cell Anemia

Nursing Diagnosis	Expected Outcomes	Nursing Interventions
1. Potential for knowledge deficit related to sickle cell anemia	Patient and family will verbalize the following: • understanding of transmission of sickle cell disease • the sickling process and subsequent effects • understanding of treatment regimen as management changes	Encourage initial visit and follow-up at a sickle cell comprehensive clinic. Provide genetic counseling on sickle cell transmission. Encourage testing of other family members. Encourage parents to express feelings regarding transmitting disease. Instruct on the abnormality of red blood cell and result of vessel occlusions. Instruct on the potential complications of sickle cell anemia. Instruct on purpose of management strategies (for example, hypertransfusions, fetal hemoglobin stimulator agent, chelation therapy, bone marrow transplantation).
2. Potential for alteration in tissue perfusion related to sickle cell crisis	Child participates in lifestyle that avoids physical and emotional stress.	Instruct in avoidance of the following factors that promote crisis: • strenuous physical activity • infection • low-oxygen environment • prolonged exposure to heat and cold • emotional stress • dehydration Calculate daily recommended oral hydration. Encourage drinking every 30 to 60 minutes:

Nursing Diagnosis	Expected Outcomes	Nursing Interventions
		• Make drinking enjoyable (for example, games, using paper cups with pictures on the bottom, giving the child a sticker after drinking)
		• Allow child to select fluid preference.
		• Have child carry large drinking container in school.
		• Promote understanding that drinking will make child feel better.
		Increase child's fluid intake during warm weather, increased exercise, pain crisis, and fever.
		Dress the child to stay warm.
		Keep temperature in home comfortable.
		Instruct on observation of the following signs and symptoms of dehydration:
		• irritability
		• dark, concentrated urine
		• dry, oral mucosa
		Report symptoms to physician that may lead to dehydration (for example, vomiting).
	Child has adequate rest.	Instruct on importance of rest periods and minimizing strenuous activities. (Inform gym teachers and coaches.)
		Encourage initial visit and follow-up at a sickle cell comprehensive clinic.
		Provide genetic counseling on sickle cell transmission.
		Encourage testing of other family members.
		Encourage parents to express feelings regarding transmitting disease.
		Instruct on the abnormality of red blood cells and result of vessel occlusions.
		Instruct on the potential complications of sickle cell anemia.
		Instruct on purpose of management strategies (for example, hypertransfusions, fetal hemoglobin stimulator agent, chelation therapy, bone marrow transplantation).
	Child remains free of infection.	Instruct on following methods to avoid infection:

Nursing Diagnosis	Expected Outcomes	Nursing Interventions
		• good hygiene • compliance in taking prophylactic penicillin and obtaining pneumococcal vaccine, annual flu shot, and routine immunizations
	Parents report symptoms of crisis immediately to physician	Stress that all febrile episodes need to be immediately reported to the physician. Instruct on how to take temperature, read thermometer, and keep thermometer available Instruct parents on the following signs and symptoms of crisis episodes: • dactylitis—swelling of fingers and toes, irritability • bones—painful (pain may be migratory) extremities • abdomen—pain and cramping of abdomen. Occasional nausea and vomiting. • spleen—"splenic sequestration"—dramatic increase in spleen size or abdominal girth, abdominal pain, paleness, marked fatigue • central nervous system—headaches, convulsions, aphasia, change in motor, strength, and movement, blindness • lungs—progressive shortness of breath and chest pain • kidney—hematuria, dysuria, enuresis • extremities—leg ulcers
3. Alterations in comfort due to sickle cell pain crisis	Child states pain is within adequate comfort range.	Teach older children to use consistent tool or scale to describe location and intensity of pain. Help child and family develop a home and school pain control regimen for mild, moderate, and severe pain (without fever) using "around-the-clock" analgesia. Instruct on the following nonpharmacologic methods for pain control: • warm compresses or baths • massage

Nursing Diagnosis	Expected Outcomes	Nursing Interventions
		• relaxation and self-hypnosis techniques • distraction activities Encourage passive or slow active range of motion. Discuss hospital management of pain control for optimizing comfort and promote early discharge. Encourage carrying a card that outlines optimal pharmacologic and nonpharmacologic pain regimen (pain control contract).
4. Potential alteration in nutrition related to megablastic disorders	Child will eat a well-balanced meal.	Emphasize importance of eating well-balanced, high-calorie, and high-protein meals. Instruct that meals should not be skipped. Provide nutritional counseling on foods high in folic acid and vitamin B_{12}. Encourage compliance in taking daily folic acid.
5. Health maintenance	Child will receive routine care management. Child will be routinely screened for complications of sickle cell disease.	Routine well-child care visits should include the following: • routine laboratory tests • routine immunizations • routine evaluation of growth and development Annual evaluations (older child) should include the following: • dental evaluation • ophthalmology evaluation • audiology evaluation • PFTs and oximetry • electrocardiogram and echocardiogram • laboratory evaluations: complete blood count, platelet, differential, reticulocyte, ferritin, total iron-binding capacity, blood chemistries
6. Disturbances in self-concept due to sickle cell disease	Child will develop a positive self-esteem.	Provide child and parents with resources for support. Encourage discussion with day care and

Nursing Diagnosis	*Expected Outcomes*	*Nursing Interventions*
		school personnel on methods to enhance academic and social success. Instruct older child on reason for shorter stature and delayed physical changes due to sickle cell. Encourage the child as he or she grows older to take responsibility for self-care.

The Child with Thalassemia Major

Nursing Diagnosis	Expected Outcomes	Nursing Interventions
1. Potential for knowledge deficit related to thalassemia	Patient and family will verbalize the following: • understanding of transmission of thalassemia • understanding of disease, complications, and treatments	Encourage initial visit and follow-up visits to a pediatric hematology center. Instruct on genetic transmission of thalassemia. Instruct on red blood cell abnormality. Instruct on purpose and frequency of red blood cell transfusions. Discuss potential of bone marrow transplantation and purpose of HLA-testing of family. Discuss purpose and process of chelation therapy. Instruct on administration of home chelation. Instruct on signs and symptoms related to thalassemia, particularly anemia. Encourage early reporting of complications of thalassemia, such as the following: • congestive heart failure • cirrhosis of liver—jaundice, easy bruising • endocrine abnormalities—hypothyroidism, hypoparathyroidism, diabetes mellitus, osteoporosis and spinal cord compression Avoid or report symptoms of splenomegaly. • Avoid rough contact sports to prevent spontaneous rupture. • Report easy bruising, petechiae, or spontaneous bleeding of nose, gums,

Nursing Diagnosis	Expected Outcomes	Nursing Interventions
		urine, stool, etc. (platelet sequestration). • Report febrile episodes (leukocyte sequestration). Instruct on care after splenectomy including the following: • pneumococcal vaccination • daily bid dosing of penicillin
3. Potential alterations in nutrition related to thalassemia	Child will eat a well-balanced meal.	Instruct on importance of a diet low in iron. Provide list of high-iron foods to avoid. Encourage intake of foods with folic acid if on hypertransfusion therapy (and supplemental folic acid vitamins daily).
4. Health maintenance	Child will receive routine health care.	Maintain routine well-child visits including the following: • routine laboratory tests • routine immunizations • growth and development evaluation • routine dental care
5. Disturbances in self-concept due to thalassemia	Child will develop a positive self-esteem.	Provide child and parents with resources for support. Encourage discussion with day care and school personnel on methods to enhance academic and social success. Instruct children on reason for changes in appearance due to disease (for example, changes in facies, shorter stature, delayed puberty, etc.) and encourage expression of feelings and coping strategies.

Also refer to the following Appendixes in this chapter (as applicable):

• Appendix 12–B, The Anemias in Childhood (General)
• Appendix 12–J, The Child after Bone Marrow Transplantation

The Child with Aplastic Anemia

Nursing Diagnosis	Expected Outcomes	Nursing Interventions
1. Knowledge deficit related to aplastic anemia	Patient and family will verbalize the following: • understanding of disease • treatment • side effects of therapy and potential complications	Explore potential source of child's development of aplastic anemia (for example, chemicals, toxin exposure in environment). Instruct on disease, purpose of blood cells, normal levels of blood cells, and problems associated with low levels. Review symptoms to report associated with low levels of blood cells. Instruct on meaning of laboratory results and frequency of tests. Discuss interventions for low levels of blood cells (for example, transfusion and antibiotic therapy). Encourage expression of feelings about receiving chronic transfusion therapy. Reinforce purpose of specific treatment options, such as the following: • bone marrow transplantation • ATG/ALG infusions • steroid therapy • cyclosporin-A therapy Review home medications, schedule, dose, and side effects of the following: • steroids • cyclosporin-A • TMP-sulfa • antifungals

Nursing Diagnosis	*Expected Outcomes*	*Nursing Interventions*
2. Disturbances in self-concept due to aplastic anemia treatment.	Child verbalizes feelings and concerns about disease and treatment.	Provide opportunities for child to discuss feelings about disease, treatment, and impact on self and social interactions (for example, mood swings, chronic fatigue, etc.). Provide strategies to cope with change in appearance (for example, cushingoid appearance due to steroids and hirsutism due to cyclosporin-A) Encourage parents to promote independence and child's participation in activities that he or she is successful performing.
3. Potential for ineffective coping related to guilt and potential chronic or fatal course of disease	Patient and family will verbalize feelings and concerns.	Discuss parents' expectations on outcome of treatment. Encourage discussion of impact of illness on all family members. Encourage parents to express feelings regarding disease and transmission. Encourage open, honest communication regarding treatment failures and options and fears.

Also refer to the following appendixes in this chapter (as applicable):

- Appendix 12–B, The Anemias in Childhood (General)
- Appendix 12–H, The Immunosuppressed Child
- Appendix 12–F, The Child with Thrombocytopenia
- Appendic 12–J, The Child after Bone Marrow Transplant

Note: ATG, antithymocyte globulin; ALG, antilymphocyte globulin; TMP-sulfa, trimethoprim-sulfamethoxazole.

The Child with Thrombocytopenia

Nursing Diagnosis	Expected Outcomes	Nursing Interventions
1. Potential for bleeding related to thrombocytopenia	The nurse assesses the status of child. The nurse performs interventions while minimizing risk of bleeding. Parents and older children verbalize knowledge of disease, treatment, and side effects of therapy. Child shows no signs or symptoms of bleedings. Parents and older children initiate protective measures to prevent bleeding.	Assess for signs and symptoms of bleeding. Avoid use of tourniquet or pad tourniquet and apply loosely. If an injection is necessary, use the smallest needle possible and apply pressure for five minutes after needle removal. Avoid pumping up blood pressure cuff above usual systolic range. Instruct parents in cause of disorder and treatment measures. Review schedule of home medication and side effects. Instruct parents (if applicable) on corticosteroid therapy. • Avoid high-sodium diet. • Limit snacking; provide low-calorie snacks. • Anticipate mood swings. • Taper medication slowly after prolonged use. • Take corticosteroids with meals to prevent gastrointestinal ulceration. Review the following common signs and symptoms of bleeding to report to the health care provider • bruising and petechiae • bleeding from nose or gums • hematemesis, "coffee ground" emesis • hematuria

Nursing Diagnosis	Expected Outcomes	Nursing Interventions

		• gross blood or tarry stools
		• increase in menstrual blood flow
		• change in level of consciousness
		• blurred vision
		• unexplained vomiting
		Instruct on protective measures to minimize bleeding.
		  • Use soft toothbrush; rinse toothbrush under hot water before brushing to soften fibers; avoid flossing
		  • Measures to keep stools soft
		  • Avoid rectal temperatures, suppositories, and enemas.
		  • Avoid vaginal douching.
		  • Avoid tight, constrictive clothing.
		  • Use electric razor for shaving.
		  • Avoid use of aspirin, aspirin-containing cold preparations, or nonsteroidal analgesics. Use acetaminophen for pain.
		  • Menstruating females should consult with physician about use of birth control pill or progestational agent to prevent bleeding.
		  • Avoid activities that carry risk of injury (e.g., contact sports, sledding, rollerblading).
		  • Wear bicycle helmet while cycling.
		Assist parents in acquisition of Medic-Alert tag for child.

2. Potential for injury related to thrombocytopenia	The child participates in activities that minimize trauma. Parents demonstrate correct procedure when bleeding occurs.	Instruct parents to pad side rails of infant's bed. Assist parents in structuring activities that avoid trauma, especially falls and contact with hard objects. Assist in acquiring a helmet for active young children. Assist parents in teaching child to wipe nose rather than blowing. Instruct school personnel in precautions, especially regarding physical activity (gym, recess). Instruct parents in steps to take if bleeding occurs.

Nursing Diagnosis	Expected Outcomes	Nursing Interventions
		Apply pressure to site or to nose (in case of epistaxis) for 5 to 10 minutes. If bleeding continues, call physician and maintain pressure. Contact physician immediately in the event of any falls, trauma, or blows to the head.
3. Potential for infection related to splenectomy	Parents help child to take prophylactics daily if ordered by physician.	Instruct parents in the importance of compliance in taking antibiotics (penicillin) daily to avoid sepsis.
4. Disturbance in self-concept of child related to restricted activities, evidence of bruises, weight gain, or corticosteroid therapy.	Child verbalizes feelings and concerns about disease, treatment, and restrictions in activities.	Assess child's social interaction with peers. Encourage the child to verbalize feelings and concerns. Instruct parents to provide activities that promote independence and challenges while not initiating trauma. Discuss with teacher, coach, or gym teacher methods to encourage participation in activities with peers (for example, make the child "junior coach," "official scorekeeper") Offer suggestions on discipline, such as limit setting and "time out."
5. Potential for ineffective family coping regarding fears of spontaneous bleeding, hemorrhagic signs on child, restrictions on siblings to avoid rough contact with brother or sister	Family members verbalize their fears and concerns.	Encourage family members to express feelings and concerns. Provide suggestions to parents on how to cope with strangers who stare at child with bruises because they may think parents are abusive to child. Assist parents to instruct other care providers on care of child so they can feel comfortable leaving the child with others. Assist parents to instruct siblings on types of behavior (no hitting) and activities with ill child. *Note:* Siblings should report to parents if child takes advantage of disorder (e.g., "I can hit you, but you can't hit me back.").

The Child with Hemophilia/ von Willebrand Disease

Nursing Diagnosis	Expected Outcomes	Nursing Interventions
1. Potential for injury related to deficiency of clotting factor	Child has few bleeding episodes. Parents recognize early signs of bleeding. Parents initiate appropriate treatment when signs of bleeding are observed. Parents recognize and report early signs of bleeding.	Make the child's environment as safe as possible by doing the following: • Pad infant's crib. • Supervise activities of toddlers and young children. • Set age-appropriate limits. • Pad elbow and knee areas of clothing of young children. • Assist older children in selection of activities in which they can safely participate. • Consult with school personnel on participation in physical activities and appropriate management of bleeds. • Encourage use of Medic-Alert bracelet or necklace. • Encourage good oral hygiene using soft toothbrush and regular flossing. • Use only electric razor for shaving, not blades. • Avoid use of aspirin and aspirin-containing cold preparations. Consult with physician regarding use of nonsteroidal anti-inflammatories. • Notify hemophilia treatment center before surgery or dental extractions. • Participate in physical activities that maintain strong musculature and support joints (for example, swimming, biking, walking).

Nursing Diagnosis	Expected Outcomes	Nursing Interventions
		Teach child to eat a well-balanced diet to prevent weight gain and extra stress on joints.
		Inform parents and primary care providers that all immunizations are to be given subcutaneously followed by pressure applied for 5 to 10 minutes to avoid intramuscular bleed.
		Instruct parents and children to recognize the following symptoms of bleeding: <ul><li>stiffness, tenderness, warmth, and swelling in joints and muscles</li><li>pain in groin, on flexion of thigh and resistance to extension of extremity</li><li>change in level of consciousness, headaches, blurred vision, or unexplained vomiting</li><li>nasal or oral mucosal bleeding</li><li>unexplained discomfort or pain</li><li>hematuria</li></ul>
		Instruct parents and children to immediately infuse for all major bleeding episodes and then report to hemophilia treatment center, especially those involving the head, throat, neck, or central nervous system.
		Instruct parents and child on initial interventions for bleeding episodes including the following: <ul><li>Skin abrasions—apply pressure for 5 to 10 minutes with clean gauze.</li><li>Nosebleed—apply firm pressure for 5 to 10 minutes. Keep child upright with head tilted forward.</li><li>Muscle and joint bleeds—follow RICE—Rest the site or extremity, Infuse with factor concentrate, apply Cold compress, Elevate the extremity.</li><li>Hematuria—infuse with factor concentrate, drink 6–8 ounces of fluid every 2 hours.</li></ul>
		Discuss methods to assist parents to remain calm and supportive to child during bleeding episode.

Nursing Diagnosis	Expected Outcomes	Nursing Interventions
		Instruct parents and child (as appropriate) in the home administration of factor concentrate:
		• Assess ability and readiness to learn procedure
		• Assess knowledge of type, brand, and dose of factor concentrate used for minor and major bleeds
		• Assure access to refrigeration for factor storage
		• Observe ability to reconstitute and draw up factor concentrate accurately
		• Observe ability to perform venipuncture following aseptic technique
		• Observe administration of infusion
		• Apply pressure to site for 5–10 minutes following removal of needle
		Instruct child and family to keep log documenting bleeding episodes:
		• Date and site of episode
		• Infusion dose including lot # from manufacturer's packaging
		• Results of treatment and any follow up infusions needed
		• Pain management
2. Alteration in comfort related to painful effusions and arthropathy	Child is free of pain.	Instruct family in administration of analgesics; acetaminophen is the most common analgesic of choice. Follow RICE (rest, infuse, cold, elevate until bleeding stops). Initiate physical therapy program after acute bleeding episode and following surgery.
3. Disturbance in self-concept related to disruption in normal activities, joint deformities, previous threat of AIDS	Child expresses feelings and concerns. Child particpates in appropriate activities. Child develops social relationships with peers.	Provide age-appropriate information about hemophilia, treatment, and complications. Encourage child and family to express concerns about hemophilia and actual or potential restrictions on activities. Instruct parents to encourage their child's independence and decision-making skills by offering age-appropriate choices.

Nursing Diagnosis	Expected Outcomes	Nursing Interventions
		Encourage active participation in school and peer activities and competition in appropriate sports.
		Help child and family to learn stimulating activities for use during periods of immobilization.
		Encourage the child's active participation in treatment plans and therapies.
		Assist older children in career decisions.
4. Potential for ineffective family coping related to guilt of transmission, fear of hemorrhage, loss of "healthy" child, financial burden, and other stressors	Family members discuss their feelings and concerns.	Provide instruction to child and family members on genetic transmission, special needs of teatment, and potential complications.
		Encourage parents to express feelings of guilt or grief.
		Allow for discussion of issues related to alterations in family budget or routine.
		Provide access to support organizations.
		Encourage regular follow-up with area hemophilia treatment center and annual comprehensive clinic visits.

The Immunosuppressed Child

Nursing Diagnosis	Expected Outcomes	Nursing Interventions
1. Potential for infection related to immunosuppressive disorders	Patient and family will do the following: • verbalize knowledge of disease and treatment • verbalize signs and symptoms • identify potential sources of infections • verbalize precautions to reduce infection • provide a safe environment • perform correct central line catheter care • demonstrate postural drainage • verbalize dosage and schedule of medications	Assess child's medical history, past infections, especially contagious diseases (e.g., chickenpox, mumps, measles), allergies, immunization status. Obtain information about home environment—telephone, electricity, home hygiene system, kitchen and bathroom facilities, sleeping arrangements, pets, etc. Assess pattern of daily living of home occupants. Obtain information on child's diet, pattern of daily living, school, and hobbies. Obtain history on siblings—immunization status, exposure to contagious diseases, pattern of daily living. Assess knowledge of disease, prognosis, and treatment. Review purpose and schedule of prophylactic medications. Review dose and administration technique for growth factors (if receiving). Review laboratory tests and meaning of values. Assess instructional needs of significant caregivers—relatives, home care aides, sitters, and school personnel.

Nursing Diagnosis	*Expected Outcomes*	*Nursing Interventions*
		Instruct on the following:

Instruct on the following:
- method and times to obtain child's temperature.
- the following symptoms to report to physician: temperature greater than 101°F (38.3°C), persistent cough, shortness of breath, congestion, pain anywhere in body, rashes, skin breakdown, sores, persistent irritability, malaise, diarrhea (stools more than three per day), constipation for longer than two days, decreased food and fluid intake, headaches, increased incoordination, speech difficulties, change in level of consciousness, white patches in mouth, pain with urination, incontinence, hematuria, cloudy urine, dental swelling, or gum pain

Instruct on the following precautions to minimize contracting infections from foods:
- Avoid unpasteurized milk and milk products.
- Avoid raw fish.
- Cook all raw vegetables and fruits or wash and peel vegetables and fruits.
- Cook all meats well.
- Avoid buying prepared foods such as tuna salad, egg salad, or coleslaw.
- Do not send child to bed with bottle of juice or milk.

Instruct on how the child can avoid contagious diseases.
- Have child avoid contact with other persons with infectious disease.
- Request school to notify parents if outbreak of contagious diseases occurs in child's classroom. School should receive specific instruction on how to handle child's exposure to infections, especially chickenpox.

Instruct on avoiding using rectal thermometers, enemas, or suppositories.

Instruct parents to notify physician before dental visits.

Nursing Diagnosis	*Expected Outcomes*	*Nursing Interventions*
		Instruct on exposure to pets.
		• Avoid touching pets' excreta (feces, urine, emeses, litter box, aquariums, bird cages).
		• Discuss with physician types of pets allowed.
		• Pets should have routine health shots.
		Instruct on proper hygiene of home environment, including hot and cold running water, Proper storage of foods, and electricity.
		• Clean bedside vaporizer daily when in use with germicidal and antifungal cleaner.
		• Clean household humidifier system frequently.
		• Change air conditioner filters often.
		• Clean used utensils in hot soapy water and rinse well.
		• Dispose of garbage frequently.
		• Vacuum when child is gone for several hours.
		• Maintain good home hygiene, especially in kitchen and bathroom.
		• Do not share utensils or toothbrushes with other persons.
		• Avoid exposure to blowing dust and straw.
		Inform parents of immunization precautions.
		• Child should not receive live immunizations (measles, mumps, rubella, and Sabin polio).
		• Child may receive inactivated or killed vaccines but may be unable to elicit an effective response.
		• Annual immunization with inactivated influenza vaccine is recommended in children older than six months, and one-time administration of pneumococcal vaccine is recommended for children older than two years.
		• For direct exposure to measles and varicella, the child should receive

Nursing Diagnosis	Expected Outcomes	Nursing Interventions
		passive immunization with immune globulin and varicella-zoster immunoglobulin, respectively. *Note:* Exposure to chickenpox includes two days before outbreak of vesicles until scabbing of all lesions. Varicella-zoster immunoglobulin must be given within 72 hours after exposure to be effective.

- Other children in the home should receive only Salk polio, not Sabin polio, vaccine.
- Stress importance of receiving globulin injections or infusions; instruct in correct technique of administration if performed in home.

Instruct in importance of personal hygiene of child, including the following:

- Take a daily bath or shower.
- Use liquid soap instead of bar soap.
- Inspect skin for infection, rash, or skin breakdown.
- Apply lubricating cream (nonalcohol base) to dry, irritated skin and lip balm or petroleum jelly to dry lips.
- Apply SPF 15 (or stronger) waterproof sunscreen for sun exposure longer than 30 minutes.
- Instruct on good oral hygiene—brush teeth after meals with fluoride toothpaste and soft toothbrush and rinse with chlorhexidine mouthwash (must not swallow—swab on with sponge stick)
- Inspect oral mucosa for sores or candidiasis.
- Clean rectal area gently but well after toileting.
- Wash hands well after toileting, before eating, and after playing with pets or working or playing in dirt.

Instruct parents to provide for child's safety (for example, safe toys and activities).

Nursing Diagnosis	Expected Outcomes	Nursing Interventions
		Instruct on proper care of central line catheter.
		Instruct parents on postural drainage technique to be started daily with pulmonary congestion (should be avoided if platelet count is less than 20,000 cu mm).
		Review home medications, schedule, dose, and potential side effects of the following:
		• Trimethoprim-sulfamethoxazole (TMP-sulfa)
		• antifungals
		• Intravenous antibiotics (if ordered) by physician
2. Potential for alteration in nutrition: less than body requirements related to increased demand with infection	Child maintains appropriate weight.	Instruct on the following:
		• providing diet high in protein and calories
		• obtaining daily or weekly weight
		• providing frequent small meals
		• making meals a pleasant experience
		• providing mouth care before eating if child takes oral acidic foods and liquids with oral soreness
		• allowing child to suggest favorite foods
		• reporting diarrhea, nausea, or oral sores immediately to prevent dehydration and malnutrition
		• providing daily vitamin with iron
		• consulting nutritionist for additional suggestions and supplemental preparations
		• providing financial support to obtain groceries
		Instruct parents on procedure for home nasogastric or gastrostomy feedings or total parenteral nutrition.
3. Potential for activity intolerance related to frequent infections, especially pulmonary infections	Child participates in activities to level of tolerance.	Assess degree of activity intolerance.
		Identify source of activity intolerance.
		Encourage regular and frequent rest periods.

Nursing Diagnosis	Expected Outcomes	Nursing Interventions
		Provide activities, games, and toys appropriate for age and physical development. Provide occupational, physical, and speech therapy in home and school if required. Arrange daily schedule for tolerance level.
4. Disturbance in self-concept related to special precautions and frequency of hospitalizations	Child verbalizes fears and concerns about disorders.	Encourage child to express concerns and feelings about disease and treatment. Explain disorders and treatment at child's level of understanding. Explain disorder, treatment, and special precautions to school personnel.
5. Potential for ineffective family coping related to special needs of child, feelings of guilt, and anticipatory grief	Parents and family members verbalize fears and concerns.	Involve child in decision making related to his or her activities. Promote independence and avoid overprotection. Encourage expression of fears and concerns of all family members. Introduce family to another family whose child has a similar diagnosis. Provide genetic counseling if appropriate. Provide resource and organizational support. Provide respite care. Encourage parents to spend quality time with other children in the family.

The Child with HIV/AIDS

Nursing Diagnosis	Expected Outcomes	Nursing Interventions
1. Potential for infection: related to immunodeficiency		(*See Appendix 12–H—The Immunosuppressed Child*) Inform parents of immunization precautions (same as for immunosuppressed child). In addition, do the following: • Ensure that child is vaccinated, following American Academy of Pediatric guidelines, against diphtheria-pertussis-tetanus (DPT), hepatitis B, and haemophilus influenza B (HIB). • Because of significant risk of fatality from measles infection, ensure that child with human immunodeficiency virus (HIV) receives live measles, mumps, and rubella vaccine (MMR).
2. Potential for alteration in nutrition: less than body requirement related to increased demand		(*See Appendix 12–H.*)
3. Potential for activity tolerance related to frequent infections and immune status		(*See Appendix 12–H.*)

Nursing Diagnosis	Expected Outcomes	Nursing Interventions
4. Potential for disturbance in self-concept related to HIV/acquired immune deficiency syndrome (AIDS) diagnosis, special procedures and precautions, and frequent clinic and hospital visits	Child verbalizes feelings and concerns about diagnosis and treatment. Parents demonstrate awareness of developmental and emotional needs of child.	Encourage child to express concerns and feelings about diagnosis and treatment. Provide simple, honest, age-appropriate information on disease and treatment. Explain disorder, treatment, and special precautions to day care providers and school personnel, with written parental consent only. Involve child in decision making. Continue to set limits and provide discipline. Enable child's participation in family activities.
5. Knowledge deficit related to HIV/AIDS	Parents and children (as appropriate) verbalize understanding of disease, transmission, and treatment.	Assess prior knowledge, attitudes, and fears related to HIV and AIDS. Assess other family members for HIV infection; offer HIV testing. Provide information on HIV and its effect on the immune system. Instruct on importance of antiretroviral. and prophylactic medication dosing and schedule. Discuss risk and benefits of investigational therapy.
6. Potential for transmission of HIV to others	Family members, caregivers, and health care providers follow precautions to prevent accidental exposure to HIV. Family members, caregivers, and health care providers can verbalize that 99 percent of HIV is transmitted through sexual contact with an infected partner, by sharing needles with an infected drug partner, or from an infected mother to her child during pregnancy and delivery.	Counsel that playing, kissing, hugging, feeding, bathing, and otherwise casual contact while caring for an HIV-infected child do not expose the caregiver to HIV. Instruct in the following: • Wear disposable gloves when handling blood or body fluids or objects in contact with these fluids. • Place disposable contaminated materials (gloves, dressings, tissue, diapers) in a tied plastic bag and dispose of bag in a plastic-lined trash container with a lid. • Blood, body fluid, and soiled tissues may be disposed of in the toilet. Close lid when flushing. Clean toilet weekly.

Nursing Diagnosis	Expected Outcomes	Nursing Interventions
		• A surface in contact with blood, bloody fluids, or such spills should be cleaned with paper towel followed by a bleach solution ($1/2$ cup household bleach to 4 cups water).
		• Wash hands with soap and warm water before and after donning gloves, changing diapers, or coming into contact with body fluids.
		• Linens and clothing soiled with blood and body fluids may be laundered separately from other laundry in hot water, detergent, and common bleach. Other laundry may be washed with family laundry
		• Do not share toothbrushes, razors, or other items that may be contaminated with blood.
		• Dishware and utensils may be shared. Wash with hot soapy water or in an automatic dishwasher after use.
		• Discard needles and syringes in appropriately labeled "sharps" container. Keep out of reach of children. Bring container to hospital or clinic for proper disposal.
		• Exposure occurs through direct contact with blood or body fluid through a cut, rash, or sore on the skin. Wash the area thoroughly with soap and water and report the incident.
		• In the event of a needlestick exposure, immediately squeeze the wound to encourage bleeding, wash with soap and water, and report the incident.
7. Potential for ineffective family coping related to social isolation, feelings of guilt, and anticipatory grief	Family members verbalize sources of stress and assist in problem solving. Family members verbalize awareness of	Encourage open expression of feelings and concerns. Inform parents of their child's legal right to confidentiality. Obtain written permission before disclosing HIV diagnosis to anyone.

Nursing Diagnosis	Expected Outcomes	Nursing Interventions
	support services and legal rights. Parents demonstrate ability to assist family members in coping with stress and grief.	Inform parents of child's legal right to an education. Provide family with information regarding AIDS service organizations (ASOs) in the area, family network, national organizations, and AIDS hot lines. Ensure child's access to health care, special services, and medication. Provide financial counseling. Assist family in identifying respite care. Discuss the special needs and normal reactions of siblings to a child with chronic illness. Provide special time just for siblings. Assist siblings with understanding the reactions of others and suggest appropriate response. Provide bereavement counseling as appropriate. Initiate hospice referral as needed with family's consent.

The Child after Bone Marrow Transplantation

Nursing Diagnosis	Potential Problems	Expected Outcomes	Nursing Interventions
1. Potential for infection related to immunosuppression	• Bacterial infection • Fungal infections • *Pneumocystis carinii* • Herpetic infections • Cytomegalovirus (CMV) infections	Child and family will do the following: • verbalize understanding of avoidance of infection • promptly report signs and symptoms of infection	Instruct on avoidance of crowds. Assist with obtaining a home-based tutor. Instruct on when to wear a high-filtration mask. Instruct on foods to avoid while on a neutropenic diet. Assess for any signs and symptoms of infection. Instruct on dose and schedule of prophylactic medications. • TMP-sulfa • acyclovir • fluconazole • immunoglobulin infusion (weekly) Monitor for immune recovery by checking results of immunoglobulin levels. Assist with devising plan for updating vaccinations after immune recovery. (Also see: The Immunosuppressed Child, Appendix 12–H)

Nursing Diagnosis	Potential Problems	Expected Outcomes	Nursing Interventions
2. Potential for impairment in skin integrity related to chemoradiation effects and GVHD	Skin: • desquamation • dryness • dermal thickening • pigmentation changes • poikiloderma • telangiectasia • lichen planus • rash • herpetic shingles • skin breakdown Hair: • coarse, brittle texture • premature graying • partial alopecia Nails: • slow growth • brittle • loss of nails	Child and family will do the following: • verbalize any changes in skin • provide skin care as instructed	Assess skin integrity or problems at daily examination. Encourage prompt reporting of any skin problems to health care team. Encourage wearing loose-fitting, soft clothing. Instruct on use of nonabrasive soaps, detergents, and lotions. Encourage to apply sunblock frequently when in bright sunlight and cover exposed areas with light clothing. Recommend adding bath oil to bathwater daily. Applying water-based (nonalcohol-containing) lotion to areas of dryness two to three times a day. Recommend applying any special creams or lotions (for example, steroid creams, antibiotic ointment, etc.) as prescribed. Recommend use of oral antipruritic medication for itching. Discourage scratching. Have young children who have a tendency to scratch wear mittens. Recommend keeping nails trimmed short. Advise avoidance of tape directly to skin. Instruct on keeping open areas of skin clean, applying antibiotic ointment, and dressing as instructed. Report any area of redness, drainage, or skin

Nursing Diagnosis	*Potential Problems*	*Expected Outcomes*	*Nursing Interventions*
			breakdown, and ask whether culture should be obtained and sent. Discuss potential for dermatology consultation to diagnose skin problem. Discuss potential for skin biopsy to diagnose GVHD. Instruct on importance of maintaining schedule and dose of GVHD medications.
3. Potential for impaired physical mobility related to chemoradiation effects, prolonged period of decreased mobilization, or GVHD	• Muscular atrophy and dystrophy • Contracture • Polymyositis • Aseptic osteonecrosis	Child will participate in rehabilitative program.	Assess baseline muscle strength, coordination, and degree of range of motion. Instruct on frequency of exercise program and periodic occupational and physical therapy evaluation. Consult with adaptive physical education (PE) in school to assist in exercise program.
4. Potential for alteration in nutrition due to chemo-radiation effects and GVHD	Oral cavity: • taste loss and changes • lichen planus • candidiasis • mucositis • herpetic lesions • keratinization • xerostomia • dental cavities • dry lips Esophagus: • candidiasis • stenosis	Child and family will verbalize methods.	Assess integrity of oral mucosa daily. Instruct on good oral hygiene regimen. Instruct on frequent liquid intake or use of artificial saliva for xerostoma. Instruct on application of topical oral anesthetics for pain control, especially before eating. Obtain daily calorie log of solid intake and also oral intake.

Nursing Diagnosis	Potential Problems	Expected Outcomes	Nursing Interventions
	• mucositis • sicca Gastrointestinal: • malabsorption syndrome • diarrhea (GVHD and infection) • nausea and vomiting		Obtain twice weekly weights. (Use same amount of clothing and same scale.) Keep accurate record of losses from urine, diarrhea, and emesis. Advise reporting any blood noted in emesis or stool. Monitor results of laboratory tests (for example, electrolytes, albumin). Provide dietary counseling regarding types of cooking or food selection to enhance taste, decrease nausea and vomiting (N/V), control diarrhea, etc. Encourage frequent snacking of foods throughout the day (may need special permission for school). Encourage drinking fluids that have calories. Discuss potential for bacillary rectal biopsy to diagnose GVHD. Instruct on procedure for administration of alternative nutrition sources, such as total parenteral nutrition, nasogastric feedings, etc. Encourage reporting any difficulty in swallowing. Encourage routine dental visits (may require prophylactic antibiotics before dental work). Instruct on dose and schedule of medications to control gastrointesti-

Nursing Diagnosis	Potential Problems	Expected Outcomes	Nursing Interventions
			nal acidity, nausea, or diarrhea. Instruct on importance of administration of any medications for GVHD.
5. Potential for alterations in sensory perception related to chemo-radiation effects and GVHD	• Keratoconjunctivitis sicca • Corneal stripping • Cataracts • CMV retinitis	Child will have maximal eyesight.	Instruct on importance of reporting blurred vision, burning, or dryness of eyes. Encourage routine ophthalmology examinations for potential complications. Advise proper cleaning of contact lenses. Encourage frequent use of artificial tears.
6. Potential for neurologic impairment related to chemo-radiation effects, neurotoxic drugs, central nervous system (CNS) infections, use of mind-altering drugs, or CNS metastasis	Leukoencephalopathy: • personality changes • difficulty in abstract thinking, dementia, headaches, nausea and vomiting, marked fatigue Meningeal irritation Cyclosporine • tremors • headaches • lethargy Learning deficits Elevation of ammonia level in veno-occlusive disease	Child will have appropriate orientation. Child will be in a safe environment. Child will be able to achieve his or her maximal potential academically.	Assess for signs and symptoms of neurologic changes for baseline. Monitor levels of cyclosporine to prevent toxicity. Assess use of mind-altering drugs that may influence alertness (for example, dyphrahydramine, narcotics, relaxant, etc.). Review dose and schedule of medications to treat leukoencephalopathy (for example, steroids). Encourage periodic neuropsychometric testing and use findings to help structure educational program to meet the child's needs. Provide a safe environment for child especially if neurologically impaired.

Nursing Diagnosis	Potential Problems	Expected Outcomes	Nursing Interventions
7. Potential for problems with urinary elimination related to chemo-radiation effects or nephrotoxic drugs	Hemorrhages Cystitis Kidney failure • dysuria • oliguria Fanconi's syndrome (electrolyte wasting) Dehydration	Child will have adequate kidney output and normal electrolytes.	Encourage oral fluid intake. Encourage reporting of the following: • pain or difficulty in urination • blood in urine Monitor I & O. Monitor electrolyte levels, BUN, and creatinine. Encourage reporting edema of extremities. Monitor levels of nephro-toxic drugs (may need to reduce dose based on kidney function).
8. Potential for ineffective breathing pattern related to chemo-radiation effects, GVHD, or infection	Nonbacterial interstitial pneumonitis Restrictive decrease in vital capacity total lung capacity due to fibrosis Obstructive bron-chopulmonary sicca Infectious pneu-monitis Pulmonary edema secondary to capillary leak Pulmonary hemor-rhage	Child will be able to maintain adequate tissue oxygen-ation.	Assess pulmonary status. Report SOB, anxiety, chronic cough, wheezes, tachypnea, etc. Encourage good pulmo-nary hygiene by inspirometry exercises Recommend no smoking around the child. (The child or adolescent should not smoke.) Avoid being in dusty environment (barn, fields, etc.). Instruct on proper use of oxygen in the home (if used). Monitor pulmonary function tests and pulse oximetry.
9. Potential for impairment in cardiac function due to chemo-radiation	Congestive heart failure Abnormal ECG changes Pericardial effusions	Child will maintain adequate cardiac output.	Assess for signs and symptoms of cardiac problems (for example, SOB, tachycardia, irregular heart rate, evidence of poor

Nursing Diagnosis	Potential Problems	Expected Outcomes	Nursing Interventions
effects and electrolyte disturbances			perfusion, chest pain, etc.). Encourage to promptly report any problems. Advise to avoid strenuous physical activity shortly after transplantation and get advice from physician before beginning an exercise program. Monitor electrolytes closely.
10. Potential for impairment of liver function related to: Chemoradiation effects, GVHD, hepatotoxic drugs, or infection.	Hepatitis infection Hepatotoxic drugs TNA Veno-occlusive disease GVHD of liver	Child will have normal liver function.	Assess for jaundice. Assess for signs and symptoms of bleeding. Monitor LFTs, coagulation studies, and ammonia level. Report increase of abdominal girth or RUQ abdominal discomfort. Monitor levels of hepatotoxic drugs (for example, antibiotics, methotrexate, narcotics, etc.).
11. Potential for abnormalities in endocrine function related to chemoradiation effects.	Hypothyroidism Growth hormone deficiency Gonadal • sterility • delayed onset • early menopause • azoospermia	Child and family will verbalize understanding of potential endocrine late effects and seek evaluation and supplementation when required.	Assess for signs and symptoms of potential endocrine problems. Chart height and weight on a growth chart monthly. Monitor endocrine tests for abnormalities. Recommend fertility counseling when appropriate.
12. Potential for sexual dysfunction related to chemoradiation effects	Decreased libido Vaginal sicca Inflammation Infection Sicca	Young adult will report any concerns related to sexual organ function.	Instruct to report any concerns regarding sexuality issues.

Nursing Diagnosis	Potential Problems	Expected Outcomes	Nursing Interventions
13. Potential for disturbance in self-concept	Changes in appearance, for example the following: • chronic GVHD • steroid cushingoid symptoms • cyclosporine hirsutism Changes in physical abilities, for example the following: • weakness • muscle atrophy • contracture • unable to play usual games Isolationism and dependency on others, for example: • separation from family, friends, and classmates • dependency on parents • frustration in getting behind on schoolwork Fear of relapse, for example: • fear of experiencing death • anxiety over breaking ties with medical center • fear of acute problems continuing after discharge	Child or adolescent will do the following: • express concerns and fears • develop a behavioral program for coping	Assess for disturbances in self-concept related to potential and actual problems. Advise continued therapeutic interventions and assist in finding qualified therapist in the community. Discuss methods to reintegrate child into home, school, and community. Encourage open communication among family members to discuss the hospital and post-hospital experiences.

Nursing Diagnosis	*Potential Problems*	*Expected Outcomes*	*Nursing Interventions*
	Depression, for example: • insomnia • chronic pain • poor appetite • flat personality		

Note: I&O, intake and output; BUN, blood urea nitrogen; SOB, shortness of breath; ECG, elctrocardiogram; LFT, liver function tests; RUQ, right upper quadrant; GVHD, graft-versus host disease.

CHAPTER 13

Care of the Child Post-Transplant

Susan D. Wheeler and Christine Mudge

With the advent of cyclosporine during the early 1980s, the survival rate for children undergoing organ transplantation has improved significantly. Many programs now report a one-year patient survival rate of between 80 and 98 percent depending upon the organ transplanted. Table 13–1 lists the survival rates for pediatric patients and their grafts (United Network for Organ Sharing [UNOS] Bulletin 1996a). Although the shortage of organ donors continues to be a major problem for infants and small children, more than 1,500 children undergo organ transplantation in the United States every year (UNOS Bulletin 1996b,c). Organ transplantation in children has evolved from an experimental surgical procedure to an accepted therapeutic modality for end-stage disease.

Organ transplantation is the complex surgical procedure performed in children with life-threatening conditions as a result of failure of a particular organ. The three most prevalent organ transplant procedures available for children are heart, liver, and kidney replacement, although lung transplant procedures in the pediatric population are increasing, especially in those patients with cystic fibrosis. The clinical manifestations for end-stage heart, lung, kidney, and liver disease in children are listed in Table 13–2. Bone marrow and peripheral stem cell transplants are discussed in Chapter 12.

The purpose of this chapter is primarily to discuss the home care needs of children who have undergone the most common organ transplants.

It begins with a brief overview of the transplant evaluation process, discusses current immunosuppressive agents, and concludes with the general nursing care plan for the child post-transplant.

TRANSPLANT EVALUATION

The evaluation process for organ transplantation is relatively similar for all transplants, with a slight variation among organs (Table 13–3). The primary purpose of the evaluation process is to identify which patients would benefit from organ transplantation and to confirm the child's diagnosis. Indicators for pediatric organ transplantation are listed in Table 13–4. In addition to the clinical manifestations as indicators for organ transplantation, the decision to transplant must be further evaluated regarding the natural history of the disease and natural timing for the transplant, at what point the patient was referred to the transplant center, the severity of the illness, the availability of donors, the patient's support systems, and the patient's and family's ability to comply with the post-transplant regimen (Lake 1993; Roberts et al. 1989).

Contraindications to pediatric organ transplant are controversial and may vary among transplant centers. In general, contraindications are divided into two categories—absolute and relative contraindications. Absolute contraindications typically include human immunodeficiency virus (HIV) seropositivity, systemic ma-

Table 13–1 One-Year Survival Rates for Patient and Graft, Total Number of Pediatric Transplants Performed, and Number of Pediatric Patients on the United Network for Organ Sharing Waiting Lists as of June 30, 1996

Organ	One-Year Survival Rates for Pediatric Patients (1993)	One-Year Pediatric Survival Rates for Graft (1993)	Total Number of Pediatric Transplants Performed in 1995	Total Number of Pediatric Patients on Waiting Lists as of June 30, 1996
Kidney			700	589
cadaveric	94.1%	83.2%		
living donor	97.3%	91.9%		
Liver	81.6%	73.4%	492	653
Heart	82.3%	81.5%	275	195
Lung	76.9%	75.9%	66	722
Pancreas	91.9%	73.8%	0	10

lignancy, inability to comply with the immuno-suppressive regimen after the transplant, active substance abuse, active infection, sepsis, and documented anatomic anomalies that preclude transplantation. Relative contraindications are highly variable among organs transplanted. In general, relative contraindications might include advanced cardiac or pulmonary disease, acute renal failure, advanced malnutrition, localized malignancy, hepatitis B virus infection, chronic hepatitis C infection, or severe psychosocial problems.

Because decisions regarding indications, timing, and appropriateness of organ transplantation are complex and often controversial, most programs use a multidisciplinary selection committee to assist in the patient selection decisions (Klintmalm and Moore 1985). The purpose of

Table 13–2 Comparative Clinical Manifestations of End-Stage Heart, Lung, Kidney, and Liver Disease

Heart	Lung	Kidney	Liver
Tachypnea	Cyanosis	Electrolyte imbalances	Hepatomegaly
Congestive heart failure	Severe respiratory distress	Hyperkalemia	Portal hypertension
Respiratory distress	Growth retardation	Hypokalemia	Jaundice
Growth retardation	Pulmonary fibrosis	Sodium retention	Ascities
Arrhythmias	Primary pulmonary hypertension	Metabolic acidosis	Hypoalbuminemia
Heart murmurs		Congestive heart failure	Hypoprothrombinemia
Possible cyanosis		Anemia	Splenomegaly
Cardiomegaly		Hyperlipidemia	Hypoglycemia
Tachycardia		Hyperglycemia	Hormone imbalance
		Growth retardation	Hepatic encephalopathy
(see Chapter 7)		Renal osteodystrophy	Puritis
		Peripheral neuropathy	Dyspnea
			Increased liver function tests
		(see Chapter 10)	Leukopenia

Note: This list contains some of the common manifestations of end-stage disease. The list is not all inclusive.

the multidisciplinary process is often three-fold—(1) to confirm the etiology of the disease, assess disease progression, and determine whether medical therapy is available; 2) to verify indications for organ transplant, and the patient's and family's desire for transplantation; and 3) to identify any related disorders or contraindications to transplant. During the evaluation process, it is imperative that time be allowed to provide the patient and family with education and support regarding organ transplantation, long-term management, follow-up, and expectations. Although the evaluation process may be conducted on an outpatient basis, many children are hospitalized because of the severity of their illness or the need for additional testing.

Before organ transplantation and during the evaluation process, attempts are made to optimize the child's clinical status with particular attention to growth and achievement of developmental milestones. It is not uncommon for infants and children on waiting lists to require supplemental nutrition (for example, tube feedings).

The transplant candidate is generally presented to the multidisciplinary selection committee after the evaluation is completed. If the committee decides the individual is an acceptable candidate, the patient will be activated on the UNOS transplant list and wait for a donor. Patients are placed on the list for the transplant based on the priority system established by UNOS. This list varies among organs and takes into consideration the organ to be transplanted, clinical status of the child, blood type, length of time the child has been on the list, and immunologic markers. Table 13–1 shows the number of pediatric patients waiting for organ transplantation.

A general immunologic evaluation consists of two broad categories—typing and crossmatching. Typing procedures allow for pretransplant identification of specific antigens and human leukocyte antigen (HLA) typing. Matching procedures allow donor and recipient antigens to in-

Table 13–3 General Pediatric Evaluation for Potential Organ Transplant

Complete History and Physical	Routine Laboratory Tests	Immunologic Tests
Etiology of disease	Complete blood count with	Blood type (ABO)
Associated disorders	differential PT, PTT, platelets	Tissue typing
Previous illness and surgeries	Electrolytes, calcium,	Crossmatching
Height, weight, head circumference (infants and children)	phosphorus, magnesium, BUN, creatinine, uric acid, total protein, albumin, AST, ALT, GGT, alkaline,	
Medications	phosphatase, bilirubin, glucose,	
Diet history and nutritional evaluation	ammonia, amylase, serum vitamin A, D, E levels	

Note: Evaluations vary at all transplant centers. HIV, human immunodeficiency virus; CMV, cytomegalovirus; EBV, Epstein-Barr virus; RPR, rapid plasma reagin, syphilis; PPD, purified-protein derivative; PT, prothrombin time; PPT, partial prothromboplastin time; BUN, blood urea nitrogen; AST, asparte aminotransferase; ALT, alanine aminotransferase; GGT, gamma-glutamyl transpeptidase; ECG, electrocardiography.

teract before transplantation to ascertain the degree of compatibility. Crossmatching can be performed between recipient and a specific donor or a panel of random donors (Smith 1991). Matching procedures include white-cell crossmatch, mixed lymphocyte crossmatch, and mixed leukocyte culture.

The transplant evaluation process is often a difficult and stressful time for many children and their families. The type of support and education may depend on whether the child has had a long history of illness or presents with an emergent condition. Many of these children will be receiving some type of home health intervention (for example, oxygen, peritoneal dialysis, nutrition support, etc.).

IMMUNOSUPPRESSIVE AGENTS

The primary function of the human immune system is to protect the host against foreign substances. If an invader is identified by the host, the immune system mounts a response that at-

tacks and eliminates the intruder. If the foreign invader is a transplanted organ, this response can lead to rejection of the transplanted graft. Therefore, the success of organ transplantation depends upon the successful alteration of the immune system.

Currently, immunosuppressive medications are administered to alter the immune response and preserve graft function. Thus, rendering the immunosuppressive therapy post-transplant is critical to patient and graft survival. However, because immunosuppressive agents alter the immune response, the ability of the host to respond to other invading foreign substances, such as pathogens, is also compromised. As a result, immunosuppressive drugs are often considered double-edged swords, in that they are able to modulate the immune system to prevent rejection, yet they also can place the host at risk for infection and/or malignancies.

The goal in organ transplantation is to attain immunologic tolerance of the allograft in an immunocompromised host. Immunologic toler-

Infectious Disease Evaluation	Radiologic Procedures	Additional Studies	Additional Consults
Blood, urine, throat, sputum, stool, ascites fluid for bacterial, viral, fungal, and parasitic organisms	Chest radiograph Magnetic resonance imaging (MRI) Computerized tomography (CT) Angiography Ultrasound	ECG Cardiac catheterization Echocardiogram Endoscopy and colonoscopy Pulmonary function test Arterial blood gases Organ biopsy	Anesthesia Transplant nurse coordinator Financial counselor Exercise physiologist or physical therapist Dental Gynecology (sexually active adolescents) Social worker Psychiatrist Child life services Religious counselor
HIV Hepatitis screen A, B, C, B delta Serologies (CMV, EBV, toxoplasmosis, herpes simplex/zoster, varicella) RPR (syphilis) PPD			

ance is a state in which the host does not recognize a specific antigen as foreign—in this case, the transplanted organ (Bartucci and Seller 1990). Although methods of immunologic tolerance post-transplant are currently being investigated, it has yet to be achieved.

Immunosuppressive protocols vary among transplant centers, considering organs transplanted, physician preference, and the specific considerations for each child. However, most centers use a combination of the following agents for induction and long-term maintenance therapy: antithrombocyte globulin (ATG), muromonab-CD3 (Orthoclone OKT3), prednisone, azathioprine (Imuran), cyclosporine (Sandimmune), Neoral, mycophenalate moffitil (Cellcept), and tacrolimus (Prograf).

Rejection is typically treated with prednisone, solu-Medrol, tacrolimus, ATG, or OKT3. Antibiotics, antivirals, and antifungals are also administered post-transplant to prevent the risk of infection. See Table 13–5 for individual immunosuppressive agents and common medications administered after transplantation.

Before discharge, parents should be able to discuss medications regarding purpose, administration, side effects, and missed doses. This educational process should be continued by the home care nurse. Discharge teaching varies from center to center. The child's length of stay, the parent's availability for teaching, and the particular therapy will affect the process.

DISCHARGE PLANNING AND HOME CARE NEEDS OF THE PEDIATRIC PATIENT RECIPIENT

When a child is discharged from the hospital after transplantation, collaboration and communication among the primary pediatrician, transplant center, and the home health and infusion agency are mandatory to ensure optimal care and outcome for the child and family. Although the child's length of stay in the hospital varies among centers and considering organ transplanted, the general overall considerations are the same. Some transplant centers in heavily managed care markets have instituted early discharge programs for pediatric organ transplant patients. Although there are many aspects of care regarding the child post-transplant, two of the most important considerations are rejection and infection. Signs and symptoms of rejection and routine surveillance vary among organs. The following is a brief overview of rejection and infection in the child after the transplant.

Rejection Post-Transplant

Rejection post–organ transplant is an immunologic response that is not completely understood. It generally does not occur when genetically identical individuals are involved, only when genetically nonidentical participants are involved (Smith 1991). Rejection is initiated by the recognition of foreign antigens on the membranes of transplanted tissue (Ascher, Hanto, and Simmons, 1989). The host recognizes these antigens expressed on donor cells as foreign by recipient lymphocytes and antibodies. After this recognition, the host attacks and damages the antigen-expressing graft, the donor organ.

Rejection is often classified according to the primary cell type mediating the response and the histopathologic characteristics of the donor organ observed on biopsy. There are three main types of rejection—hyperacute, acute, and chronic (Table 13–6). Acute rejection is the most common type of rejection occurring in transplant recipients. Diagnosis varies depending upon the organ transplanted; however, it is usually based on graft dysfunction as demonstrated by laboratory findings, clinical manifestations, and biopsy results. Treatment varies among organs transplanted, patients, and transplant centers. Depending upon the severity and organ involved, acute rejection is often initially treated with additional corticosteroids.

Chronic rejection develops months to years post-transplant and is histologically and clinically characterized differently in different organs transplanted. Chronic rejection has an insidious onset that progresses over time. In most cases, there is no treatment with the exception of retransplantation. However, kidney transplant patients may consider resuming dialysis.

Table 13–4 Comparative Disease Indications for Transplantation in Children by Organ (Heart, Lung, Kidney, Liver, and Combined Transplant)

Heart	Lung	Kidney	Liver	Combined Transplant
Congenital heart defects (see Chapter 7)	Cystic fibrosis (see Chapter 5)	Metabolic disorders	Cholestatic disease	Heart and liver Intrahepatic biliary atresia and dilated Cardiomyopathy
		Primary oxalosis	Biliary atresia	
		Cystinosis	Primary biliary cirrhosis	
	Bronchopulmonary dysplasia (see Chapter 4)	Nephrocalcinosis		
Cardiomyopathy (idiopathic, viral, valvular)		Amyloidosis	Secondary biliary cirrhosis	
			Primary sclerosing cholangitis	Heart and lung
		Congenital disease	Familial cholestatic syndrome	Cystic fibrosis
Coronary artery disease	Congenital lung defects	Hypoplasia		Primary pulmonary Hypertension
		Dysplasia		Congenital heart defects with increased pulmonary vasular resistance
		Obstructive uropathy	Alagille syndrome	
Myocardial tumor	Idiopathic pulmonary fibrosis		Byler's syndrome	
		Acquired disease	(also see Chapter 8)	
Heart failure (chemotherapy or radiation therapy induced)	Eisenmenger's disease	Toxic nephropathy (lead and drugs)		Liver and kidney
		Glomerulonephritis		Cystinosis
	Bronchiolitis obliterans		Acute fulminant Hepatic failure	Oxalosis
		(also see Chapter 10)		
	Bronchiectasis		Hepatitis	Kidney and pancreas End-stage renal disease
Life-threatening arrhythmias				Chronic dialysis and Type I diabetes mellitus (also see Chapter 9)
			Metabolic disorders	
Intractible angina			Wilson's disease	
			Reye's syndrome	
Thromboembolic events			Glycogen storage disease	
			Tyrosinemia	
			Vascular disease Budd-Chiari syndrome	

Note: This list contains some of the common indications for organ transplant. The list is not all inclusive.

Infection Post-Transplant

Although there have been many advances in organ transplantation, infection continues to be a major problem. Approximately 75 percent of all organ transplant patients will experience one infectious episode during the first year after transplant, and infection remains the principal cause of death in the transplant population (Rubin and Young 1994). The high incidence of infection post-transplant is largely related to the administration of immunosuppressive therapy.

Table 13–5 Immunosuppressive Agents Used in Transplantation[*]

Immunosuppressive Agent	Primary Mechanism of Action	Use	Oral or IV	Major Side Effects (All Increase Risk of Infection and Rejection)
Azathioprine (Imuran)	6-Mercaptopurine antimetabolite, which interferes with DNA and RNA synthesis; inhibits proliferation of cells	Induction and maintenance	Oral and IV	Bone marrow suppression, leukopenia, anemia, thrombocytopenia, alopecia, hepatic dysfunction, gastric upset
Cyclophosphamide (Cytoxan)	Interferes with DNA, RNA, and protein synthesis; is an alkylating agent	Maintenance	Oral	Leukopenia, thrombocytopenia, gastric disturbance, hemorrhagic cystitis
Prednisone Prednisolone (Deltasone)	Inhibits production of IL-1 and IL-2; inhibits lymphocytes' ability to mount an immune response; inhibits inflammatory response	Induction and maintenance; treat rejection	Oral and IV	Early: cushingoid, hyperglycemia, increased appetite, sodium and water retention, delayed healing, acne, night sweats, hypertension, diaphoresis, pancreatitis, emotional disturbances, mood alterations, headache, insomnia
				Later: ulcer disease, growth retardation, easy bruising, steroid-induced diabetes, avascular joint necrosis, osteoporosis, muscle weakness, cataracts, fragile skin
Methylprednisolone (Solu-Medrol)	Same as prednisone, more potent	Treat rejection	IV	Same as prednisone
Cyclosporine (Sandimmune)	Inhibits synthesis of IL-2; inhibits cytotoxic T-cell precurers; prevents gamma-interferon	Induction and maintenance	Oral or IV	Nephrotoxicity, hyperkalemia, hypomagnesemia, hypertension, hepatoxicity, headaches, gingival

[*] Immunosuppressive management varies between transplant center protocol and organ transplanted.

continues

Table 13–5 continued

Immunosuppressive Agent	Primary Mechanism of Action	Use	Oral or IV	Major Side Effects (All Increase Risk of Infection and Rejection)
	secretion and B-cell activating factors			hyperplasia, hirsutism, nausea, vomiting, diarrhea, mild anemia, flushing, tremors, paresthesias, muscle weakness, seizures
Tacrolimus (Prograf/FK506)	Inhibits IL-1 lymphocyte proliferation, cytotoxic T-cell generation, IL-3, and gamma-interferon	Induction and maintenance; treat rejection	Oral or IV	Renal insufficiency, diarrhea, nausea, vomiting, hyperglycemia, hyperkalemia, hypertension, alopecia, anorexia, anemia, thrombocytopenia, headaches, tremor, insomnia, seizures
Cellcept (mycophenalate moffitil)	Inhibits 5'-monophosphate dehydrogenase (IMPDH), which regulates the growth rate of rapidly proliferating cells	Induction and maintenance	Oral	Gastrointestinal: nausea/vomiting/diarrhea, recurring ulcers, anorexia; slight elevation of alkaline phosphatase; does not cause nephrotoxicity, hepatotoxicity, or bone marrow depression
Antithrombocyte globulin (ATG)	Polyclonal preparation; inhibits activity and number of lymphocytes	Induction; treat rejection	IV with pre-meds	Thrombocytopenia, leukopenia, anemia, serum sickness, hypersensitivity response, arthralgias, myalgias
Muromonab-CD3 (Orthoclone OKT3)	Monoclonal preparation binds to CD3 complex on the surface of T cells; inhibits activity and increases removal of T lymphocytes	Induction; treat rejection	IV push with pre-meds	Flulike symptoms, fever, chills, arthralgias, myalgias, nausea, vomiting, dyspnea, wheezing, chest pain, pulmonary edema, aseptic meningitis, hypersensitivity response

* Immunosuppressive management varies between transplant center protocol and organ transplanted.

continues

Table 13–5 continued

Immunosuppressive Agent	Therapeutic Class	Use	Oral or IV	Major Side Effects
Common Medications Administered after Transplantation				
Ganciclovir (Cytovene)	Antiviral	CMV infection induction and maintenance	IV	Neutropenia, thrombocytopenia, anemia, eosinophilia, retinal detachment, headache, confusion, increased liver function tests
Acyclovir (Zovirax)	Antiviral	HSV 1 and HSV 2 infections; herpes zoster; varicella-zoster; induction and maintenance	Oral and IV	Nephrotoxicity, phlebitis at the injection site, headache, lethargy, tremulousness, dizziness, nausea and vomiting, increased liver function, enzymes, bone marrow depression
Nystatin (Mycostatin)	Antifungal	Cutaneous, monocutaneous, and oral cavity fungal infections	Cream, ointment, powder, oral suspension, troches	Irritation, contact dermatitis, nausea, vomiting, diarrhea
Clotrimazole (Lotrimin, Mycelex)	Antifungal	Fungal infections	Cream, lotion, troches	Mild burning, irritation, stinging to skin or vaginal area, abnormal liver function tests, nausea, vomiting
Nifedipine (Procardia)	Antihypertensive	Hypertrophic cardiomyopathy and hypertension	Capsule (liquid fill), tablet	Dizziness, flushing, hypotension, tachycardia, palpitations, peripheral edema, nausea, diarrhea, thrombocytopenia, leukopenia, anemia
Ranitidine (Zantac)	Antacid/ histamine blocker	Duodenal ulcers and gastric hypersecretory states	Oral, IM, and IV	Headache, dizziness, sedation, malaise, constipation, nausea and vomiting, rash, hepatitis, arthralgias, increased serum creatinine

* Immunosuppressive management varies between transplant center protocol and organ transplanted.

continues

Table 13–5 continued

Immunosuppressive Agent	Therapeutic Class	Use	Oral or IV	Major Side Effects
Furosemide (Lasix)	Antihypertensive/diuretic	Edema associated with CHF, liver or kidney disease, hypertension	Oral suspension, tablets, IM and IV	Hypokalemia, hyponatremia, hypochloremia, alkalosis, dehydration, potential ototoxicity, nausea, diarrhea, dizziness
Hydralazine hydrochloride (Apresoline)	Antihypertensive	Moderate to severe hypertension and CHF	Oral, IM, and IV	Headache, palpitation, flushing, tachycardia, anorexia, nausea and vomiting, diarrhea, weakness, fever, rash, malaise, arthralgias, salt and water retention, dyspnea on exertion
Metronidazole (Flagyl)	Anti-infective, antiprotozoal	Anaerobic and protozoal infections	Oral and IV	Headache, metallic taste, nausea, dry mouth, diarrhea, peripheral neuropathy, dizziness, confusion, rash, thrombophlebitis, "furry" tongue, leukopenia, seizures

* Immunosuppressive management varies between transplant center protocol and organ transplanted.

Note: DNA, deoxyribonucleic acid; RNA, ribonucleic acid; IL-1, interleukin-1; IL-2, interleukin-2; IL-3, interleukin-3; CD3 complex, subset of total T-cell count; HSV 1, herpes simplex virus 1; HSV 2, herpes simplex virus 2; CHF, congestive heart failure; IM, intramuscular; IV, intravenous; CMV, cytomegalovirus.

Immunosuppressive therapy, for the prevention and treatment of rejection, alters the immune system, leaving the host vulnerable to infection. The goal in organ transplantation is to provide adequate immunosuppression to prevent rejection and simultaneously maintain host defense mechanisms. There is an inverse relationship between rejection and infection, and the balance of this relationship must be weighed carefully for each child. For example, the more immunosuppressive therapy administered to prevent rejection, the greater the risk of infection. Less immunosuppressive therapy decreases the chance of infection but promotes the risk of rejection.

Transplant patients are at the greatest risk for acquiring opportunistic infections. Opportunistic refers to the ability of a mildly virulent organism to cause disease in the presence of an altered immune state (Young 1994). Most of these organisms are naturally present on the skin and in the gastrointestinal tract, or are innocuous substances in the environment.

The risk of infection and the "break down" in protective mechanisms for the organ transplant recipient is based on a number of considerations, the most important being immunosuppressive therapy. Other factors that contribute to the transplant recipient's risk of infection include exposures to microorganisms in the home and

Table 13–6 Types of Transplant Rejection

Type of Rejection	Etiology
Hyperacute: occurs in the surgical suite, graft prognosis poor	• Primary humoral B lymphocyte response • Caused by preformed cytotoxic antibodies against donor HLA antigens
Acute: occurs five days to four months. Treatment is with corticosteroids	• Primary cellular T-lymphocyte response with accompanying B-lymphocyte response
Chronic: occurs months to years after transplant. No treatment, graft failure ensues	• Primary humoral B-lymphocyte response with accompanying T-lymphocyte response

hospital environment, alteration in normal microbial flora, break in the skin or mucous membranes, administration of antibiotics or antacids, decreased gastric motility, poor nutritional status, hyperglycemia, preexisting disease, diminished or absent splenic function, invasive tubes, intravenous devices, procedures, length of time on a ventilator, and the presence of one of the immune modulating viruses (Epstein-Barr virus [EBV], cytomegalovirus [CMV], hepatitis B or C, and HIV) (Rubin and Tolkoff-Rubin 1993; Rubin and Young 1994; Smith, 1991). Infections in organ transplantation are classified considering the following: type of infection, time of infection, and site of infection. Types of infections are categorized as bacterial, viral, fungal, and parasitic (Table 13–7). Time of infection is classified by considering when the infection is likely to occur post-transplant (for example, the first month, one to six months, or six months, as outlined in Table 13–8) (Johnson and Flye, 1989; Rubin 1988; Rubin and Young 1994). Fre-

quent sites of infection in the child post-transplant are listed in Exhibit 13–1. The following is a review of the more common infections found in children post-transplant.

Clostridium difficile is a common cause of diarrhea and abdominal cramps in most organ transplant recipients. Although diarrhea can be the result of many etiologies (for example, antibiotics, cyclosporine, and other infections), *C. difficile* must be considered. Diagnosis is based on a stool specimen or *C. difficile* toxin and culture. Treatment consists of oral vancomycin or Flagyl for 10 to 14 days with a follow-up including study of a stool specimen.

Viral infections can be a serious complication post-transplant. Viral infections commonly observed include the herpes group of viruses, herpes simplex 1 and 2, CMV, varicella-zoster, EBV, and viral hepatitis.

Viruses enter the host by close cell-to-cell contact. Upon entering the host, viral deoxyribonucleic acid (DNA) penetrates host nuclei and begins viral protein synthesis and replication. Viral maturation and proliferation occur in host nuclei, rendering viruses dependent on host cells for survival. Once an individual has experienced a primary viral infection, he or she is infected for life even after there is no longer active replication or clinical symptoms. Viruses generally enter the host through the mucous membranes, proliferate, cause active infection, and then set up permanent residence. Viruses usually remain latent in either the lymphocyte pool or sensory ganglia. Viruses are protected from antiviral antibodies because antibodies do not permeate host cells (Smith and Ciferni 1990).

CMV is the most common viral infection affecting organ transplant recipients and is a major cause of all morbidity and mortality. Although all viruses can be considered potentially oncogenic, EBV has specifically been associated with EBV-mediated lymphoproliferative disease (Ho et al. 1988; Nalesnik et al. 1988).

Most viral infections present with fluctuating fever, malaise, fatigue, arthralgias, myalgias, and anorexia. On physical examination, lymphadenopathy is generally observed; however,

Table 13–7 Comparative Infections Observed Post-Transplant

Viral	Bacterial	Fungal	Parasitic
Cytomegalovirus (CMV)	Pseudomonas	Candida	Toxoplasmosis
Epstein-Barr virus (EBV)	*Escherichia coli*	Aspergillus	*Strongyloides*
Herpes (HSV 1, HSV 2)	Klebsiella	Histoplasmosis	*stercoralis*
Varicella-zoster (VSV)	Legionella	Coccidioides	
Hepatitis	*Clostridium difficile*	Cryptococcus	
Human immunodeficiency	Tuberculosis	*Pneumocystis*	
virus (HIV)	*Streptococcus pneumoniae*	*carinii*	
Influenza A and other RNA	Staphylococcus	Nocardia	
viruses			
Papovavirus			
Adenovirus			
Influenza virus			

there is an absence of splenomegaly. Laboratory evaluation may reveal leukopenia, thrombocytopenia, or superinfection. Viruses also can have a suppressive effect on host defense mechanisms that can render the host susceptible to opportunistic superinfection, rejection, and may subsequently cause allograft damage.

Diagnosis is often based on clinical manifestations, serology, and viral culture. Viremia can be detected several days before clinical symptoms appear. Management of the post-transplant recipient with viremia has two approaches—the prevention of infection and disease, and the treatment of disease. Strategies used to prevent

Table 13–8 Timetable Approach to Infection Post-Transplant

One Month Post-Transplant	One to Six Months Post-Transplant	Six Months or More Post-Transplant
Exacerbation of infection before transplant (for example, herpes)	High immunosuppressive dosages enhance onset of opportunistic infections	Most infections acquired from community (for example, respiratory viruses)
Acquisition from the donor (for example, CMV)	Acquisition of viruses, fungi, or antibiotic-resistant bacteria	Opportunistic infections from excessive acute or chronic immunosuppression
Technical complications (for example, pneumonia, line sepsis)	Technical complications (for example, drains, line sepsis) and risk of superinfection	Infections in patients afflicted with recurrent problems (for example, cholangitis, URI)

Note: URI, upper respiratory infection.

Source: Adapted from Rubin and Young 1994.

Exhibit 13–1 Frequent Sites of Infection in the Pediatric Patient Post-Transplant

Respiratory tract	Heart
Gastrointestinal tract	Biliary tree
Surgical wound	Bladder
Blood	

viruses, particularly CMV, vary considerably among transplant centers. Generally, prevention involves one or a combination of the following: (1) using seronegative blood products, (2) minimizing the use of seropositive donors in seronegative recipients, (3) administering prophylactic intravenous ganciclovir during the immediate postoperative period and during rejection episodes, (4) administering high-dose oral acyclovir for two to six months post-transplant, and (5) administering prophylactic intravenous immunoglobulin (IVIG). Occasionally, granulocyte colony–stimulating factor (GCSF) may be prescribed to enhance cell development in the severely leukopenic child.

EBV is the same virus responsible for infectious mononucleosis. In a normal host, EBV disease is initiated by infecting epithelial cells of the upper respiratory tract and B lymphocytes. Immunologic surveillance in a normal host provides EBV-specific cytotoxic T cells that prevent lymphoproliferation. After transplant, this immune mechanism has been suppressed in recipients and an outgrowth of B lymphocytes occurs, resulting in lymphoproliferation. Thus EBV is not only associated with persistent infection, it is also strongly associated with lymphoproliferative malignancies (lymphoma). Clinical disease states range from asymptomatic infection, to symptoms associated with mononucleosis, to fatal lymphoproliferative disease (Rubin and Young 1994). Diagnosis of viral reactivation is generally based on clinical manifestations, serial increases in antibody titers, and biopsy findings. Treatment for EBV infection is intravenous acyclovir or ganciclovir.

EBV-mediated lymphoproliferative disease (LPD) can be one of the most devastating complications post-transplant. Approximately 10 to 15 percent of all malignancies that develop in post-transplant recipients are a form of lymphoma (Rubin 1988). Those children who have intense immunosuppressive therapy including antilymphocyte antibody preparations in conjunction with triple therapy (prednisone, azathioprine, and cyclosporine) are generally considered to be at risk for developing this complication. Home health care of these children should incorporate close monitoring for this complication, which would include assessment for the following: clinical manifestations of unexplained fever; mononucleosis-like symptoms demonstrated by fever, arthralgias, myalgias, malaise, and lymphadenopathy; persistent upper respiratory congestion similar to allergies; gastrointestinal (GI) manifestations (for example, GI bleeding, abdominal pain and cramps, splenomegaly, perforation, or obstruction); hepatic dysfunction; and central nervous system symptoms such as seizures, alteration in consciousness, and focal disease (Ho et al. 1988; Rosenthal et al. 1994).

Diagnosis of LPD is generally made by biopsy to the transplanted organ and/or affected tissue. Pathologic observations of LPD occur in a range of histologic findings. These findings are classified as polymorphic B-cell lymphoma and range from nonspecific reactivity to malignancy (for example, nonspecific reactive hyperplasia, polymorphic B-cell hyperplasia, polymorphic B-cell lymphoma, and immunoblastic sarcoma). Although computerized tomography (CT) or magnetic resonance imaging (MRI) scanning can be helpful in making the diagnosis of LPD, the absence of adenopathy on scan does not rule out the presence of LPD, because this disease can occur completely extranodally (Stephman et al. 1991; Hanto et al. 1981).

Treatment of LPD usually consists of strictly reducing or withdrawing immunosuppressive therapy. High-dose intravenous acyclovir or ganciclovir is typically added to the treatment regimen. Other treatment approaches have included one or a combination of the following: B-cell monoclonal antibody, interferon alpha and intravenous immunoglobulin, radiotherapy, surgical resection, and antilymphoma chemotherapy. Emphasis must be placed on prevention including antiviral prophylactic therapy and antiviral therapy during intensive immunosuppression (for example, rejection episode) to minimize the evolution of EBV-mediated LPD (Rubin and Young 1994; Fisher et al. 1990). In stable children, long-term (up to a year) intravenous therapy may be necessary. Home nursing considerations include parent and patient education and return demonstration for the preparation and administration of the medication, including instruction of the electronic infusion device, venous access device care and maintenance, troubleshooting, and signs and symptoms that warrant contacting the physician.

Candidal species are the most common fungi observed after transplant in patients, with *Candida albicans* being the most frequently observed organism. *Candida* fungi prefer moist, warm areas and are ordinarily found on diseased skin, throughout the gastrointestinal tract, and in the perianal area (Rubin and Young 1994). The most frequently observed manifestation of candidal infections in the transplant recipient is from monocutaneous overgrowth secondary to immunosuppressive therapy. Clinical examples of candidal infections include oropharyngeal thrush, candidal esophagitis, vulvovaginitis, urinary tract candidiasis, and disseminated fungal infections.

The most common manifestations of *Candida albicans* in children is thrush, which occurs as a white, plaquelike covering over the mucous membranes either in the mouth or in the diaper area. Surrounding areas, such as the gums or vulva, may become erythematous and painful. If severe, thrush can interfere with oral intake and nutritional status, particularly in young children and infants. Treatment includes a topical antifungal agent such as nystatin or clotrimazole troche three to four times daily. It is imperative that the patient be instructed to swish and swallow nystatin or allow clotrimazole troche to dissolve in his or her mouth. Generally, oral thrush can be avoided with the prophylactic administration of these antifungal agents during episodes of high-dose immunosuppressive therapy (for example, immediately after transplant and during rejection episodes).

NURSING CONSIDERATIONS REGARDING THE CHILD POST-TRANSPLANT

The goals in caring for the child post-transplant are the same for all the members of the multidisciplinary team. They are the following: (1) maintain optimal graft function, (2) prevent infection, (3) prevent rejection, (4) promote adequate nutritional intake and optimal growth, (5) support the family's and child's coping skills, (6) empower parent and patient to provide care, and (7) support the child in achieving his or her developmental milestones.

Patient assessment and parent and patient education are the most important components of home care nursing. Table 13–9 provides a comprehensive general care plan for the child post-transplant. Nursing assessment should include a complete review of all major body systems with particular emphasis placed on the organ transplanted, parent and patient coping responses, and the child's growth and development. Education should include information related to the short- and long-term post-transplant course, prevention of infection and rejection, tests and procedures, home management, oral or intravenous medications, venous access devices, wound care if indicated, individual patient problems (for example, diarrhea, hyperglycemia, hypertension, etc.), and how to access community resources.

With the advent of managed care and the hospital's need to reduce costs, early discharge programs for the pediatric organ transplant patients have begun to emerge. Discharge criteria in such programs are decided upon by the physician and nursing staff, and the home care and infusion agency to appropriately deliver home care services to these patients. The patient is discharged to an alternative site arrangement (a

Table 13-9 Nursing Care Plan for the Child Post-Transplant

Assess	Assessment — Potential Observations
General	Febrility, pain and discomfort, agitation, complaints of feeling ill, changes in emotional response from euphoric to depressed
Renal	Decreased urine output, pain over the kidney (kidney transplant), weight gain, peripheral edema, hypertension, increased serum BUN and creatinine, alteration in electrolytes
Urinary tract	Urine cloudy with possible foul smell, hematuria with/without clots, complaints of lower abdominal pain
Cardiovascular	Hyper/hypotension (check pretransplant BP), changes in heart sounds, peripheral edema, tachycardia
Pulmonary	Decreased breath sounds with crackles in the posterior bases, O$_2$ saturation 92%–94% on room air, increase in respiratory rate and effort
Gastrointestinal	Decreased or absent bowel sounds, mild abdominal distention, pain, nausea, vomiting, diarrhea, constipation, decreased or increased appetite, weight loss or gain
Immune	Wound site has serosanguinous, slightly purulent drainage, change in WBC count, fever, change in laboratory data related to tranplanted organ
Endocrine	Hyper/hypoglycemia

continues

Table 13-9 continued

Nursing Diagnosis	Supportive Findings	Patient Goals	Intervention	Rationale	Expected Outcome	Data
Potential for fluid volume excess: inadequate urinary elimination, steroids	Decreased urine output, increased respiratory effort, pulmonary infiltrates and congestion on radiograph, restlessness, hypertension, peripheral edema, increased weight, intake greater than output	The patient will demonstrate normal fluid balance and remain euvolemic.	Monitor total daily intake and output. Document daily weight with same scale. Monitor blood pressure. Assess jugular distention. Assess and monitor skin turgor and edema. Assess heart sounds. Assess breath sounds.	Provides fluid balance and status that facilitates easy recognition of fluid volume overload	Patient remains euvolemic.	Intake and output are balanced; weight is stable; blood pressure is within normal limits; there is absence of edema; and mucous membranes are moist.
Potential for fluid volume deficit: related to excessive output, diuretic therapy, inadequate fluid administration, vomiting and diarrhea and/or bleeding	Orthostatic or hypotensive, decreased weight, output greater than intake, elevated BUN, poor skin turgor, dry mucous membranes	The patient will obtain adequate fluids to maintain body function.	Monitor total daily intake and output. Document daily weight with same scale. Monitor blood pressure. Assess and monitor skin turgor. Offer fluids if patient on oral diet.	Provide fluid balance and status that facilitate easy recognition of fluid volume deficit.	Patient remains euvolemic.	Intake and output are balanced; weight is stable; blood pressure is within normal limits; there is absence of edema; mucous membranes are moist.

Table 13–9 continued

Nursing Diagnosis	Supportive Findings	Patient Goals	Intervention	Rationale	Expected Outcome	Data
Potential for electrolyte imbalance: related to level of renal function, metabolic disorders associated with acidosis and hyperglycemia, side effects of medications (cyclosporine, steroids)	Elevated BUN and creatinine, elevated potassium, decreased magnesium, decreased urine output, cardiac arrhythmias	Electrolyte balance will be maintained.	Monitor changes in serum electrolytes. Monitor ECG for changes. Assess for physical symptoms of electrolyte imbalance (for example, irritability, hypo/hyperreflexia, weakness, cardiac arrhythmias, seizure activity).	To determine electrolyte imbalance	Electrolytes remain normal; there are no complications related to electrolyte abnormalities.	Electrolytes are maintained within normal limits.
Altered patterns of urinary elimination: related to kidney transplant, infection, diabetic neurogenic bladder	Decreased urine output; inability to void spontaneously; hematuria; cloudy, foul-smelling urine; pain on urination	The patient will resume normal bladder function.	Measure urine output and record. Monitor temperature. Assess catheter; assess wound.	To ensure adequate urination, to avoid bladder distention, identify obstruction and lymphocele, prevent infection	Urine output and patterns of urination are normal.	Patient is able to void spontaneously without pain; there is no evidence of infection.
Potential for ineffective breathing pattern: related to lung transplant	Complaints of shortness of breath, dyspnea, fatigue, decreased breath sounds and crackles on auscultation,	The patient's breathing pattern will be effective without fatigue.	Measure lung breath sounds. Assess for shortness of breath, dyspnea, rales. Assess O_2 saturation	To ensure adequate functioning of the lungs	Pulmonary functions will be WNL.	Patient breathes without difficulty; O_2 saturation is normal; breath sounds are normal.

Nursing Diagnosis	Expected Outcomes	Nursing Interventions	Rationale	Evaluation
pain, excess fluid volume, hypoxemia, decreased lung expansion Late complication: bronchiolitis obliterans; decreased O_2 saturation by arterial blood gas or pulse oximetry	Oxygenation and blood gases will be within normal limits.	by observing nailbeds and mucous membranes.		
Potential for injury: related to organ rejection; Alteration in laboratory results related to the transplanted organ, abnormal biopsy findings, clinical manifestations related to organ transplant	The patient will have no signs of organ rejection.	Monitor for signs and symptoms of graft rejection. Administer immunosuppressive therapy as ordered and monitor patient response. Prepare patient for diagnostic procedures that may indicate rejection (for example, biopsy, echocardiogram). Provide emotional support.	Promotes early detection of graft dysfunction and facilitates prompt intervention that prevents further complications	Injury related to rejection has been minimized or prevented. Patient exhibits no clinical manifestations of rejection and is tolerating immunosuppressive therapy.
Potential for infection: related to alterations in the immune system secondary to; Monitor for signs and symptoms of infection (steroids may mask symptoms of infection) (for example, fever, elevated WBC,	Patients will have no signs and symptoms of infection.	Monitor vital sogns frequently. Monitor and assess CBC and differential. Collect cultures as ordered.	To provide prompt detection of infection and facilitate proper intervention,	There are no signs or symptoms of infection. Patient remains afebrile; vital signs and laboratory work are within normal limits; cultures are

continues

Table 13-9 continued

Nursing Diagnosis	Supportive Findings	Patient Goals	Intervention	Rationale	Expected Outcome	Data
immunosuppressive therapy, presence of invasive lines, and procedures.	decreased platelets, redness, swelling, purulent drainage from incision, pain, increased respiratory effort, cough).		Encourage patient to cough and deep breathe. Assess presence of sputum. Assess and monitor IV lines. Practice universal precautions. Staff caring for immunocompromised patients should not be ill.	and to prevent the patient from infection		negative; chest radiograph is clear; patient does not have a cough; IV lines are free of redness or drainage.
Potential for diarrhea: related to inadequate dietary fiber, medications, or infection	Child is irritable; stools are loose and frequent; there is perianal discomfort; signs and symptoms of dehydration are present.	Stool will be of normal consistency.	Assess abdomen for the presence of distention. Auscultate bowel sounds. Assess appetite. Assess and document episodes of nausea, vomiting, or diarrhea. Encourage adequate fluid intake to prevent dehydration; document frequency and consistency of stool. Assess temperature. Take stool culture.	To promote normal stool formation and minimize dehydration in the infant or child	Patient will resume normal bowel function.	Patient resumes pretransplant bowel function; there is no evidence of bloating, nausea, or vomiting.
Potential body image disturbance: related to medication effects and transplantation	Concerns regarding changes in weight (loss or gain), acne, moon facies, facial hair or loss of hair, incorporation of	The patient will have a positive accepting, realistic body image.	Assess and monitor self-concept. Provide a supportive environment for the patient to discuss concerns and anxieties.	To guide therapeutic intervention and referrals; to establish trust and	Patient has positive accepting, and realistic body image.	Patient expresses integration of body image into sense of self, demonstrates and understand-

	donor organ into sense of self		Prepare patient for medication side effects that may alter his or her appearance. Acknowledge body changes, assist patient to focus on identifying strengths. Direct patient to appropriate resources.	confidence in improving self-image; to minimize "surprises" with physical changes; and to promote positive self-image		ing of physical changes, discusses strategies to improve body image, and reports "feeling better" about physical appearance.
Potential for knowledge deficit: Related to short- and long-term post-transplant course, unfamiliar tests and procedures, home management, medications, venous access devices, rejection, and risk of infection	Patient and family are unable to state medications (side effects, dose schedule, purpose), signs of rejection, how to protect themselves from infection, routine tests and procedures, and care of venous access device.	The patient will have an increased knowledge regarding organ transplantation and be able to perform all activities required to maintain health after transplant.	Establish baseline assessment of cognitive and developmental levels of patient and family readiness and ability to learn. Identify teaching goals and record patient and family responses. Mobilize appropriate community resources as indicated.	To determine patient's pre-existing level of knowledge for development of a realistic teaching plan; to ensure patient and family are able to participate in care in the home, and to provide additional resources to facilitate transition to home care	Patient and family are knowledgeable regarding post–organ transplant care	Patient and family are able to accurately self-administer all medications; state signs and symptoms of rejection and appropriate action to take; demonstrate ability to take temperature, weight, blood pressure, heart rate, blood glucose level as indicated; and provide venous access line care. Patient states post-transplant activities and limitations.

continues

Table 13–9 continued

Nursing Diagnosis	Supportive Findings	Patient Goals	Intervention	Rationale	Expected Outcome	Data
Potential for noncompliance: related to psychosocial problems, adolescents' need to "fit in," body image changes	Adolescents may stop taking the medications that have altered their body images.	Patient will be compliant in post-transplant care	Provide a supportive environment for the patient to discuss concerns and anxieties. Prepare patient for medication side effects that may alter his or her appearance. Acknowledge body changes; assist patient to focus on identifying strengths. Direct patient to appropriate resources.	To determine if the patient is compliant with post-transplant care in the face of peer pressure	Patient has positive, accepting, and realistic body image and all aspects of care post-transplant are being followed, especially in the adolescent.	Patient medications are accounted for; no signs of infection or rejection are present.
Potential for IV line problems: related to immunosuppressive therapy and the increased risk of infection	Redness, drainage, swelling, and pain at IV site	Patient and family will understand and demonstrate aseptic technique with all line care.	Instruct patient and family in line care maintenance (flushes, dressing changes) (see Chapter 8). Instruct patient and family in taking patient's temperature. Instruct patient and family in signs and symptoms of infection and whom to contact if observed.	To provide prompt detection of infection and to facilitate proper intervention, and to prevent infection	The intravenous line will be free of signs and symptoms of infection.	Patient and family are able to discuss and demonstrate aseptic line care (flushing the intravenous line with normal saline before and after the administration of a medication and/or flushing the intravenous line with heparin

to keep it patent between uses, and changing dressings to the intravenous site), state signs and symptoms of infection, and demonstrate ability to take temperature and appropriate actions to take.

Note: BUN, blood urea nitrogen; BP, blood pressure; WBC, white blood cell; ECG, electrocardiogram; WNL, within normal limits; O_2, oxygen; CBC, complete blood count; IV, intravenous.

Patient Teaching Plan

1. Teach patient and family the post-transplant routine.
2. Teach patient and family all medications including purpose, side effects, dose schedule, route of administration, and frequency.
3. Teach patient and family the basic laboratory values that will be monitored (for example, BUN, creatinine, electrolytes, liver function tests).
4. Teach patient/family the signs and symptoms of rejection, and appropriate actions to take.
5. Teach patient/family the signs and symptoms of infection, importance of monitoring and actions to take.
6. Teach patient/family type and purpose of dietary restriction, if any.
7. Teach patient/family the amount and type of fluid to drink.
8. Teach patient/family the importance of skin care, sunscreen, and acne prophylaxis in preventing complications.
9. Teach patient/family the importance of routine dental care.
10. Teach family planning, use of contraceptives and birth control, and risks of pregnancy.
11. Teach the importance of exercise and encourage regular activity.
12. Teach health maintenance skills and encourage a return demonstration (e.g., temperature, weight, pulse, BP, glucose monitoring, wound care).
13. Teach patient/family venous access device care, troubleshooting line problems, and infusion device.
14. Teach the patient/family the importance of regular follow-up health care and laboratory tests.
15. Provide the family with information about organ transplantation and local agencies.
16. Teach the usefulness in keeping a log of the disease course, treatment, and other disease related information.
17. Teach the patient/family the importance of carrying medical alert information at all times.
18. Provide the patient/family with information regarding financial, psychological, and rehabilitative resources.

combination of clinic, home and hotel, and infusion center) and receives infusion therapies (for example, total parenteral nutrition, antibiotics, anti-rejection medications, etc.) by parent or nurse, depending on several criteria (for example, blood products should be given by the nurse). Appropriate assessment and teaching skills of patient and family are essential for comprehensive care. In many cases, the patient or family member can be taught to administer intravenous therapies at home. It is of paramount importance that the home care nurse be skilled in the care of pediatric organ transplant patients. The clinical signs of organ rejection may be minimal or subtle, and it can be difficult to distinguish rejection from infection; in some cases, rejection and infection may coexist (Paradis et al. 1992).

Infection

One of the primary nursing care goals is to protect the child post-transplant from infection. This includes safeguarding the patient from possible sources of infection (for example, ill visitors, construction sites), consistent good handwashing technique, never coming into contact with anyone's blood, pulmonary toilet, consistent patient mobilization, maintaining aseptic technique during dressing changes (see Chapter 8), bladder irrigations and other procedures, knowledge of absolute neutrophil count and instructions to follow when the count is low, administration of antipyretics and antibiotics as ordered, and monitoring fluid status to prevent dehydration, especially in infants. Prompt reporting of the signs and symptoms of infection (for example, fever, swelling, redness, and pain) supports early intervention and management. Communication with personnel from the child's school is important in the identification of potential problems. In situations when the patient has a confirmed infection, educating the patient and family is essential. Wound care may involve teaching aseptic care of drain sites, wound irrigation, wet to dry dressing changes, use of a shower head directed at the wound for circulation, and removal of debris.

Fever

The two causes of fever in the child post-transplant are infection and rejection. To determine the cause, routine cultures are obtained from the urine, sputum, and blood. Laboratory tests and possible biopsy of the transplanted organ are also ordered. If diarrhea is present, stool cultures will be ordered. If there are prominent pulmonary manifestations, a chest radiograph and possibly a bronchial wash may be indicated. Identification of the causative organism before the initiation of antibiotics is the optimal approach to therapy. Because most post-transplant patients are already taking medications that can adversely affect their kidneys, caution must be taken to avoid nephrotoxic antibiotics, if possible.

Pulmonary Complications

Pulmonary complications are often manifested in the early post-transplant period. Atelectasis and pleural effusions result in poor ventilation and oxygenation, increasing the risk of pneumonia. Pulmonary complications are attributed to prolonged anesthesia, paralysis of the diaphragm, and pain. Vigorous pulmonary toilet, pain management, and early and consistent mobilization assist in reversing the effects of pleural effusion and atelectasis, thus preventing pneumonia. The home health nurse should encourage the patient and family in continued mobilization and should assess the pulmonary system regularly to identify potential pulmonary problems.

Hypertension

Hypertension is a common problem that affects the child post-transplant. It may be related to volume, catecholamines, or a side effect of cyclosporine or tacrolimus. Many patients will be placed on oral antihypertensive therapy. The home care nurse plays a vital role in ensuring that patients and parents know how to monitor blood pressure and what actions to take when the blood pressure falls outside the acceptable limits. Blood pressure monitoring should occur at each home care and clinic visit.

Metabolic Complications

Metabolic complications in the child post-transplant can occur during the early or late postoperative period. Hyperglycemia is a common complication early post-transplant, usually secondary to high-dose corticosteroids causing an increase in glucose from the liver. Cyclosporine and tacrolimus (Prograf) also contribute to hyperglycemic states. These patients often need initial insulin therapy, which may be discontinued as high-dose corticosteroids are tapered. The home care nurse is instrumental in monitoring blood glucose levels and instructing the patient and parents to monitor blood glucose levels to facilitate insulin taper schedules. Late complications of high corticosteroid use include metabolic bone disease in the form of osteoporosis and compression fractures.

Growth and Development

Many children who undergo organ transplantation are small for their size because of the effects of their chronic illnesses and the long-term effects of corticosteroids after transplant. The ability of the body to grow post-transplant is influenced by many factors, including the following: the child's age at transplant, the child's potential for growth, the physiologic condition of the child, the dose of corticosteroids, and the adequate functioning of the graft.

Research efforts are focused on growth and development outcomes for children post-transplant. Linear growth and a marked increase in weight have been noted in patients who have undergone heart and kidney transplantation and who survive longer than one year (Pahl et al. 1988; Tejani et al. 1989; Trento et al. 1989). Accelerations in growth after liver transplantation have been reported in children who receive low-dose corticosteroid therapy and cyclosporine (Urbach et al. 1987).

All children post-transplant should have height and weight documented on growth charts at each physician visit to ensure that the child's growth potential is maximized. Table 13–10 is an example of a health maintenance screening schedule for the child after transplant.

Dietary Considerations

End-stage organ failure, regardless of the organ, causes changes in the way the body handles physical and emotional stress. Many children experience excessive weight gain post-transplant. All children should have a dietitian consultation before leaving the hospital to "sketch out" a balanced meal plan that includes all the basic food groups.

Appetites may be significantly affected by medication. Prednisone greatly increases the appetite and causes both sodium and water retention and a redistribution of muscle and fat. Cyclosporine may decrease the appetite and can cause children to be hypertensive. Mouth and throat lesions caused by azathioprine may make eating and/or swallowing painful or difficult.

The post-transplant diet is usually a "no-added salt" diet. Modified or restricted fats are suggested in heart transplant recipients because of the incidence of atherosclerosis. Children younger than two years would be an exception because they need fat for normal tissue and neurologic development.

The child's preferences and dislikes should be noted, and the focus for the patient and family should be on a normal, healthy, and well-rounded diet rather than on strict guidelines. The home care nurse should complete a nutritional assessment at each visit. Teaching the family is especially important so that suggested and acceptable foods and snacks will be brought into the home to help increase compliance with new eating patterns.

Psychosocial Considerations

Short stature, delay in development of secondary sexual characteristics, and other body alterations due to medication can be difficult to devastating for some children and teenagers. Psychosocial support and education regarding

Table 13–10 Health Maintenance Screening Examination Schedule

Type	Frequency
Vision	Yearly examinations should be completed for changes in eyesight, blurred vision, cataracts, or glaucoma from corticosteroids.
Hearing	Audiograms should be completed on an annual basis to evaluate hearing loss from ototoxic drugs.
Dental	Dental examinations should be completed at a minimum of biannually, with prophylactic antibiotics used. Cyclosporine may cause gum hyperplasia.
Blood pressure	Blood pressure should be monitored by the patient and family on a daily basis and at each visit.
Height and weight	Assessments of height and weight should be completed at each visit. Long-term corticosteroids can affect growth.
Breast and testicular examinations	Instruction should be initiated at Tanner stage II.

strategies in managing altered body image can help facilitate coping and social adjustment and minimize the risk of noncompliance.

Weight gain can be significant and can create devastating problems for some children after transplantation. Severe weight gain can result in the loss of positive body image and cause significant depression and noncompliance.

Psychosocial problems after transplantation are often manifested as noncompliance, particularly among teenagers. In general, the adolescent's developmental need to "fit in" with peers and not be "different" is in direct conflict with the continued reminder of his or her chronic illness (for example, daily medications, special precautions). Teenagers may find their appearance disturbing and stop taking their medications.

Anxiety and depression can occur as a result of the transplant, immunosuppressive therapy, or changes in family functioning. The adolescent may experience additional anxiety when there is a transition from the pediatric service to the adult service. Most children post-transplant return to school and work.

Immunizations

Whenever possible, all required immunizations should be given to children before organ transplant surgery because it is not clear whether immunocompromised children can respond adequately to routine vaccines post-transplant (Addonzio and Rose 1987). Post-transplant patients should not receive any live virus vaccine, such as measles, mumps, rubella (MMR), smallpox, or oral polio (OPV). However, inactivated poliovirus vaccine (IPV), diphtheria, tetanus toxoid, pertussis, and hepatitis B vaccines may be given to the child post-transplant.

Children who are exposed to chickenpox must be treated with human varicella-zoster immune globulin (VZIG) within 72 to 92 hours if they do not have a history of varicella as demonstrated by antibody titers. Children who develop lesions after VZIG administration should also receive acyclovir intravenously within 24 hours of eruption of the skin rash and continued for 7 to 10 days (McGregor et al. 1989). The treatment varies among transplant centers, and some centers are treating patients with oral acyclovir for four to six weeks after exposure.

Hepatitis B and *Haemophilus influenzae* are two of the significant causes of decreased graft survival, serious infection, and patient death post-transplant. Patients waiting for organ transplant should be vaccinated with inactivated Hib vaccine (Heptavax-B, Recombivax HB, or Engerix-B) (Committee on Infectious Diseases 1991).

If the child post-transplant is planning a trip to a foreign country that requires immunizations, a

Table 13–11 Immunizations in the Child Post-Transplant

Immunization	Important Information
Measles, mumps, and rubella (MMR)	Transplant recipients should never receive MMR after transplant. It may be given to household members.
Oral polio vaccine (OPV)	Transplant recipients and household members should not receive OPV because vaccine strains are transmissible in stool.
Inactivated poliovirus vaccine (IPV)	Transplant recipients and household members may receive IPV instead of OPV.
Diphtheria, tetanus, toxoid, pertussis (DPT)	Transplant recipients and household members may receive DPT. They can resume interrupted schedule of treatment after transplant.
Hepatitis A and B vaccine	Transplant recipients and household members may receive hepatitis A and hepatitis B vaccine.
Tetanus shot	Transplant recipients and household members may receive tetanus shot. It is generally given every 10 years.
Haemophilus influenzae B (Hib)	Transplant recipients may receive Hib.
Pneumococcal or flu shots	Transplant recipients may receive flu shots.
Tuberculosis (TB) testing using a purified protein derivative (PPD)	Transplant recipients may receive testing using PPD.
Varicella	Transplant recipients should not receive the vaccine. Household members may receive it.

letter may need to be written to the passport bureau stating that the patient cannot receive certain vaccines. Table 13–11 provides information regarding common vaccines in the child post-transplant.

Teen Sexuality and Pregnancy

Surgical interventions before transplant and transplant surgery can leave significant incisional scars on the body. Medication side effects can also result in altered physical appearance (for example, obesity, hirsutism, cushingoid face, and teeth discoloration), which may result in long-term alterations of body image. These changes are especially difficult for the older school-age children and adolescents who are also experiencing the hormonal changes of puberty.

Adolescents after organ transplant are often thinking about what will happen to their new organs when they have sex, and they have concerns about their bodies, with all their scars, and how their sexual partners will feel when they see them. This is of less concern to the younger adolescent than to the older and sexually active adolescent. General sex education and information about pregnancy should be given to all adolescents. Sexually active adolescents should be referred to a teen clinic or gynecologist. Most transplant centers recommend that condoms and a spermicidal gel be used as contraceptives rather than birth control pills, intrauterine devices (IUDs), or Norplant. There is a greater risk associated with birth control pills that can potentially cause thrombus formation, and IUDs can potentially cause endocarditis.

If the patient who has undergone transplantation becomes pregnant, it is imperative that the transplant center be notified. Pregnant transplant recipients may need to have their immunosuppression reduced and will require intense, close monitoring. Care monitoring is done in collaboration with the primary physician and gynecologist.

Recent reports suggest that women have successful pregnancies after renal transplant (Potter et al. 1986) and that women are able to safely have children after liver transplant, although the incidences of prematurity and small-for-gestational-age babies are greater (Scantlebury et al. 1990).

FAMILY CONCERNS

Parents often fear that their child's body will reject the new organ, that there will be an unsuccessful search for another donor, and that their child may die. In addition, parents are concerned about the effect of the transplant on the entire family and the possibility of life returning to "normal." Another concern for parents and families is the financial burden from the transplant procedure. Financial support is usually obtained through third-party payers; however, it is not adequate for all the "unseen" incurred costs (for example, loss of work, housing). Families require support from the transplant team, the primary care provider, and the home care nurse as they make the transition to home. Resource organizations can often assist families in finding emotional support and empowerment by referral to local community chapters (see Exhibit 13–2).

Exhibit 13–2 Resources—Organizations

American Heart Association
National Center
7320 Greenville Ave.
Dallas, TX 75231
(214) 373-6300

American Kidney Fund
6110 Executive Blvd., No. 1010
Rockville, MD 20852
(301) 881-3052

American Liver Foundation
998 Pompton Ave.
Cedar Grove, NJ 07009
(800) 223-0179

American Lung Association and local or state affiliates
(check your telephone book for the local chapter)

Children's Liver Foundation
76 South Orange Ave., No. 202
South Orange, NJ 07079
(201) 761-1111

National Association of Patients on Hemodialysis and Transplantation
211 East 43rd Street, No. 310
New York, NY 10017
(212) 867-4486

National Heart Assist and Transplant Fund
P.O. Box 163
Haverford, PA 19041
(215) 527-5056

National Kidney Foundation
2 Park Ave.
New York, NY 10016
(212) 889-2210

Transplant Recipient's International Organization
244 North Bellefield Ave.
Pittsburgh, PA 15312
(412) 687-2210

United Network for Organ Sharing
3001 Hungary Spring Road
P.O. Box 28010
Richmond, VA 23228
(804) 289-5380

REFERENCES

Addonzio, L., and E. Rose. 1987. Cardiac transplantation in children and adolescents. *Journal of Pediatrics* 111: 1034–38.

Ascher, N., D.W. Hanto, and R.L. Simmons. 1989. Immunobiology of allograft rejection. In *Principles of organ transplantation,* ed. M.W. Flye, 91–104. Philadelphia: W.B. Saunders.

Bartucci, M.R., and M.C. Seller. 1990. The immunology of transplant rejection. In *Nursing care of the transplant recipient,* ed. K.M. Sigardson-Poor and L.M. Haggerty. Philadelphia: W.B. Saunders.

Committee on Infectious Diseases. 1991. *Report of the Committee on Infectious Diseases.* 22d ed. Elk Grove Village, IL: The American Academy of Pediatrics.

Fisher, A., et al. 1990. Anti-B-cell monoclonal antibodies and the treatment of severe B-cell lymphoproliferative syndrome following bone marrow and organ transplantation. *New England Journal of Medicine* 324:1451–56.

Hanto, D., et al. 1981. The Epstein-Barr virus in the pathogenesis of post transplant lymphoproliferative disorders. *Surgery* 90:204–13.

Ho, M., et al. 1988. The frequency of Epstein-Barr virus infection and associated lymphoproliferative syndrome after transplantation and its manifestations in children. *Transplantation* 45:719–27.

Johnson, M., and M.W. Flye. 1989. Infectious complications in renal transplant patients. In *Principles of organ transplantion,* ed. M.W. Flye, 307–34. Philadelphia: W.B. Saunders.

Klintmalm, G., and A.E. Moore. 1985. Organization of a new liver transplant center. *Seminars in Liver Disease.* 412–17.

Lake, J. 1993. Changing indications for liver transplantation. *Gastroenterology Clinics of North America.* 22:213–29.

McGregor, R.S., et al. 1989. Varicella in pediatric orthotopic liver transplant recipients. *Pediatrics* 83:256–60.

Nalesnik, M.A., et al. 1988. The pathology of post transplant lymphoproliferative disorders occuring in the setting of cyclosporine A-prednisone-amino suppression. *American Journal of Pathology* 133, no. 1:173–92.

Pahl, E., et al. 1988. Late follow-up of children after heart transplantation. *Transplant Proceedings* 20 (suppl. 1): 743–46.

Paradis, J.L., et al. 1992. Distinguishing between infection, rejection, and the adult respiratory distress syndrome after human lung transplantation. *Journal of Heart and Lung Transplant* 11:S232–S236.

Potter, D., et al. 1986. Twenty years of renal transplantation in children. *Pediatrics* 77:465–70.

Roberts, J.P., et al. 1989. Liver transplantation today. *Annual Reviews in Medicine* 400:287–303.

Rosenthal, P., et al. 1994. Liver transplantation in children. *American Journal of Gastroenterology* 89:480–92.

Rubin, R. 1988. Infectious disease problems. In *Current topics in gastroenterology transplantation of the liver,* ed. W.C. Maddrey. New York: Elsevier Science.

Rubin, R.H., and N.E. Tolkoff-Rubin. 1993. Antimicrobial strategies in the care of the organ transplant recipient, antimicrobial agents in chemotherapeutic. *Chemo Therapeutics* 37:619–24.

Rubin, R., and L. Young. 1994. Clinical approaches to infection and the compromised host. In *Infection in the organ transplant recipient,* 3d ed., ed. R. Rubin and L. Young, 629–86.

Scantlebury, V., et al. 1990. Childbearing after liver transplantation. *Transplantation* 49:317–21.

Smith, S.L., and S. Ciferni. 1991. Liver transplantation. In *Tissue and organ transplantation: Implications for professional nursing practice,* ed. S.L. Smith. St. Louis: C.V. Mosby.

Smith, S.L. 1991. Immunologic aspects of transplantation. In *Tissue and organ transplantation: Implications for professional nursing,* ed. S.L. Smith. St Louis: C.V. Mosby.

Stephman, E., et al. 1991. Post transplant lymphoproliferative disorders. *Transplant Review* 5:120–29.

Tejani, A., et al. 1989. Strategies for optimizing growth in children with kidney transplants. *Transplantation* 47:229–33.

Trento, A., et al. 1989. Lessons learned in pediatric heart transplantation. *Annals of Thoracic Surgery* 48:617–23.

The United Network for Organ Sharing Update. 1996a. 12, no. 2:8–14.

The United Network for Organ Sharing Bulletin Update. 1996b. 12, no. 4, April, 26–27.

The United Network for Organ Sharing Bulletin. 1996c. 1, no. 3, July.

Urbach, A.H., et al. 1987. Linear growth following pediatric liver transplantation. *American Journal of Diseases in Children* 141: 547–49.

Young, L.S. 1994. Opportunistic infections in the immunocompromised host. In *Basic and clinical immunology,* 8th ed., D.P. Stitts, A.I. Terr, and T.G. Parslo.

CHAPTER 14

Care of the Terminally Ill Child

Belinda Barry Mitchell

It is often stated that there is nothing more difficult for a parent to face than the untimely death of a child. When the death is due to a catastrophic disease, the process usually followed a long and difficult path that included the stages of diagnosis, treatment, the terminal phase, and the grief and bereavement period. Health care providers have directed significant attention toward providing optimal support to families of terminally ill children during these most difficult times. One way to assist these families is to offer the option of caring for their children at home with the support of a home care team.

Research studies have shown that families who elect to care for their children at home during the terminal phase have reported many positive experiences (Benson et al. 1993; Martinson et al. 1983; Lauer and Camitta 1980), including improved satisfaction of the child, return of control to the parents, reunification of the family in its own environment, and the ability of the siblings to participate in the care of the sick child and feel part of the family unit again (Martinson 1979).

DISCHARGE PLANNING

Hospital discharge planning for the terminally ill child is critical. It requires a thorough assessment of patient and family needs and the availability of community resources (Walker et al. 1993). Several factors need to be determined in preparation for discharge before meeting with the family. These include the following: the geographic location of the family residence, extent of medical insurance benefits to the patient, and the type and expertise of home care services available in the community where the family lives. These determinations will allow the health care team to present a realistic home care plan to the family.

Due to the significant growth of the home care industry, an increasing number of patient care needs can now be met at home. Home care services may include the support of an interdisciplinary home team as well as the provision of appropriate medical and pharmaceutical supplies and equipment. If home care is the option selected, the health care team must assist the family in determining the most appropriate methods of care to support the child in the final stages of life (Dragone 1996).

SELECTION OF THE HOME CARE TEAM

Certain criteria should be considered when selecting a team to provide support to the family at home. Factors to consider when selecting the home care team are outlined in Exhibit 14–1.

HOSPICE SERVICES

The concept of hospice care has developed in response to advances in technology and the application of these advances to terminally ill pa-

Exhibit 14–1 Criteria for Selection of Home Care Team

- Use of other support systems
- Language, spoken by staff, and cultural background
- Expertise in pediatric pain management
- Distance from home—30-minute response time including who takes call and how far away they are
- Psychosocial skills in death and dying
- 24-hour availability to respond
- Philosophy of care—willingness to permit aggressive therapy and longer, more questionable prognosis
- Support staff—volunteers, medical director if home consultation seems appropriate and hospital physician not available
- Financial—accept Medicaid or Children with Special Health Care Needs reimbursement, hospice funds, awareness of family's stress related to expenses
- Physical, occupational, speech therapists to enhance quality of life
- Awareness and relationship of community resources—American Cancer Society, Make-A-Wish Foundation, mental health clinics, culturally related systems

Exhibit 14–2 Hospice Services

- Medically directed interdisciplinary team
- 24-hour availability of nursing care
- Experts in pain and symptom management
- Trained volunteers
- Bereavement follow-up services

tients and their families (Exhibit 14–2). Hospice care, usually provided in the home setting, is the implementation of a philosophy that places the primary focus on comfort rather than cure (Humphrey and Milone-Nuzzo 1991). The hospice care plan is designed with emphasis on the management of pain and symptom control (Balinsky 1994). Hospice standards require an interdisciplinary approach to home care. Twenty-four–hour availability of the home care nurse is also required (Fetsch and Miles 1986). This is necessary to provide optimal support to the family, particularly when sudden changes in condition or death of the patient occurs.

Hospice programs have traditionally limited enrollment to patients with a prognosis of less than six months to live and those who have refused further aggressive treatment. These two limitations must be eliminated when caring for pediatric patients. A pediatric hospice program must allow the parents and patient the choice of continuing aggressive treatment and be prepared to accept a child who appears to be terminally ill even though the prognosis is not clearly defined as less than six months to live (Exhibit 14–3). This approach provides terminally ill children and their families with the benefits of hospice support even when they elect to continue aggressive treatment or the prognosis is not clear. This approach also gives parents the right to hospice support when the child's condition is high risk while providing the necessary assurance that they will be allowed to try any medical intervention they believe is necessary to save the life of their child. The freedom to make these decisions is critical to the parents' future mental health.

If a hospice program will be available to the family as the option for home support, it is extremely important how the hospice concept is introduced. The emphasis needs to be placed on living rather than dying. All too often well-intentioned staff members ask the parents if they would like to take their child home to die. It is much more appropriate to determine if they would like to take their child home in an effort to *maximize* the quality of their lives. Later, it can be determined if it will be appropriate to plan for the death to occur at home. This approach will eliminate the unnecessary anxiety produced by forcing consideration of managing the death at home prematurely.

Hospice services will usually be the program of choice when selecting from the home care options available to parents with a terminally ill child. This is primarily because of the expertise

Exhibit 14–3 Hospice Concepts

- Focus on comfort and pain and symptom management.
- Patient is the family; address physical, psychological, and spiritual needs.
- Attempt to allow family to regain control.
- Goal is to achieve maximum quality of life.
- Patient may continue with aggressive treatment.
- Prognosis is not limited to six months.

in symptom management and the 24-hour availability of staff, which hospice services offer. However, it is important to examine the skills of the hospice caregivers who would be assigned to a particular family to determine if they would be comfortable and skilled enough to meet the needs of the child and family. Under certain circumstances, a home health care team may be more appropriate than the local hospice provider in meeting the needs of the family. These circumstances may include language barriers, a hospice provider's discomfort with caring for children, or the child's complex clinical needs. If the home care team is selected rather than hospice, it is essential that a member of the home team with pediatric experience accept the responsibility of being on call 24 hours a day so that the family has support on a continuous basis. It is also important to continue to provide psychosocial support to the family through the hospital and/or the home care providers.

PATIENT AND FAMILY ASSESSMENT

Once the resources required for home care support have been identified, it is necessary to meet with the parents to discuss the option of taking their child home. Home care always needs to be presented as another option of care (Goldman et al. 1993). This eliminates the idea of abandonment often introduced by a physician's statement that "there is nothing more we can do for your child so we are sending you home." It is much more supportive to suggest to parents when appropriate that even when further treatment may not be available that will arrest the child's disease, the health care team can offer support in caring for their child at home, if desired.

Financial coverage for home care is a major concern for families of children with catastrophic diseases. Many of these children have been receiving complex medical care for a long period, and most families' financial resources are drained. The discharge planner must act as the family advocate with the third-party payer before discharge. A family may be insured by a company who contracts for all home care services from one provider. This provider may not have the specialists (for example, pediatricians, hospice) required to meet the needs of a particular child. The discharge planner must be responsible for assessing these skills and negotiating with the third-party payer to ensure maximum quality of care. For additional information about home care financing, see Chapter 3.

Initially, home care could be introduced (Exhibit 14–4) as an alternative to hospitalization. However, because of the recent changes in reimbursement patterns, rehospitalization after discharge may not always be an option (Schweitzer et al. 1993). Health care providers must work with the third-party payer to define insurance benefits and advocate on behalf of the family to achieve the care plan requested by the family, particularly if readmission to the hospital is requested by the family (Adams 1984). Frequent and thorough monitoring of the patient's status will be required in addition to the ongoing communication with the third-party payer and the family.

It is often difficult for the parents to accept the idea of additional professionals becoming involved in the care of their child or entering their home. They may also feel incompetent when the idea of a home team is introduced. The parents need to be assured that the home care team is offered as a support service available if and when the parents need it. It is a "consultation" service, designed to intervene only when re-

Exhibit 14–4 Introductory Concepts of Home Care

- Alternative to hospitalization
- Rehospitalization as an option
- Staff members act as "consultants" to parents
- Staff members are an *addition* to hospital team, not *replacement*
- Patient's physician directs care
- Support available 24 hours a day, 7 days a week
- Cost covered by third-party payer
- Flexibility to meet family needs
- Focus on *comfort* of child
- Visit by appointment, never unannounced

quested and as necessary to reassure the parents that they are doing the best possible job. The parents also need to be reassured that the home care team is respectful of their need for control in caring for their child at home.

The family needs to understand that a home care team works under the direction of the family's physician in the same way as the hospital team (Goldberg, Gardner, and Gibson 1994). In addition, the family needs to know that any out-of-pocket costs experienced as a result of home care services will be discussed with the family in advance to enable the family to authorize or deny any costs. This will alleviate the concern of many families regarding their ability to afford needed services without causing them the embarrassment of asking.

Most parents are extremely anxious about taking their children home, and this anxiety can be significantly reduced through an informative conference. The home care nurse, the most significant member of this team, plays a key role in establishing home care as a viable option by participating in planning before hospital discharge. This also helps the home care nurse to become familiar with the needs of the child and family in an effort to ensure continuity of care in the home setting.

At the onset of the care conference, it is important to identify who will be the primary caregiver in the home. Whenever possible, both parents should be encouraged to share this role. The daily responsibilities of the primary caregiver(s) need to be determined, and these must include nonclinical areas such as care of other siblings, employment, and self-care, along with the specific care needs of the sick child. All of these factors need to be placed within a 24-hour time frame to determine the reasonableness of the parents being able to manage at home and to identify the amount of supplemental support needed to define a realistic plan (Perrin, Shayne, and Bloom 1993). For example, a plan for a single parent with three children younger than five years with one child who requires frequent suctioning around the clock would not be viable without supplemental care. This care may be provided through a friend, relative, or hospice volunteer or combination of all three. It is the responsibility of the health care team to make these determinations as an effort to send a family home with a reasonable plan for management. This type of advanced planning would prevent future problems, such as overwhelming fatigue, neglect of the siblings, or the parent's feeling of failure should the need for readmission of the child arise. Supporting the caregiver is essential to maintaining the patient in the home (McMillan 1996).

The care conference should also be used to determine the family's fears and concerns regarding caring for their child at home. The most common concerns are related to breathing or bleeding problems, unmanageable pain, and fear of the death process. Before discharge, the specific symptoms that may occur due to disease progression can be discussed along with methods of management. These potential symptoms can be determined by the physician in relation to the child's specific disease. This information can be extremely helpful in reducing the family's anxieties regarding its ability to cope at home and the impending death of the child.

The family will need to be constantly reassured that the major focus of the home care team will be the child's comfort and that measures can be quickly initiated to maintain optimal symptom management whenever necessary. Interventions focused on maintaining the child's comfort should be determined when symptoms are discussed. This planning should include the availability of the proper type and amount of resources in the home needed to control the symptoms that may occur. A "care package" of items such as an antiemetic, nose packing, and the stronger drug of choice for pain may be prepared and sent home at the time of discharge. The family can be instructed to place the care package in a safe place out of the reach of children. When the parent observes a new or increased symptom, it can be reported to the physician or home care nurse, who can refer the parent to the care package for intervention. This will enable parents to provide the needed symptom control without unnecessary delays.

Flexibility regarding the frequency of home care involvement is another important issue to consider. Most children have an irregular pattern of "good" and "bad" days. Family members who expect a child to die may witness improvement and stabilization. Emotional reactions can be erratic because of frequent and constant changes in the child's condition. Planning on an hour-to-hour basis is often difficult; planning days or weeks at a time is virtually impossible. It is critical that the home care team members be flexible: they must make themselves available as needs arise, and they must also be able to "pull back" on the good or stable days to allow the family as much normal, uninterrupted time as possible.

After the parents have been presented with all of the options available to them, it is helpful to allow them some private time to think about and discuss alternatives between themselves. The ill child should be included in this discussion in a manner appropriate for his or her age (Jackson 1975).

COMFORT CARE

One major role of the health care team is to help the family focus on keeping the child comfortable. Current technology makes it possible to implement almost any kind of intervention in the home setting. Families often become confused and unsure about how aggressive they should be in caring for their children. Members of the health care team, particularly the physician, need to help the family focus on the philosophical and psychosocial issues related to interventions. For example, if a child is decreasingly able to ingest food or fluid, the idea of total parenteral nutrition or intravenous feedings may be considered as an appropriate option for one patient but not for another. Selected options need to focus on maintaining comfort and quality of life without prolonging the dying stage.

Symptom management is most effectively achieved through the design of a detailed care plan addressing the needs of each child and his or her family. An example of this type of care plan is described in Table 14–1. Symptom management is the key to the success of home care. If the child is comfortable, the family usually remains cohesive and functional. Once the child becomes symptomatic, the family becomes distressed and coping becomes difficult. The home care nurse needs to be readily available to assist the family in the management of any symptoms that may occur. In some situations, admission to the hospital may be an option and should be offered to the family when indicated. Some readmissions may require only a brief period to determine appropriate measures for symptom control followed by discharge and resumption of home care.

Fear of the child suffering is probably the most common and serious concern of parents as well as the ill child and other family members (Miles and Warner 1992). Measures are now available to assess and control pain much more effectively than in the past. Families need to be reassured that pain management is a constant concern of the health care team, who will always be available to intervene to maintain the maximum comfort possible.

The first significant step to successful pain management is a thorough and explicit assessment of the child's pain (McCaffery and Beebe 1989). This must include an assessment tool that

Table 14–1 Generalized Care Plan for Symptom Management

Symptom	*Goal/Objective*	*Intervention*
1. Pain resulting in alterations in comfort	Pain free Activity to tolerance Decrease anxiety Maximum level of independence	Assessment for location/intensity Administration of medication Assessment of interventions Use of behavioral interventions Consult with physician
2. Ineffective breathing pattern resulting in dyspnea/respiratory distress	Nonanxious breathing pattern	Assess etiology. Use medication related to cause (morphine, scopolamine). Position patient with head of bed elevated. Use oxygen. Consider transfusions.
3. Altered respiratory function resulting in wet respirations (near death)	Quiet breathing Decrease family anxiety	Instruct family in process. Give medication to decrease secretions (scopolamine patch). Provide gentle suctioning if required to prevent choking. Position to decrease noise.
4. Nausea and vomiting resulting in alteration in nutrition	Control to level of comfort to patient	Reassure family that child is comfortable. Use prescribed medications. Give small portions, dry foods; rest after eating. Provide mouth care.
5. Anorexia resulting in alteration in nutritional status	Acceptance of family as part of dying process	Instruct family in "slowing down" process of dying, allow them to offer favorite foods but encourage not to pressure child. Provide oral hygiene.
6. Constipation resulting in alteration in elimination	Maintenance of normal bowel pattern Prevention of impaction	Make diet interventions as permitted by child's ability to eat. Initiate bowel program when using narcotics. Use least invasive measures if medication is ineffective—suppositories to enema to digital (caution when platelet levels are decreased).
7. Seizures resulting in high risk for injury	Prevention of seizures Protect the patient Decrease family's anxiety	Assess for etiology. Obtain and administer prescribed drug if indicated. Instruct parent in management, detection. Implement plan for home management whenever possible.

continues

Table 14–1 continued

Symptom	Goal/Objective	Intervention
8. Potential for infection	Maximize patient comfort	Discuss options with physician, team. Present options to family with goals of comfort as primary focus. Use support measures for related symptoms such as fever, anxiety, respiratory symptoms.
9. Skin breakdown resulting in alteration in skin integrity	Maximize patient comfort	Position as comfortable. Use egg-crate or alternating-pressure mattress. Treat as family desires with minimal interruption to patient. Consult with an enterostomal therapist for appropriate interventions.
10. Potential for bleeding	Prevention when appropriate Maximum patient comfort	Discuss platelet transfusion option with physician and family. Apply ice pack over area or pressure if appropriate. Use packing (Gelfoam or gauze). Have towels or blue pad available. Use oral hygiene for bleeding gums.
11. Fever with alteration in comfort level	Maximize patient comfort with minimal intrusion	Reassure family regarding comfort of patient. Initiate cooling measures. Use medication as indicated. Instruct family in use of cooling measures and control of environment and temperature.
12. Eye dryness	Maximize patient comfort	Use artificial tears. Instruct family in care. Keep area clean and moist.
13. Overall weakness resulting in decreased level of life	Maximize quality of activity	Provide continual assessment of level of function. Maximize pain control. Use physical or occupational therapist for evaluation to obtain maximal function. Obtain equipment to assist such as reclining wheelchair, bars in bathroom, ramps. Instruct family in transfer.

continues

Table 14–1 continued

Symptom	Goal/Objective	Intervention
14. Sleep pattern disturbance resulting in insomnia	Improved rest pattern	Decrease anxiety about being alone and impending death. Encourage daytime activity to tolerance, range-of-motion exercises, body massage. Provide maximal pain and symptom control. Give prescribed medication as needed. Use night light, soft music.
15. Anxiety	Reduce to minimum	Instruct parents in potential causes for anxiety. Obtain and maintain maximal pain and symptom control. Encourage to ventilate. Use psychosocial treatments to intervene. Provide reassurance of constant support.
16. Alteration in family coping	Decrease anxiety. Family verbalizes understanding of impending death process. Family understands function of home care team intervention, 24-hour availability. Family feels in control. Appropriate use of coping mechanisms. Prevent sense of being overwhelmed, exhaustion.	Instruct in physiologic process of impending death. Instruct in function of home care team; reinforce focus on comfort and 24-hour availability. Listen to family members; meet their needs; act as consultant. Provide information. Do not force response. Allow family members to use coping mechanisms (denial, anger) and help direct in appropriate expression. Offer ministerial support. Encourage psychosocial intervention from social worker, psychologist. Encourage acceptance of outside support from church, neighbors, etc. Use hospice volunteers.

is appropriate for the child's cognitive level. Visual analog scales can be easily adopted for children who have numerical ability. The nurse or parent can draw a line with numbers equally spaced including one to five. The nurse explains to the child that one is "no hurt" and five is the "worst hurt" and asks the child to select the number for the current amount of pain. The Eland Color Tool, shown in Appendix 14–B, is an ex-cellent assessment tool that describes location and intensity of pain (Eland 1985). It can be useful in children as young as three years old. Once a tool is selected, the same tool must be used after any intervention to determine the degree of success.

Once the type and intensity of pain have been determined, a pain management plan can be designed. Research has determined that intervention usually requires an integrated or multimodal approach (National Institutes of Health 1986). The most common component of the multimodal approach is the use of analgesic medications with progression from nonnarcotic drugs such as aspirin or acetaminophen to narcotics such as methadone or morphine. These drugs can be delivered through a variety of routes, including oral, nasogastric tube, intravenous, subcutaneous, epidural, or intrathecal.

The oral method can include liquid or tablet forms that may be swallowed or absorbed sublingually or through the buccal membranes (Pitorak and Kraus 1987). If oral medications are not an option, the child must be carefully assessed to determine which route will be most efficient and easily managed at home. Tubes that may already be in place, such as nasogastric tubes, are another simple option. If a central line is in place, continuous intravenous infusions may be the choice. If there is no central line, continuous subcutaneous infusion may be the best method (Coyle et al. 1986). Epidural or intrathecal catheter methods may also be considered when other systems are not an option (Moulin and Coyle 1986). In addition, there are a variety of portable infusion pumps available for home use and excellent protocols available for continuous infusion of drugs (Burlich 1988; Goldman et al. 1993).

Medications used for control of chronic pain need to be administered on a "round the clock" basis for maximal pain control. Parents need to be instructed to record the intervention and related pain rating on a pain flowchart (Meinhart and McCaffery 1983). An example of such a flowchart is given in Appendix 14–A.

Options other than analgesic medications should be considered in the integrated approach to pain management (Appendix 14–C). One of these options is the use of drugs to decrease the pain caused by the inflammatory process. These include corticosteroids and nonsteroidal anti-inflammatory drugs.

Nonpharmacologic interventions may also be an effective approach to pain management. These include modalities such as acupuncture, biofeedback, transcutaneous electrical nerve stimulation, hypnosis, and physical therapy. Some interventions that can be easily initiated in the home include distraction techniques such as music, stories, television programs, or visitors (Klein and Winkelstein 1996). Guided imagery, relaxation exercises, and self-hypnosis are also effective in reducing the degree of pain.

In addition to managing symptoms related to pain, other symptoms must also be monitored to maintain maximum comfort and quality of life. An example of this type of care is described in Table 14–1. Interventions need to be determined through consultation with the primary physician and the hospital team. The home care nurse needs to be readily available to assist the family in the management of any symptoms that may occur. In some situations, admission to the hospital may be an option and should be offered to the family when indicated. Readmission may be necessary for a brief period to determine appropriate measures for symptom control followed by discharge and resumption of home care.

FUNERAL ARRANGEMENTS

Families whose children have died have reported that funeral arrangements should be made before the child's death. Although it is extremely difficult for families to face this issue before death, some parents are able to plan together and include the child when appropriate. Parents will experience numbness and shock after the death, and it will be extremely difficult for them to accomplish this kind of planning at that time (Benson et al. 1993). The home care team needs to encourage the family to make funeral arrangements before the child's death whenever possible.

Families that plan to have a child home until death also need to decide if an autopsy will be performed. This may be at the family's request or the request of the physician. The family needs to discuss this with the physician and be given time to think about the decision. If an autopsy will be performed, the body will need to be transported to the appropriate facility. Frequently, the mortuary will agree to do this for the family. It is helpful if these arrangements are also made before the death of the child.

THE DEATH EVENT

Parents whose children have died have also expressed how frightening the impending death can be. They have stated that preparing them by describing possible symptoms that might cause death had been most helpful. They also have stated that it can be tremendously reassuring to know that help from the home care nurse will always be available. The home care nurse needs to assist the family in planning where the death will occur. Many families have elected to keep children who remain in symptom control at home. Others have readmitted their children for more treatment or symptom control, and death occurs during hospitalization. Many times, the child will determine if he or she wants to be in the hospital or at home. These decisions can also be considered tentative, allowing the parents and child the freedom to vacillate according to the condition of the child and coping skills of the family.

GRIEF AND BEREAVEMENT

The grieving process for the family actually begins at the time the child is diagnosed and continues indefinitely. Care of the family must always include not only parents but siblings as well who may experience profound effects (Davies and Martinson 1989). Anticipatory grieving before the death creates feelings of sadness, anxiety, and anger; a need to deny and/or seek information; and a need to seek emotional support. The intensity of these feelings is directly proportionate to the medical status of the sick child. Remember that the process of denial, anger, guilt, shock, bargaining, and acceptance are fluid stages. Family members will move back and forth among these stages. Members of the health care team must be able to discern where family members are in their coping cycle to effectively provide support to them (Wass and Coff 1984; Rando 1988). After the death of the child, the family will experience intense feelings that can be categorized into three stages. The first stage can be described as a period of numbness and disbelief. The next stage is one of intense grief, which includes feelings of yearning, helplessness, anger, behavioral changes, physical symptoms, and a search for meaning. The third stage is a period of reorganization, which can be measured by criteria such as renewed bursts of energy, greater ease in making decisions, and a return to regular eating and sleeping patterns (Wass and Coff 1984; Rando 1988).

Professionals need to be aware of the intensity and length of grief and ensure continued support to families. Support may be provided through measures such as home bereavement visits, attendance at support groups made up of other families who have suffered similar losses, or professional counseling. Professionals also need to be aware of signs of pathologic grief and facilitate referrals to mental health therapy resources when indicated.

REFERENCES

Adams, D. 1984. Helping the dying child. In *Childhood and death*, ed. H. Wass and C. Coff, 95–112. Washington: Hemisphere Publishing Company.

Balinsky, W. 1994. *Home care: Current problems and solutions.* San Francisco: Jossey-Bass Inc.

Benson, P., et al. 1993. Home and hospice care for the child or adolescent with cancer. In *Nursing care of the child with cancer,* 2d ed., ed. G. Foley, D. Fochtman, and K. Mooney, 435–39. Philadelphia: W.B. Saunders.

Burlich, R. 1988. Guidelines for subcutaneous infusion of morphine. Poster session presented at the Second International Conference on Cancer Pain, New York, July 14–17.

Coyle, N., et al. 1986. Continuous subcutaneous infusions of opiates in cancer patients with pain. *Oncology Nursing Forum* 13:53–57.

Davies, B., and I. Martinson. 1989. Care of the family: Special emphasis on siblings during and after death. In *Pe-*

diatric hospice care: What helps? ed. B. Martin, 186–99. Los Angeles: Childrens Hospital Los Angeles.

Dragone, M.A. 1996. Cancer. In *Primary care of the child with a chronic condition,* 2d ed., ed. P. Jackson, and J. Vessey. St. Louis: C.V. Mosby.

Eland, J. 1985. The child who is hurting. *Seminars in Oncology Nursing* 1:116–22.

Fetsch, S., and M. Miles. 1986. Children and death. In *Nursing care of the terminally ill,* ed. M. Amenta and N. Bohnet, 199–226. Boston: Little, Brown and Company.

Goldberg, A., H. Gardner, and L. Gibson. 1994. Home care: The next frontier of pediatric practice. *Journal of Pediatrics* 125:686–90.

Goldman, A., et al. 1993. Pain in terminal illness (home care). In *Pain in infants, children, and adolescents,* ed. N. Schecter, C. Berde, and M. Yaster, 425–33. Baltimore: Williams & Wilkins.

Humphrey, C., and P. Milone-Nuzzo. 1991. Special home care practice. In *Home care nursing, an orientation to practice.* Norwalk, CT.: Appleton & Lange.

Jackson, P.L. 1975. The child's developing concept of death: Implications for nursing care of the terminally ill child. *Nursing Forum* 14:204–15.

Klein, S., and M. Winkelstein. 1996. Enhancing pediatric health care with music. *Journal of Pediatric Health Care* 10:74–81.

Lauer, M., and B. Camitta. 1980. Home care for dying children: A nursing model. *Journal of Pediatrics* 97:1032–35.

Martinson, I., et al. 1983. Home care for children dying of cancer. *Pediatrics* 62:106–13.

Martinson, I.M. 1979. Caring for the dying child. *Nursing Clinics of North America* 14:467–74.

McCaffery, M., and A. Beebe. 1989. *Pain: Clinical manual for nursing practice.* St. Louis: C.V. Mosby.

McMillan, S. 1996. Quality of life of primary caregivers of hospice patients with cancer. *Cancer Practice* 4:191–98.

Meinhart, N.T., and M. McCaffery. 1983. *Pain: A nursing approach to assessment and analysis.* Norwalk, CT: Appleton & Lange.

Miles, M., and J. Warner. 1992. The dying child in the intensive care unit. In *Nursing care of the critically ill child,* ed. M. Hazinski, 1011–16. St. Louis: C.V. Mosby.

Moulin, D.E., and N. Coyle. 1986. Spinal opioid analgesics and local anesthetics in the management of chronic cancer pain. *Journal of Pain and Symptom Management* 1:179–86.

National Institutes of Health Consensus Development Conference Statement. 1986. *The integrated approach to the management of pain* (syllabus). 6, no. 3:1–18.

Perrin, J., M. Shayne, and S. Bloom. 1993. *Home and community care for chronically ill children.* New York: Oxford University Press.

Pitorak, E.F, and J. Kraus. 1987. Pain control with sublingual morphine: The advantages for hospice care. *American Journal of Hospice Care.* 4, no. 2:39–41.

Rando, T. 1988. *Grieving: How to go on living when someone you love dies.* Lexington, MA: Lexington Books.

Schweitzer, S., et al. 1993. The costs of a pediatric hospice program. *Public Health Reports* 108:37–44.

Walker, C., et al. 1993. Nursing management of psychosocial care needs. In *Nursing care of the child with cancer,* 2d ed., ed. G. Foley, D. Fochtman, and K. Moorey, 397–434. Philadelphia: W.B. Saunders.

Wass, H., and C. Coff. 1984. *Childhood and death.* New York: Hemisphere Publishing.

Flowsheet—Pain

Patient _____ Date _____

Pain rating scale used* _____

Purpose: To evaluate the safety and effectiveness of the analgesic(s).

Analgesic(s) ordered: _____

Time	Pain rating	Analgesic	R	P	BP	Level of arousal	Other†	Plan and comments

*Pain rating: A number of different scales may be used. Indicate which scale is used and use the same one each time. Two common examples:
- 0 to 10 with 0 being no pain and 10 being as bad as it can be.
- Melzack's scale: 0 = no pain; 1 = mild; 2 = discomforting; 3 = distressing; 4 = horrible; 5 = excruciating

†Possibilities for other columns: bowel function, activities, nausea and vomiting, other pain relief measures. Identify the side effects of greatest concern to patient, family, physician, nurses, etc.

Source: Reprinted with permission from *Seminars in Oncology Nursing,* Vol. 1, No. 2, pp. 119–122, © 1985, W.B. Saunders Company.

Eland Color Tool

Name of Nurse _____

Date _____

INTERVIEW PROTOCOL

Ask the child, "What kind of things have hurt you before?" If the child does not reply, ask the child, "Has anyone ever stuck your finger for blood? What did it feel like?" After discussing several things that have hurt the child in the past, ask the child, "Of all the things that have ever hurt you, what has been the worst?"

1. Present eight crayons to the child in a random order.
2. Ask the child, "Of these colors, which color is like . . . ?" (the event identified by the child as hurting the most).
3. Place the crayon away from the other crayons (represents severe pain).
4. Ask the child, "Which color is like a hurt but not quite as much as . . . ?" (event identified by the child as hurting the most).
5. Place the crayon with the crayon chosen to represent severe pain.
6. Ask the child, "Which color is like something that hurts just a little?"
7. Place the crayon with the others.
8. Ask the child, "Which color is like no hurt at all?"
9. Show the four crayon choices to the child in order from their worst hurt color to the no hurt color.
10. Ask the child to show on the body outline where they hurt using the crayon for worst, middle, little, or no hurt. Then ask if the hurt is "right now" or "from earlier in the day." Ask why the area hurts.
11. Record the colors identified by the child for:
    Worst pain color
    Middle pain color
    Little pain color
    No hurt color

Source: Reprinted from *Seminars in Oncology Nursing,* Vol. 1, No. 2, pp. 119–122, with permission of Grune & Stratton, Inc., May 1985.

Medications Commonly Used for Symptom Control

Fever

- Acetaminophen (Tylenol)

Nausea/Vomiting

- Diphenhydramine (Benadryl)
- Promethazine (Phenergan)
- Metoclopramide (Reglan)
- Chlorpromazine (Thorazine)
- Trimethobenzamide (Tigan)

Seizures

- Phenytoin (Dilantin)
- Phenobarbital

Increased Intracranial Pressure

- Dexamethasone (Decadron)
- Prednisone

Constipation

- Docusate sodium (Colace, Peri-Colace)
- Bisacodyl (Dulcolax)
- Glycerine suppositories (if not platelet risk)
- Senna concentrate (Senokot)

Restlessness/Sleep

- Diphenhydramine (Benadryl)
- Chloral hydrate
- Phenobarbital
- Diazepam (Valium)
- Hydroxyzine (Vistaril)

Oral Hygiene/Sores

- Hydrogen peroxide
- Nystatin (Mycostatin)
- Lidocaine 2% viscous (Xylocaine)
- Dyclonine (Dyclone)
- Nystatin, lidocaine, diphenhydramine 1:1:1

Mood Elevators

- Diazepam (Valium)
- Alprazolam (Xanax)

Skin Care

- Povidone-iodine (Betadine)

Pain Control (Analgesics)

- Acetaminophen (Tylenol)
- Acetaminophen with codeine
- Hydromorphone (Dilaudid)
- Methadone (Dolophine)
- Morphine sulfate (elixir, rectal, long acting, sublingual, intravenous/subcutaneous)

Pain Control (Nonsteroidal Anti-Inflammatory Drugs)

- Choline magnesium trisalicylate (Trilisate)
- Indomethacin (Indocin)
- Naproxen (Naprosyn)
- Piroxicam (Feldene)
- Ibuprofen (Motrin)

Dry Eyes

- Methylcellulose

CHAPTER 15

Cognitive Development

Joanne K.H. Howard

The pediatric home care nurse has an important role in providing explanations and instructions to children and/or adolescents about their nursing and medical care. Having an understanding of the cognitive developmental level of these patients makes it possible to present information more closely suited to their needs. In this chapter, terms and principles of Piaget's cognitive developmental theory are presented (Piaget 1952). Piaget's stages of cognitive development (sensorimotor, preoperational, concrete operations, formal operations) are discussed for five age groups (infants, toddlers, preschoolers, school-age children, and adolescents). In addition, concepts of illnesss causation and conceptions of internal body parts and functions are discussed for children or adolescents in the preoperational, concrete operations, and formal operations stages. Finally, criticisms of Piagetian theory are discussed.

TERMS AND PRINCIPLES OF PIAGETIAN THEORY

The focus of Piaget's cognitive developmental theory is the understanding of the growth of knowledge, particularly the characteristics or quality of children's and adolescents' knowl-edge. The growth of knowledge is viewed as a process along with psychological growth.

Piaget viewed children as active constructionists of their knowledge. Through interactions with environment, children gain knowledge. Meaning is not in the objects of the knower's experiences nor in the knower alone but is derived from interaction of the knower with the object. This interaction is a process and is biased in the sense that it is dependent on the knower's interpretation (Miller 1983).

Intelligence consists of two functions—organization and adaptation. Organization and adaption are called functional invariants because they function in the same manner throughout all development. Organization refers to the person's integration of schemas that form the basis of one's underlying mental or cognitive structures. Specifically, schemas represent thoughts and patterns of behavior used in interaction with the environment (Miller 1983). Adaptation refers to the dynamic process in which the person interacts with the environment and includes two processes—assimilation and accommodation.

Assimilation is the taking in of new information and adding it to existing knowledge. For example, the child sees that a table is brown and adds it to his or her preexisting knowledge of other brown objects. Assimilation guarantees order (Ausubel, Sullivan, and Ives 1980). *Accommodation* is the taking in of new information that requires that preexisting knowledge be altered in some way. For example, the child learns that the table is brown because it is made from wood.

Note: The author wishes to thank Margaret L. Young, Binghamton University, State University of New York, Binghamton, New York, for her review of this chapter.

The child must accommodate this new information by altering his or her understanding of all brown objects such that some brown objects may be brown because they are made from wood or some may be brown for other reasons. Accommodation leads to new schemas and guarantees adaptation (Ausubel, Sullivan, and Ives 1980). Equilibration is the self-regulating process or motivating force for assimilation and accommodation. When both assimilation and accommodation are in balance, equilibrium exists. The equilibrium state can refer to a moment-by-moment equilibrium, a final level of achievement at a given stage, or to the entire course of cognitive development (Miller 1983).

Cognitive development includes the following four factors: (1) physical maturation; (2) experience with the environment; (3) social experience; and (4) equilibration. Physical maturation refers to central nervous system maturation and provides, in part, for the child's interaction with the environment. Experience with the environment refers to the child's physical manipulation of objects as well as his or her reflections of these actions or objects. Social experience refers to the child's cultural and educational experiences and includes the experience of play. Equilibration, as discussed previously, serves as a force in the processes of assimilation and accommodation in which the other three factors have a role.

Piaget identified four stages of cognitive development that characterize changes in the mental or cognitive structures of children and adolescents—the sensorimotor stage, the preoperational stage, concrete operations, and formal operations. The stages are universal, have an invariant sequence, reflect primarily qualitative changes, and cover the life span. Each stage is derived from the prior stage, transforms the prior stage, and serves as preparation for a more advanced stage (Miller 1983). The rate of progression through the stages may vary, but the sequence and formal characteristics of the stages do not vary. Piaget did not attend to the transitional mechanisms from one stage to another.

In summary, children and adolescents are active knowers of their world and, through interaction with the environment, construct knowledge. This interaction is dependent on the child's physical maturation and includes the experience of acting on objects and reflecting on one's actions with those objects. Through this interaction, the child gains knowledge (assimilation) and changes the form of what is known (accommodation). These processes lead to a balanced state or equilibrium. Throughout life, these changes in the form of what is known are typified by stages that are universal and do not vary in sequence. Therefore, children's cognitive development does not reflect merely varying and limited abilities from those abilities seen in adults but entirely distinctive characteristics.

A summary of the Piagetian stages of cognitive development for various age groups is presented in Table 15–1.

INFANTS

Infants between birth and 12 months of age are in the sensorimotor stage. Four substages of the sensorimotor stage characterize the infant's cognitive development. As the name of the stage implies, infants begin to know their world through use of their senses and motor activities. During the first year, infants develop primitive concepts of space, time, causality, and intentionality (Ausubel, Sullivan, and Ives, 1980).

Substage 1: Reflexes

Infants from birth to one month of age are in the first substage of the sensorimotor stage. Through reflexive activity stimulated by needs (for example, hunger), infants begin to assimilate perceptual information about the world. A reflex according to Piaget is a hereditary reaction and not acquired through experience (Gruber and Voneche 1977). Reflexive activities include vision, hearing, sucking, and grasping. Repetition and rhythmicity of these experiences serve as a basis of cognitive predictability (Maier 1979). Infants do not have the notion of

Table 15–1 Summary of Piagetian Stages for Various Age Groups

Age Group	Stage	Characteristics
Infants (0–1½ years)	Sensorimotor (substages 1–4)	Begins to know world through the use of senses and motor activities; primitive concepts of space, time, causality, and intentionality develop.
Toddlers (1–2 years)	Sensorimotor (substages 5–6)	Learns about characteristics of objects and interrelationships among objects through trial and error; onset of the ability to mentally represent objects.
Preschoolers (2–4 years)	Preoperational (symbolic substage)	Internally represents the world in their minds as they have seen it; egocentric view; dominated by perceptions; transductive reasoning
School-age children (5–7 years)	Preoperational (intuitive substage)	Develops qualitative identity; understanding of seriation begins; decreased egocentricity somewhat
School-age children (7–11 years)	Concrete operations	Reasons logically with objects or events based in reality; capable of mental operations, including transitivity, seriation, classification, conservation
Preadolescents and adolescents (11+ years)	Formal operations	Capable of abstract thought, hypothetico-deductive reasoning

objects existing apart from themselves and are able to respond only to an aspect of an object that is associated with a need (for example, mother's breast for feeding). Causality is not known by infants in the first substage because they do not have an understanding of objects apart from themselves and no notion of time between two events.

Substage 2: Primary Circular Reactions

Infants between one and four months of age are in the second substage of the sensorimotor stage. During this substage, the infant's reflexive activity begins to be replaced with voluntary activity. Circular reactions refer to the infant's repetition of an activity that was discovered by chance. Primary circular reactions refer to activities that are focused on the infant's body, rather than on objects. Actions are repeated for the mere pleasure of the activity. For example, the infant may repetitively bring the hand toward

the mouth for sucking. Thus, activities that were noted as separate events during the first substage (for example, sucking, grasping) become coordinated in the infant's activities during the second substage. This coordination of activities represents the beginning notions of causality with two events in a sequential relationship. Pseudoimitation also emerges in which the infant repeats an action the adult has just performed that mimicked the infant's initial action.

Substage 3: Secondary Circular Reactions

Infants between four and eight months of age are in the third substage of the sensorimotor stage. During this substage, infants perceive themselves as acting on things. Infants have a greater understanding of objects as separate from themselves and try to recover an object as long as it remains in their visual field. Again, the infant repetitively performs actions that have been discovered by chance for the mere pleasure of the activity. However, the actions are centered on the objects, rather than on the infant's body. Infants try to make fascinating environmental events occur again and again (for example, swinging a mobile). The causes of all events are still viewed as related to the infant's action. Pure imitation emerges at this substage. Only behaviors that infants can see or hear themselves produce are imitated (Caron and Caron 1982).

Substage 4: Coordination of Secondary Schemata

Infants between 8 and 12 months of age are in the fourth substage of the sensorimotor stage. During this substage, the infant intentionally coordinates schema (thoughts and patterns of behavior) developed within prior substages as the means to produce a desired goal. In addition, the infant's acquired schema can be applied to novel situations. An example of infants' ability to apply acquired schema to novel situations is their imitation. Now infants can imitate the behaviors of others that they have not heard or seen themselves perform.

Object permanence, which is the understanding that an object exists despite not being present in one's visual field, develops within this substage. With the development of object permanence, infants are able to remove barriers when trying to accomplish a task. For example, the infant will attempt to search for a toy when it is placed under a blanket. The infant recognizes that the self is separate from objects. However, the infant's view of objects existing in space separate from himself or herself is still tied to action schemas (Caron and Caron 1982). Infants cannot understand that objects exist in space with no relationship to themselves. For example, a toy is placed under a blanket, removed, and then placed under a pillow while the infant observes. The infant will search for the toy under the object in which the toy was placed when initially taken from the infant (i.e., the blanket). This search error is referred to as place error (Caron and Caron 1982).

TODDLERS

Toddlers between the ages of one and two years are in the sensorimotor stage. Two substages of the sensorimotor stage characterize toddlers' cognitive development. The onset of the toddler's ability to mentally represent objects marks the end of the sensorimotor stage.

Substage 5: Tertiary Circular Reactions

Toddlers between 12 and 18 months of age are in the fifth substage of the sensorimotor stage. During this substage, the toddler experiments in a trial-and-error fashion to discover multiple means to achieve a goal. These behaviors are seen in the toddler's ritualistic play. Through these repetitive trials, the toddler learns about the characteristics of objects and interrelationships among objects. Objects are viewed as distinct from the self. Place error as seen in substage 4 no longer occurs. Toddlers search for an object in the last place in which it was seen hidden. Toddlers also recognize that they, as well as others or objects, can be causes of events and they may be recipients of causes. Toddlers imitate both animate and inanimate objects.

Substage 6: Invention of New Means through Mental Combination

Toddlers between 18 and 24 months of age are in the sixth substage of the sensorimotor stage. During this substage, toddlers are capable of determining a cause after observing an effect or predicting an effect when observing a cause within the limits of their prior experiences without actually acting out the scenario. The toddler internally represents schemas that are used in these mental tasks. The beginning of symbolic representation has its roots in the sixth substage. This is evident in the toddler's use of pretense or make-believe in play. Toddlers also demonstrate deferred imitation, which is the imitation of actions that they have not seen performed in the past. In the final substage of the sensorimotor stage, toddlers recognize that objects exist apart from themselves and exist even when they are not observable. Thus, toddlers will search for objects that they have not seen.

PRESCHOOLERS

Preschoolers between the ages of two and four years are in the symbolic substage of the next stage of Piaget's cognitive developmental theory, the preoperational stage. During the symbolic substage, preschoolers use signs and symbols such as words and images to represent objects that may not be present. Thus, preschoolers are capable of internally representing the world in the mind as they have seen it. The preschoolers' view of the world is egocentric and is dominated by their experiences. Preschoolers believe that others view the world in the same manner as they do. This egocentrism is evident in preschoolers' language and play. Rosen (1985) cites qualities of the preschooler's language that reflect egocentrism: "The child does not bother to construct sentences which will provide the information which the listener needs for comprehension. He uses pronouns without explanatory referents, he leaves out necessary causal connections, and he does not offer logical proof of his assertions."

The mental representations or preconcepts that preschoolers have are dominated by their perceptions of an object or event and thus are very literal and concrete. In addition, preschoolers are able to focus on only one characteristic of an object or event at one time (referred to as "centration"), which leads to preconcepts that are fairly global. An example of centration is a preschooler's ability to see his or her mommy as only a mommy and not as a wife to his or her father. Preschoolers also judge persons on the basis of one characteristic. The child who receives a shot from a nurse may view that nurse as mean because the child has associated the nurse with a painful event.

The preschoolers' mental representations, as stated previously, are near copies of their experiences. Therefore, the preschooler's understanding of an experience is only in the direction in which the events occurred. Preschoolers cannot understand reversibility and therefore cannot retrace their steps from the end to the beginning of an event. Preschoolers who are ill may not understand that their health can return.

The preschoolers' thinking is also static in the sense that they cannot understand transformations. The preschooler who observes water being poured from a short, squatty glass to a tall, thin glass believes that the tall, thin glass contains more water. The preschooler focuses on the change in status, rather than the process.

Transductive reasoning, rather than inductive or deductive reasoning, is used by preschoolers. The preschoolers' thinking proceeds from particular to particular. Two events that occur closely in time are thought to be related. For example, the preschooler who yells at a younger brother just before the brother's accident may think that his or her yelling caused the accident.

Preschoolers are unable to delineate between physical or mechanical causes and psychological or moral ones. Preschoolers often believe that humans or supernatural beings make things happen or events occur by magic. Along with these beliefs, preschoolers believe that anything that moves is alive. Animism or "life" is attributed to things such as the clouds and the sun.

SCHOOL-AGE CHILDREN

Two stages constitute the cognitive development of children of school age. Young school-age children (younger than seven years) are in the intuitive substage of the preoperational stage. Older children (older than seven years) are in the stage of concrete operations. By the time of preadolescence these children have developed a conceptual system that is both logical and coherent.

Preoperational Stage: Intuitive Substage

School-age children between five and seven years of age are in the intuitive substage of the preoperational stage. Children in the intuitive substage are still governed by their perceptions.

Increases in young children's social experience serve to decrease their egocentricity by providing other points of view. Young children observe objects for their many different characteristics such as color, shape, and size. However, the young school-age child is able to reason only on the basis of one characteristic at a time.

Two abilities that are qualitative and develop in children in the intuitive substage are identities and functions (Rosen 1985). The child who observes water being poured from a short, squatty glass to a tall, thin glass recognizes that the water in the tall glass is the same water that was previously in the short glass. This is evidence of qualitative identity. Young school-age children also develop a logic of functions evident in their understanding that a change in one variable may be related to a change in another variable. For example, the child observes a scarf being pulled through a ring. The child recognizes that the scarf on the right side of the ring (though longer on that side after being pulled through the ring somewhat) is still the same scarf that was used before the action. However, the child cannot recognize that the length of the scarf has remained the same.

An understanding of seriation or ordering of events begins in the intuitive substage. The young school-age child may be able to recognize two events in a series when they are in consecutive order. For example, the child understands her third birthday follows her second birthday but does not understand her third birthday also comes after her first birthday.

Concrete Operations

Children between the ages of 7 and 11 years are in the stage of concrete operations. Piaget believed that this stage represented the first stage of rational thinking in the child.

Piaget borrowed the terms or language of mathematics and logic to describe the cognitive structures of the child in concrete operations. His model is referred to as the logico-mathematical model and consists of nine groupings. Groupings are cognitive structures that are logically organized. Each grouping contains multiple sets of elements (for example, objects, actions, ideas). Four rules apply to the relationships among these elements when an operation (an internalized mental action) is performed on two of the elements. These four rules include the rule of closure, the rule of associativity, the identity rule, and the inverse or reversibility rule. Definitions for these four rules are given in Table 15–2.

As the name of the stage implies, Piaget believed that children in concrete operations perform operations or internalize mental actions on the objects of their experiences. Children are able to reason logically with those objects or events based in reality. Children in the stage of concrete operations are not able to reason logically on abstract concepts or hypotheses.

The many operations or mental actions children develop in concrete operations serve to order and relate their experiences into an orga-

Table 15–2 Rules for Relationships among Two Elements

Rule	Definition
Closure	Any operation combining two elements in the set must result in an element within the set.
Associativity	The combination of elements within the set must hold irrespective of the order in which they are treated.
Identity	There must be one element only that in combination with any other element leaves it unchanged.
Inverse	For each element in the set there must be another that in combination with it results in the identity element.

Source: Piaget's Theory: A Psychological Critique by G. Brown and C. Desforges, p. 33, Routledge and Kegan Paul, © 1979.

nized whole (Maier 1979). These operations emerge gradually. Four of the operations include transitivity, seriation, classification, and conservation. *Transitivity* means that children understand the A − B = B − C when A is longer than B by the same amount as B is longer than C (Pulaski 1980). *Seriation* means that children can order objects according to magnitudinal dimensions such as length, weight, and color. Reversibility of thought is an inherent aspect of the operation of seriation. The child is able to think in both directions from point A to point B or from point B to point A. Transitivity has been found to be more difficult than seriation (Murray and Youniss 1960; Achenbach and Weisz 1975; Kingma 1983).

With the operation of classification, the child is able to recognize that the class does not change despite recognition of a subclass. For example, the child is shown six yellow beads and four white ones and is asked about the number of yellow beads. The child responds appropriately. Then the child is asked about the number of total beads. Again, the child responds appropriately. The child's response indicates that he or she can perceive the existence of a subclass and still recognize the total class appropriately.

Decentration is evident in the emergence of the operation of conservation. The child is able to understand that an object may change in its perceptual characteristics without a change in the actual quantity of the object. Before concrete operations, the preoperational child was able to center on only one characteristic of an object at a time, and, thus, when the object changed in appearance, the child believed the object had also changed in quantity. Conservation of number occurs initially followed by conservation of substance, area, weight, and volume.

With the use of these various concrete operations, school-age children are able to classify their knowledge, order it hierarchically or sequentially, and allow for transformations in their thinking. They use these operations to conduct trial-and-error experiments on the objects of their experiences. They try to determine which means create which ends and try to relate themselves to the outcome. This is referred to as deductive logic.

Along with the logicomathematical operations, Piaget also identified infralogical operations. These operations deal with continuous wholes, rather than discrete objects. An example of a continuous whole is a block of space. With infralogical operations, the integrity of the whole is not maintained when a part is removed from it. Piaget's work on space and geometry is the basis of the infralogical operations.

The ability of school-age children to take more characteristics of objects within their experience into account is also related to their ability to take other viewpoints into account. Their social experience leads to this loss of egocentrism. They are able to separate their views from others and coordinate multiple viewpoints. Within these social experiences there is strict adherence to rules. The child in concrete operations believes that justice is accomplished when the punishment equals the misdeed.

Piaget stated that true causality does not appear until the child is seven or eight years of age (Piaget 1951). True causality may be defined as a physical explanation for a natural phenomenon. Children in concrete operations explain causes less in terms of themselves, can understand intermediary steps in causality, can order the events, and can understand the reversible nature of cause and effect.

PREADOLESCENTS AND ADOLESCENTS

Preadolescents at 11 or 12 years of age enter the final stage of Piaget's cognitive developmental theory—formal operations. While the child in concrete operations is capable of mental operations with objects or experiences in the real world, the preadolescent or adolescent in formal operations is capable of thinking about the real world as well as the world of possibilities. The adolescent's thinking extends beyond the present to what is possible in the future. Adolescents use hypothetico-deductive reasoning, which means that they take into account all of the variables within a situation, form hypotheses about their interrelationships, and test each of them to derive multiple alternative solutions to a given problem. Exploration of all possible combinations of variables is referred to as combinatorial analysis. Within this problem-solving process, one variable may be held constant or neutralized while the others are examined. Before this stage, the child in concrete operations was only capable of negating a variable so as not to consider it within a problem-solving situation. Through the process of integrating variables, adolescents form theories. In the early stage of formal operations, these theories are simplistic and lack originality (Billingham 1983).

Along with reflecting or thinking about the content within a given problem-solving situation, the adolescent is capable of examining the probelm-solving process used within the specific situation. The adolescent recognizes that a solution may be valid when it is logically derived from assumptions regardless of its factual truth. Meta-thought refers to the adolescents' thinking about their thinking.

With the development of the ability to conjecture and create, adolescents form ideals of themselves, others within their immediate experiences, and society. Adolescents are egocentric to the extent that they sometimes cannot distinguish between their ideals and those of the world. They often give unlimited power to their views. During this time of idealism and introspection, adolescents become very critical of their appearance and behavior and think the world is focused on them as much as they are on themselves. From mentally testing their ideals, often in the context of peer groups, adolescents lose their egocentrism. Toward late adolescence, they gain perspective over their ability of abstract thought, so that insight and problem solving can be accomplished with objectivity. Adolescents can then take many perspectives into account, differentiate their own from others, and derive a solution to the problem.

A fifth stage has been postulated by some researchers for cognitive development beyond formal operations. Problem solving or novel thought has been suggested as the foci for a stage beyond formal operations (Riegel 1973; Arlin 1975; Langford 1975).

CONCEPTIONS OF ILLNESS CAUSATION

Studies that have been conducted to examine children's and adolescents' conceptions of illness causation have focused on the subjects' cognitive developmental level or chronologic age as a function of their conceptions. Sequences for the conceptions of illness causation have been described, along with particular causes of illness named by children and/or adolescents in different cognitive developmental stages or age groups. These conceptions of illness causation are discussed for children or adolescents in three stages of Piaget's cognitive developmental theory—properational, concrete operations, and formal operations.

Preoperational Stage

Bibace and Walsh (1980) identified two themes of illness causation for children in the preoperational stage. These themes are phenomenism and contagion, with the former theme being the most cognitively immature one. Before the use of these themes to explain the cause of illness, children name irrelevant or incomprehensible causes (Redpath and Rogers 1984). Children whose explanations for illness causation are phenomenistic attribute illness to an external concrete phenomenon (often a sensory phenomenon within their immediate experience) that may exist with the illness but is not related spatially or temporally. For example, children may name the sun as the cause of a cold (Bibace and Walsh 1980). Explanations are derived from the child's own experience, focus on a specific detail of the experience as the cause, and do not specify a causal link. The theme contagion refers to the child's belief that the cause of illness is in objects or persons nearby but not touching the child or with an event that occurs just before the illness onset. The causal event is often more closely related to the actual illness than causal events given by children who have a phenomenistic explanation. The causal event also does not represent just a single experience. For example, the child may answer, "You catch it, that's all," when asked about how a person gets a cold (Bibace and Walsh 1980).

In conjunction with these themes by Bibace and Walsh (1980) and Blos (1978) found that preschool children attributed illness to contiguous temporal and spatial cues. Potter and Roberts (1984) studied 112 healthy five- to nine-year-old children. They found that children within the preoperational stage viewed themselves as significantly more vulnerable to contagion than children in concrete operations.

Concrete Operations Stage

Two themes for illness causation identified by Bibace and Walsh (1980) for children in concrete operations are contamination and internalization. Contamination refers to the cause of illness as another person, object, or external action. The child either touches the contaminated object or person or is involved in an action and becomes contaminated. The child does not differentiate between the mind and body, and, therefore, a harmful action by the child can result in illness. For example, the child may attribute a cold to taking off his or her jacket outdoors (Bibace and Walsh 1980). There is a qualitative shift from the theme contagion to the theme contamination. The cause as defined in the latter theme is located at the surface of the body.

Numerous studies with school-age children that serve to confirm the theme of contamination for illness causation have found that the children attribute illness to their actions; as punishment specifically for their actions, such as violating a rule; to human agents; and to factors within the environment (Richter 1943; Brazelton, Holder, and Talbot, 1953; Schechter 1961; Lynn, Glaser, and Harrison, 1962; Palmer and Lewis 1976; Perrin and Gerrity 1981; Wood 1983; Gratz and

Piliavin 1984). These studies have been conducted with healthy children, children with either acute or chronic illness, or hospitalized children.

Other findings from studies with school-age children are in conflict with the attribution of punishment for the cause of illness. Instead, causes of illness named included chance and natural phenomenon (Gofman, Buckman, and Schade 1957; Brodie 1974; Williams 1979).

Internalization, another theme of illness causation for children in concrete operations, refers to the child's recognition that the illness is located inside the body whereas the cause may be external. Swallowing or inhaling are two common processes of internalization. For example, the child may attribute a cold in the winter to breathing in too much cold air (Bibace and Walsh 1980). A cause of illness named by school-age children that is related to this theme is germs or microorganisms (Nagy 1951; Palmer and Lewis 1976; Perrin and Gerrity 1981).

These two themes for concrete operations represent the child's distinction between internal and external events, although the child focuses on real, concrete external events as the cause of illness. The child is still confused about the function of internal organs with the illness experience.

Formal Operations Stage

Physiologic and psychophysiologic themes have been identified by Bibace and Walsh (1980) for persons in formal operations. The physiologic theme refers to the malfunctioning or nonfunctioning of an internal organ or system as the cause of illness. A step-by-step sequence may be given as an explanation for the events culminating in illness. Both the host and casual agent are recognized as factors leading to the illness onset. The cause may be an external event. Multiple causes may be named, or causes may have a cumulative effect. Others have reported that children at 11 or 12 years of age name multiple causes for illnesses (Nagy 1951; Perrin and Gerrity 1981).

The psychophysiologic theme represents a more mature cognitive explanation for illness causation. The cause of illness is described as a combination of physiologic and psychological factors. The relation between thoughts and feelings and body functioning are recognized by persons who explain illness causation within the psychophysiologic theme.

CONCEPTIONS OF INTERNAL BODY PARTS AND FUNCTIONS

Children's and adolescents' understanding of internal body parts and functions is discussed for three stages of Piaget's cognitive developmental theory—preoperational, concrete operations, and formal operations. For the clinician working with ill children, it is important to remember that accurate understanding of body parts does not necessarily mean that the child understands the illness and its effects on body functioning.

Preoperational Stage

When asked to name body parts, young children often include nonorgans such as foods, blood, feces, and urine or noninternal body parts such as skin and the belly button (Tait and Ascher 1955; Gellert 1962; Porter 1974; Smith 1977; Williams 1979; Crider 1981). Gellert (1962) and Williams (1979) noted that young children conceive of the interior of the body as containing those substances that go in and come from it. Schilder and Wechsler (1935) suggested that the child can be certain only that the body contains those substances that have gone into it, such as food.

Crider (1981) developed a sequence for the levels of conceptualization for children's conceptions of internal body parts. At the first level, which may represent children in the preoperational stage, children focus on global and observable activities of the body such as breathing without any understanding of its purpose or connection with a specific body part. The child may label specific body parts differentiated by their spatial locations without any understanding of their purpose or function.

Concrete Operations Stage

The child in early concrete operations can name several body parts, which often include bones, the brain, the heart, blood, and blood vessels (Gellert 1962; Williams 1979). Later in concrete operations, the child may also include the intestines, stomach, muscles, liver, and lungs (Williams 1979). Systems that are frequently mentioned include the musculoskeletal and cardiovascular systems (Gellert 1962; Porter 1974; Smith 1977).

According to Crider (1981), the child at six or seven years of age identifies a global function that is a perceived activity or state (for example, working, playing) for every body part named. Next, the child more specifically labels a particular attribute (for example, shape, substance, motion) of the body part, and this attribute is related to activities. For example, the child states that the heart pumps so that he or she can move around (Crider 1981). At the next level of conceptualization, the child conceives of the organ as a container in which things are displaced from it. For example, blood is pumped though the body by the heart (Crider 1981). Followed by this understanding, the child conceptualizes organ functions as having coordinated and reversible properties. The child understands that blood comes into the heart and also leaves from it. Finally, the child recognizes that a transformation of body substances takes place as a function of the organ. These transformations may have animistic or moral qualities. For example, the lungs are viewed as something that changes good air, which is inhaled, to bad air, which is exhaled (Crider 1981).

Formal Operations Stage

Persons in formal operations name body organs that represent their understanding of the coordinated and reversible functions of the organs, along with the organ's ability to transform substances at the cellular level (Crider 1981). Other body parts that are named include nerves, kidneys, and reproductive organs (Porter 1974; Crider 1981). Adolescents can also relate one organ's function to another organ's function and can hierarchically arrange organ functions from a cellular or systems' perspective (Gellert 1962).

CRITICISMS OF PIAGETIAN THEORY

Three major criticisms of Piagetian theory should be kept in mind when applying this theory to practice. Piaget has been criticized for his harsh standards and conservatism used to evaluate the child's cognitive level. Piaget has been particularly concerned with false-positive results that overestimate the child's ability (Miller 1983). Thus, the age levels given for the stages should be applied with caution. Children's cognitive levels may be more advanced than their age indicates according to the age parameters given for the stages.

The issue of regression is also not addressed in depth by Piaget. He does not offer an explanation for the child's use of formerly acquired mental operations when the environment is overwhelming. Piaget attributes the use of these operations to the lack of more efficient operations that will develop later.

Cross-cultural studies have provided insight regarding individual differences that are not explained by Piaget. Although the qualitative aspects of Piaget's theory have been verified, the rate of development has been found to be influenced by cultural factors (Dasen 1972). Marked individual differences have been found among different ethnic groups where physical and social environments, child-rearing practices, and health conditions are relatively homogeneous (Dasen 1972).

REFERENCES

Achenbach, T.M., and J.R. Weisz. 1975. A longitudinal study of development synchrony between conceptual identity, seriation, and transitivity of color, number and length. *Child Development* 46:840–48.

Arlin, P.K. 1975. Cognitive development in adulthood: A fifth stage? *Developmental Psychology* 11:602–06.

Ausubel, D.P., E.V. Sullivan, and S.W. Ives. 1980. Theory and problems of child development. 3d ed. New York: Grune & Stratton.

Bibace, R., and M.E. Walsh. 1980. Development of children's concepts of illness. *Pediatrics* 66:912–17.

Billingham, K.A. 1983. *Developmental psychology for the health care profession. Part 1—Prenatal through adolescent development.* Boulder, CO: Westview Press.

Blos, P. 1978. Children think about illness: Their concepts and beliefs. In *Psychologic aspects of pediatric care,* ed. E. Gellert. New York: Grune & Stratton.

Brazelton T.B., R. Holder, and B. Talbot. 1953. Emotional aspects of rheumatic fever in children. *Journal of Pediatrics* 43:339–58.

Brodie, B. 1974. Views of healthy children toward illness. *American Journal of Public Health* 64:1156–59.

Caron, A.J., and R.F. Caron. 1982. Cognitive development in early infancy. In *Review of human development,* ed. T.M. Field, et al. New York: John Wiley & Sons.

Crider, C. 1981. Children's conceptions of the body interior. In *Children's conceptions of health, illness, and bodily functions,* ed. R. Bibace and M.E. Walsh. San Francisco: Jossey-Bass.

Dasen, P.R. 1972. Cross-cultural Piagetian research: A summary. *Journal of Cross-Cultural Psychology* 3:23–39.

Gellert, E. 1962. Children's conceptions of the content and functions of the human body. *Genetic Psychology Monographs* 65:293–405.

Gofman, H., W. Buckman, and G.H. Schade. 1957. The child's emotional response to hospitalization. *American Journal of Diseases of Children* 93:157–64.

Gratz, R., and J. Piliavin. 1984. What makes kids sick: Children's belief about the causative factors of illness. *Children's Health Care* 12:156–62.

Gruber, H.E., and J.J. Voneche, eds. 1977. *The essential Piaget.* New York: Basic Books.

Kingma, J. 1983. Seriation, correspondence, and transitivity. *Journal of Educational Psychology* 75:763–71.

Langford, P.E. 1975. The development of the concept of development. *Human Development* 18:321–32.

Lynn, D.B., H.H. Glaser, and S.G. Harrison. 1962. Comprehensive medical care for handicapped children: III. Concepts of illness in children with rheumatic fever. *American Journal of Diseases of Children* 103:42–50.

Maier, H.W. 1979. Three theories of child development. 3d. ed. New York: Harper & Row.

Miller, S.A. 1983. Cognitive development: A Piagetian perspective. In *Strategies and techniques of child study,* ed. R. Vasta. New York: Academic Press.

Murray, J.P., and J. Youniss. 1960. Achievement of inferential transitivity and its relation to serial ordering. *Child Development* 39:1259–68.

Nagy, M.H. 1951. Children's ideas of the origin of illness. *Health Education Journal* 9:6–12.

Palmer, B.B., and C.E. Lewis. 1976. Development of health attitudes and behaviors. *The Journal of School Health* 46:401–02.

Perrin, E.C., and P.S. Gerrity. 1981. There's a demon in your belly: Children's understanding of illness. *Pediatrics* 67:840–49.

Piaget, J. 1951. *The child's conception of physical causality.* New York: Humanities Press.

Piaget, J. 1952. *The origin of intelligence in children.* New York: International Universities Press.

Porter, C.S. 1974. Grade school children's perceptions of their internal body parts. *Nursing Research* 23:384–91.

Potter, P.C., and M.C. Roberts. 1984. Children's perceptions of chronic illness: The roles of disease symptoms, cognitive development, and information. *Journal of Pediatric Psychology* 9:13–27.

Pulaski, M.A.S. 1980. *Understanding Piaget.* New York: Harper & Row.

Redpath, C.C., and C.S. Rogers. 1984. Healthy young children's concepts of hospitals, medical personnel, operations, and illness. *Journal of Pediatric Psychology* 9: 29–40.

Richter, H. 1943. Emotional disturbances of constant pattern following nonspecific respiratory infection. *Journal of Pediatrics* 23:315–25.

Riegel, K.F. 1973. Dialectical oprations: The final period of cognitive development. *Human Development* 16: 346–70.

Rosen, H. 1985. *Piagetian dimensions of clinical relevance.* New York: Columbia University Press.

Schecter, M. 1961. The orthopedically handicapped child. *Archives of General Psychiatry* 9:247–53.

Schilder, P., and D. Wechsler. 1935. Short communication. What do children know about the interior of the body? *International Journal of Psychoanalysis* 16:355–60.

Smith, E.C. 1977. Are you really communicating? *American Journal of Nursing* 77:1966–68.

Tait, C.D., Jr., and R.C. Ascher. 1955. Inside-of-the-body test: A preliminary report. *Psychosomatic Medicine* 27: 139–48.

Williams, P.D. 1979. Children's concepts of illness and internal body parts. *Maternal Child Nursing Journal* 8: 115–23.

Wood, S.P. 1983. School-aged children's perceptions of the causes of illness. *Pediatric Nursing* 9:101–04.

CHAPTER 16

Motor Development

Joanne K.H. Howard

In this chapter, normal motor development is described for the following five age groups: infants, toddlers, preschoolers, school-age children, and adolescents. The understanding of normal motor development can aid the home care nurse in assessing the pediatric patient's motor skills and in instituting appropriate interventions based on the patient's motor abilities. Further assessment is necessary when children or adolescents do not demonstrate motor skills appropriate for their developmental level.

Principles that govern motor development are initially discussed, followed by a short summary of central nervous system maturation. Motor development is discussed in terms of gross motor and fine motor development for the five age groups. Gross motor development includes patterns of posture and locomotion, and fine motor development refers to the development of prehension (that is, grasping or manipulation of objects) (Di Leo 1977). Infant reflexes are discussed before the description of gross and fine motor development in infants. In addition, self-care skills of each age group are presented.

PRINCIPLES OF MOTOR DEVELOPMENT

Several principles have been identified that govern motor development. The first principle is

Note: The author wishes to thank Margaret L. Young, Binghamton University, State University of New York, Binghamton, New York, for her review of this chapter.

that motor development is dependent on central nervous system maturation. This principle is significant when considering the child's readiness for a particular motor task. For example, when beginning toilet training with a child, the child's central nervous system must be sufficiently mature for the child to recognize physiologic cues necessary for bowel and bladder control.

The second principle is that motor development progresses in an orderly sequence. The rate may vary with the individual, but the sequence does not vary. The differences in children's rates for achievement of developmental milestones are evident in a study by Neligan and Prudham (1969), who studied the age (in months) at which more than 3,000 children were able to sit unsupported and walk. They recorded the number of months in which 3, 10, 25, 50, 75, 90, and 97 percent of the subjects achieved the skill. The number of months for between 50 and 97 percent of the subjects was nearly twice the number of months for between 3 and 50 percent of the subjects.

The third principle of motor development is that development progresses in a cephalocaudal (that is, head to toe) direction. The child generally gains control of the head and neck before upper trunk control and, later, lower body control.

The fourth principle, the proximodistal principle, is that motor development generally progresses from the central part of the body to the periphery. The child gains relatively more control over the trunk before control over the extremities. This principle has been challenged by Loria (1980), who studied reaching and prehensile skills of 12 normal infants at 30 weeks of age. She found that proximal ability (that is, visually guided reaching) was not related to distal ability (that is, prehensile skills) in the infants, and she suggested that there may be two different motor control systems that govern proximal and distal abilities.

Differentiation is the fifth principle of motor development. Development proceeds from simple to complex or from general to specific. For example, children are able to wave their arms before they are able to have fine motor control with their fingers.

CENTRAL NERVOUS SYSTEM MATURATION

At birth, the newborn's motor activity is primarily reflexive. The cerebral cortex is half its adult thickness. As the child ages, motor activity is governed more and more by the cerebral cortex. Myelinization facilitates the conduction velocity of the axons of nerve fibers. Myelinization of sensory pathways occurs first and is almost entirely completed at birth. Myelinization of motor pathways follows that of sensory pathways. Myelinization ends with myelinization of the cerebral cortex and thalamus (Lowrey 1986).

INFANTS

Reflexes

Infant reflexes that are discussed here include oral reflexes, eye reflexes, general reflexes, and reflexes involving the extremities (Table 16–1).

Oral Reflexes

Oral reflexes that are present in the full-term infant include swallowing, gag, cough, yawn, sucking, rooting, and extrusion. The swallowing, gag, cough, and yawn reflexes are present throughout a normal lifetime. An intact glossopharyngeal (ninth cranial) nerve is responsible

for the gag reflex when stimulation of the posterior pharynx is elicited by food or a foreign object. The cough reflex is evoked by irritating substances to the mucous membranes of the upper respiratory tract. In response to decreased oxygen, the yawn reflex occurs and leads to an increase in inspiration. To elicit a sucking reflex, one need only put a finger in the infant's mouth. Vigorous sucking should occur. The sucking reflex may persist through seven months. The rooting reflex is elicited by brushing or stroking the infant's cheek near the mouth. The infant will turn the head to the side that is stroked and begin to suck. This reflex may be difficult to elicit at times other than feeding times. The rooting reflex should disappear by three or four months of age but may continue until the child is one year old (Whaley and Wong 1994). The extrusion reflex is present until approximately four months of age and consists of the tongue being forced outward when it is touch or depressed.

Eye Reflexes

Reflexes that involve the eyes and are present in full-term infants include the blink reflex, pupillary reflex, and doll's eye reflex. The third (oculomotor), fourth (trochlear), and fifth (abducens) nerves are responsible for the blink reflex, which continues throughout a lifetime and can be elicited by many stimuli. A blink reflex occurs with a bright light (visuopalpebral reflex), sharp noise (cochleopalpebral reflex), painful touch (cutaneous-palpebral reflex), tapping the bridge of the nose (nasopalpebral reflex), stroking they eyelashes (cilliary reflex), or approaching or touching the cornea (corneal reflex) (Illingsworth 1987). The pupillary reflex consists of pupillary constriction when a light shines toward the eye. A bright light should not be used to test this reflex because it may evoke a blink reflex. The length of light exposure may have to be prolonged with some full-term infants to elicit the reflex (Illingsworth 1987). This reflex also persists throughout a lifetime. The doll's eyes reflex is tested by moving the infant's head slowly to the right or left. During the first 10 days of life when the reflex is present

Table 16–1 Summary of Infant Reflexes

Reflex	Elicitation	Response	Duration of Reflex
Oral			
Swallowing	Substance in mouth	Swallow	Birth → LIfetime
Gag	Stimulation of posterior pharynx with food or foreign object	Gag	Birth → Lifetime
Cough	Stimulation of mucous membranes of upper respiratory tract by irritating substances	Cough	Day 1 → Lifetime
Yawn	Decreased oxygen intake	Yawn	Birth → Lifetime
Sucking	Finger in infant's mouth	Suck	Birth → 7 months
Rooting	Brushing or stroking of infant's cheek near mouth	Head turns to side that is stroked, and infant begins to suck.	Birth → 3 or 4 months or 1 year
Extrusion	Tongue touched or depressed	Tongue is forced outward	Birth → 4 months
Eye			
Blink	Bright light, sharp noise, tapping bridge of nose, painful touch	Blink	Birth → Lifetime
Pupillary	Bright light	Pupil constricts.	Birth → Lifetime
Doll's eye	Infant's head moved slowly to right or left	Eyes do not move when head is turned.	Birth → Fixation
General			
Moro	Head at midline; infant held at 45° angle; head dropped back somewhat	Arms abduct and extend; hands open with fingers curved; then adduction of arms occurs.	Birth → 3 or 4 months
Startle	Loud noise, sternum tapped	Adduction of arms; elbows flexed; hands closed	Birth → 4 months
Perez	In suspended position, pressure is applied along spine from sacrum to neck.	Flexion of both arms and legs, lifting of the pelvis, and extension of the neck	Birth → 4 or 6 months
Tonic neck			
Asymmetrical	In supine position, head is turned to one side.	Arm on the side to which the head is turned extends; other arm flexes.	Birth → 3 or 4 months
Symmetrical	Child's head is raised.	Arms extend and legs flex.	3 or 4 months → crawl

continues

Table 16–1 continued

Reflex	Elicitation	Response	Duration of Reflex
Reflexes involving the extremities			
Palmar grasp	Head is midline; object is placed in ulnar side of palm.	Fingers flex around object; muscles tense from wrist to shoulder when object is moved upward in hand.	Birth → 3 or 4 months
Plantar grasp	Stimulation of sole of foot behind toes.	Flexion of toes	Birth → 8 months
Babinski	Stroking of outer edge of sole of foot from heel upward.	Big toe dorsiflexes; other toes fan out.	Few days after birth → 1 year
Walking	In upright position, soles of feet are pressed against a surface.	Reciprocal flexion and extension of legs	Birth → 5 or 6 weeks
Placing	Anterior side of tibia is brushed against a table.	Lifts leg to "place" it on the table	Birth (except breech delivery) → 6 weeks
Crossed extension	One leg is held extended while pressure is applied to sole of foot.	Other leg attempts to push away stimulating force.	Birth → 1 month

and before the development of fixation, the infant's eyes do not move when the head is turned (Illingsworth 1987).

General Reflexes

Reflexes that involve both upper and lower extremities that are present in full-term infants include the Moro, startle, Perez, tonic neck (asymmetrical and symmetrical), and tonic labyrinth reflexes.

Moro Reflex. The Moro reflex (Figure 16–1) is a vestibular reflex present in the child until three to four months of age. To test this reflex, the infant's head should be at midline. The infant is held at a 45° angle, and then the head is allowed to suddenly drop back somewhat. With this movement, the infant's arms become abducted and extended, the hands open although the fingers may be curved inward, and then ad-

duction of the arms occurs. Crying often occurs with this reflex.

Startle Reflex. When a loud noise occurs or the infant's sternum is tapped, the startle reflex is elicited. Abduction of the arms occurs with the elbows flexed and hands closed. The reflex generally disappears by four months of age.

Perez Reflex. The Perez reflex is present in infants until four to six months of age. To evoke this reflex, the infant is held in a suspended prone position and pressure is applied along the spine from the sacrum to the neck. The reflex consists of the infant's flexion of both arms and legs as well as lifting of the pelvis and extension of the neck. Crying as well as urinating often occurs with this reflex.

Tonic Neck Reflexes. Both the asymmetrical (Figure 16–2) and symmetrical tonic neck re-

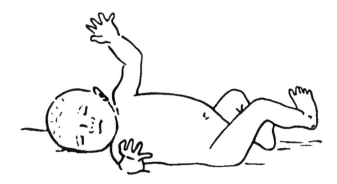

Figure 16–1 Moro reflex. *Source:* Reprinted with permission from N.S. Streeter, *High-Risk Neonatal Care,* p. 367, © 1986 Nan Streeter.

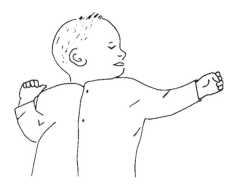

Figure 16–2 Asymmetrical tonic neck reflex. *Source:* Reprinted with permission from N.S. Streeter, *High-Risk Neonatal Care,* p. 367, © 1986 Nan Streeter.

flexes are discussed. The asymmetrical neck reflex is present in infants until three or four months of age. When the infant is placed in a supine position and the head is turned to one side, the arm on the side to which the head is turned extends while the arm on the other side flexes. The legs follow the movement of the arms for their respective sides of the body but may have a reduced response. The symmetrical tonic neck reflex emerges after the disappearance of the asymmetrical tonic neck reflex. It occurs with extension or raising of the child's head. The arms extend and the legs flex. This reflex disappears when the child begins to crawl.

Righting Reflexes. The righting reflexes include the neck righting reflex, the labyrinth righting reflex, and the body righting reflex. These reflexes are responsible for the child's ability to roll from back to stomach and stomach to back, to get on the hands and knees and sit up, and to maintain normal posturing of the head, trunk, and limbs during motor activities (Illingsworth 1987). The neck righting reflex consists of the infant (in a supine position) moving the shoulders, trunk, and pelvis toward the side to which the head is turned. The reflex is strongest at 3 months of age and disappears by 10 months of age. The labyrinth and body righting reflexes do not occur during the neonatal period. The labyrinth reflex occurs at 1 to 2 months of age and is strongest at 10 months of age. Initially, the reflex allows for the young child to lift the head while in a prone position, and later it allows the child to maintain normal head position in space while supine. The body righting reflex does not occur until 7 to 12 months of age after the neck righting reflex disappears. This reflex enables the child to rotate one part of the body before another, which are activities that are important when the child attempts to sit or stand.

Reflexes Involving the Extremities

One reflex that involves the upper extremities is the palmar grasp reflex. Reflexes that involve the lower extremities include the plantar grasp,

Babinski, walking, placing, crossed extension, withdrawal, anal, hip, heel, and leg-straightening reflexes.

Palmar Grasp Reflex. Illingsworth (1987) identified the following two components of the palmar grasp reflex: (1) the reflex and (2) the response to traction. With the infant's head in midline, the reflex is evoked by putting an object into the ulnar side of the palm of the hand. The fingers flex around the object when the palm is stimulated (the reflex) (Figure 16–3). After the grasp, the infant continues to tense the muscles from the wrist to the shoulder when the object in the palm is moved upward in the hand (the response to traction). The palmar grasp reflex disappears around three to four months of age.

Plantar Grasp Reflex. Stimulation of the sole of the foot behind the toes causes the plantar grasp reflex (Figure 16–4). This reflex consists of flexion of the toes and disappears around eight months of age.

Babinski Reflex. The Babinski reflex is initially present a few days after birth and exists until the child walks (usually around one year of age). The reflex is evoked by stroking the outer edge of the sole of the foot from the heel upward. In response, the infant's big toe dorsiflexes and the other toes fan out or hyperextend.

Walking Reflex. The walking reflex is present in the infant until five or six weeks of age. When the infant is held in an upright position with the soles of the feet pressing against a surface, the infant reciprocally flexes and extends the legs. The legs may cross, and there is no movement of the trunk or arms (Figure 16–5).

Placing Reflex. The placing reflex is present at birth in full-term infants weighing over 1,800 g (Illingsworth 1987). It may not be present in infants who are born breech (Chow 1984). The reflex disappears around six weeks of age (Chow 1984). The placing reflex consists of the child lifting the leg up to "place" it on the table in response to the anterior side of the tibia being brushed against the table. Placing of the arm on the table may also be elicited by brushing the ulnar side of the arm against the table.

Crossed Extension Reflex. The crossed extension reflex is present only during the first month of life. The reflex occurs when one leg is held extended while pressure is applied to the sole. The leg that is not extended appears to push away the stimulating force by flexing, adducting, and extending.

Withdrawal Reflex. The withdrawal reflex is shown by the infant's quick flexion of the leg when it has been stimulated by a noxious agent

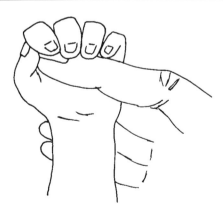

Figure 16–3 Palmar grasp. *Source:* Reprinted with permission from N.S. Streeter, *High-Risk Neonatal Care,* p. 367, © 1986 Nan Streeter.

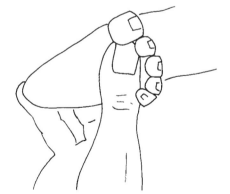

Figure 16–4 Plantar grasp. *Source:* Reprinted with permission from N.S. Streeter, *High-Risk Neonatal Care,* p. 369, © 1986 Nan Streeter.

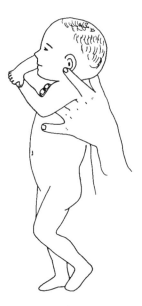

Figure 16–5 Supporting reaction and stepping. *Source:* Reprinted with permission from N.S. Streeter, *High-Risk Neonatal Care,* p. 368, © 1986 Nan Streeter.

such as a pinprick. This response may also occur in the upper extremities.

Anal Reflex. The anal reflex is present in infants at birth. The response is elicited when the infant is lying in a supine position with both legs vertical and the perianal area is touched. The anus contracts with stimulation.

Hip Reflex. The hip reflex is evident with flexion of one leg at the hip in the infant. The other leg flexes in response.

Heel Reflex. The heel reflex is elicited by tapping the heel or applying pressure on the sole of the foot. When this is done, the limb extends.

Leg-Straightening Reflex. The leg-straightening reflex is elicited by pressing the sole of the foot on a hard surface. The infant straightens the legs and body in response.

Gross Motor Development

During infancy, dramatic changes occur rapidly in the infant's gross motor abilities. The newborn's motor activity is primarily reflexive. By the end of the first year, voluntary control of movement has advanced to the point that the child can stand upright and walk.

One Month Old

During the first month of life, reflexive activity dominates the newborn's motor activity. Flexor patterns are evident with the newborn's posture. Development of slight head control is a predominant factor in gross motor development. In a prone position, the neonate can turn the head to the side and can lift the head off its resting surface momentarily. The knees are tucked under the abdomen with the hips and/or pelvis held high. In the supine position, the newborn's shoulders and hips are externally rotated and the elbows and knees are flexed. The asymmetrical tonic neck reflex is seen when the infant's head is turned to one side. When the one-month-old infant is pulled to a sitting position there is almost complete head lag and the back is rounded. The walking reflex occurs when the infant is held standing with the feet against a hard surface.

Two Months Old

The two-month-old infant has increasingly greater head control by being able to hold the head in midline with the rest of the body. While prone, the infant can lift the chin off the resting surface so that the infant's face is at a 45° angle from the surface. Extensor tone generally increases as flexor tone decreases. The infant's hips are extended slightly more than the hips of the one-month-old infant. When the child is held in a sitting position, the back is less rounded and the head is held in midline, although it bobs forward. The asymmetrical neck reflex is present when the infant is in the supine position.

Three Months Old

At three months of age, the infant is able to hold the head up for longer periods. Upper body control is beginning to develop. In the prone position, the infant can bear weight on the forearms, raising the chin and shoulders so that the face is between a 45° and a 90° angle from the resting surface. The infant's pelvis is flat against the resting surface with the hips straight and the knees bent. The asymmetrical tonic reflex disappears, and symmetrical posture dominates. The child is able to bring the hands to midline because of the disappearance of the asymmetrical tonic reflex. Reflexive rolling due to the neck righting reflex may occur when the infant is in the supine position. When the infant is pulled to a sitting position, there is only slight (if any) head lag, although the head may bob forward when the infant is held sitting. The infant may bear weight momentarily when held standing.

Four Months Old

The four-month-old infant does not yet have complete head control under all conditions. When the infant is moved or rocked, the head still wobbles. However, when the infant is held in a sitting position, the head is held steady, enabling the infant to examine the environment. The lumbar region remains as the only curved area of the back. When the infant is prone, the infant is able to raise the face at a 90° angle from the resting surface. Another skill that the four-month-old infant is able to do is roll from a prone (stomach) to a supine (back) position.

Five Months Old

Head control in all positions is evident with the five-month-old infant. There is no head lag when the child is pulled to a sitting position and the infant can hold the head erect and steady. In the prone position, the infant is able to bear weight on the forearms with both elbows extended raising the upper trunk. Patterns of extension and flexion are diminishing. When lying on the back (supine), the infant may extend the legs high in the air, as well as bring the feet to the mouth. When held in a standing position, the infant can bear most weight with the legs somewhat flexed while maintaining shoulder positioning.

Six Months Old

During the sixth month of life, the child gains further control of the upper trunk. In the prone position, the child is able to raise the chest and abdomen off the resting surface, bearing weight on the hands. The infant is also able to roll from a supine (back) to a prone (stomach) position. The child anticipates being pulled to sit by lifting the head. The infant is able to sit unassisted with the trunk erect when in a chair. When sitting on the floor, the infant leans forward on the hands for support. Six-month-old children can bear almost all of their weight on their legs and will bounce when held in a standing position.

Seven Months Old

Until seven months of age, the infant's gross motor development has primarily been centered on head and upper body control. Further gains are made in these areas as well as gains in lower body control during the seventh month. The infant can now sit without support for short periods and puts the hands closer to the sides of the body for balance. In the prone position, the infant is able to bear weight on one hand at a time. Lower body control is evident when the child begins to crawl (moving with the abdomen parallel to the floor). Children do not involve their legs in their first attempts with crawling, but instead they slide forward using their arms to pull themselves along. Some children may also go backward with their first attempts to crawl. Later, the legs are used with the arm movements. When the child begins to crawl, the symmetrical tonic neck reflex disappears. While held standing, children bounce and make walking movements while supporting all of their weight. These walking movements are the first stage in walking.

Eight Months Old

The eight-month-old child is able to sit steadily without support. In addition, the child can lean forward reaching for objects while maintaining postural control. The labyrinth righting reflex is responsible for the child's ability to maintain the head in a normal position in space. The child continues to crawl. Bearing all of their weight on their legs, children may stand by holding onto a table or a crib rail. When standing, the child's trunk is slightly forward and the hips are flexed.

Nine Months Old

Further gains are made in locomotion during the ninth month. Creeping (moving on the hands and knees with the abdomen parallel to the floor) develops after the child's crawling. The child's posture when first beginning to creep consists of bent-elbow posturing with the feet drawn under the hips. The child who creeps well moves contralateral extremities. The nine-month-old child is able to sit unassisted for long periods. When sitting, the hips are flexed and the legs are extended. Maneuverability from one position to another also is evident in the nine-month-old child. The child is able to sit up from a supine position by rolling onto the stomach, bending the legs, and pushing upward. The child is also able to go from a sitting to a prone position without difficulty.

Ten Months Old

The child continues to creep during the 10th month. Holle (1976) cites the following five advantages of the child's increasing mobility: (1) the child has practice holding the head up; (2) eye fixation develops with the eyes becoming used to moving to extreme positions; (3) the arm muscles are trained; (4) the leg pattern becomes more advanced; and (5) the child gains body balance with the cross pattern movement. Ten-month-old children are able to pull themselves to a standing position and cruise along furniture, holding on with both of their hands.

Eleven Months Old

The child's capability in upright posturing continues to develop within the 11th month. The child is able to maintain balance momentarily without assistance. The child also cruises using only one hand to hold onto the furniture. Walking with assistance (both hands held) is possible. In addition, 11-month-old children are able to pivot while in a sitting position so that they can pick up objects anywhere in near proximity.

Twelve Months Old

The most dramatic achievement near or shortly after the child's first birthday is the child's first independent steps. The child is now able to stand independently and walk several steps without assistance. The child's stance is very wide, providing a wide base of support. The child's feet are turned outward with the knees flexed (Cratty 1979). The child's hands are held at shoulder level or above for balance. Initially, the child's arm movements are not reciprocal and the steps are not regular (Cratty 1979). The one-year-old child is also able to stoop and pick up objects from the floor and climb into a small chair to sit. Creeping is still evident when the child goes up stairs.

Fine Motor Development

Fine motor development in infancy proceeds from the newborn's grasp reflex to the one-year-old child's ability to use a superior forefinger grasp and pick up small objects deftly. Hohlstein (1982) cites three major phases of the development of prehension in infancy. In phase one, infants do not use their hands in specialized movements. The infant's fingers are extended and abducted when the infant attempts to grasp an object. When the object is grasped, the fingers are flexed and adducted. Infants during this phase are beginning to develop shoulder stability and cannot always maintain postural control when upright. In the second phase, infants have shoulder stability as well as stability in the elbow joints. Infants use more precise hand movements in grasping objects. Before phase three, infants develop stability at the shoulder, elbow, wrist, and carpometacarpal joints. Infants in phase three are able to use the fingers in highly specialized movements.

Preference for various types of fine motor activities may vary among infants at a given stage in development. Kopp (1974) studied the fine motor abilities of 26 full-term and 10 preterm infants at 32 to 36 weeks of age (age corrected for the preterm infants). The infants were classified as having coordinated or clumsy movements based on clinical judgment, developmental norms, and Halverson's (1932) study of grasping. The clumsy group spent almost one-half of the observed time in visual exploration of objects, whereas the coordinated group spent only one-third of the time in visual exploration and over one-half of the time in manipulation of the objects. Kopp (1974) concluded that the "most important developmental issue is not what type of object interaction is used by infants but rather that the preferred style does not distract the infant from attending to relevant events occurring in his environment."

One Month Old

The newborn's hands are usually closed or fisted. The palmar grasp reflex is evident. With the grasp reflex, the infant's thumb and fingers are flexed and adducted.

Two Months Old

The hands of the two-month-old infant are often open, although the grasp reflex is still present. The child may have swiping movements toward objects without any grasp of them.

Three Months Old

The three-month-old infant's hands are more loosely open (Illingsworth 1987). Hand regard is present. The palmar grasp reflex begins to disappear and will be replaced by ulnar and radial grasps over many months. The infant does not reach for an object before eye contact is made and cannot hold an object unless it is placed in the hand.

Four Months Old

The infant is able to hold objects indefinitely but cannot retrieve them when dropped. The four-month-old infant is yet unable to pick up or grasp objects despite attempts of reaching for them. The infant is able to bring the hands together in midline for play as well as bring the fingers to the mouth.

Five Months Old

The child is now able to secure objects voluntarily using a primitive squeeze grasp or raking movement. The child pulls or "corrals" the object toward the body and then holds it there "squeezing" it against the other hand or the body. The infant often brings objects to the mouth with both hands.

Six Months Old

The six-month-old infant uses a palmar or squeeze grasp. The thumb is extended and the child grasps the object with the other four digits holding the object against the heel of the palm. The child "scoops" up the objects in this fashion. In addition, six-month-old children enjoy grabbing and playing with their feet.

Seven Months Old

The grasp of the seven-month-old infant changes to an emphasis on the radial, rather than ulnar, side of the hand. The child uses a radial-palmar or whole-hand grasp in which the fingers are curled downward over the object like a paw and the thumb is slightly adducted when the object is held against the palm. The child is able to transfer objects from hand to hand, holding onto one when another is offered.

Eight Months Old

The eight-month-old infant uses an inferior scissors grasp or a superior palm grasp. The radial side of the palm is placed over the object, the fingers press downward on the object, and the thumb opposes the first two fingers. The object is still held against the palm of the hand, rather than by the fingers alone.

Nine Months Old

The grasp of the nine-month-old infant is referred to as an inferior forefinger or a radial-digital grasp. The grasp is similar to the superior palm grasp except the last three digits of the hand move more medially than downward, thus moving toward an eventual fingertip grasp in months to come (Halverson 1932).

Ten Months Old

The inferior pincer grasp, which consists of grasping an object with the thumb and index finger, develops during the infant's 10th month. The infant's thumb presses the object against the first joint of the index finger. The child also begins to voluntarily release objects.

Eleven Months Old

The 11-month-old infant enjoys putting objects in and taking them from containers. These actions involve both grasping and releasing. A neat pincer or forefinger grasp develops. A small object can be held by the infant's fingertips of the thumb and index finger. The child must rest the hand on the surface where the object is lying to use this grasp. Slight extension of the wrist occurs with this grasp. In addition, the child is able to release an object with slight force forward.

Twelve Months Old

The superior forefinger grasp is evident in the 12-month-old child. The grasp is similar to the one that precedes it, except that the child does not need to rest the hand on the surface where the object is lying to grasp the object. The child's wrist is extended and deviated to the ulnar side (Erhardt 1974). The child can release large objects well but has difficulty releasing smaller objects smoothly.

Self-Care Skills

The infant's self-care skills center around feeding activities. Before four months of age, the extrusion reflex is present, which makes feeding solid foods somewhat difficult. After this reflex has disappeared, solids can be introduced into the infant's diet with greater ease. The six-month-old infant is able to use a bottle or cup with handles to drink. By seven months of age, the child can chew solids. Children at seven months of age are able to feed themselves larger food items such as crackers or cookies. Once the inferior pincer grasp begins to develop (at approximately 10 months of age), children are able to feed themselves a multitude of different kinds of finger foods. By one year of age, children are able to deftly feed themselves small bites of food.

TODDLERS

Toddlers include children who are between 12 and 36 months of age (one and three years). Gross motor activity in the toddler is characterized by greater stability in walking, as well as the ability to climb and descend stairs. The toddler's fine motor activity is characterized by the child's ability to handle small objects in play.

Gross Motor Development

In the beginning of toddlerhood, the child's walk is characterized by widely spaced feet with the toes turned outward, the arms elevated, and no rotation of the back or hips. By 18 months of age, the child develops a hurried walk that resembles running. At 21 months of age, the child is able to run.

The child's ability to master stairs changes dramatically during the first year of the toddler years. Before 15 months of age, the child creeps up stairs. At 15 months of age, the child is able to walk up stairs with one hand held and creep down stairs. At 18 months of age, the child can walk down the stairs with one hand held. By 21 months of age, the toddler is able to walk up or down stairs by holding the rail.

When attempting to jump in play, the young toddler keeps one foot in contact with the ground. When playing with a ball, the 15-month-old toddler is able to hurl the ball, the 18-month-old toddler attempts to kick the ball by walking into it or stepping on it, and the 21-month-old toddler can kick the ball.

The two-year-old child's feet when walking are less widely spaced than the younger child's, and the child's arms are down at the sides. Children put the heel of one foot in front of the toes of the other when walking and visually watch their steps (Cratty 1979). The child's steps are approximately one-half the length of the adult's step. In the second year, the child is able to walk sideways, on tiptoes, and occasionally backward (Cratty 1979). The two-year-old child can run but cannot start and stop abruptly. At 30 months of age, the child is able to alternate feet going up stairs. In terms of balance, the toddler can stand on one foot briefly (one second) without holding on.

In jumping activities, the two-year-old toddler jumps with both feet off the floor at the same time and can jump from a bottom step to the ground (Knobloch, Stevens, and Malone 1980). The arms are retracted when jumping.

When playing with a ball, the two-year-old toddler is able to throw a ball either forward or backward, although there is little weight shift. The two-and-a-half-year-old child can throw a small ball four to five feet (Cratty 1979). The larger the ball, the less distance the child can throw it (Wellman 1935). Between the second and third year of age, the child is also able to pedal a tricycle.

Fine Motor Development

Before the child's first birthday, the child plays with small cubes or objects by collecting them in piles. Soon after the first year, the child is able to stack two one-inch cubes and insert a large object through a container that has an appropriately matched hole for the object. By 15 months of age, the child can stack three cubes; at 18 months of age, the child can stack four cubes; and by 21 months of age, the child can stack six cubes. The child at 18 months of age is also able to turn two to three pages of a picture book and can put small objects of various shapes into a container with appropriately matched holes for the objects.

During the second year, the child's fine motor skills become further refined. At 24 months of age, the child is able to build a tower of seven cubes, thread a shoelace through a large hole (such as safety pin size), and insert small and large objects swiftly into containers with appro-priately matched holes. At 30 months of age, the child can turn single pages in a book, build a tower of nine cubes, and drop small objects such as raisins into a bottle using a neat superior fore-finger grasp.

With writing or drawing, young toddlers (18 months of age) hold their crayons with a suppinate grasp (holding the crayons in their fists) (Rosenbloom and Horton 1971). The child scribbles in circular, undefined patterns. Near-ing the end of the toddler years (30 months of age), the child holds the crayon in a pronate manner (Rosenbloom and Horton 1971). The child holds the distal part of the crayon with the index finger straight and along the top of the crayon. The two-year-old child can draw single lines.

Self-Care Skills

During the toddler years, the child gains some skills necessary for independent feeding. The superior forefinger grasp is developed in one-year-old children, which enables children to fin-ger-feed themselves with small bites of food. The young toddler also begins to use a spoon. When first attempting to use a spoon, the arm is pronated. The child does not have good control over the spoon, such that it may easily tip, spill-ing the food before reaching the mouth. During the second year, the child gains further control with a spoon, but spills are still common. During the young toddler's years, the child also devel-ops the ability to use a cup. Initially, the child can hold a cup by the handles but may tip the cup when trying to drink from it. The child is then able to drink well from the cup but may drop it when trying to release it onto the table. By the second year, the child can control a cup well and release it appropriately.

The toddler also develops skills in dressing. The young toddler helps in dressing by holding out a foot to have a shoe put on or by holding out the arms to have them put through the sleeves of a shirt. The young toddler can take off shoes, hats, mittens, and socks as well as unzip clothing (Coley 1978). During the second year, the child helps in dressing by pushing down or pulling off clothes and removing the shoes. Children are also able to put their arms through large sleeve holes and button a large front button (Coley 1978).

A major self-care skill that is initiated within the toddler years is bowel and bladder control, much to the relief of the parents or caregivers. A number of physiologic as well as psychological cues for toilet training readiness must be evident before toilet training is attempted. Physiologic cues include voluntary control of the anal and urethral sphincters (Whaley and Wong 1994), an awareness of the characteristics of the sensations before elimination (Scipien et al. 1975), an awareness of the discomfort when incontinent (Scipien et al. 1975), the ability to hold a specific amount of urine in the bladder up to two hours (Whaley and Wong 1994), the ability to walk to go to and leave the toilet (Brazelton 1962), and the ability to sit down, get up, and maintain balance (Brazelton 1962). Psychological cues include the ability to understand simple directions (Chow 1984), the ability to communicate a desire, the absence of a terribly negative period (Brazelton 1962), and the wish to please the caregiver(s) and behave like others (Brazelton 1962).

Toilet training is most often begun between 18 and 30 months of age depending on the readiness of the child and caregiver. Brazelton (1962) studied the toilet training efforts of 1,170 children in a 10-year period; 80 percent of the children achieved bowel and bladder control simultaneously, 12 percent achieved bowel control before bladder control, and 8 percent achieved bladder control before bowel control. The mean age for first achievement (bladder, bowel, or bladder and bowel control) was 27.7 months. No significant differences were found between boys and girls. Daytime control was achieved on the average at 28.5 months of age. Nighttime control was achieved on the average at 33.3 months of age. The girls achieved night-time control about 2$^1/_2$ months before the boys. For urinary night-time control, the bladder must be able to retain 300 to 350 mL of urine. Brazelton (1962) found that 40 percent of the children were bedwetting at age four years and 30 percent were still bedwetting at age five years.

PRESCHOOLERS

Preschoolers include children between 36 and 60 months of age (three to five years). Increasing balance and coordination are apparent in the preschooler's gross motor activity. Preschoolers further develop fine motor skills necessary with intricate movements of the hands during writing.

Gross Motor Development

Children at three years of age have increasing balance and do not visually watch their steps. Bayley (1935) found that 50 percent of the three-year-old children tested could walk 10 feet on a one-inch wide line without falling from the line. The three-year-old child is also able to walk heel to toe for 10 feet and balance with one foot off the ground for three to four seconds (Bayley 1935). The child between three and four years of age is able to descend stairs with alternating steps (Knobloch, Stevens, and Malone 1980). At four years of age, the child can walk on a circular line (Wellman 1935). At five years of age, the child can maintain balance between three and five seconds standing on one foot with the arms folded (Cratty 1979).

In running activities, the preschooler gains both coordination and speed. By five years of age, the child demonstrates smooth reciprocal arm movements and can run reasonably fast (11.5 feet/second) (Cratty 1979).

The ability to skip is not fully attained during the preschool years. The four- or five-year-old child skips on one foot while walking on the other foot.

The child's ability to jump develops further in the preschool years. The three-year-old child can broad-jump 8 to 10 inches (Cratty 1979). By five years of age, the child can broadjump 2 to 3 feet with a 2-foot takeoff (Cratty 1979).

The child's ability to hop changes during the preschool years. The three-year-old child is able to hop on one foot 1 to 3 steps without accuracy of rhythm or distance; the four-year-old child can hop 4 to 6 steps on one foot; and the five-year-old child can hop 8 to 10 steps (Cratty 1979).

When throwing a ball, the three-year-old child throws overhand, rotating the body but not shifting weight (Cratty 1979). The child can throw a ball about 6 or 7 feet (Wellman 1935). The four-year-old child demonstrates reasonable weight shift when throwing a ball. When catching a ball, the three-year-old child holds the arms straight with the elbows stiff (Cratty 1979). The four-year-old child opens the hands in an attempt to catch a ball, although the elbows are kept stiff (Cratty 1979). During the child's fifth year, the arms are held at the side of the body, allowing for some "give" when catching a ball (Wellman 1935). The five-year-old child can catch a large ball about 75 percent of the time when it is bounced to the child from 15 feet (Cratty 1979).

Fine Motor Development

The three-year-old child can build a tower of 10 cubes. By the later preschool years, the child is able to construct complex structures with cubes and blocks. The child during the preschool years is also able to drop small objects into a container (such as a piggy bank) with reasonable speed.

Fine motor skills become further evident in the preschooler's writing and drawing behaviors. Between four and six years of age, the child develops the dynamic tripod finger posture (Wynn-Parry 1966), which consists of the child's ability to use the thumb, index, and middle fingers as a tripod in holding a crayon or pencil with the fourth and fifth fingers providing added stability (Rosenbloom and Horton 1971). The writing utensil is held in the posture as most adults hold a writing utensil. This finger posture allows for highly coordinated writing movements.

The three-year-old child is able to copy a cross, and by four or five years of age the child is able to copy a square and circle. Cutting with scissors is attempted by the preschooler but is not a refined skill until the early school-age years.

Figures appear in the drawings of preschoolers. The three-year-old child may draw two figures together; crude drawings of human figures and objects appear in the four-year-old child's drawings; and more refined human figures and objects appear in the five-year-old child's drawings (Cratty 1979). The five-year-old child may also draw recognizable letters.

Another fine motor skill that the five-year-old child can demonstrate with slow speed is finger opposition. The child touches each finger in turn to the thumb.

Self-Care Skills

During meals, the preschooler learns to distinguish between finger foods and foods requiring a spoon. The child at five years of age is able to hold a spoon with the fingers when either liquid or solid foods are eaten. The child is also able to use a fork. Initially, the fork is held in the fist and then by the fingers.

With dressing activities, the three-year-old child can manage to remove pants or a skirt by pulling them down but requires help with pulling a shirt over the head to remove it. The child can open front or side buttons or zippers. When putting on clothes, the three-year-old child needs help in distinguishing the front from the back of clothes and may need help putting on clothes. The child can manipulate buttons and close snaps and may attempt to put on a shoe, although it may be on the wrong foot. By the fifth year of age, the child can dress independently with simple clothing. The child can put on and tie shoes, pull clothing on, put a belt through loops, button front and side buttons, and close a front or back zipper (Coley 1978).

Self-care skills in bathing develop in the following order during the preschool years: (1) the child can dry the hands; (2) the child can wash the hands; (3) the child can dry the body with help; (4) the child can wash the body including the face; and (5) the child can dry the body. Preschoolers are also able to brush their teeth independently.

As described previously, toilet training occurs within the toddler and preschool years. Three-year-old children will attempt to wipe themselves after toileting without success. By five years of age, children can wipe themselves after toileting, flush the toilet, and wash and dry their hands.

SCHOOL-AGE CHILDREN

School-age children are between 6 and 11 years of age. Greater speed, strength, versatility, and accuracy become evident in the school-age child's gross motor activities (Ausubel, Sullivan, and Ives 1980). School-age children develop the fine motor skills necessary for cursive writing.

Gross Motor Development

Throughout much of the literature for gross motor skills of school-age children, boys' performances exceed those of girls (Ausubel, Sullivan, and Ives 1980). Sex differences are postulated to occur, in part, due to socialization.

The school-age child runs with more coordinated and reciprocal arm and leg movements. Running speed increases about 1 foot per second during each of these years (Cratty 1979). The young school-age child is also able to skip with both feet.

Balance improves in both static and dynamic activities. The 6-year-old child can walk on a two-inch beam (dynamic), and the 7-year-old child can maintain balance when immobile and both eyes are closed (static) (Cratty 1979). The early school-age child is also able to hop rhythmically in place from one foot to the other, as well as hop into small squares on one foot

(Cratty 1979). The child is also able to ride a bicycle.

The 7-year-old child can jump 7 inches vertically using arm action with the jump (Cratty 1979). By 7 years of age, the child can also jump rope and do jumping jacks. By 9 years of age, girls can vertically jump $8^{1}/_{2}$ inches and boys can vertically jump 10 inches (Cratty 1979). Boys and girls can jump approximately 20 inches in the standing broad jump (Cratty 1979).

Increases in eye-hand coordination are evident when these children throw and catch balls. In the early years, the child has reasonable throwing skill by shifting the weight and stepping with the opposite foot from that of the throwing arm. Distances improve for boys by 11 to 23 feet between 9 and 10 years of age (Cratty 1979). For girls, distances improve between 10 and 11 years of age by 7 or 8 feet (Cratty 1979). The young school-age child can catch a ball when it is thrown waist high from 15 feet (Cratty 1979).

Fine Motor Development

Sex differences tend to be small in fine motor skills of school-age children (Ausubel, Sullivan, and Ives 1980). Whereas the 5-year-old child can do the finger opposition task slowly, the 7- to 8-year-old child can do the task quickly (Cratty 1979). The child is also able to use scissors.

The school-age child's writing and drawing abilities increase. Hand preference is established by 6 years of age (Ausubel, Sullivan, and Ives 1980). The 6-year-old child can draw a triangle; the 7-year-old child can draw a diamond; and the older school-age child can draw three-dimensional figures. Cursive writing is usually not possible before the child is 8 or 9 years of age.

Self-Care Skills

At 6 to 8 years, the child gains the ability to use a knife in both spreading and cutting food. Few spills occur when eating. With dressing, the 6-year-old child gains the skills to button back buttons or snap back snaps (Coley 1978). Thus, the child has all of the abilities to be independent in dressing.

Personal hygiene skills are evident in the self-care activities of school-age children. The child can anticipate appropriate times to wash hands, brush teeth, and bathe and/or shower and can carry out these tasks independently.

ADOLESCENTS

Adolescents include persons between 12 and 18 years of age. Sex differences in gross motor activities become apparent in adolescence, with adolescent males excelling beyond adolescent females in most activities. Increases in speed and accuracy occur in the fine motor development of adolescents.

Gross and Fine Motor Development

Until the preadolescent years (10 or 11 years of age), the growth rate for males and females is fairly equal. The growth spurt for females begins at between 10 and 14 years of age and ends near 17 years of age. Females grow between 2 and 7.9 inches during these years (Whaley and Wong 1994). The growth spurt for males begins at between 12 and 16 years of age and ends near 20 or 21 years of age. Males gain between 4 and 12 inches in height (Whaley and Wong 1994). The growth spurt begins with the growth of the extremities and neck, followed by the growth of the hips, chest, shoulders, and trunk. The head circumference also increases during the pubertal growth spurt. Awkwardness may temporarily develop because of these rapid skeletal changes. In general, girls are smaller than boys, have arms and legs that are proportionately shorter, have a larger trunk, and have a broader pelvis (Carpenter 1938).

The relationship between gross motor performance and age, anatomic growth, and physiologic maturity has been studied. Gross motor performance in adolescent males was positively related to age, anatomic growth, and physiologic maturity (Atkinson 1924; Espenshade 1940). Increases in motor performance were found to

cease between 17 and 18 years of age for adolescent boys (Espenshade 1940). Gross motor performance in adolescent females was only slightly positively related to height (Atkinson 1925). A slightly negative relationship between weight and gross motor performance was found for adolescent females (Atkinson 1925). The relationship between physiologic maturity and gross motor performance in adolescent females was task specific (Atkinson 1925). Increases in motor performance for female adolescents were found to cease between 13 and 16 years of age (Espenshade 1940).

In addition to skeletal changes, muscle mass increases during adolescence, particularly in male adolescents. Muscular individuals generally excel in gross motor activities (Tanner 1964). Strength was found to be positively related to gross motor skill in adolescent males but only slightly related to gross motor skill in adolescent females (Bliss 1927). The most rapid increases in strength for adolescents occur between 13 and 16 years of age for adolescent males and between 12 and 14 years of age for adolescent females (McCloy 1935). Dimock (1935) found that adolescent males' increases in strength were slightly related to their physiologic maturity. Strength was most marked after the first year after the postpubescent stage.

Cardiac and pulmonary changes occur that lead to the adolescents' increased endurance during physical activity. Overall, male adolescents' greater muscle mass and capacity to carry oxygen as well as their superior height, weight, limb length, and shoulder breadth lead to better performances in gross motor activities compared with female adolescents (Ausubel 1954).

Literature attending to fine motor skills in adolescence is primarily concerned with coordination and reaction time tasks. The speed and accuracy of these tasks increase with age during adolescence (Goodgold-Edwards 1984). Gross motor ability was not found to be highly related to fine motor ability in adolescence (Espenshade 1940). (Table 16–2 is a summary of gross motor, fine motor, and self-care skills of children and adolescents within each age group.)

Table 16–2 Summary of Gross Motor, Fine Motor, and Self-Care Skills for Five Age Groups

Age Group	Gross Motor Skill	Fine Motor Skill	Self-Care Skill
Infants			
1 month	Pulled to sit: slight head control	Palmar grasp reflex is evident.	
2 months	Prone: lifts head so face is at 45° angle from resting surface	Makes swiping movements toward objects.	
3 months	Prone: supports self on forearms	Hands are more loosely open.	
4 months	Rolls stomach to back	Hands are brought together in midline.	
5 months	Head control is evident in all positions.	Primitive squeeze grasp or raking movement	
6 months	Rolls back to stomach	Scoops objects; palmar or squeeze grasp	Drinks from cup with handles; holds bottle
7 months	Sits without support; crawls	Transfers objects; radial-palmar or whole-hand grasp	Chews solids; feeds self large food items
8 months	Stands holding onto furniture	Inferior scissors grasp or superior palm grasp	
9 months	Creeps	Inferior forefinger or radial-digital grasp	
10 months	Cruises along furniture	Voluntarily releases objects; inferior pincer grasp	Feeds self small bites of food
11 months	Walks with both hands held	Neat pincer or forefinger grasp	
12 months	Walks independently	Superior forefinger grasp	
Toddlers	Walks sideways and backward	Stacks two to nine cubes	Uses spoon
	Runs	Turns pages in book	Drinks from small cup
	Climbs and descends stairs	Scribbles	Pushes down or pulls off simple pieces of clothing
			Gains bowel and bladder control
Preschoolers	Rides tricycle	Builds complex structures with cubes	Uses fork
	Balances on one foot	Copies cross, square, and circle	Dresses independently with simple clothing by age five
	Alternates feet when descending stairs	Can perform finger opposition task slowly	Brushes teeth

continues

Table 16–2 continued

Age Group	Gross Motor Skill	Fine Motor Skill	Self-Care Skill
School-age children	Skips Rides bicycle Running speed increases. Distance in throwing a ball increases.	Has dynamic tripod finger posture[*] Uses cursive writing Copies triangle, diamond, and draws three-dimensional figures Uses scissors	Uses knife Dresses independently Bathes/showers independently
Adolescents	Increases in strength and endurance	Increases in speed and accuracy	Independent in eating, dressing, and personal hygiene activities

[*]*Rehabilitation of the Hand*, 2d ed., by C.B. Wynn-Parry, p. 26, Butterworth Publishers, © 1966.

REFERENCES

Atkinson, R.K. 1924. A motor efficiency study of eight thousand New York City high school boys. *American Physical Education Review* 29:56–59.

Atkinson, R.K. 1925. A study of athletic ability of high school girls. *American Physical Education Review* 30: 389–99.

Ausubel, D.P. 1954. *Theory and problems of adolescent development.* New York: Grune & Stratton.

Ausubel, D.P., E.V. Sullivan, and S.W. Ives. 1980. *Theory and problems in child development.* 3d. ed. New York: Grune & Stratton.

Bayley, N.A. 1935. The development of motor abilities during the first three years. *Monographs in Social Research and Child Development* 1:1–26.

Bliss, J.G. 1927. A study of progression based on age, sex, and individual differences in strength and skill. *American Physical Education Review* 32:11–21.

Brazelton, T.B. 1962. A child-oriented approach to toilet training. *Pediatrics* 29:121–28.

Carpenter, A. 1938. Strength, power and "femininity" as factors influencing the athletic performance of college women. *Research Quarterly American Physical Education Association* 9:120–27.

Chow, M.P. 1984. *Handbook of pediatric primary care.* 2d ed. New York: Delmar Publishers.

Coley, I.L. 1978. *Pediatric assessment of self-care activities.* St. Louis: C.V. Mosby Co.

Cratty, B.J. 1979. *Perceptual and motor development in infants and children.* 2d ed. Englewood Cliffs, N.J.: Prentice-Hall, Inc.

Di Leo, J.H. 1977. *Child development: Analysis and synthesis.* New York: Brunner/Mazel.

Dimock, H. 1935. A research in adolescence: I. Pubescence and physical growth. *Child Development* 6:176–95.

Erhardt, R.P. 1974. Sequential levels in development of prehension. *American Journal of Occupational Therapy* 28:592–96.

Espenshade, A. 1940. Motor performance in adolescence including the study of relationships with measure of physical growth and maturity. *Monographs of the Society for Research for Child Development* 5:1–126.

Goodgold-Edwards, S.A. 1984. Motor learning as it relates to the development of skilled motor behavior: A review of the literature. *Physical and Occupational Therapy in Pediatrics* 4:5–18.

Halverson, H.M. 1932. An experimental study of prehension in infants by means of systematic cinema records. *Genetic Psychology Monographs* 10:107–284.

Hohlstein, R.R. 1982. The development of prehension in normal infants. *American Journal of Occupational Therapy* 36:170–76.

Holle, B. 1976. *Motor development in children: Normal and retarded.* Oxford: Blackwell Scientific Publishers.

Illingsworth, R.S. 1987. *The development of the infant and young child: Normal and abnormal.* 9th ed. Secaucus, NJ: Churchill.

Knobloch, H., F. Stevens, and A.F. Malone. 1980. *Manual of developmental diagnoses.* New York: Harper & Row.

Kopp, C.B. 1974. Fine motor abilities of infants. *Developmental Medicine and Child Neurology* 16:629–36.

Loria, C. 1980. Relationship of proximal and distal function in motor development. *Physical Therapy* 60:167–72.

Lowrey, G.H. 1986. *Growth and development of children.* 8th ed. Chicago: Year Book Medical Publishers.

McCloy, C.H. 1935. The influence of chronological age on motor performance. *Research Quarterly American Physical Educational Association* 6:61–64.

Neligan, G., and D. Prudham. 1969. Norms for four standard developmental milestones by sex, social class and place in the family. *Developmental Medicine and Child Neurology* 11:413–22.

Rosenbloom, L., and M.E. Horton. 1971. The maturation of fine prehension in young children. *Developmental Medicine and Child Neurology* 13:3–8.

Scipien, G.M., et al. 1975. *Comprehensive pediatric nursing.* New York: McGraw-Hill Book Co.

Tanner, J.M. 1964. *Physique of the Olympic athlete.* London: Allen & Unwin.

Wellman, B.L. 1935. Motor achievements of preschool children. *Child Education* 13:311–16.

Whaley, L.F., and D.L. Wong. 1994. *Essentials of pediatric nursing.* 4th ed. St. Louis: C.V. Mosby.

Wynn-Parry, C.B. 1966. *Rehabilitation of the hand.* 2d ed. London: Butterworth.

CHAPTER 17

Communication Intervention

*Mary Lou Fragomeni-Nuttall, Nancy Williams, and
Jennifer Casteix*

This chapter provides information on the sequence of communication development and suggestions for treating the child who has disordered communication. Emphasis is placed on determining the most functional means of communication and the most functional means of promoting the normal developmental sequence of language. The skills needed for communication are explained to help determine the initial phase of intervention.

Children hospitalized for extended periods experience both motor and communicative developmental delays. These children then being cared for in the home vary in age, medical etiology, and extent of intervention requirements. There is one factor that is evident in a child who demonstrates delays in communicative development—a breakdown in the ability to express wants, needs, thoughts, and difficulty showing how much is understood. The information presented here can be used to give caregivers the means to increase the child's ability to participate with the environment and to reduce the frustration of those desperately trying to understand.

Communication is a process of developing and refining the rudimentary skills of hearing and vocalizing into listening and verbalizing. This process involves receptive and expressive skills that integrate with other thinking skills. Hearing and seeing are receptive skills that are complemented by the expressive skills of gesturing and talking. Understanding of motor and sensory input from the environment, which leads to the ability to manipulate and adapt, is the cognitive process that integrates thought into expression. In a normal child, this sequence can be viewed by developmental guidelines. For the child who demonstrates language delays, the correlation to chronologic age may vary but the sequence of skills should progress in a manner similar to normal development.

When a child's ability to communicate is impaired, a referral to a certified speech/language pathologist (SLP) is recommended. The SLP is qualified to assess the child's ability to communicate and express language and to recommend appropriate measures to enhance communication. Information about the child's hearing acuity is also needed, which may result in a referral to a certified audiologist. The following guidelines should be considered when considering a referral to an SLP:

- The child has never received a complete speech/language assessment by a certified SLP.
- The child and/or family demonstrates frustration in the communicative process.
- Little or no progress has been demonstrated with the present recommendations.

- The child has achieved all previous recommendations and the course for further improvement of communication is unclear.

NORMAL DEVELOPMENT

The natural process of sequenced changes in communication that occur in "normal" children also occur in children demonstrating delays. These delays may change the timing of the acquired skills, but the sequence is typically not altered. Disordered language differs in that the sequence of development is disrupted by sensory or motor difficulties. It is important to focus on each child's skill level and needs rather than to correlate his or her abilities to those of other children at the same chronologic age.

Periodic plateaus commonly occur in language development. Each child develops at a different rate. When a child remains at one level for a period, it may be because gains are being made in other developmental areas. Each child, whether of normal development or with communication deficits, progresses at an individual pace. Therefore, children may not demonstrate skills exactly parallel to those on normal development charts.

Communication is often associated with a means of requesting a desired activity or object. This is one of the many roles of language in normal communication. Other functions are to obtain information, indicate notice of an event or object, display displeasure, gain relief from an undesirable situation, and acknowledge the presence of others as well as bringing them into contact.

Language development is outlined in Exhibit 17–1 to assist the home care nurse in reviewing the progression of language skills and should be used as a guideline, recalling that each child is unique in his or her strengths and rate of development. Used as a checklist, Exhibit 17–1 can help determine how well the communication is meeting the child's cognitive skill level and the current and future environmental needs.

EARLY COMMUNICATION BEHAVIORS

Early communication behaviors involve a variety of skills that allow a child to interact with the environment. From birth through the first years of life, a child uses many skills to play, communicate, investigate, and relate to his or her surroundings. These skills are necessary for initiating the communication process for the younger child learning language or for the older child who needs to redevelop these skills to be retrained in communication techniques.

The importance of these early behaviors may be understood more clearly with examples. Without the understanding that a particular behavior may achieve a desired end result, the language learner may never use communications (means) to achieve a result (end). The development of functional communication would be hindered by the lack of other behaviors as well. Without initiation skills, the language learner would not repeat new gestures or words. The failure to comprehend the functional use of objects would not allow for more complex conceptualization to relate to others about the child's daily life. The behaviors needed are sensorimotor skills that occur before more sophisticated language development.

The following skills can be observed or stimulated and, if absent, can be taught as the most basic skills in communication. Some age ranges are included, but, as with all developmental ranges, these are approximate. The sequencing of events within each area is the expected developmental ordering. Many of the skills overlap into various areas and, as teaching and learning commence, the early items common to several areas should be emphasized.

The most concrete skill of the behaviors presented is *object permanence*. The concept that objects exist even when out of sight for periods is basic to communication development and to cognitive awareness. In normal development the following sequence exists:

Exhibit 17–1 Developmental Communication Scale

1–2 Months

- Cries, random vocal play
- Makes "animal-like" sounds
- Stops activity when looking at a face
- Follows movement with eyes
- Is alert
- Has startle response when loud sounds are made
- Makes rudimentary head turn
- Opens eyes to voice

3–4 Months

- "Coos" one-syllable vowel-like sounds
- Cries less
- Begins vocal-social response (talks back)
- Inspects own hand
- Smiles or face "brightens" in response to talking
- Regularly localizes speaker with eyes
- Is frightened by angry voices
- Recognizes and responds to name
- Usually stops crying when someone talks to him or her
- Laughs, repeats own vocalizations
- Babbles, vocalizes strings of syllable-like sounds
- Moods of pleasure last up to 30 minutes

5–6 Months

- Vocalizes spontaneously to self
- Tries to imitate inflection
- Babbles sounds with more consonants
- Babbles back, experiences "belly" laughs
- Imitates social play by smiling and vocalizing
- Talks to mirror image
- Looks and vocalizes to own name
- Appears to recognize words such as "daddy," "bye-bye," "mama"
- Stops or withdraws in response to "no" about 50 percent of the time

7–8 Months

- Has defined syllables—ma, da, mi, my
- Attention more concentrated; looks for toy that disappears
- Repeats oral-motor sounds—cough, raspberry, tongue-click
- Babbles in more adultlike manner for fun
- Uses defined two-syllable utterances—"mama," "choo-choo," "dada"
- Regularly stops activity when name called
- Will sustain interest in pictures if they are named

9–10 Months

- Signals emphasis and emotions by vocalizing distinct intonation patterns
- Vocalizes to gain attention
- Combines words with gestures—"no-no" with head shake, "bye-bye" with wave
- May repeat same word for many meanings
- Understands commands with gestures

11–12 Months

- Speaks more gibberish
- Imitates inflections, gestures, and speech rhythms
- Speaks jargon with occasional meaningful word
- Practices words that are known; produces more sounds specific to the child's language
- Aware of expressive function of language—may repeat "damn, damn"
- Babbles short sentences
- Uses appropriate intonation patterns
- Uses two to three words meaningfully
- Follows one-step command without gesture
- Appears to understand simple questions such as—"Where's the ball?"
- Shows more intense attention and response to speech over prolonged periods

continues

Exhibit 17–1 continued

- Demonstrates understanding by responding with appropriate gestures to several kinds of verbal requests

13–18 Months

- Names one object on request
- Names one black-and-white picture on request
- Appears to understand some new words each week
- Points to more than one body part
- Identifies more than one picture in a book
- Responds to action verb request
- Brings object from another room on request
- Identifies two or more objects from a group of familiar objects

19–24 Months

- Uses one- and two-word phrases
- Puts two words together
- Names at least three familiar objects or pictures
- Has vocabulary of 10–15 words by age 2
- Identifies several pictures

- Understands possessor-possession relationships (for example, mama's shoe)
- Follows a number of simple requests

25–36 Months

- Points to smaller body parts, such as chin and elbow
- Points to pictures showing action
- Points to objects described by use
- Understands most common verbs
- Responds to two related actions (run fast)
- Likes to listen to simple stories
- Uses words "on" and "in"

37–48 Months

- Responds to primary seriation of categorization such as "Put them in order."
- Follows simple commands with two objects
- Follows "in, on, under, beside" when asked to do so
- Names item when cued by function (for example, when asked "What do you sit on?"
- Uses more adultlike language

- Visual tracking observed: 1–4 months
- Visual search of where object disappears: 1–4 months
- Finds partially covered object: 4–8 months
- Finds completely covered object: 8–12 months

Objects that can encourage looking, tracking, and finding include brightly colored noisemakers and toys. The use of toys with both visual and audible characteristics provides at least one mode of input for visually or hearing impaired children. If a child is not visually or hearing impaired, the toy can be limited to using either sound (hidden bell) or visual input (flashing light) to make tracking or finding more difficult, making it more challenging for the child. At later stages, toys can be hidden under cups, scarves, or blankets. If needed, have the child watch you

hide the toy (or hide it in the same place) and let the child discover it independently.

The second behavior is an awareness of *cause and effect*. This is the recognition that specific actions give specific results and is observed as the early development of initiating communications. The expected progression is as follows:

- Focuses on interesting objects: 0–1 month
- Watches hands: 1–4 months
- Indicates desire for the recurrence of an event by touching an adult's hands: 4–8 months
- Pushes away an interfering hand: 8–12 months
- Requests the activation of an object after its demonstration: 12–18 months
- Activates a mechanical object: 18–24 months

The third skill is "means/end." This can be observed in motor responses that bring about a desired occurrence. Acting out of the thought process can be seen. The progression of this expected skill is as follows:

- Reaches and grasps: 1–8 months
- Releases one object to grasp another: 8–12 months
- Uses props to get desired object: 12–18 months
- Uses a mallet to pound in pegs: 18–24 months

A child reaching to make a mobile swing demonstrates the early use of means/end. This purposeful movement brings about the desired change. A more active child may pull a toy by its string or hit the pegs on a toy bench to cause a specific occurrence. The child then demonstrates greater manipulation of the environment.

Imitation, the fourth language behavior, is the most important skill in learning to communicate. It is manifested in verbal or gestural fashion, possibly both. By following another's lead, communication often begins. The following developmental levels are expected:

- Mutual imitation: 1–4 months
- A skill within the child's repertoire is imitated: 4–8 months
- Child imitates new behavior: 8–12 months
- Child imitates unfamiliar and subtle gestures: 18–24 months

Activities that encourage imitation range from sound or melody imitation to mirroring the "so big" gesture. Pat-a-cake and peek-a-boo games, at the appropriate developmental level, give appropriate redundancy to early imitation.

Expecting an event to recur describes the fifth behavior, *anticipation*. Recognition that a certain environment surrounds the occurrence involves memory of details, as well as a response that prepares a person for the next event. The sequence of skills that develop is shown in the following:

- Sucks before external excitement: 1–4 months
- Looks for an object dropped in front of him or her: 4–8 months
- Holds hands out to catch a ball: 12–18 months

During feeding, a child may suck just at the sight of the bottle. Repeated play with a familiar toy can bring about an anticipation response. Often, when daily events occur routinely, this response will be seen before a favored activity.

Relating to objects for purposeful use in the environment is the sixth early communication behavior. The child demonstrates more purposeful control of surroundings as his or her experience expands. His or her interest and need to communicate also grow. The order of development for functional relating is as follows:

- Mouths, holds object: 1–4 months
- Waves, visually inspects, hits, stabs objects: 8–12 months
- Demonstrates object function: 12–18 months
- Labels objects: 18–24 months

When a child puts a spoon in his or her mouth during feeding, purposeful use of the object is shown. All activities of daily living (washing, brushing teeth, putting on shoes) provide excellent opportunities for the use of objects as tools.

The seventh and final early behavior in language development is *construction of objects in space*. Spatial relations develop as a function of motor and visualization skills. Recognizing that objects can combine in "novel" ways is a complex skill that progresses as follows:

- Focuses on single object: 1–4 months
- Glances between two objects: 4–8 months
- Localizes to sound: 4–12 months
- Stacks two blocks, rings on stick: 18–24 months

The home care nurse or caregiver can observe how the child interacts with the environment and can encourage increased interactions by providing the child with different opportunities. In the following section, a similar idea to that discussed previously is presented—of stimulating the senses with specific items. Once it is determined that a certain object achieves a response through a specific sense, try to combine it with another object so that learning is occurring. An example of this combination might be a simple mobile that attracts the child visually when it moves. Bells can then be added so the child associates the sounds with the mobile. Then, when the child hears the bells, he or she will look for the moving mobile.

SENSORY STIMULATION

Multisensory stimulation may be indicated for the child who is severely impaired or in a persistent vegetative state (PVS). Some specialists believe that the child in a persistive vegetative state may develop increased responsiveness and increased quality of life and may even regain consciousness if given controlled and persistent stimulation (Smith 1983).

Stimulation is more effective when done at the same time of the day each day and in the same sequence. As these activities are used, it may become apparent that they stimulate early communication. Family participation, using this treatment modality, should be encouraged.

Sensory stimulation can be provided through auditory, visual, tactile, taste, and olfactory senses. The variety of the presentation can change from session to session. Rarely should a presentation last longer than 10 seconds, and the whole sequence may take only 20 minutes. It may be completed in two sessions. Suggestions for each modality are provided in Exhibit 17–2.

The goal of sensory stimulation is to bring about increased awareness of the environment. This change in awareness may be observed as greater intensity in responses, more variety of responses, or an improved level of consciousness. Examples of cause/effect toys are listed in Exhibit 17–3.

A limited form of sensory stimulation is also effective with a very young child or toddler who has spent much of his or her early life in the hospital. Even though staff in nursery intensive care units and special care nurseries are becoming more aware of the needs of a fragile infant, they cannot provide a home environment with the accompanying sensory experiences. A child requires slow introduction to a variety of sensations on his body, face, and in his mouth. Introducing various sensations in his mouth is especially important if this child is not an oral feeder. Encourage mouthing of a variety of different types of safe objects. Toys made of various viscosities of rubber and plastic, with various textures and of different sizes make for good oral stimulation. Provide gentle stimulation on the tongue or teeth and gums using a cloth-swathed finger or a beginning toothbrush.

Any oral stimulation program should be advanced by a speech/language pathologist or occupational therapist along with the parents/caregivers of the child. Progression should be steady, and involved persons should always follow the lead of the child so as not to overstimulate him or her. Other activities incorporating movement and exploration are discussed in Chapter 18.

AUGMENTATIVE COMMUNICATION

Verbal communication may not be a sufficient or viable mode of expression for some older infants, toddlers, children, and adolescents. It is then necessary to determine how to augment existing skills and create improved communication potential. The augmentative device may consist of a system of eye blinks for communicating yes or no responses, a simple alphabet board for spelling out words, or a laser beam connected to a headband that makes a computer "talk." Infants as young as 8 months can develop gestures to indicate specific items, "milk" being a favorite. Establishing the need and motivation to express one's thoughts is, however, the important first step in providing an

Exhibit 17–2 Types of Stimulation

Auditory

- Bell
- Clicker
- Hemisynchronized music
- Television (never longer than 30 to 60 minutes so as not to become background noise)
- Recording of family or friend
- Loud clapping

Visual

- Light on/off, flashlight
- Sunlight
- Pictures of family, pets, friend
- Mobile (moving)
- Tinsel
- Black and white drawing of face

Taste

Place on tongue for taste only. Precautions should be taken to use only small amounts and that no substance should be left in the child's mouth. Cleaning the mouth before and after these presentations can be included as part of the stimulation program.

- Lemon
- Candy stick

- Catsup
- Chicken soup
- Ice/popsicle
- Salty breadsticks

Tactile

- Rough/smooth (washcloth)
- Wet
- Warm/cool (water, ice)
- Shaving brush
- Cotton
- Lotion (vanilla scented)

Olfactory

Pleasant or familiar odors

- Vanilla
- Cinnamon
- Nutmeg
- Perfume (family's)
- Fruit
- Chicken soup

Alerting odors

- Ammonia
- Onion
- Garlic

appropriate system of augmentative communication.

A child who has not developed an expressive communication system requires a different strategy from the child who has lost the means of communication. The first child must establish the precursors of language and then a system that works within his or her abilities. The child who loses the means of communication may not lose the precursors but now needs a new means of self-expression. Both of these children must be provided with stimulation that will develop language intent. The child who has been long term on a ventilator may not even understand that voicing is available, how it is available, and why he or she would even begin to use it. This child has learned to get attention by not breath-

Exhibit 17–3 Cause/Effect Toys

1. Objects that make noise or move by manipulation—music boxes, toy radios, or squeeze toys
2. Objects that stimulate reach—mobile, tactile materials that are suspended (tissue paper streamers, aluminum foil, yarn)
3. Objects that stimulate grasp—cloth-covered blocks that make noise, Nerf balls, squeeze bulb, squeeze animals, or visual tracking rattle
4. Objects that stimulate finger movement—finger paints, sand and water play, nontoxic clay, push-button jack-in-the-box, touch-me books, or finger play rattles

ing to set off alarms; to vocalize, the child must now use controlled breathing to vibrate the vocal chords.

The key step in developing augmentative communication is determining the best response available to the child. Motor abilities may be a significant factor; therefore, a consultation is recommended with occupational and physical therapists. Considerations when establishing the best possible communication system are

- need for communication
- cognitive skills
- motor abilities
- visuoperceptual abilities
- psycholinguistic abilities

A simple, flat on/off switch hooked up to a tape recorder with music can aid the child in understanding cause/effect, as well as be an early form of communication.

Once a response mode has been determined and a method of operation developed, the actual use of the augmentative system requires training. When selecting vocabulary be sure to consider the persons, foods, toys, and other objects or needs the child may have. Concentrate on what the child regularly attempts to communicate and what is perceived as enjoyable. When an evaluation is not available, use the previous suggestions and consider using an illustrated language board (Figure 17–1) and/or sign language (Figure 17–2). The communication board can be simple; for example, you can use the provided example placed on poster board. More sophisticated language boards with more space between pictures or additional elements appropriate for the child's skills may also be used. Be sure that the pictures are large enough for the child to see, placed where the child can reach

them, and closely represent what they are to symbolize. It is also important that the child's posture is stabilized for the best support of fine motor skills for sign language.

Vocabulary selection for a communication board or sign language requires input from those persons who regularly interact with the child. The following should be considered when selecting vocabulary: include items that are important to the user, can be used in a variety of contexts, can be demonstrated easily, have potential usefulness, and are within the child's experiences. Nouns, verbs, pronouns, words denoting emotions, and attributes can be used if they are commensurate to the child's language skills.

Visuoperceptual skills, posture, and ambulation potential are important factors in the physical construction of the communication board. Consider the child's vision when determining the size of the board. It may be more appropriate to use photographs of both objects and persons when photographs are available. The designed portability of the board and the arrangement of the pictures should cater to both the child's posture and ambulation potential.

HEARING

Determine early on if a hearing screening or evaluation was completed on the child. This could be in the form of an auditory-evoked brain stem response, otoacoustic emission, or behavioral audiometry. Middle ear function can be impacted by middle ear infection (recurrent otitis media). Sensory function can be impacted by ototoxic drugs. If ototoxic drugs are being administered or recurrent ear infections are occurring, a hearing evaluation by an audiologist is recommended.

REFERENCE

Smith, R. 1983. Treatment of communication disorders. In *Rehabilitation of the head-injured adult,* ed. M. Rosenthal, et al. Philadelphia: F.A. Davis.

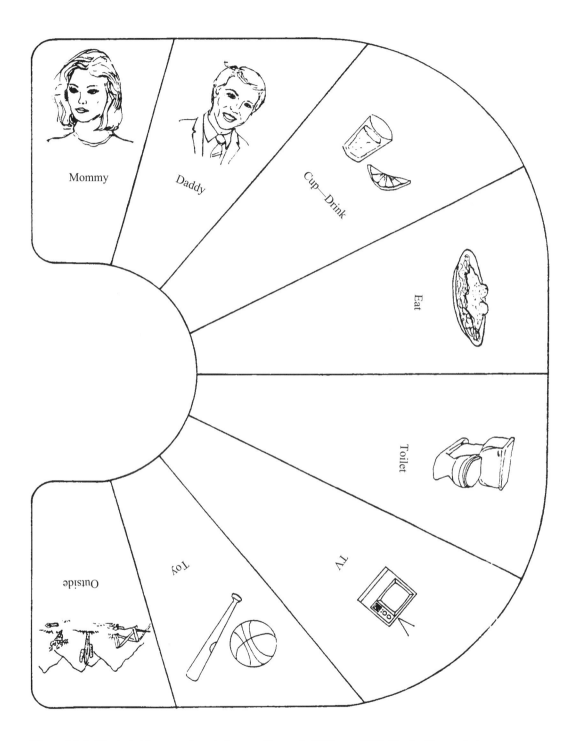

Figure 17–1 Illustrated language board. *Source:* Steven A. Williams, 1987. Used with permission.

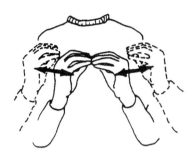

More
Holding hands in flat O-shape with palms and tops facing lap together once or twice.

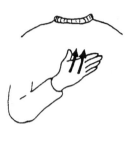

Happy
Brush up and out twice with an open B on chest.

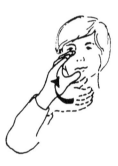

Drink
With a C hand on mouth as if drinking.

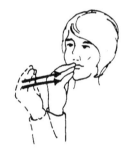

Eat
Repeating several times, place tips of right flat O on lips.

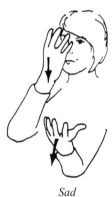

Sad
With both five shape and palms up and slightly curved fingers, hold hands in front of face and drop slowly.

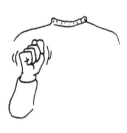

Toilet
Shake right T from left to right.

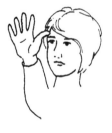

Daddy
Place thumb of right five hand on forehead.

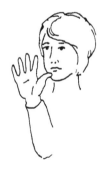

Mommy
Place thumb of right five hand on chin.

Figure 17–2 Examples of sign language. *Source:* Steven A. Williams, 1987. Used with permission.

CHAPTER 18

Physical Therapy and Occupational Therapy Interventions

Nancy Harris Ossman and Jill K. Martindale

The major roles of physical and occupational therapists are evaluation of sensorimotor functioning, implementation of therapeutic interventions, and training of caregivers in home programming. These therapists use specific treatment techniques to minimize the effects of sensorimotor impairment and provide the child with more normal sensorimotor experiences to maximize independence and normal development. These roles often overlap in pediatrics, not only in educational training but also in evaluation and treatment techniques used. In this chapter, the disciplines of physical and occupational therapy are combined when appropriate and separate specialty areas are also described. Those aspects of a home therapy program that are most often expected of pediatric home care nurses when therapists are not available are included. Strongest emphasis is placed on increasing one's awareness of the needs of the sensory- and motor-impaired child and how to respect those needs in all aspects of the child's daily routine, including handling, positioning, activities of daily living (ADLs), mobility, and use of adaptive equipment. Guidelines are included that indicate when referral to a therapist is appropriate, noting which pediatric therapist(s) could best address the particular condition or problem (Table 18–1). Range of motion (ROM) techniques are also included in Appendix 18–A.

REFERRAL TO A THERAPIST

An evaluation from a therapist can be helpful in determining the appropriateness, type, frequency, and duration of treatment required. The child's diagnosis, medical history, family and social situation, degree of impairment, intelligence, age, developmental readiness, and motivation are several factors that may affect the outcome of treatment.

Therapy disciplines that would most likely be involved in evaluations and treatment when the specific conditions or problems are identified are indicated in Table 18–1. Those conditions or problems that are appropriate for referral to a pediatric physical or occupational therapist are listed in Table 18–2. A physician's referral may be required depending on local, state, or agency practice regulations.

MANAGEMENT STRATEGIES FOR THE PEDIATRIC HOME CARE PATIENT

Based on the therapist's assessment, a number of therapeutic interventions for managing abnormal muscle tone, sensory deficits, posture and mobility, range of motion, and self-help skills may be appropriate. Some of the important management strategies that the home care nurse would be required to implement follow.

Table 18–1 Commonly Used Therapy Services per Condition or Problem

Condition/Problem	Occupational Therapy	Physical Therapy	Speech Pathology
Congenital/genetic abnormalities	X	X	X
Perinatal high-risk factors	X	X	X
Neurologic impairments	X	X	X
Orthopedic conditions	X	X	
Trauma/abuse	X	X	X
Minimal cerebral dysfunction/learning disabilities	X		X
Cardiopulmonary disorders	X	X	X
Metabolic/endocrine disorders	X	X	X
Neuromuscular disorders	X	X	X
Sensory impairments	X	X	
Burns	X	X	
Mental retardation	X	X	X
Emotional problems	X		
Developmental delays	X	X	X
Spinal trauma	X	X	
Feeding disorders	X		X
Cognitive delays	X		X
Language/communication delays/disorders	X		X
Perceptual disorders	X		
Fine motor difficulties/delays	X		
Gross motor difficulties/delays	X	X	
Dressing difficulties	X		
Bathing difficulties	X	X	
Grooming difficulties	X		
Toileting difficulties	X	X	
Ambulation difficulties		X	

Abnormal Muscle Tone

Abnormal muscle tone adversely affects all aspects of a child's development and subsequently his or her health care maintenance. Most commonly, it is characterized by either high tone or low tone, although many variations exist. One may find that there is both high and low tone present or that tone may fluctuate. Emotional and physical state (for example, crying, being excited, or having a fever or runny nose) can also influence a child's tone. Management of tone during all activities must be incorporated into the nursing care plans. Intervention strategies for managing each type of abnormal tone are discussed in Table 18–3. Figure 18–1 should help clarify these strategies.

Sensory Deficits

Sensory stimuli are crucial to learning. An inability to perceive incoming sensory information accurately or process internal sensory cues can greatly diminish the efficiency of the "feedback loop" of learning (Figure 18–2). Certainly, this is an oversimplified description of how we learn; current motor learning theory is much more complex regarding how systems interrelate and impact our learning.

Table 18–2 Appropriate Referral Conditions

Condition/Problem	Occupational Therapy	Physical Therapy
Loss of range of motion	X	X
Skin breakdowns due to equipment, splints, positions, decreased mobility, etc.	X	X
Significant change in muscle tone	X	X
Development of, or significant increase in, asymmetry of posture or movement (for example, scoliosis)		X
Equipment changes needed due to growth, wear and tear, surgery, changing tone, social appropriateness, etc.	X	X
Mastery of skill or therapy goal	X	X
Difficulty implementing therapy plans	X	X
Changing eating habits, needs, or behaviors (for example, transitions from liquids to purees to solids; increased gagging; coughing or vomiting during feeding; significant weight loss; increase in time needed to feed; decrease in quantity of food taken)	X	
Loss of sensation	X	
Significant behavioral response to therapeutic programs or routines	X	X
Changing activities of daily living needs (for example, puberty, increase or decrease in functional ability, age appropriateness)	X	
Change in mobility		X
Increase in deformity	X	X
Need for environmental adaptation	X	X
Change in caregiver's ability to manage home program	X	X
Need for caregiver training	X	X
Change in day program or living situation	X	X

Sensory perception includes vision, hearing, taste, smell, touch and pressure, gravity and movement, position and direction, pain and temperature, vibration, discrimination, and localization. Determining which of the senses or perceptual-cognitive areas have been impaired is not always "clear-cut" and may require thorough evaluation. Children who have had a neurologic insult may manifest motor, learning, and/or behavioral problems. Decreased sensory functioning may cause, or compound, the observable deficit behavior. General guidelines to consider when working with a child with sensory deficits are shown in Table 18–4. The most common problems observed in the child receiving home care are included. Remember that each person processes and perceives sensory infor-

mation differently. It is a subjective experience, and tolerance levels must be respected. The amount, type, and duration of stimulation tolerated can vary daily depending on mood, health, fatigue, and emotional conditions.

Auditory and visually impaired children have special needs. The materials and resources available to address those needs are extensive. Most states have specialized programs designed to specifically serve these special needs.

Posture and Mobility

The developmental areas of posture and mobility are most often associated with ambulatory patients; however, they are much broader—they encompass the multihandicapped nonambula-

Table 18–3 Dos and Don'ts for Handling the Child with Abnormal Muscle Tone

Type of Muscle Tone	Dos	Don'ts
High Tone: Hypertonicity or spasticity may be present in any or all parts of the body, including lips, face, and tongue. Spasticity is manifested by resistance to passive movement. Tone is strongly influenced by mood, stress, general health condition, and position. The caregiver's handling of the patient with high tone is crucial to the management of this tone and the effective-ness of any nursing care plan. Spasticity is often found in patterns of flexion or extension synergies.	Range of motion (ROM) should be included as a daily routine and can be incorporated into dressing, diapering, bathing, playtime, and positioning activities. Support the joint you are moving and hold the body part at the point of resistance to achieve maximal range possible. At this point, you may feel a relaxation of tone and can then move the point to its fullest range. This may be more easily facilitated during water play (bath or pool) and at times of the child's greatest relaxation. (Refer to Appendix 18–A for further ROM details.)	Range of motion should not be done quickly or in a stressed or negative atmosphere. Try not to stimulate the spastic muscle groups by your hand place-ments. Rotational movements and proximal joints (pelvis, scapula, neck, and spine) should not be neglected, but the caregiver will need specific instructions by the therapist to perform these motions safely. It is also important to include areas of skin contact and/or creases such as the axilla, groin, and palm of the hand.
	Synergies need to be "broken." The client with flexor spasticity needs to be positioned more "open," and likewise the extensor synergy requires more containment. Key points of control are usually at the thumb, scapula, neck, trunk, hips, and ankles. Carrying and positioning strategies can be incorporated with the neonate through the adult. Tone can be managed in most activities and needs to be considered carefully during feeding and toileting as well. Improved attention and social interaction can also be gained with control of muscle tone.	Do not position and carry the child in ways that reinforce the synergies of spastic flexion or extension. For example, the child with increased extension should not be positioned supine or carried with legs scissored. Do not allow abnormal movement patterns. They will become stronger with "practice" and become even more difficult to inhibit.
Low Tone: Hypotonicity is character-ized by a lack of stability and, often,	Give enough support so that the child does not fatigue com-pletely while trying to maintain	Although it is important to provide adequate support, do not oversupport to the point

continues

Table 18–3 continued

Type of Muscle Tone	Dos	Don'ts
hypermobility of the joints. This patient usually has trouble working against gravity, and hence positioning supports and facilitating dynamic motor activity are primary goals.	a position. The child will not be able to attend or interact with the environment if primary effort is used for seeking stability. Support in alignment and symmetry of body with particular attention to optimizing eye-hand interactions and preventing deformities. See Figure 18–A1. Care of head/neck positioning during feeding is crucial to encourage oral-motor control and to prevent aspiration (Figures 18–A3 and 18–A4). Provide proximal support to achieve distal functioning. Controlled dynamic weight bearing can be a method to improve muscle tone and stability (Figure 18–A6). Working in more upright positions such as sitting, standing, and kneeling (devices can be used to assist) is often more successful than prone lying.	where the child does not have to actively "work" to improve stability. Do not allow asymmetrical positioning with poor postural alignment. A soft, flexible support such as a beanbag chair is contraindicated and only reinforces the child's tendency to "sink" into gravity. Positioning and handling should not reinforce joint hypermobility. Lying supine with arms out to the sides and legs spread is to be avoided. "W" sitting (Figure 18–A2) and transfers in and out of sitting by spreading legs wide open to each side should be avoided. "Bird-feeding" with the child's head tipped back and neck extended is not only poor positioning but also extremely dangerous (Figure 18–A5). Do not place play/work materials at a level such that the child has no way to stabilize the upper extremities or to reach them when the trunk is given adequate support.
Athetoid/Mixed Tone: Fluctuating tone is characterized by an increase of mobility over a lack of stability. Mobility is often involuntary and uncontrolled. This child often knows where and how he or she wants to do something but has a great deal of difficulty executing coordinated purposeful activity. In efforts to achieve stability, the athetoid	Follow the general guidelines for increasing stability and providing adequate support as described for the child with low muscle tone. However, you must also incorporate the suggestions for decreasing excess tone as described previously for the child with high tone. Remember that increased effort and frustration will increase tone and incoordination for the athetoid child. Provide proximal stability as well as light resistance to distal	Again, follow previously outlined suggestions so as to not reinforce either the poor stability of the child with low tone or movement limitations of the child with high tone. Do not allow the child to use extraneous movements to the point at which he or she becomes fatigued, frustrated, and even less stable. In addition, do not restrict the child to the point at which he or she is frustrated or is

continues

Table 18–3 continued

Type of Muscle Tone	Do's	Don'ts
child often fixates distally. Over time, this can produce joint deformities.	movements to improve efficiency of movement. The use of weighted wrist or ankle cuffs, utensils, or bilateral holding often helps. Keep work surfaces in close proximity to the child. Particular attention, as it relates to safety, must be given to this child, especially during feeding and transferring. Remember that the child's muscle tone and control can change rapidly.	constantly "fighting" or working against physical restraints.

tory child as well as the child who is developing postural control and mobility in lower positions such as prone, quadruped, and sitting. Posture not only includes the standing position, but also alignment in all antigravity positions such as prone, supine, and side-lying positions. Mobility includes any means of changing or moving between positions (for example, rolling, supine to sit, creeping and crawling, knee walking, sit to stand, ambulation). In the home care population, mobility also includes transfers, movement in bed, and wheelchair mobility.

Posture and mobility are greatly affected by abnormal muscle tone. Specific orthopedic and neuromuscular conditions such as arthrogryposis, osteogenesis imperfecta, congenital hip dislocation, muscular dystrophy, cerebral palsy, and Guillain-Barré syndrome have an obvious effect on the child's development of normal postural alignment and mobility. The development of hip dislocations, asymmetry, and spinal curvatures, such as scoliosis and kyphosis, are of great concern. Many children have problems in these areas because of imbalances in muscle tone and strength and the tendency to assume preferred, but usually not optimal, positions that reinforce abnormal patterns.

The effect that limitations in cardiopulmonary capacity (for example, as with cystic fibrosis,

congenital heart defects, and bronchopulmonary dysplasia) have on posture and mobility cannot be neglected. The child with limited energy and endurance or who relies on equipment, such as supplemental oxygen or ventilators, will also have greater difficulty in achieving antigravity postures and developing mobility. Interventions for achieving posture and mobility goals are provided in Table 18–5. Optimal interventions should be dynamic rather than static positioning. The consulting therapist can help use the guidelines in Table 18–5 to achieve dynamic activities.

Self-Help Skills

Performance of self-help skills or ADLs is often affected in the child who is ill or has a sensory, motor, cognitive, or perceptual impairment. ADLs are the basic skills essential to everyday living. They include dressing, eating, toileting, bathing, and grooming. ADLs for the older patient may also include homemaking and functional skills for living more independently (for example, money management, shopping, cooking, cleaning, child care, banking, leisure and social skills, and handling emergencies).

ADLs are a narrow specialty area within the broader confines of occupational therapy. The

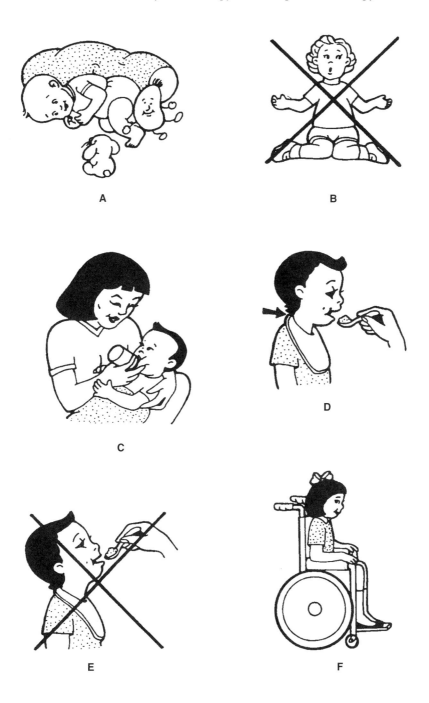

Figure 18–1 A. Assisted side lying with midline flexion tuck. **B.** "W"-sitting. **C.** Infant feeding position with cheek support. **D.** Correct feeding presentation with head and neck in slight forward flexion. **E.** "Bird feeding": Head and neck hyperentension. **F.** Proper body alignment in sitting. *Source:* Reprinted with permission of Therapy Skill Builders, San Antonio, Texas.

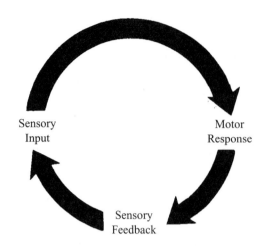

Figure 18–2 Feedback loop of learning.

occupational therapist can help by (1) recommending or developing adaptive equipment to facilitate the caregiver or the child regarding the task at hand; (2) recommending ways to modify the task or the position of the child; (3) guiding the amount, type, and timing of assistance needed during the activity; and (4) determining the readiness (or lack of readiness) to move to the next step toward maximizing the child's independence. An occupational therapist can show the caregiver how to integrate range of motion, flexibility, exercise, activity, or language programs into the daily routine of self-help skills. Some guidance on interventions for some of the most common problems in the areas of feeding, dressing, bathing, and toileting is provided in Tables 18–6 and 18–7.

It may not be necessary to consult only an occupational therapist to perform these functions. The reader should be aware that a speech therapist specializing in feeding techniques or a physical therapist familiar with bathing equipment and programs may be available.

Feeding

The following guidelines should be considered during mealtime. Make it a relaxed, social time with the family; allow for imitation; allow

for age- or stage-appropriate exploration of foods; give the child choices; don't rush the child; keep the stress level down and try to make eating a pleasant experience. The child who is tube fed should be included at the family table, and some form of oral stimulation should be paired with the tube feeding if possible. Feeding should always occur with the infant or child in proper position. Generally, the head is slightly forward, the body is upright with the pelvis tilted forward (or semireclined for infants) and in good alignment, the feet are supported, and the arms and shoulders are slightly forward. Avoid extremes of flexion and extension postures with the neuromuscularly involved child. These positions may make the control of breathing, chewing and sucking, and swallowing more difficult. There are many issues that can arise regarding feeding, including nutritional adequacy, failure to thrive, constipation or chronic diarrhea, and behavioral or emotional concerns that require support of additional professionals.

Suggestions for each of the basic problem areas are given in Table 18–6. If the problems persist, consult a physician and seek out a feeding therapist.

Bathing and Toileting

Bathing is a necessary activity of daily living that can be fun as well as therapeutic. Toileting is a skill that one hopes to teach the child with special needs. There are special concerns to be addressed for both the child with neuromuscular impairments and the caregiver during bathing and toileting. It is critical to assess the space available and ease of use before any equipment is ordered. Some of these concerns and helpful suggestions are discussed in Table 18–7.

Dressing

Some general guidelines should be followed to ease the dressing process. These guidelines apply whether the child is dressing indepen-

Table 18–4 Dos and Don'ts for Handling the Child with Sensory Deficits

Sensory Problem/Condition	Dos	Don'ts
1. Hypo/hypersensitivity to touch	Verbally prepare the child before touching Use firm pressure. Limit the amount of stimuli presented at a time and give the child time to adapt before changing it. Allow the child to use another sensation or another body part. Try to incorporate it into a whole body image. Pair verbal descriptions with sensory stimulation.	Don't tickle or use light feathery strokes. Avoid going against the direction of hair growth. Don't overstimulate. Don't surprise the child. Don't restrict use of compensation skills during concept formation tasks. Don't ignore the impaired body part.
2. Proprioception/kinesthesia: impairments in the perception of joint position and direction of movement can influence a child's body concept and his or her accuracy and quality of movements in space.	Provide weight bearing in proper body alignment. Work against resistance to provide increased stimulation to joint receptors. Increase graded, bilateral activities (for example, playing catch with various sized and weighted balls, wheelbarrow walking).	Don't allow the child to use only the body parts or side of the body that he or she can perceive. Don't overdo resisted input to joints. Pain reception at joints may also be impaired. Don't encourage rapid movements.
3. Visual perception: visual perception can include ocular motor skills; depth perception; figure-ground, spatial, and position perceptions; form constancy; visual discrimination; and memory and sequencing skills.	Place materials in child's visual fields. However, it is important to encourage and provide opportunities to explore beyond the visual fields. Minimize the confusion. Avoid "busyness" of visual presentations. Give the child alternative sensory modes to learn from. Move, touch, or talk to the child through the activity. Work on form constancy and object permanence first. Directionality, laterality, position, and spatial concepts develop first on oneself, then with oneself in relationship to each other, and, last, in two dimensions (on paper). Use functional, experiential tasks that are repeated and familiar (for example, eating. dressing, bathing).	Don't allow the child to ignore deficit sides. Don't assume the child sees things the same way you do even if visual acuity is reported to be normal. Don't assume the "blind" child has no vision at all. Responses to light or movement may be present. Don't work on higher-level visuoperceptual skills until basic concepts are mastered.

continues

Table 18–4 continued

Sensory Problem/Condition	Dos	Don'ts
4. Vestibular movement and gravity: movement and changes in position are an integral part in early development. The formation of body concept, motor planning, body in space, cause-and-effect concepts, spatial relationships, and ocular motor skills and the development of balance and equilibrium are dependent on experiencing movement and the effect of gravity.	For the child with limited movement experiences, introduce passive movement slowly and gradually. Observe for any signs of stress or discomfort including nausea or increased muscle tone. Begin with slow, rhythmical rocking and provide postural security or support throughout the experience. Gradually change planes and direction of movement and know that responses to linear and rotary movements may be very different. Whenever possible, allow this stimulation to be self-directed.	Don't overstimulate. Don't ignore signs of stress or discomfort. Don't allow excess tone or movement in abnormal postures.
5. Smell and taste: these are often overlooked sensations, especially for the child receiving nonoral feedings.	Identify, describe, and present smells and tastes (avoiding swallowing for the nonoral feeder) that are familiar in the home environment. Pair them with other sensations to round out concept formation. Allow choices.	Don't forget the importance of these sensations. Teach appropriate safety responses of certain smells or tastes to avoid. Never force unpleasant foods or smells.

dently or being assisted. The guidelines and related information are as follows:

- Start instruction early and establish a routine and sequence for dressing and undressing.
- The child will begin to anticipate and assist and should be given time to react.
- Consider the child's balance and mobility skills required for each phase of dressing.
- Undressing is learned before dressing.
- Use clothes that are a little too large.
- Elastic-waisted pants and scoop-necked shirts are easier to don and doff.
- Velcro can be used to replace most fasteners.

- Hemiplegics should dress the affected limb first and undress it last.
- Elastic thread can be used for sewing on cuff buttons of the affected arm side.

There are a multitude of adaptive devices for dressing. These include trouser pulls, stocking aids, long-handled shoe horns, elastic or zippered laces, button hooks, zipper pulls, and dressing sticks. Choosing aids should be done carefully: using the wrong device could make it more difficult for the child instead of easier.

Before dressing or undressing the child with increased muscle tone, consider the child's best positions and your best hand placements for the most controlled movements and tone man-

Table 18–5 Dos and Don'ts for Posture and Mobility Goals

Goal	Dos	Don'ts
1. Improved head control	Position prone on forearms on wedge or over roll. Position propped kneeling or propped side sitting over a support. Use fully supported standing as with a prone, supine, or upright stander. Work on midline positioning.	Don't allow the child to "hang" over the wedge/roll or on the shoulder girdle in sitting or when propping in prone. Watch for fatigue. Don't inadvertently develop or reinforce a preference for head turning to one side.
2. Increased eye-hand coordination and bilateral arm usage	Side lying promotes bilateral upper extremity use and visual awareness. Provide upper extremity weight bearing in prone and propped kneeling. Leave a "window" space between the arms and the trunk. Provide a work surface in sitting and standing. Place materials to promote neck flexion and visual gaze toward hands. Provide scapular support to avoid retraction of upper extremities.	Avoid supine because this position increases upper extremity retraction. Don't always position side lying on one side. Don't allow the upper extremities to be positioned in internal rotation and adduction with weight bearing on the radial (thumb) side of the hand.
3. Improved alignment and symmetry	Use towel rolls, foam rolls, etc. to provide trunk support in sitting. External supports such as "H"-strap harnesses and butterfly chest supports can be used. Use corner or saddle-chairs combined with a tray. Use standing devices (for example, prone boards, standers) to achieve proper standing position.	Don't allow asymmetry or lateral trunk flexion when sitting. Don't oversupport to the point where the child does not actively "work" to maintain balance and posture. Do not work in unsupported standing if alignment is poor. Do not allow the child to ignore or favor the more involved side.
4. Increased postural extension and sitting balance	Position sitting on a firm flat surface. Try short sitting (stool, bench, booster seat, elevated corner chair) or straddle sitting (bench, roll, saddle seat, push trike).	Don't position in unsupported floor sitting with legs in front of body if significant postural rounding occurs or if balance is precarious. Don't sit the child on a soft, cushioned, or prefabricated molded seat.

continues

Table 18–5 continued

Goal	Dos	Don'ts
	Use an elevated work surface for upper extremity supporting. Provide assistance, as needed, to balance upright in long, ring, half-ring, tailor, and side sitting.	Avoid "W"-sitting. Don't allow the child to always assume a habitual sitting position.
5. Increased weight bearing and stability	Provide optimal surface contact required to support the child in the activity (for example, feet flat on floor, thighs resting on chair, forearms on supporting surface). Use kneeling at a support as an alternative to standing. Position in standing using a prone board, flexi-stand, or similar standing device. Use footrests in sitting or a seat low enough for feet to securely rest on.	Don't allow feet to hang unsupported in sitting. Do not use a "Johnny Jump-Up" and infant walkers unless approved by a therapist. Do not allow "locking" of joints or "hanging" on bones.
6. Improved lower extremity and trunk mobility	Incorporate a variety of sitting positions (long, tailor, ring, half-ring, side sitting). Encourage rotating between sitting and kneeling, sitting and quadruped to change position. Place toys to the side to encourage weight shift and trunk rotation with reach. Have child play in side lying and practice turning from supine to each side. In supine, elevate pelvis with a wedge or pillow to encourage lifting legs to bring hands and feet together. Have child practice riding a "push trike." In diapering and dressing, incorporate mobility exercises such as alternate flexion and extension of legs ("bicycling" legs), abduction of flexed lower extremities, and rotation of pelvis and trunk.	Don't allow transfers in and out of sitting by spreading the legs to the sides and doing the "splits." Discourage abnormal patterns of movement such as scooting in supine or sitting or "bunny-hopping" on hands and knees.

Table 18–6 Suggestions and Equipment for Common Feeding Problems

Problems	Suggestions To Assist	Equipment To Try
1. Taking too long to take too little may indicate poor suck control.	Try providing jaw stability by placing a finger under the chin. Support the cheeks during sucking. Try putting an extra hole in the nipple, but watch that the fluid does not flow too quickly, causing the infant more distress.	Try different size, shape, and firmness of nipples. A natural nipple may help facilitate tongue elevation whereas a round nipple may encourage more tongue curl and sucking. Consider using a Haberman feeder.
2. The infant or child pulls away or withdraws from stimulation around the mouth and face or shows a lack of awareness when food is presented. This may indicate a hyper/hyposensitivity to touch in and around the mouth.	Let the child self-direct. Encourage hand-to-mouth play. Make mealtime fun—get creative and "open the hanger and let the airplane in." Use a washcloth and napkin frequently and firmly. Explore temperature and textures of food.	Try different size, shape, and firmness in nipples. Feed in an infant seat or high chair to minimize extraneous sensory stimulation and to provide stability and containment.
3. Poor lip closure around the nipple or spoon may be indicated by excessive dripping and loss of food.	Cold can facilitate puckering, but watch for adverse reactions. Offer cheek support. Try thicker foods and liquids. Place food on spoon in the mouth and wait for the upper lip to draw it off. Place formula or food on lips and encourage tongue play or lip drawing in to remove it. *Never* use honey to stimulate this with an infant.	Various infant pacifier shapes, sizes, and circumferential mouthpieces can be tried to help stimulate lip closure away from mealtime. Proper seating and positioning with head in slight forward flexion Short durable straws Cups with spouts
4. Hyperactive gag reflex may make food presentation, swallowing textures, or keeping foods down a problem.	Present small amounts of food at a time. Present the spoon to the forward portion of the child's mouth and gradually "walk" it midway back and apply a firm pressure to stimulate tongue retraction. Reduce stress or changes in routines.	Nipples of various size, shape, length, firmness, and flow speed Coated spoon Flatter or rounded spoons may make a difference.

continues

Table 18–6 continued

Problems	Suggestions To Assist	Equipment To Try
	Check food preferences and give the child a choice. Consult child's physician if you suspect the possibility of food allergies or structural or neurologic complications.	
5. Reflux that occurs closer to the next feeding should be of concern.	Add cereal to the formula or food. Sometimes heavier food stays down better. Feed smaller amounts more frequently. Discuss with the physician any need or indications for metoclopramide (Reglan), cimetidine (Tagamet), or nutritional supplements.	"Danny sling" for maintaining prone lying after feeding on a bed with the head elevated to a 30° angle
6. The transition from liquids to purees and solids may be difficult. Increases in gagging, spitting up, avoidance behaviors, and oral-motor incoordination may be observed.	Gradually add yogurts, custards, applesauce, mashed fruits, etc. to drinks. Change from a bottle or cup to a bowl and spoon in the thickened liquids. Ask child to remove purees from your fingers or toys. Make eating fun. Proceed to mashed, semisolids keeping lumps "together" (cottage cheese) vs. floating in liquid (soup). Allow finger play exploration of foods. Combine liked and disliked foods. Let child hold and mouth solid foods and do assisted teaching of biting. Watch carefully.	Try various-shaped cups, spoons, and bowls for specific sensorimotor problems or deficits and to encourage self-feeding and self-image and socialization. There are many items to choose from in the many books and catalogues available (see Appendix A at the end of this book for a directory of resources).
7. The transition to cup drinking is normally awkward. However, the child with special needs may require assistance and take longer to develop smooth, coordinated	Start with thicker liquids. Use yogurt, applesauce, cereal, or pureed foods. Provide jaw stability. Assist with lower lip seal as needed.	Try cups with lids, preferably without spouts. Start with somewhat flexible plastic cups (nonbreakable). "Cut-out cups" prevent excess neck and trunk extension and allow the caregiver to monitor the fluid flow.

continues

Table 18–6 continued

Problems	Suggestions To Assist	Equipment To Try
skills with minimal dripping and spills.		
8. One-handed eating	Depending on the age and ability of the child, this may require more or less manual assistance or adaptive equipment.	A damp cloth or piece of rubber matting can be placed under the plate to prevent sliding. Use suction bowels. A universal cuff or foam builtup handles can be used for those patients with decreased grasping ability. A rocker knife can be used for one-handed cutting. Bowls or plates with a lip can be used for ease of scooping food onto the spoon or fork. Food guards used with standard plates serve the same purpose.
9. Decreased motor control of the mouth and face, as well as the trunk and limbs, may interfere with effective independent feeding.	Position well. Stabilize proximally. Allow elbows on the table or lap tray. Decrease the distance the food has to travel. Add weighted resistance to limbs or utensils.	Try previously stated suggestions but concentrate on stability. Weighted utensils and wrist cuffs may decrease extraneous movements. Teflon-coated utensils help prevent injuries. The "C.P. Feeder" device minimizes motions necessary for self-feeding. Swivel spoons may help keep the food on the spoon. Use two-handed drinking cup with a lid, preferably with nonspout lid. Straw drinking with the cup in a cup holder decreases spilling.
10. The child with a cleft palate needs special feeding considerations.	Feed this child in an upright position. Assist manually with closing the lips together. Regulate fluid flow. Let the infant or child be in charge of the rate of feedings as well as his or her readiness	Mead-Johnson cleft palate set is a soft, longer nipple with a squeeze bottle. Consider using a Haberman feeder. Try crosscutting a nipple to increase flow rate but don't "drown" the child.

continues

Table 18–6 continued

Problems	Suggestions To Assist	Equipment To Try
	for strained, pureed, or lumpy foods. Present spoon foods in small amounts. Some foods may "escape" through the nose. Don't overreact. Clean the infant and resume feeding when the child has recovered.	Do not use the lamb's nipple. It is usually much too big and awkward.

agement. Side lying is often a more neutral position. Lying prone over your lap may work well for the smaller child with extensor spasticity. Symmetrically supported sitting maintains hips, neck, and shoulders in slight forward flexion and allows the child to participate more actively.

Patience is the key to a smooth dressing process. Remember, it takes longer to allow the child to do it for himself or herself than to do it for the child. Allow yourself the needed time!

BEHAVIORAL CUES AND MANAGEMENT STRATEGIES FOR INFANTS

The following tables and exhibits are based on the neurobehavioral research of Dr. T. Berry Brazelton and Dr. Heidelise Als, who have developed the Neonatal Behavioral Assessment Scale (NBAS) and the Assessment of Premature Infant Behavior (APIB) (see Table 18–8 and Exhibit 18–1). All caregivers working with sick or fragile infants must be able to recognize when a child is displaying approach and self-regulating or avoidance and stress behaviors and understand appropriate interventions. Caregivers must effectively control the environment and the amount and type of stimulation these infants receive. Appropriate responses to the infant's behavioral cues make all interactions easier and

enhance growth and development. Parent teaching in this area is invaluable.

Interrelating systems that have been defined by Brazelton and Als are physiologic (autonomic), motor, and state. The ability to achieve and maintain attentional-interactive and self-regulatory behaviors demonstrates the presence or absence of integration between these systems.

Physiologic control, the most basic and vital area of concern, refers to the functioning of the autonomic nervous system, including the ability to maintain heart rate, respirations, temperature, and color. The development of motor control is characterized by the infant's ability to maintain a posture (initially flexion) or to move in and out of it with smooth actions. This control takes time to develop, especially for the premature infant, and is greatly influenced by adult interactions. State control is an infant's ability to achieve and maintain various levels of sleep and wakefulness with smooth transitions between states.

It is difficult for an infant to reach and maintain an alert state with the ability to interact or attend to the environment if the child cannot regulate his or her physiologic, motor, or state systems. Normal growth and development rely on the integration of these systems. Table 18–8 describes the approach and self-regulatory behaviors that indicate maturation of these systems, as well as the avoidance and stress behaviors that indicate the need for an intervention or reduction in stimuli. When an infant is showing

Table 18–7 Bathing and Toileting Concerns and Suggestions

Concerns	*Suggestions*
1. Making the bathtub area safe is of great importance. Most of these suggestions can be done easily. Special grab bars and seats are available for children with neuromuscular problems through catalogues, drugstores, or medical supply companies.	Use nonskid mats or strips in and around the bathtub and floor to decrease chances of slipping. Faucet covers can be purchased or made to protect the child from accidental bumps. Use safety rails and grab bars, transfer benches, tub seats, foam pads, shower chairs, bath pillows, etc. as needed. Do not make the water too hot or cold. Besides any skin or thermoregulation changes that may occur, muscle tone is greatly affected by temperature and may make management of the child more difficult. Tub toys should be chosen carefully. Watch for mouthing of toys or soaps. Don't *ever* leave the child alone in the bathtub. Monitor the water level as well. Use "no tears" shampoos and soaps. Use soap on a rope or wash mitts with soap holder pockets, or place soap in a nylon stocking that has one end tied to a fixed point so that soap does not get lost in the bathtub area.
2. Lifting, carrying, transferring, and /or holding a child for bath care can be a physical strain on the caregiver. Always follow good principles of body mechanics. Making the transition into and out of the water smoothly is important for both you and the child.	Keep the child "collected." Use special bath seats as needed. They can help maintain a good seating posture to control tone and still leave a hand free for washing. They may also raise the child, reducing the amount of leaning or bending over into the tub. An extended shower hose can ease washing and rinsing care. Use a short stool to sit on during bath time. Use transfer aids for bath time (for example, hydraulic or pump lifts and chairs, transfer benches). Control the child's tone. Keep the child close to your body. Do not lean over with the load! Bend your knees and let your legs do the work. Half-kneeling may be a more comfortable transition position for you while transferring the child in and out of the tub. Prepare the environment and the child. Have everything where you want it and within reach.
3. Sensory stimulation can affect autonomic functions, behavior, and motor tone and control. The hypertonic child may become more spastic, or the hypotonic child may become more flaccid.	Keep the water temperature moderate. Try keeping the infant or child wrapped in towel or a T-shirt during the transition into the water. These can be removed and replaced as tolerated or needed during bath time. Have towels ready that are large enough for wrapping the child up. Rubbing the towel over the body may be too much stimulation—rub your hands over the towel-wrapped body. This also helps maintain body warmth. Change to a dry towel to avoid chilling.

continues

Table 18–7 continued

Concerns	Suggestions
4. There are several programs available for toilet training special populations. Whatever method is used for bowel and bladder care, the toilet area must be a safe environment as well. Please consult an enterostomal nurse for specialized bowel and bladder concerns.	Safety rails may be fastened or placed over the standard toilet. Make sure the feet are supported. Child-sized commodes with attachable positioning aids, safety bar, footrests, and head supports are available. Get assistance from occupational and physical therapists regarding the amount and types of support needed. Deflection shields are available for toilet seats or urinals and can be used for boys who will not be standing up.

signs of stress, particularly physiologic stress, it is important that the caregiver stop what is being done and let the infant recover! Assist with the recovery if necessary. Intervention strategies and suggestions for caregivers are discussed in Exhibit 18–1.

EQUIPMENT ISSUES

There are many types of therapeutic equipment available for home care. The pediatric physical and occupational therapist will be valuable in determining what equipment will best meet the child's needs and will help facilitate the most normal development possible. Equipment resources are listed in Appendix 18–B.

It is advisable to use caution when dealing with suppliers of therapeutic equipment. Many vendors are experienced in working with the pediatric population, but others have had little or no exposure. The following questions can help in the selection of a vendor:

- Does the vendor specialize in rehabilitation equipment and does the vendor have a salesperson who services primarily the pediatric clientele?
- Does the vendor prefer to involve the child's therapist in choosing and fitting the equipment?

- Does the vendor have the capacity to individually modify the equipment?

A therapist's input and consultation should be sought before using the following:

- positioning wedges
- rolls and bolsters
- side-lyers (cushions that support side lying)
- positioning chairs such as corner chairs, molded Tumble Forms or feeder seats, "bucket"-type seats, saddle chairs
- therapy balls
- beanbag chairs

A therapist should always be involved with choosing certain types of equipment to ensure correct fit, features, and adaptations, such as the following:

- prone boards and standing devices
- wheelchairs
- ambulation devices
- orthotic and prosthetic devices
- transportation-positioning chairs

If consulting a therapist is not possible when selecting a wheelchair or positioning chair, the prescriptive guide shown in Figure 18–3 will assist in obtaining the best fit. Remember that a lap

Table 18–8 Identifying Approach and Self-Regulatory Behaviors and Avoidance and Stress Behaviors

	Approach Behaviors	*Avoidance Behaviors*
Physiologic	Maintained heart rate (140–160 beats per minute, premature), (100–120 beats per minute, term) Sustained well-coordinated respiration Maintain "pink" color	Changes in heart rate Changes in respiratory rate Fluctuations in muscle tone Decreased oxygenation Seizures Hiccuping Yawning Sneezing Coughing Gagging, gasping Sighing Spitting up Bowel movement training
Motor	Hands-to-mouth maneuvers Hands-to-face Hand clasp Foot clasp Finger fold Grasping Tucking Leg/foot bracing Mouthing Suck search Sucking Handholding Smooth, well-modulated posture tone and movements	Facial grimaces Arching/opisthotonus Finger/toe splay Prolonged tremor, twitches Arm/leg extension: "saluting," "sitting on air," "airplane" Flaccidity or "tuning out" Hypertonicity Frantic, diffuse activity Tongue thrustings Hands over face High guard arm position Hypertonic fetal tuck
State	Clear, robust sleep states Rhythmic, robust crying Able to self-quiet, self-console Focused alertness with intent Animated facial expressions Frowning Cheek softening "Ooh" face Attentional smiling Smooth transitions between states	Diffuse sleep or awake states accompanied by whimpering and twitching Eye floating Averting gaze Closed eyes while awake and reacting Strained fussing Crying Staring Strained alertness, glassy-eyed Irritability and diffuse arousal

belt is always necessary, not only for safety purposes but also to maintain correct sitting positions.

Positioning adaptations will be needed if you answer "no" to any of the following five questions:

1. Can the child hold his or her head upright for extended periods? Is the head secure enough during transportation? If no, consider some type of headrest or head control device that may be removable depending on need.

Exhibit 18–1 Strategies and Suggestions for Caregivers To Assist with Infant Stress Reduction

Reduce or Eliminate Stimulation

- Turn the light down/off.
- Put the infant down (decrease touch and movement).
- Stop rocking.
- Turn off music or play rhythmical or soothing music quietly as tolerated.
- Leave a blank wall or side of crib for the infant to turn and "escape" to.
- Decrease/eliminate mobiles, mirrors, toys from infant's direct view until infant is ready.

Provide Containment and Postural Stability

- Swaddle
- Position toward a flexor tuck and midline orientation; "nesting"—use assist toward flexion and getting hands together near the face.

- Give the hands something to grasp.
- Use a pacifier or fingers to suck on.
- Perform gentle manual assist of limbs in a contained range to prevent flailing, diffuse movements—do not restrain forcibly!
- Perform slow and gentle rhythmical tapping, stroking, or rocking to tolerance.
- Hold and carry infant securely. Contact on the infant's frontal surface is often soothing.
- Give the feet something to brace against.
- Approach and remove contact gradually, giving the infant time to adjust.
- Prepare infant by increasing, decreasing. or substituting your tactile pressures (for example, with a toy or blanket roll).

WHEELCHAIR SPECIFICATIONS

Age _____
Weight _____
Height _____

Measurements

Figure 18–3 Guide for choosing the best wheelchair fit.

2. Can the child sit upright with good symmetrical posture? If no, consider a tray, lateral trunk supports, an "H"-strap harness, a butterfly chest support, a firm seat and back cushion, lumbar support, or combinations of the devices listed above.

3. Do the child's lower extremities maintain neutral alignment? If no, consider using an abductor component to control adduc-

tion and internal rotation and lateral thigh supports to control excessive abduction and external rotation. Often, the two are used in conjunction to optimally position the lower extremities.

4. Do the child's feet remain on the footrests? If no, consider some type of Velcro straps, heel-toe loop device, ankle strap, or foot trough to ensure placement on footrests.

5. Does the child easily maintain sitting without sliding forward or moving into extensor patterns? If no, examine seats where the degree of hip flexion can be adjusted, chairs with varying degrees of inclination, a wedge-shaped seat cushion, or a lap/hip belt rather than a seat waist belt.

A word of caution: The more supports and devices used, the more difficult it is to free the child in a medical emergency. Try to use "quick-release" strapping and attachments if at all possible.

While the provision of adequate support is necessary, it is also important to give the child less restrictive seating opportunities to work on active postural control.

Range of Motion

Range of motion (ROM) is the extent to which a particular joint is capable of being moved. Not everyone is capable of moving a joint through the same ROM. A person's range is affected by many factors, such as genetic makeup and developmental pattern, the presence or absence of disease processes, and the amount and type of physical activity in which he or she normally engages.

A ROM program is designed to meet each patient's needs and capabilities. The purpose is to preserve present joint range, thus preventing deformity and further loss of motion. If the goal is to increase joint range, consultation with a therapist is required. ROM is often a form of passive mobilization, but it can and should be incorporated when possible into an active exercise program.

The following is a list of "points to remember" used in ROM:

1. When doing ROM, use good body mechanics to conserve your energy and avoid unnecessary strain.
2. Move slowly, smoothly, and rhythmically.
3. Repeat each motion approximately three times, moving through as full a range as possible.
4. Use a firm but comfortable grip. If spasticity is present, try to keep your hands on the surface of the extremity you want to facilitate (for example, when trying to straighten the patient's elbow, try not to place your hands on the muscles that bend the elbow).
5. When moving an extremity, try to stabilize all proximal joints so as to make the patient feel secure and comfortable.
6. Generally, side lying is the best position for doing ROM because there will be less interference from postural reflexes in this position. Have the patient lie with his or her back toward you, head bent forward, and hips and knees in flexion.
7. Move from proximal to distal when doing each extremity because you will be less likely to forget any motions.
8. When noting ROM limitations, it is sometimes useful to compare the right and left sides. This is particularly true if the patient has more involvement on one side than the other.
9. Talk to the patient when doing ROM so that the child can be an active participant. Explain what you are doing when appropriate.

Definition of Terms

- *abduction*—lateral movement away from midline
- *adduction*—movement toward midline
- *active*—patient performs motion independently, no assistance given

- *active-assistive*—patient performs motion with assistance
- *DIP joint*—distal interphalangeal joint, last joint of finger
- *distal*—farthest from the body (for example, hand)
- *dorsiflexion*—bending ankle so foot comes toward body
- *eversion*—turning the foot outward toward the little toe
- *extension*—movement bringing a limb into or toward a straight condition
- *flexion*—condition of being bent
- *inversion*—turning the foot inward toward the big toe
- *MP joint*—metacarpophalangeal joint of the hand ("knuckle")
- *opposition*—movement of thumb toward little finger
- *passive*—patient does not actively move extremity
- *PIP joint*—proximal interphalangeal joint of finger (middle joint of finger)
- *plantarflexion*—pointing foot down
- *pronation*—turning forearm so that palm faces downward
- *proximal*—nearest to the body (for example, shoulder)
- *supination*—turning forearm so that palm faces upward

The illustrations in Figures 18A–1 through 18A–56 show each movement involved in ROM. These pictures are included to help you learn the individual motions and optimal hand placement. Remember, you will usually have the patient with abnormal tone in the side-lying position and the motions will be performed in that position, rather than as pictured.

Stretches

When stretching a spastic muscle, move it to the point where you meet resistance. Hold the extremity at this point until you feel it relax or "give." You can then continue the motion through the pain-free range. When the end of the range is reached, hold for several seconds to give a sustained stretch. Do not give a quick stretch because this will only increase spasticity.

A contracture is also a condition of muscle tightness, but it is caused by actual bony change in the joint and shortening of the connective tissue structures around the joint. Therefore, it is difficult to stretch out a contracture. Remember, stretching should be done just to the end of the pain-free range.

1. Hamstring stretch: reach for toes in long sitting position, keeping knees straight.
2. Hip flexor stretch:
   a. Bend both knees to chest. Hold one knee up and slowly straighten the other leg down to the floor. Hold in extended position for several seconds.
   b. Lie in prone position.
3. Adductors:
   a. Hold one leg straight and push the other leg out to the side, keeping it straight.
   b. With legs bent and feet resting on floor, spread knees apart.
4. Heel cord stretch:
   a. With leg straight, place your hand so that the patient's heel is in your palm and the ball of the foot rests against your forearm. Pull heel down while slowly pressing the foot up toward the body by leaning against the foot with your arm. Make sure to keep the knee straight while stretching the heel cord.
   b. If the patient is able to stand independently, he or she can stand facing a wall and support himself or herself on extended arms. By leaning forward on his or her arms, keeping flat on the floor and body straight, the patient can actively stretch the heel cords.

Hip and Knee Flexion and Extension

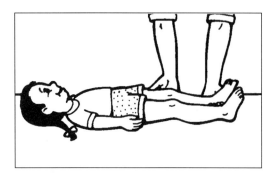

Figure 18–A1 Support under the child's knee and foot.

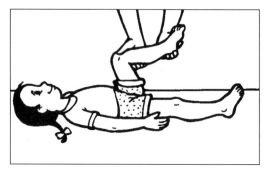

Figure 18–A2 Bend the knee toward the chest and return to a straight position. Stabilize opposite leg so it does not simultaneously lift.

Hip Abduction and Adduction

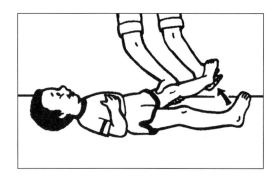

Figure 18A–3 Maintaining your support under the child's knee and foot, hold the leg in neutral rotation and move it away from midline. For the child with higher tone, do this in side lying by lifting the leg up rather than in supine as pictured. Make sure to stabilize the other leg so it does not move along with the leg you are moving. If this occurs, effectiveness of the exercise decreases.

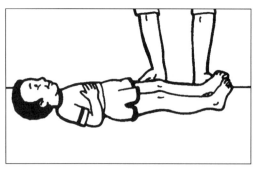

Figure 18–A4 Return to midline position.

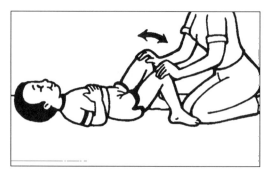

Figure 18–A5 Another way to abduct the hips is to bend both legs up and apply gentle pressure to spread legs apart.

Hip External and Internal Rotation

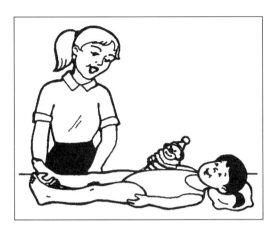

Figure 18–A6 Support under the child's knee and foot.

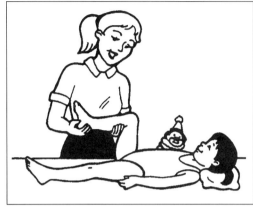

Figure 18–A7 Bend knee toward chest to a right (90°) angle.

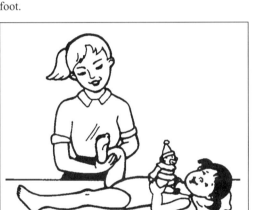

Figure 18–A8 Externally rotate the leg at the hip by moving knee away from midline and foot toward the opposite leg.

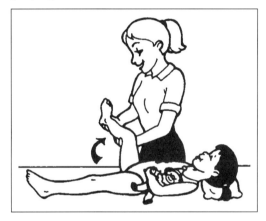

Figure 18–A9 Internally rotate by moving the foot away from midline and knee toward the opposite leg. With internal rotation it is important to move only within the easily available range. This is contraindicated in children who have hip subluxation and dislocation problems.

Straight-Leg Raising

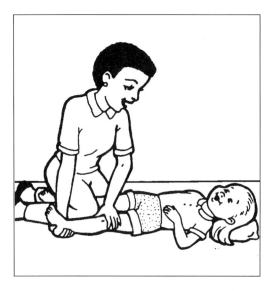

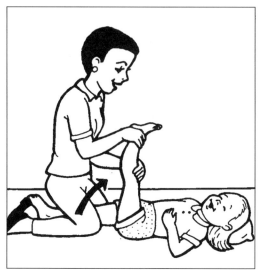

Figure 18–A10 Support over the knee and under the foot, being careful not to hyperextend knee. Again, remember to stabilize opposite leg so it does not simultaneously lift.

Figure 18–A11 Lift leg up toward chest while keeping the knee straight. Stop when you meet resistance or when you reach a 90° angle.

Ankle Dorsiflexion and Plantarflexion

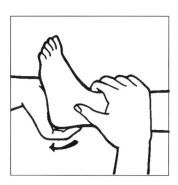

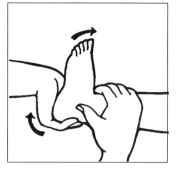

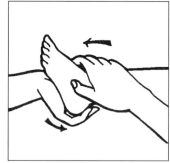

Figure 18–A12 Use your fingers to securely grasp the child's heel.

Figure 18–A13 Dorsiflex the ankle by pulling the heel toward you while the heel of your hand pushes the foot up and back toward the child. Make sure to maintain straight alignment by not allowing the foot to turn in or out.

Figure 18–A14 Plantarflex the ankle by pushing down on the fore-foot (toes toward the floor) and bringing heel up toward leg.

Ankle Inversion and Eversion

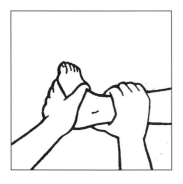

Figure 18–A15 Hold the foot above and below the ankle in neutral alignment.

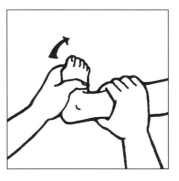

Figure 18–A16 While stabilizing above and below the ankle, evert the foot by moving it away from the midline.

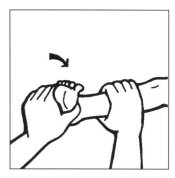

Figure 18–A17 While stabilizing above and below the ankle, invert the foot by moving it toward the midline.

Toe Flexion and Extension

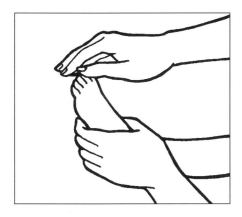

Figure 18–A18 Hold foot with one hand.

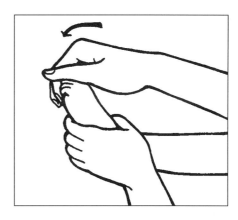

Figure 18–A19 Flex toes and then return to neutral starting position.

Shoulder Flexion and Extension

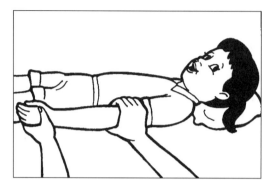

Figure 18–A20 Support at elbow and wrist with arm in neutral ("thumb-up") position. With high tone and/or decreased shoulder mobility it will be more important to support the shoulder blade from behind with one hand while you move the arm and the humerus with the other (not pictured).

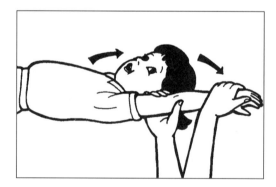

Figure 18–A21 Maintain your support and lift the arm overhead until you meet resistance or see the child compensate by arching the low back. Return to starting position.

Shoulder Abduction and Adduction

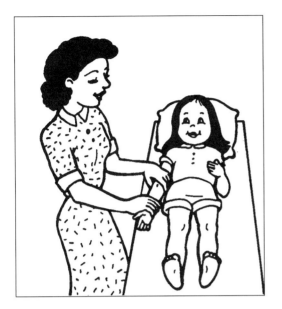

Figure 18–A22 Use same supporting position as described in Figure 8–A20.

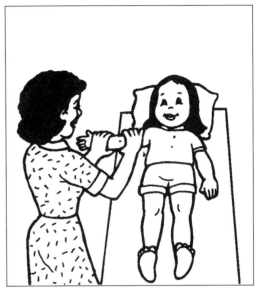

Figure 18–A23 Maintain your support and move the arm to the side away from the body, keeping it on the surface.

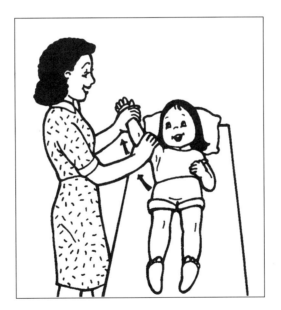

Figure 18–A24 Continue moving arm overhead until you meet resistance, feel very taut tendons in the axilla (armpit), or see compensation by arching of the low back. Return to starting position.

Shoulder Horizontal Adduction and Abduction

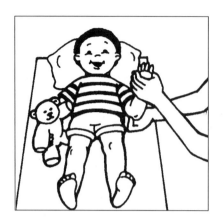

Figure 18–A25 Support arm at elbow and wrist.

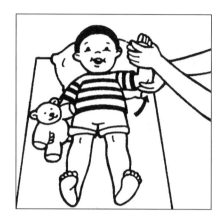

Figure 18–A26 Move arm away from body to shoulder height.

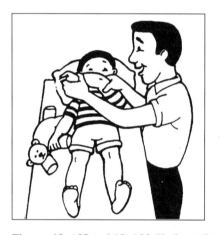

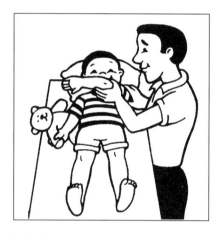

Figures 18–A27 and 18–A28 Horizontally adduct shoulder by bringing arm across the body, being careful not to overstretch arm at shoulder joint.

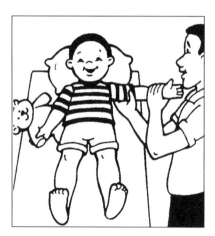

Figure 18–A29 Horizontally abduct shoulder by returning the arm to neutral position and bringing it back across the body and then down alongside.

Shoulder Hyperextension

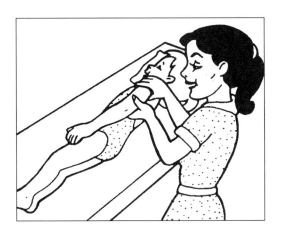

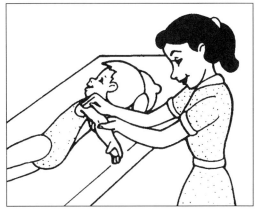

Figure 18–A30 In side lying, support in front of shoulder with your hand over the joint and your other hand on the arm above the elbow. This will help you feel the movement and protect the shoulder from dislocation.

Figure 18–A31 Maintain this support position and bring arm behind body, keeping it in neutral alignment and not allowing internal or external rotation.

Shoulder External and Internal Rotation

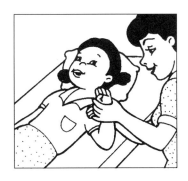

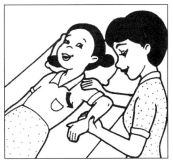

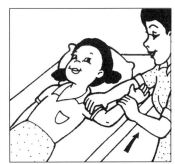

Figure 18–A32 Position arm out to side at right angle to body. Support at front of shoulder joint and at wrist.

Figure 18–A33 Internally rotate by bringing palm of hand toward the surface. Stop when you meet resistance or when shoulder lifts off surface. Return to starting position.

Figure 18–A34 Externally rotate by bringing back of hand toward the surface. Stop when you meet resistance. Return to starting position.

Elbow Flexion and Extension

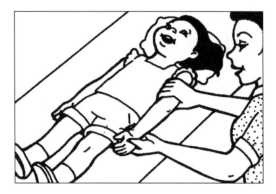

Figure 18–A35 Support arm in neutral ("thumb-up") position above elbow and at wrist.

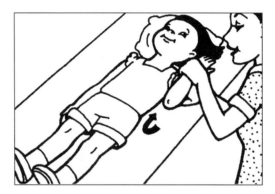

Figure 18–A36 Flex elbow by bringing hand toward shoulder. Extend by returning to neutral starting position.

Forearm Pronation and Supination

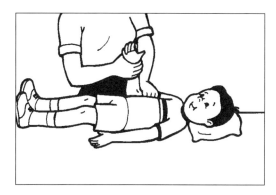

Figure 18–A37 Start with elbow bent to 90°, stabilizing upper arm and holding wrist.

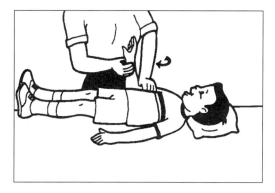

Figure 18–A38 Pronate by turning forearm so palm is down. Return to neutral.

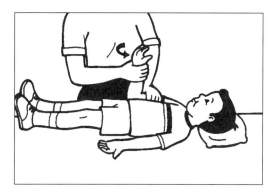

Figure 18–A39 Supinate by turning forearm so palm is up. Return to neutral.

Wrist Flexion (Palmar Flexion) and Extension (Dorsiflexion)

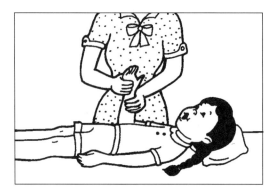

Figure 18–A40 With elbow bent, stabilize above and below the wrist.

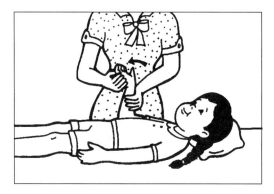

Figure 18–A41 Extend wrist by moving hand back; finger curl may increase due to natural tenodesis action of the hand.

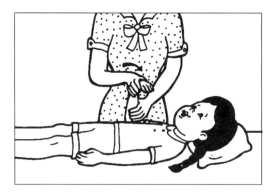

Figure 18–A42 Flex wrist by moving hand forward; fingers may extend.

Wrist Radial and Ulnar Deviation

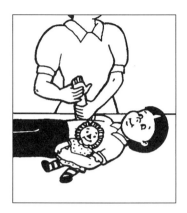 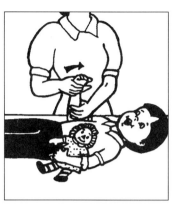 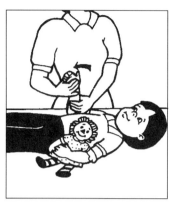

Figure 18–A43 With elbow bent, stabilize above and below wrist.

Figure 18–A44 Radially deviate by moving hand sideways in the direction of thumb.

Figure 18–A45 Ulnarly deviate by moving hand sideways in the direction of the little finger.

Finger Flexion and Extension

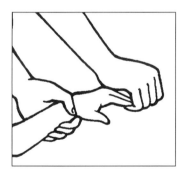 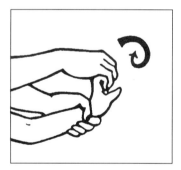

Figure 18–A46 Extend fingers by bringing them out into a straightened position. Wrist position can be neutral or slight flexion.

Figure 18–A47 Flex fingers by bending them into hand. Wrist position can be in neutral or slight extension.

Finger Abduction and Adduction

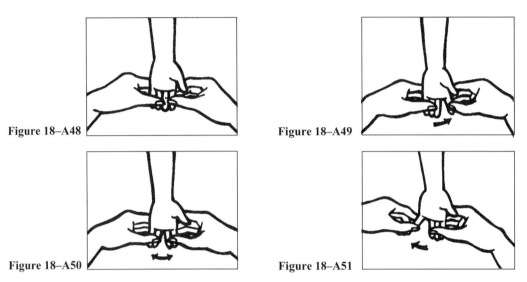

Figure 18–A48

Figure 18–A49

Figure 18–A50

Figure 18–A51

Figures 18–A48 through 18–A51 Abduct by spreading the fingers apart moving them away from the middle finger. Adduction is returning to neutral. Remember to move the middle finger side to side in both directions.

Thumb Flexion and Extension

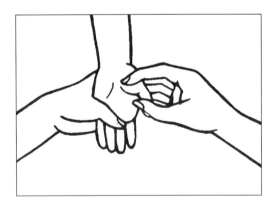

Figure 18–A52 Hold hand comfortably. If child has a subluxed or unstable thumb joint, give additional support at base of thumb to keep the bones in alignment before bending or straightening.

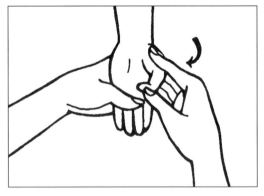

Figure 18–A53 Flex by bending thumb into palm, making sure both joints bend.

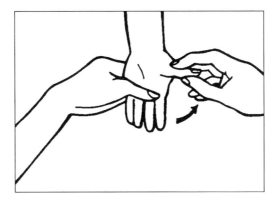

Figure 18–A54 Extend by straightening thumb. Do not hyperextend and allow the base of the thumb to sublux.

Thumb Abduction and Opposition

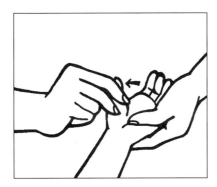

Figure 18–A55 Abduct thumb by moving it perpendicularly in from the index finger, not to the side, which is extension. You should form the letter "L" with the thumb in the air.

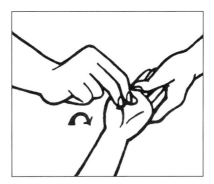

Figure 18–A56 Opposition is moving the thumb from the abducted position across the palm toward the base of the little finger.

Equipment Resources

Self-Help Aids

Comfortably Yours
52 West Hunter Avenue
Maywood, NJ 07607

Enrichments Catalog for Better Living
P.O. Box 579
Hinsdale, IL 60521

Fashion Ease
Division of M & M Health Care Apparel Co.
1541 60th Street
Brooklyn, NY 11219

Sammons/Preston, Inc.
P.O. Box 5071
Bolingbrook, IL 60440-5071
1-800-323-5547

Smith & Nephew Roylan, Inc.
P.O. Box 1005
Germantown,WI 53022-8205
800-558-8633

Special Clothes
P.O. Box 4220
Alexandria, VA 22303

Pediatric Rehabilitation Therapy Equipment

Achievement Products for Children
P.O. Box 547
Mineola, NY 11501

Community Playthings
Rifton, NY 12471

Danmar Products
2390 Winewood
Ann Arbor, MI 48103

Flaghouse
150 N. MacQueston Parkway
Mt. Vernon, NY 10550
1-800-793-7900

G.E.R. Devices, Inc.
"Danny Sling"
14 Fairfield Street
Lowell, MA 01851

Haberman Feeders: Medela, Inc.
P.O. Box 660
McHenry, IL 60051-0660
1-800-435-8316

Kaye Products, Inc.
1010 E. Pettigrew Street
Durham, NC 27701-4299

Sammons/Preston, Inc.
P.O. Box 5071
Bolingbrook, IL 60440-5071
1-800-323-5547

Ways and Means
The Capability Collection
2800 Citrin Drive
Romulus, MI 48174

Educational/Institutional Materials

Abilitations
One Sportime Way
Atlanta GA 30340
1-800-850-8602

Constructive Playthings
1227 E. 119th Street
Grandview, MO 64030-1117

Developmental Learning Materials
P.O. Box 4000
One D.L.M. Park
Allen, TX 75002

Discovery Toys
400 Ellinwood Way, Suite 300
Pleasant Hill, CA 94523

Lakeshore Curriculum Materials Co.
2695 E. Dominguez Street
P.O. Box 6261
Carson, GA 90749

Therapy Skill Builders
555 Academic Court
San Antonio, TX 78204-2498
1-800-228-0752

Children with Special Health Care Needs in School, Child Care, and Early Education Programs

Christine O. Perreault

The primary goal for schools is to provide education, but schools must also address the complex health needs of a new population of students. The current trend is to include students with many diverse needs, including children with special health care needs, into school, child care, and early education programs. Schools must find new ways to provide medications and special health care procedures and adjust teaching for students who have health care needs that often result in frequent, illness-related absences.

Recent legislation, in combination with social pressures for inclusion, is supporting efforts to have children with special health care needs attend school, child care, and early education programs. The trend toward inclusion comes in the aftermath of expanded home-based services for severely ill children. The following three forces powered the expansion in home-based services: (1) greater awareness of the rights of families; (2) technologic advances improving the survival rate of children, allowing out-of-hospital treatments; and (3) emphasis on health care cost containment (Perrin, Shayne, and Bloom 1993).

The length of hospitalization for children with complex health needs and/or who are technology dependent has steadily decreased over the past 20 years. Escalating costs and improved technology have resulted in early discharge of even very young children who require complex health care (Urbano 1992). Children are usually discharged into the care of their families.

Parents, family members, and friends have learned to care for the child with special needs including how to perform special procedures at home and how to respond to the child's complex health needs. If a parent or family member is able to perform these procedures and respond to the health care needs, often the question becomes "Why can't school personnel do the same?" (Krajicek and Steinke 1995).

Data from the 1988 National Health Interview Survey indicate that 31 percent of children younger than 18 years (about 20 million) have one or more chronic health conditions, excluding chronic mental health problems and learning disabilities. Twenty percent of U.S. children experienced mild chronic conditions, 9 percent experienced chronic conditions of moderate severity, and 2 percent of children experienced severe chronic conditions (Newacheck and Taylor, 1992). Other investigators have found that 17 percent of children in the United States were reported to have had a developmental disability (Boyle, DeCouflé, and Yeargin-Allsopp, 1994). The proportion of children who have had to limit their usual activities because of chronic illness and impairments has doubled since 1960 (Department of Health and Human Services 1995).

Many children with complex health needs have benefited from advances in health care that have increased the survival rates for children of low birth weight, children with chronic diseases, children with congenital anomalies, and survivors of trauma. Substance use and abuse during pregnancy have increased the number of drug-exposed infants born with congenital anomalies and/or subsequent developmental delays. With advances in medical technology and treatment, at least 90 percent of children with severe illnesses now survive to young adulthood and beyond. And most dramatically, in ever-growing numbers, the children live at home (Perrin, Shayne, and Bloom 1993).

More than 200 chronic conditions and disabilities affect children, including asthma, sickle cell anemia, spina bifida, epilepsy, and autism (Ireys, Grason, and Guyer 1996). Among the chronic physical health conditions that affect children, asthma is by far the most common, affecting 2.5 million youngsters in the United States. Ten percent of children with asthma have severe forms of the illness. Asthma accounts for one-third to one-half of all severe childhood health conditions (Perrin, Shayne, and Bloom 1993).

The number of students diagnosed and treated with attention-deficit hyperactivity disorder (ADHD) has increased dramatically, by some estimates doubling between 1990 and 1995. Between 1990 and 1993, the annual number of out-patient visits for ADHD increased from 1.7 million to 4.2 million (Swanson, Lerner, and Williams 1995).

Children dependent on technology are attending schools in increasing numbers. They include those who require assisted ventilation to help their breathing, oxygen support, specialized feeding by intravenous (IV) tubes (parenteral nutrition), IV antibiotics over a prolonged period, and ongoing care or monitoring by trained personnel (Task Force on Technology Dependent Children 1988). Their portable equipment makes them sufficiently mobile to live with their families and to attend school in their communities.

Even while providing new levels of opportunities and care for children with complex health issues, schools, families, and communities are dealing with many issues directly linked to a changing population. Prominent issues include the following: child poverty, children and families with no health insurance, increasing numbers of immigrants who may arrive with undiagnosed and unmet health needs, homeless individuals, changing family structures, and societal issues including child abuse, drug abuse, teenage pregnancy, and domestic and neighborhood violence.

FEDERAL LAWS RELATING TO CHILDREN AND YOUTH WITH DISABILITIES

Twenty-five years ago, many children with disabling conditions could not attend school. Federal legislation and court cases have resulted in dramatically expanded services that include students with special health care needs in public school programs (both special education and regular education) and in private school and child care programs.

P.L. 93-112 (1973)—The Rehabilitation Act

This act provides a comprehensive plan for rehabilitation services to all individuals, regardless of the severity of their disabilities. Section 504 of this act contains a civil rights law designed to protect individuals with disabilities that limit major life activities (including self-care, performing manual tasks, seeing, hearing, speaking, breathing, learning, and walking) from discrimination in education or employment. Section 504 ensures equal opportunities for children with disabilities in schools that receive federal funding. Schools have a responsibility to locate and identify all children eligible for services. The student is not required to be eligible for special education to receive services. The school district is responsible for meeting the special needs that a student with a disability may have in the educational setting. The services provided are paid for with general education funds and not special education funds.

P.L. 94-142 (1975)—The Education for all Handicapped Children Act

This bill, related to the education of children with disabilities from ages 3 to 21 years, became effective in October 1977. State law and practice may not have provided for public school services for children 3 to 5 or 18 to 21 years old. There are several basic rights that this law promised to children with disabilities and their parents, including the following:

- the right to a "free, appropriate public education" at public expense
- the right to an educational placement that is based on assessment and evaluation of each child's own special needs
- the right for children with disabilities to receive teaching or instruction that is designed to meet their needs (These are to be clearly written and included in an individualized education plan (IEP), with statements about what services the child will receive.)
- the right to a full range of educational services that may include related services (Exhibit 19–1)
- the right for parents or guardians to be included in making decisions about their child's educational needs and to approve the educational plans for their child
- the right for parents or guardians to appeal any decisions made about the identification, evaluation, and placement of the child through a due process procedure
- the right for parents or guardians to confidentiality of information

P.L. 94-142 requires that children with disabilities be educated in the least restrictive environment, that is, in the most normal school setting possible, with special help provided (NICHCY 1991).

P.L. 99-457 (1986)

This is an amendment to P.L. 94-142. This law mandated the provisions and services outlined in P.L. 94-142 to extend to all preschoolers with disabilities (ages three to five years) and expanded funding available for developing and improving programs. The law also provided incentives for states to serve infants and toddlers with disabilities or who are at risk for having disabilities. P.L. 99-457 established the Part H Early Intervention Program for Handicapped Infants and Toddlers, which established new discretionary programs to help each state plan, design, and implement a comprehensive and coordinated interdisciplinary program of early intervention services for infants and toddlers with disabilities and their families. P.L. 99-457 required the use of the individual family service plan (IFSP).

P.L. 101-576 (1990) Reauthorized P.L. 94-142; renamed Individuals for Disabilities Act (IDEA)

It redefined the criteria for eligibility for services and established two new categories (see

---

Exhibit 19–1 Related Services That Students with Disabilities May Require To Benefit from Their Special Education Programs

Audiology
Occupational therapy
Physical therapy
Psychological services
Medical services for diagnostic or evaluation purposes only
School health services
Transportation services
Counseling services
Speech-language pathology
Social work services
Parent counseling and training
Recreation therapy
Early identification and assessment of disabilities in children

Source: Reprinted from 34 Code of Federal Regulations (CFR) Section 300.13(b)(1)–(13), 1988.

Exhibit 19–1 for a list of related services and Exhibit 19–2 for criteria for eligibility):

1. autism
2. traumatic brain injury.

IDEA expanded and created the following discretionary programs:

- a coordinated system of transition including planning, related instruction, community experience, and interagency coordination for students in special education, who are 16 years and older
- schools are responsible for ensuring that students with disabilities have access to assistive technology

- a new program to improve services for children and youth with serious emotional disturbances
- a research and information dissemination program on attention deficit disorder.

This legislation changed all terminology to "people first language." For example, the term "handicapped child" was replaced with "child with disabilities."

P.L. 101-336 (1990)—The Americans with Disabilities Act

This is a major civil rights legislation. It requires that people of all ages with disabilities have equal access to and reasonable accommodations offered regarding public and private ser-

---

Exhibit 19–2 Disabilities That Qualify Children and Youth for Special Education Services under the Individuals with Disabilities Education Act (IDEA)

The *Education for All Handicapped Children Act,* Public Law (P.L.) 94-142, was passed by Congress in 1975 and amended by P.L. 99-457 in 1986 to ensure that all children with disabilities would have a free, appropriate public education available to them which would meet their unique needs. It was again amended in 1990 and the name was changed to *Individuals with Disabilities Education Act* (P.L. 101-476), or IDEA.

IDEA defines "children with disabilities" as having any of the following types of disabilities: autism, deaf-blindness, hearing impairments (including deafness), mental retardation, multiple disabilities, orthopedic impairments, other health impairments, serious emotional disturbance, specific learning disabilities, speech or language impairments, traumatic brain injury, and visual impairments (including blindness). These terms are defined in the regulations for IDEA, as described below.

1. Autism
A developmental disability significantly affecting verbal and nonverbal communication and so-

cial interaction, generally evident before age three, that adversely affects educational performance.

2. Deafness
A hearing impairment which is so severe that a child is impaired in processing linguistic information through hearing, with or without amplification, which adversely affects educational performance.

3. Deaf-Blindness
Simultaneous hearing and vision impairments, the combination of which causes such severe communication and other developmental and educational problems that a child cannot be accommodated in special education programs solely for children with deafness or children with blindness.

4. Hearing Impairment
An impairment in hearing, whether permanent or fluctuating, which adversely affects a child's educational performance but which is not included under the definition of "deafness."

continues

Exhibit 19–2 continued

5. Mental Retardation

Significantly subaverage general intellectual functioning existing concurrently with deficits in adaptive behavior and manifested during the developmental period, which adversely affects a child's educational performance.

6. Multiple Disabilities

Simultaneous impairments (such as mental retardation/blindness, mental retardation/orthopedic impairment, etc.), the combination of which causes such severe educational problems that the child cannot be accommodated in a special education program solely for one of the impairments. The term does not include children with deaf-blindness.

7. Orthopedic Impairment

A severe orthopedic impairment which adversely affects a child's educational performance. The term includes impairments caused by a congenital anomaly (e.g., clubfoot, absence of some limb, etc.), impairments caused by disease (e.g., poliomyelitis, bone tuberculosis, etc.), and impairments from other causes (e.g., cerebral palsy, amputations, and fractures or burns which cause contractures).

8. Other Health Impairment

Having limited strength, vitality, or alertness, due to chronic or acute health problems such as a heart condition, tuberculosis, rheumatic fever, nephritis, asthma, sickle cell anemia, hemophilia, epilepsy, lead poisoning, leukemia, or diabetes, which adversely affects a child's educational performance. According to the Office of Special Education and Rehabilitative Services' clarification statement of September 16, 1991, eligible children with attention deficit disorder (ADD) may also be classified under "other health impairment."

9. Serious Emotional Disturbance

I. A condition exhibiting one or more of the following characteristics over a long period of time and to a marked degree, which adversely affects educational performance:

    A. an inability to learn which cannot be explained by intellectual, sensory, or health factors;

    B. an inability to build or maintain satisfactory interpersonal relationships with peers and teachers;

    C. inappropriate types of behavior or feelings under normal circumstances;

    D. a general pervasive mood of unhappiness or depression; or

    E. a tendency to develop physical symptoms or fears associated with personal or school problems

II. The term includes children who have schizophrenia. The term does not include children who are socially maladjusted, unless it is determined that they have a serious emotional disturbance.

10. Specific Learning Disability

A disorder in one or more of the basic psychological processes involved in understanding or in using language, spoken or written, which may manifest itself in an imperfect ability to listen, think, speak, read, write, spell, or to do mathematical calculations. The term includes such conditions as perceptual disabilities, brain injury, minimal brain dysfunction, dyslexia, and developmental aphasia. The term does not include children who have learning problems which are primarily the result of visual, hearing, or motor disabilities, of mental retardation, of emotional disturbance, or of environmental, cultural, or economic disadvantage.

11. Speech or Language Impairment

A communication disorder such as stuttering, impaired articulation, a language impairment, or a voice impairment, which adversely affects a child's educational performance.

12. Traumatic Brain Injury

An acquired injury to the brain caused by an external physical force, resulting in total or partial functional disability or psychosocial impairment, or both, which adversely affects educational performance. The term does not include brain injuries that are congenital or degenerative, or brain injuries induced by birth trauma.

13. Visual Impairment, Including Blindness

A visual impairment which, even with correction, adversely affects a child's educational perfor-

continues

Exhibit 19–2 continued

mance. The term includes both children with partial sight and those with blindness.

SERVICES FOR INFANTS, TODDLERS, AND PRESCHOOLERS WITH DISABILITIES

P.L. 94-457, the *Education of the Handicapped Amendments of 1986*, creates a new mandate for all state education agencies to serve all children with disabilities from age three by 1991–1992. The Preschool Program's purpose is to extend the P.L. 94-142 rights to children from age three, including all definitions and requirements. However, Congress made an important distinction for preschoolers: States are not required to label 3–5-year-olds in order to serve these children.

P.L. 99-457 also established the Part H. program, now known as the Early Intervention Program for Infants and Toddlers with Disabilities. This program is directed to the needs of children, from birth to their third birthday, who need early intervention services because they:

1. are experiencing developmental delays in one or more of the following areas: cognitive, physical, language and speech, psychosocial, or self-help skills;
2. have a physical or mental condition that has a high probability of resulting in delay, such as Down syndrome, cerebral palsy, etc.; or
3. at the state's discretion, are at risk medically or environmentally for substantial developmental delays if early intervention is not provided.

In addition, under this program the infant's or toddler's family may receive services that are needed to help them assist in the development of their child. State definitions of eligibility under this program vary; many states are still in the process of developing their Part H programs. Therefore, depending on the state, services may be fully available or still in the process of developing.

FOR ADDITIONAL INFORMATION

If you feel that any of the above statements accurately describe your child, we encourage you to find out more about special education and related services available in your child's public school district. Many parents have the NICHCY publication entitled "Questions Often Asked about Special Education Services" helpful. For children birth through five years, ask for the publication "A Parents' Guide to Accessing Programs for Infants, Toddlers, and Preschoolers with Disabilities." All NICHCY publications are free of charge.

The Special Education Director for your child's school district, Child Find Coordinator, or the principal of your child's school should be able to answer specific questions you may have about obtaining special education and related services for your child. In addition, the federally funded Parent Training and Information Programs across the country are excellent sources of information. For a listing of information sources in your state, NICHCY has a State Resource Sheet for each state and U.S. Territory; this sheet includes the address of the Parent Training and Information Program.

Source: Reprinted from National Information Center for Children and Youth with Disabilities, June 1995. Publication of this document is made possible through Cooperative Agreement #H030A30003 between the Academy for Educational Development and the Office of Special Education Programs of the U.S. Department of Education. The contents of this document do not necessarily reflect the views or policies of the Department of Education, nor does mention of trade names, commercial products, or organizations imply endorsement by the U.S. Government. *This publication is copyright free.* Readers are encouraged to copy and share it, but please credit NICHCY.

vices. It prohibits discrimination against individuals with disabilities because of their disabilities. The Americans with Disabilities Act is the most significant federal law, ensuring the full civil rights of all individuals with disabilities.

RELATED SERVICES: HEALTH AND MEDICAL SERVICES

Related services are those supportive services that are required by a student with a disability to benefit from his or her special education program (Exhibit 19–1). Health services are typically provided by a qualified school nurse or a specifically trained, unlicensed person who is supervised by a qualified nurse. The school district is responsible for providing these services and for the costs involved. In contrast, medical services are those services provided to a child by a licensed physician and may include prescribing of medications, therapies, surgery, or other corrective measures. A school district is not required to provide medical services.

Deciding whether a related service is "medical" or "health" has been a long-standing problem. There have been many court cases that have challenged the interpretation of "health services" and "medical services." In 1984, the issue of providing clean, intermittent catheterization as a school "health service," rather than as a "medical service" was heard by the U.S. Supreme Court in *Irving Independent School District v. Tatro. Tatro* continues to be the controlling case in point defining the issue of "medical services" versus school "health services" for children with special health care needs. The Supreme Court's decision obligated school districts to provide services related to both the health and educational needs of children with disabilities (Rapport 1996).

Since 1984, the care of children with special health needs has become more complex and the number of health care procedures has increased. Some children with special health care needs require the assistance of the nurse or other highly qualified individual at frequent intervals throughout the day. This need for direct care has caused school districts to question whether full-time (or frequent) attention to a child's medical needs is consistent with the provision of related services school districts are obligated to provide under IDEA. In the case of *Detsel v. Board of Education,* 637 F. Supp. 1022 (2d Cir 1986), the court held that private duty nursing services, which were intensive in nature and required for the student to attend school, were considered medical services, not health services, and were, therefore, not included in the related services clause of the special education laws. The same

court later ruled that the Department of Health and Human Services was responsible for providing the required services in the school setting through Medicaid. *Detsel v. Sullivan,* 895 F2d 58 (2d Cir 1990). To date, none of the cases involving children with extensive medical needs has been heard by the Supreme Court.

In the event that the care or service required will assist the child in benefiting from his or her educational program, there are several factors that can be considered when assessing whether the related service may be deemed medical or health related, including the following:

- the nature of the care or service
- the scope and intensity of care or service
- the cost of providing the care or service

Students with complex health needs who require related health services are attending school. This may be in a segregated setting or perhaps in the general education classroom. Few schools have a nurse in every building. Child care centers generally do not have access to regular nursing support or consultation. In the absence of adequate nursing support, a common dilemma is the choice between two equally unappealing alternatives—deny admission to the least restrictive environment or accept a child and make do with the resources on hand, risking personal and agency liability if the child is harmed (Krajicek and Steinke 1996).

TRENDS IN SCHOOL HEALTH SERVICES AND SCHOOL NURSING

Traditional school health services have predominantly included the following: mandated screenings, verification of immunization status, first aid, emergency care, infectious disease control, and health education and promotion. Over the years, school health services have changed and expanded to meet the needs of the increasing number of children who are coming to school with physical and emotional health conditions that prevent them from learning to their fullest potential (Passarelli 1994).

The role of the school nurse as primary care provider, case manager, and epidemiologist is now emerging and replacing outdated nursing functions (Igoe 1994). Individualized health care plans, emergency care, medication administration, specialized health care procedures, implementation of human immunodeficiency virus (HIV) infection policies, and the provision of health education and counseling to students and staff also are included, depending on state and local practice mandates (Small et al. 1995).

More than half of all states fund school-based or school-linked health clinics (Small et al. 1995). The number of school-based and school-linked health centers nationwide increased to more than 600 in 1994 from 327 in 1991 (Shriver 1996). The integration of primary care services through school-based clinics has added to activities of school health programs.

School nurses are unevenly distributed from one district to the next and from state to state (Igoe and Speer 1996). The National Association of School Nurses (NASN) recommends the following minimum standard ratio of school nurses to students: 1 nurse per 750 students for the general school population, 1 nurse per 225 mainstreamed students with special needs, and 1 nurse per 125 severely disabled students (Proctor, Lordi, and Zaiger 1993). A ratio of 1 nurse to 1,500 students is more realistic in terms of the supply of prepared nurses that is available and the costs involved (Igoe and Speer 1996). A NASN survey of membership indicated that 42 percent of the nurses report having fewer than 1,000 students under their direct care, with 85 percent stating that the nurse-to-pupil ratio was the area of most concern because of the complexity of student problems (National Association of School Nurses 1993).

The continuing shortage of nurses and increases in the need for health care in school will affect the models of care that will be used in the schools (Caldwell and Sirvis 1991). Although schools traditionally have employed their own school personnel or contracted with a public health agency for these services, new partnerships and organizational arrangements are emerging. School nurses in California and New York are forming their own school health companies and contracting directly with schools. Hospitals, both profit and nonprofit, also have begun to contract with schools to administer school health programs (Igoe and Speer 1996). The Children's Hospital School Health Program of Denver is an example of a hospital that partners with school districts to tailor a health service program balancing mandated requirements with school district resources. The program provides nursing and allied health professional services directly in the school district or provides consultation to augment existing programs (see Appendix A).

Student characteristics, student needs, and staffing patterns for student health services present a challenge for developing an objective method of identifying individual student health needs, the intensity of those needs, and the health services required to appropriately address those needs (Burt et al. 1996). The School Health Intensity Rating Scale (SHIRS) project provides valuable research-based information on individual needs and the allocation of health resources. SHIRS assesses student health status and classifies the information according to the intensity of student health service needs. SHIRS provides documentation of student needs and the potential to develop levels of needed health services (Burt et al. 1996). The SHIRS tool was published in 1997.

OBTAINING SPECIAL EDUCATION SERVICES FOR INFANTS AND TODDLERS WITH DISABILITIES UNDER PART H OF IDEA

P.L. 99-457 (1986) also established the Handicapped Infants and Toddlers Program, Part H of IDEA. Part H supports services to infants and toddlers, from birth to three years old, who meet at least one of the following criteria:

- developmental delay in cognitive, physical, communication, social or emotional, or adaptive development

- diagnosis of a physical or mental condition that has a high probability of resulting in developmental delay
- risk of developmental delays if early intervention services are not provided (Code of Federal Regulations, Title 34, Subtitle B, Chapter III, Part 303)

The intent of this legislation is to create parent-professional partnerships and to use these partnerships as a foundation for developing and implementing a system to evaluate, monitor, serve (the child), support (the family), encourage progress, and, finally, transition the child to school-age services. Parents and professionals are intended to be equal partners (The Legal Center 1993). Part H of IDEA does provide opportunities to integrate medical, health, educational, and social service needs in ways that enhance and strengthen family-centered, community-based, coordinated care (Von Rembow and Sciarillo 1993).

Part H is not mandatory in all states. Part H services are provided by a variety of agencies, coordinated through a state interagency coordinating council, and administered by a lead agency, such as the state department of education. Part H of IDEA provides funding for states to develop and implement a system of early intervention services for infants, toddlers, and their families.

Services provided under Part H are not entirely free of charge to families and children. A state can establish a sliding-scale fee schedule for the provision of some services. However, the following functions for early intervention services are to be provided at no charge to families:

- implementation of the identification process
- evaluation and assessment for the purpose of accessing the Part H system
- service coordination
- administrative and coordinated activities related to the development, review, and evaluation of the IFSP
- implementation of procedural safeguards

Health care providers, hospitals, home health care, child health clinics, social service agencies, and parents may initiate referrals for early intervention services. The families of children are an integral part of the early intervention process. It is best to discuss the referral with the parents beforehand and to encourage their participation in the referral process.

Evaluation and assessment of the child's needs consider the unique needs of the child in each of the developmental areas. An assessment of the child's level of functioning should include the following areas:

- cognitive development
- physical development, including health status, vision, and hearing
- communication development
- social or emotional development
- adaptive development

The nurse or another appropriate health representative can facilitate communication between health care providers and the multidisciplinary team, especially as it relates to the child's medical history and current health status (Von Rembow and Sciarillo 1993).

The focus under IDEA Part H is on the collaborative development of an IFSP. The IFSP offers parents and professionals an opportunity to plan coordinated and individualized services to support the development of an infant or toddler with special needs in the context of the family. Exhibit 19–3 lists the components of an IFSP.

The IFSP is a family plan. The plan reflects a cooperative effort in addressing child and family needs. The IFSP is not a form. It is a process driven by the family's values. However, family participation in the identification, evaluation, and development of an IFSP is entirely voluntary.

There are increasing numbers of infants and toddlers who need medical devices, such as gastrostomy tubes and tracheostomy tubes, that require specialized care on a consistent basis. In the past, these children were served in more re-

Exhibit 19–3 Components of an Individual Family Service Plan

The IFSP is a written plan developed by a multidisciplinary team, including the parent(s) or guardian(s), that contains the following:

- a statement of the child's present levels of physical development (this includes vision, hearing, and health status), cognitive development, language and speech development, psychosocial development, and self-help skills, based on acceptable objective criteria
- a statement of the family's strengths and needs relating to enhancing the development of the family's infant or toddler with a disability
- a statement of the major outcomes expected to be achieved for the child and family
- a statement of specific early intervention services necessary to meet the unique needs of the infant or toddler and family
- the projected dates for initiation of services and the anticipated duration of the services
- the name of the service coordinator who will be responsible for implementing the plan and coordinating with other agencies and persons
- the steps to be taken supporting the child's transition to Part B preschool services, if appropriate

Source: Federal Register, Department of Education, 34 CFR Part 303, Section 1477(d).

---

strictive environments such as a hospital setting or the home. Today, children are participating in various community settings and may be attending a family child care home, child care center, or early education program.

Subsequently, a family may need one or several early intervention services. If health services, such as medications or treatments, are needed to ensure successful inclusion of a child with complex health needs into an integrated community setting, they should be identified as needs on the IFSP. The service coordinator could assist in finding needed training and sup-

port for the service providers in that setting. The service coordinator coordinates all services across agency lines, and serves as the single point of contact in helping parents obtain the services and assistance that they and the child need (The Legal Center 1993).

For children with complex health needs, the nurse often is requested to act as the service coordinator in early intervention (Exhibit 19–4). Parents identified the following case management activities as important: locating community activities, help in understanding the child's individual education plan, periodic phone calls to assess status, direct care to the child, providing information about parent groups, and help in contacting families with similar problems (Steele 1991). A family-centered approach to early intervention is critical. The emphasis is on using the resources of the community to provide services in more natural settings to the child and family.

Families need to know about possible community program options, school, child care, or early education programs. In many situations, the transition from Part H early intervention services to child care or early education programs means the child attends school independently with peers or the child may travel by school bus for the first time. These developmental milestones can be significant for both the child and the family.

OBTAINING SPECIAL EDUCATION SERVICES FOR SCHOOL-AGE CHILDREN WITH DISABILITIES UNDER IDEA

School districts are responsible for the identification of students with disabilities. A child suspected of having a disability is evaluated by school personnel to determine the child's eligibility for services under IDEA. The child must be evaluated before program recommendations can be made.

The evaluation process should look at the "whole child" and include information about the child's total environment. Parents are an integral

Exhibit 19–4   Role of Nurse in Early Intervention Services

The role of the nurse in providing early intervention services includes the following:

- diagnosing and treating health problems of children and families at risk for or with existing special health or developmental needs
- screening and assessing the psychological, physiologic, and developmental characteristics of the child and family for early identification, referral, and intervention
- planning and coordinating with the family and interdisciplinary team
- providing interventions to the family to improve the child's and family's health and developmental status
- evaluating the effectiveness of nursing care provided to the child and family

Source: Data from Consensus Committee-Maternal Child Nursing, 1993.

---

part of the evaluation. The process should also include:

- testing and observations by a multidisciplinary team
- review of the child's medical history and the relationship with the child's development or performance in "school" (The health assessment should be done by the school nurse, especially if there are significant health issues.)
- information and observations from the family about the child's school experiences, abilities, needs, and behavior outside of school

Subsequently, the information that is gathered is used to determine whether a child is eligible for special education and related services. If it is determined that the child qualifies for special services, then the individual education plan (IEP) is developed. If the school district finds the child to be ineligible for special education services, then the school district may need to accommodate the child's special health needs and/or related disabilities by developing a plan under Section 504 of the Rehabilitation Act.

An IEP is a written statement of the educational program that is designed to meet a child's special needs. The IEP will establish the educational goals and objectives for the child as well as indicate the services the school district will provide. The provision of related services, such as health and transportation services, must be included in the IEP and indicate who will provide these services. The individual health care plan may also be a part of the IEP. The IEP may also include educational goals and objectives related to the special health needs of the child.

Parents are invited to participate in the IEP meeting, which is usually held at the school at a time that is convenient for parents and other members of the team. The school may hold an IEP if no mutually agreed-upon time can be set. The school must keep the parents informed. The signature of a parent is required to be on the IEP for the plan to be carried out.

At least once a year, a meeting is held to review the child's progress and develop goals for the following year. For a child with special health needs, an annual health assessment and a review of the individual health care plan is to be done by the school nurse with input from the family, the child as appropriate, health care providers, and other community representatives. Changes in the IEP can be made sooner at the request of parents or the school if there is a need to discuss the child's progress. Including health care providers such as community or home care staff in the meeting can be useful in assessing needs and developing goals. A full reevaluation must be done every three years.

If there is a disagreement over the evaluation, assessment, identification, or placement decision, parents can appeal the decision of the IEP team. In addition, if the parents believe that a procedural violation has occurred (for instance if the IEP is not being implemented as documented), the parent may file a complaint with the school district or the state department of Education. The local department of special education can provide parents with guidelines and information about the process. Parents may also seek advice from the state parent information and training center (see Appendix A).

IDEA incorporates the following procedural safeguards for children and parents:

- notice of school's proposed actions and of parents' rights
- consent to evaluate
- appropriate evaluation
- independent evaluation
- consent to placement
- input to the IEP
- appeal to impartial hearing officer
- the "stay put" provision (Once placement has begun, it can be changed only by the IEP committee.)
- private right of action in federal court
- attorneys' fees

These procedural safeguards are described in the U.S. Code of Federal Regulations, Title 34, Subtitle B, Chapter III, Part 300.

Under IDEA, whenever appropriate, the child with disabilities must be educated in the regular classroom. It requires the school to consider providing "supplemental aids and services" to support a child in the regular education classroom *first,* before moving the child to a more restrictive environment. Supplemental aids and services may include modifying the curriculum, providing a paraprofessional to assist a child, assistive technology or devices, training, and other support services. A child can be removed from the regular education classroom only after it is determined that even with the use of supplemental aids and services, the child cannot receive an appropriate education in the regular classroom.

IDEA's least restrictive environment requirement is not a mandate for inclusion but gives adequate support for its practice. Inclusion can be defined as the practice of educating a child with disabilities within the general education classroom, with supports and accommodations needed by that student. This inclusion typically takes place at the student's neighborhood school (NICHCY 1995). For many states, inclusion may not take place in the neighborhood school; this debate has been considered by the courts.

If the IEP team determines that the student cannot be educated satisfactorily in the general education classroom, even when appropriate aids and supports are provided, then alternative placement must be considered. Alternative placements may include special classes, special schools, home instruction, and instruction in hospitals or other facilities (NICHCY 1995). Decisions about placement must be made by the IEP staffing team on an individual basis with consideration for the student and his or her special needs.

OBTAINING SPECIAL EDUCATION SERVICES UNDER SECTION 504 OF THE REHABILITATION ACT

The school is responsible for developing a plan that addresses the individual student's needs. This plan incorporates any modifications necessary for a child with disabilities who does not qualify for special services under the eligibility requirements of IDEA. According to the Section 504 regulation, an education can consist of either regular or special education and must include any related aids or services necessary to provide a free appropriate public education designed to meet the student's needs in the least restrictive environment.

Section 504 does not require the student to be in special education to receive services. The schools are reimbursed for educational and support services provided under IDEA but do not receive funds specifically "earmarked" for students with disabilities that qualify under Section 504. This civil rights law requires the evaluation of any child who needs or is believed to need special education or related services because of a disability. The definition of a disability under

Section 504 differs from IDEA. Section 504 does not link the child's disability to a need for special education services, but rather to the existence of limitations on a major life activity such as caring for one's self, speaking, seeing, hearing, or walking. A student may have a disability that qualifies him or her under Section 504, but that disability does not affect educational performance (Exhibit 19–5).

Whenever a student's health status appears to affect educational performance, then the student should be referred to the school for further assessment to determine whether special education services may be needed.

TRANSITIONING THE CHILD WITH SPECIAL HEALTH CARE NEEDS INTO A SCHOOL, CHILD CARE, OR EARLY EDUCATION PROGRAM

An organized planning process is important for a smooth transition to occur. In addition to the child and family, there are many key players who must participate in this process.

Children and families experience many transitions. Part H of IDEA incorporates transition planning as a child and family move from receiving early intervention services and support provided through Part H. IDEA requires transition planning as part of the IEP for students 16 years of age and younger, if appropriate (Table 19–1) In addition, there are many other transitions that may occur in a child's educational experience. They can include the following transitions:

- from early childhood or child care program to kindergarten
- from kindergarten to a full-day first-grade classroom
- from elementary school to middle school
- from middle school to high school
- from high school to vocational education, college, or employment
- from hospital to home
- from home (after prolonged hospitalization, illness, or injury) to school

Exhibit 19–5 Section 504 Plans

Often, the plan under Section 504 for a student with special health care needs may be delineated in the health care plan. Some situational examples may include the following:

- a student diagnosed with ADHD who does not qualify under IDEA but requires daily use of medication at school
- a student with a chronic illness such as asthma, diabetes, seizure disorder, etc., who requires monitoring while at school and an emergency plan
- a student with a communicable disease such as human immunodeficiency virus (HIV), acquired immune deficiency syndrome (AIDS), tuberculosis (TB)
- a student with a temporary injury or illness who is recovering at home (The student could receive home tutoring, adapted assignments, etc.)
- a student with severe allergies to certain foods (Parents can request modifications of their child's meals with a written statement from their physician stating their child's disability and the special dietary needs.)
- a student with severe allergies who may need improved room ventilation and/or a modified physical education schedule
- a student who has received an organ transplant or a student with cancer who is receiving chemotherapy who may need a modified schedule that allows for rest
- a student who may require transportation as a related service (Modifications may be needed regarding access to transportation, length of bus ride, etc.)

Source: Data from The Legal Center for People with Disabilities and Older People, 1996.

Other transitions may occur if a child attends child care or a before- or after-school program, changes schools, or is enrolled in a special program.

Table 19–1 Factors in the Transition of Students with Special Health Care Needs to Adulthood and Employment

Biologic	Psychologic	Social
Continuity of primary care and preventative health service	Transition to self-management	Independent living skills
Access to appropriate specialty care	Appropriate mental health counseling	Knowledge of community resources including transportation and homemaker services
Transition into adult health care for primary, preventative service, and specialty medical care	Updated assessment of potential job placement or higher education	Recreational activities; build on physical strength and/or needs
Understanding and education of their disease or condition (process and management)	Assertiveness training	Driver education and adaptive car, if applicable
Participation in the development of the individual health care plan, as appropriate	Contact with role models	Access to financial information and aid
Reproduction education specific to the student's health condition	Understanding sexuality	Contraceptive information
Genetic counseling	Parent support in understanding transition process	Vocational training and ongoing support in job placement
Adequate third-party payment coverage	Lifestyle options	Nontraditional vocational and educational options
Availability of adaptive equipment and medications	Personal awareness and adjustment	
Nutritional training, for example, weight management		
Continuity of dental care and availability		
Safety issues		

Source: Adapted from *Procedure Guidelines for Health Care of Students with Special Needs in the School Setting,* Colorado Department of Education and Colorado Department of Public Health and Environment, 1995.

Children with special health needs also have the same needs as their peers—the opportunity to participate in an educational setting that promotes the development of each student's potential, the opportunity to make friends, and the opportunity to participate in their school and community. Plans to satisfy the special health care needs should not interfere with the child's ordinary and basic needs.

Timely notification about a prospective student with special health needs is essential. This notification is usually done by the parent. If the child is transitioning from a hospital setting or another setting that has provided health support (such as private duty home nursing or other care facility), then it is important for the appropriate health care provider(s) to be a part of the referral process in conjunction with the family. Also, parents should be recognized as experts in maintaining their child's health and conducting activities that promote health (Graff and Ault 1993).

Advanced planning is essential to ensure appropriate management of a child's special health needs. Creation of the team initiates the planning process for children with special health needs. This team may include the family, the child, health care providers, school nurse, special and/or regular education staff, and other community providers (Palfrey et al. 1992).

The school nurse is central to collecting and reviewing pertinent information; communicating with the family, various health care providers, and community representatives; and providing the team with a written health assessment. Assessment information includes the child's health history and current health status and needs, and addresses school health care and safety needs. A home visit may be useful in gathering information about a child with complex health needs. A home visit is an opportunity to develop a relationship with the child and family, observe the child in his or her environment, and determine how health care needs are being met.

Health assessment information is reviewed at the IEP meeting or, if the child is not eligible for special services, becomes part of the Section 504 plan. Through these activities and exchanges of information the team, rather than any individual, is making decisions and plans about care, while recognizing and supporting the child's and family's expressed needs and priorities. The health assessment and health care plan must be considered when determining the most appropriate school placement and what type of health service supports will be needed. Exhibit 19–6 describes the preparation for the child's transition to school, child care center, or other designated agency.

This process of assessment and planning to meet the child's health and safety needs requires that school personnel and the environment be prepared before the child's entry to school. Entry to school should be delayed only by the amount of time necessary to prepare for safe transition into school. Significant delay requires the development and implementation of an alternative education program such as homebound services.

Exhibit 19–6 Transition to School, Child Care Center, or Other Designated Agency

Preparation for the child's transition to school, child care, early education program, or other designated agency includes the following:

- development of the health care plan; including a safety plan and transportation plan, as appropriate
- determination of the child's level of participation in the management of his or her health needs
- identification of appropriate school personnel who will carry out health care plan
- training of personnel who will interact with the child or carry out the health care plan (This may include classroom teacher, office staff, playground or lunchroom supervision staff, physical education teacher, or transportation staff.)
- identification of personnel who will provide direct care or perform delegated health procedures
- training of select personnel who will provide direct care or perform delegated health procedures
- assessment of the classroom, school, or other designated environment, including the playground, and consideration for field trips or other community experiences
- determination of medications, equipment, and supplies needed and where they will be safely stored
- strategies for the child to prepare for entry or reentry into the school such as bringing the child to school for brief visits, identifying a "buddy" while at school, and/or role playing
- orientation of peers regarding a health condition or equipment (The child and parents may be involved in the planning and delivery of information.)
- plan for communication among the school or designated facility, family, school nurse, other health care providers, classroom teacher, and other school personnel
- protection of rights to confidentiality for the child and family

For some students, frequent absences or a shortened school day due to illness, medical appointments, therapy, or treatments presents unique challenges in the educational experience. All these possibilities must be taken into consideration when determining the student's needs and developing annual educational goals. Modifications for instruction need to be outlined in the IEP. An extended school year may be an option for some students.

For prolonged absences, parents need to arrange for homebound instruction. There are variations from state to state regarding the waiting period, sometimes two to four weeks, before homebound instruction can begin. There are some school districts that have responded to this need by having the student immediately become eligible for homebound instruction. The amount of instructional time that can be provided to the student while homebound is often limited to only several hours per week.

If homebound status is relatively permanent, an IEP should be written with the family, community, and home health care providers. Parents and providers who know that a particular child may need homebound instruction in the future should insist on the inclusion of a specific objective in the IEP that prepares and plans for uninterrupted school instruction. The provision of homebound services should be viewed only as a transition to regular school placement.

Careful transition allows for communication, collaboration, and training to take place. Early notification regarding a child's entry or reentry to school is critical for a child to enter a school or child care program when he or she is ready (Palfrey et al. 1992). Otherwise, additional time, personnel, or even alternative placement in a more restrictive environment may be necessary until arrangements can be made to support the individual needs of the student (Caldwell and Sirvis 1991).

CHILD CARE AND EARLY EDUCATION PROGRAM

A task force appointed by the Carnegie Corporation warned that poor-quality child care, in-

adequate health care, and increasing poverty were creating a "quiet crisis" among children younger than three years (Children's Defense Fund 1995). Reports from the Health and Human Services Office of the Inspector General and the Report on the Cost, Quality, and Child Care Outcomes in Child Care Centers indicate that significant numbers of centers were not meeting state standards and thus were placing children at risk (Children's Defense Fund 1995); most child care is poor to mediocre in quality, with almost half of the infants and toddlers in rooms with less than minimal quality, which interferes with children's emotional and intellectual development (Helburn et al. 1995).

Although this information is alarming, there have been some positive gains for young children. The federal government expanded and strengthened Head Start and created a new Early Head Start Program for children younger than three years. The number of states supporting preschool initiatives for four-year-olds considered at risk of school failure also has increased, nearly tripling between 1979 and 1992 (Children's Defense Fund 1995).

Child care centers operate in the profit, nonprofit, and public sectors. Most often, children who attend early education programs are closely linked to the public school system and have access to various resources including a school nurse or public health consultation. Direct consultation between health professionals and child care centers varies from state to state and often is not a requirement of state licensing regulations.

The Americans with Disabilities Act became effective in 1992. As a result, children can no longer be excluded from a child care setting on the basis of a disability. Child care centers must make reasonable modifications in policies, practices, and procedures to accommodate individuals with disabilities.

Early intervention for young children with disabilities has occurred in a range of different settings including clinics, hospitals, the children's homes, private preschools, and public preschools (Bailey and Wolery 1992). A majority of the early childhood programs designed for typically developing children report they enroll at least one child with a disability (Wolery et al. 1993).

Child care is essential to many families who are employed or attending school. There are few child care programs that openly accommodate children with special health needs. There have been many local and federally grant–funded projects that have focused on (1) the inclusion of children with complex health needs in child care settings and (2) training of home and child care providers on medication administration and health procedures (see Appendix A).

Numerous initiatives are advocating the need for quality child care programs and building the supply of child care. However, inadequate consumer knowledge is creating market imperfections and reducing incentives for some centers to provide good-quality care. Consumer and education efforts are needed in the public and private sectors to help parents identify high-quality child care programs and to inform the American public of the liability of poor-quality programs (Helburn et al. 1995).

There are wide variations from state to state regarding child ratios, group size, caregiver qualifications, and the minimum amount of space required for child care centers. For instance, only two states require child-to-staff ratios at levels recommended by the National Association for the Education of Young Children (NAEYC), which, for infants, is no more than 3 infants per staff person; conversely, there are several states that indicate no more than 8 to 12 infants per staff person (Casey Foundation 1996). Minimum child care licensing requirements are published in each state and can vary significantly.

The National Health and Safety Performance Standards were published in 1992 by the American Academy of Pediatrics and the American Public Health Association. These standards have been established as a guide for improving the regulation and licensing of child care programs and should be used to plan and establish a quality program of child care (American Public Health Association and American Academy of Pediatrics 1992). In addition, the NAEYC has developed standards concerning developmentally appropriate practices. For more information on how to select a quality home or child care program, please contact the National Association of Child Care Resource and Referral Agencies (see Appendix A).

High-quality child care programs provide a safe and nurturing environment that promotes the physical, social, and cognitive development of young children while responding to the needs of families (Bredekamp 1987). The steps necessary for the successful transition of a child with special health needs or a disability to a family child care home or child care center program is similar to the transition to public schools. However, the key elements of successful participation in a child care environment for a child with special health care needs are developing trusting relationships, establishing collaboration, and practicing direct communication among the child, the child's family, health care providers, and other community resources or consultants (see Exhibit 19–7).

INDIVIDUAL HEALTH CARE PLANS

The individual health care plan is designed to provide the school with written information that addresses a student's particular health needs and outlines health issues or procedures that may need to be addressed during the school day (Exhibit 19–8). Formulation of an individual health care plan helps to ensure that all necessary information, needs, and plans are considered to maximize the child's participation and performance in the school setting (Haas 1993). This plan is developed and written in cooperation with the family, school nurse, school administrator, appropriate health care providers, and the members of the school team. Exhibit 19–9 lists the components of an individual health care plan.

The individual health care plan is written for students with special health care needs, or for students who need a modification in the school environment because of individual health care needs. These may include the following: moderate to severe asthma, seizures, sickle cell ane-

Exhibit 19–7 Selecting a Quality Child Care or Early Education Program

In order to make the best decisions in selecting a quality child care or early education environment, families should spend time visiting with staff and children and observe the overall program.

"Quality" child care can be defined as that which is most likely to support children's positive development (Helburn et al. 1995).

Considerations include:

- Is the program licensed by the state licensing agency? Are references available?
- Is the center program accredited by a national accreditation program, such as the National Association for the Education of Young Children (NAEYC)
- What is the program's philosophy toward child development?
- What are the caregiver's education and experience in caring for children?
- What are the caregiver's education and experience in caring for children with special health needs?
- Are the caregivers' verbal and physical interactions with children warm and positive?
- Do the caregivers respond to disciplinary issues with redirection, positive guidance, or the setting of clear-cut limits (American Public Health Association and American Academy of Pediatrics, 1992)?
- Do the caregivers change frequently in the course of a day?
- Is there high staff turnover?
- What is the child-to-caregiver ratio? Centers enrolling children with special needs should have a ratio of one staff member for every three children with special needs (American Public Health Association and American Academy of Pediatrics, 1992).
- Are children properly supervised during indoor play, field trips, outdoor play, and nap time?
- Are there adequate, accessible physical space (indoor and outdoor) and opportunities for the children to explore and play?
- Are there a sufficient amount and variety of developmentally appropriate materials and toys?

- Is the equipment adaptable for a child to use independently or with minimal supervision?
- Is the equipment in good condition and safe for children to use?
- Are there quiet areas available for children?
- Is there a daily routine with a written planned program of activities?
- Is family involvement welcome? Is there an open door policy?
- How do caregivers and families communicate? How often?
- Does the program respect and acknowledge diversity?
- If the program provides snacks and meals, does it meet the child's individual nutritional and health needs?
- If the program provides transportation, is there a plan regarding safe pickup, transport, and drop-off? Are safety restraints or car seats used?
- What is the program's emergency evacuation plan?
- What are the diaper-changing or toileting practices?
- What are the program's infection control, health, and safety practices?
- Are program staff certified in CPR and first aid?
- What are the program policy and practice regarding medication administration and other special health procedures?
- What is the inclusion and exclusion policy for ill children?
- Is there a health consultant available to the program?
- Are other outside resources able to participate or consult with the program (such as therapists, educators, nurses, or other health care providers)?
- Can program staff actively participate in the planning, development, and implementation of the IFSP/IEP or individual health care plan?

Note: For more information on how to select a quality home or child care program, contact the National Association of Child Care Resource and Referral Agencies.

Exhibit 19–8 Planning Checklist for Individual Health Care Plan and Individual Education Plan Development for Students with Special Health Care Needs

FAMILY

Goals and priorities
Liaison
Collaboration
Communications
Other

HEALTH CARE SERVICES

Health assessment, including
    student strengths
Individual health care plan
Emergency plans
Health status monitoring
Specialized health procedure
Health teaching and
    counseling
Medication
Personnel training
Personnel supervision
Staff consultation
Family support and liaison
Physician consultation and
    orders
Parent authorization(s)
Release of information to and
    from health care provider
Other

TRANSPORTATION

Vehicle
Access
Safety
Equipment
Positioning
Emergency plan
Communications
Special assistance
Evacuation
Aid
Other

TUTORING/HOME/ HOSPITAL

Supplemental in-school tutor—
    regular, intermittent
Plan for continuous program-
    ming—school, home, and
    hospital
Extra set of books at home
Regular home and hospital
    program
Other

OTHER PROGRAM ADAPTATIONS

Curriculum and instruction
Special equipment
Activities of daily living
Scheduling of health interventions
Positioning
Mobility
Special diet
Other

ACCESS

School entrance
Hallways
Stairs and elevator
Classroom
Bathroom
Health room
Cafeteria
Library
Locker
Gym
Playground
Other

FIRE SAFETY

Evacuation plan
Evacuation practice

Backup plan
Other

SCHEDULING

Length of day
Number of days
Rest periods
Flexible schedule
Testing schedule
Other

THERAPIES

Occupational therapy
Physical therapy
Speech and language pathology
Other

OTHER RELATED SERVICES

Social work
Counseling
Psychology
Other

EXTRACURRICULAR ACTIVITIES

Special learning opportunities
Extended-day program
Clubs
Sports
Social events
Transportation
Access
Other

FIELD TRIPS

Medication plan
Emergency plan
Personnel
Transportation
Other

Note: The original version of this checklist was published by the Federation for Children with Special Needs as "Checklist of items for consideration in developing IEPs for students with physical disabilities or special health needs." This adaptation appeared in *Serving Students with Special Health Care Needs,* Connecticut State Department of Education, 1992. It is used here with permission of both sources.

Courtesy of State of Connecticut Department of Education, Hartford, Connecticut, and Federation for Children with Special Needs.

Exhibit 19–9 Individual Health Care Plan Components

- Identification of assessment data
- Source of medical care
- List of health problems, nursing diagnosis
- Description of illness or condition
- Medications (at home and school) including dosage and time
- Allergies
- Equipment, including assistive technology
- Specific precautions
- Health care treatment plan, nursing interventions
- Schedule
- Personnel trained
- Procedure
- Physician-written authorization
- Parent-written authorization
- Student-written authorization, if appropriate
- Emergency information
- Person(s) to contact
- Backup plan
- Transportation plan for health needs
- Reevaluation date
- Outcomes expected

The family is responsible for notifying the school nurse of any changes in medication, treatment plan, health care providers, or hospitalization. The school nurse will update the plan as needed.

Source: Adapted with permission from *Procedure Guidelines for Health Care of Students with Special Needs in the School Setting,* Colorado Department of Education and Colorado Department of Health and Environment, 1995.

mia, diabetes, hemophilia, cardiac disorders, an altered immune system, metabolic disorders, neuromuscular and musculoskeletal disorders, and special nutritional needs. Written health care plans also include instructions for school personnel for any health or nursing procedures. Technical assistance and training from the home health care provider, hospital, or other community health care provider may be needed when more complex health needs exist.

Emergency care plans are necessary and can be incorporated into the individual health plan process and the IEP process. The information provided includes procedural guidelines on whom to call and other information to be used when a predictable emergency occurs (Haas 1993).

It is crucial for parents to play a central role in the development of the individual health care plan and the written instructions for health procedures. Parents have tremendous knowledge about their child and their child's specific health needs. Parents should be given the opportunity to participate in the education of school personnel by sharing information about how health-related activities are performed at home, by demonstrating how health procedure(s) are done, and by providing guidance in planning and conducting these procedures at school (Graff and Ault 1993). The child's participation and input should also be invited. The child's cooperation in the development of individual health care goals and objectives can promote the student's maximum independence and self-reliance in the school setting. The plan should consider the performance of health care procedures at a time that minimizes disruptions to the student's educational process and other students present.

Knowledge of technical skills is necessary but not inclusive when providing special health care. Technical skills must be complemented by an understanding of how to work with a child and family to carry out the procedure. This should include the interpersonal or affective aspects of care (Perrin, Shayne, and Bloom 1993). Each family's unique approach to its child's health should be acknowledged and respected. Approaches to health should be considered as evolving from various perspectives including the family, geographic region, culture and ethnicity, and socioeconomic perspectives (Graff and Ault 1993).

The individual health care plan must be written in language that school personnel understand and in a format that is easy to follow. This information is confidential and should be shared only on a need-to-know basis. The plan should be kept by school personnel who may come into contact with the student or in the area where a health procedure may be performed. A copy of the plan is kept in the student's special education file, if appropriate, and in the student's health record. The parent should also be given a copy of the current plan especially because it is part of the IFSP or IEP. A list of names indicating who has copies of the plan is helpful especially when there is new information to share or the plan has been revised.

Contacting the local emergency response team may be appropriate for children with complex health needs. Contact can be made by the school nurse or other health care providers with a parent's written permission and with participation from the family. The emergency response team may not always be prepared to deal with complex pediatric emergencies and may need additional information and training. School personnel should be instructed to share a copy of the individual health care plan with the emergency response team whenever they are called to respond to an emergency at school. Permission to share this information with the emergency response team should be indicated on the health care plan. The most appropriate health care provider(s) should also have a copy of the plan.

Documentation of care that is being provided in the school is essential. Documentation also provides an avenue for communication among care providers in the school, the family, and health care providers as appropriate. The written record also offers checks and balances to ensure that school nurses and their clients have done complete assessments, made logical conclusions, developed reasonable plans, and judged the effectiveness of the results (Haas 1993). Exhibit 19–10 depicts development of the individual health care plan.

ASSISTIVE PERSONNEL IN THE SCHOOL SETTING

Students with special health care needs must be educated to the maximum extent appropriate with nondisabled students. However, this right to integrated or inclusive education extends to all students with health care needs, not just those eligible to receive services under IDEA (The Legal Center 1996). When children are educated in the regular classroom, accommodations and supports must be provided, as appropriate, to meet the child's special needs.

Greater numbers of students with disabilities are attending their neighborhood schools. Many of these students have chronic health conditions or require assistance with medications or special health procedures. Under IDEA, "a qualified school nurse or other qualified person" is the appropriate person providing school *health services.* Exactly who provides school *health services* or *medical services* is an issue that is determined by state regulations, school district policy, and collective bargaining agreements. Each state has requirements regarding what kind of services must be performed by licensed nurses (and physicians).

Many types of school employees care for students with special health care needs in schools. These employees can include the secretary, teacher, paraprofessional, health assistant, clerk, bus driver, custodian, or food service worker. Each year, more school personnel, usually paraprofessionals, are involved in providing health services, which may include medication administration and performance of health care procedures such as gastrostomy feedings, respiratory treatments, and intermittent catheterization, all under the direction and supervision of a licensed registered nurse. It is no longer unusual for a school secretary or paraprofessional to assist students in the administration of 50 to 60 medications per day and to be ready to respond to one of a dozen students with an individual health care plan if a potentially emergent health condition, such as severe allergy, asthma, or diabetes, presents.

Schools are increasingly relying on the use of classroom aides and paraprofessionals to provide needed assistance in the classroom, provide student personal assistance for daily activities, access assistive technology, or perform special health procedures. The amount of training and

Exhibit 19–10 Development of the Individual Health Care Plan

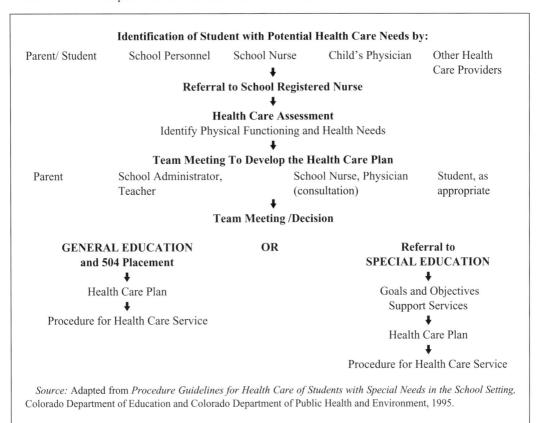

Identification of Student with Potential Health Care Needs by:

Parent/ Student   School Personnel   School Nurse   Child's Physician   Other Health Care Providers

↓

Referral to School Registered Nurse

↓

Health Care Assessment
Identify Physical Functioning and Health Needs

↓

Team Meeting To Develop the Health Care Plan

Parent   School Administrator, Teacher   School Nurse, Physician (consultation)   Student, as appropriate

↓

Team Meeting /Decision

GENERAL EDUCATION and 504 Placement   OR   **Referral to SPECIAL EDUCATION**

↓   ↓

Health Care Plan   Goals and Objectives Support Services

↓   ↓

Procedure for Health Care Service   Health Care Plan

↓

Procedure for Health Care Service

Source: Adapted from *Procedure Guidelines for Health Care of Students with Special Needs in the School Setting,* Colorado Department of Education and Colorado Department of Public Health and Environment, 1995.

supervision that is provided for the paraprofessional varies depending on state regulations, school district policy, individual school practice, and the role of the school nurse. The roles, responsibilities, and training related to health services in schools is not as well defined as the requirements for specific services (Small et al. 1995). At the least, training should take place before school personnel perform any of the responsibilities. A plan for supervision should be clearly delineated. This is important for each member of the student's educational team.

When it has been determined that the service is considered a medical service rather than a health service, then how the child receives his or her education in the least restrictive environment becomes a challenge. There are instances when a student may have a private duty nurse (provided at the parent's expense or reimbursed by health insurance) who accompanies the student to school on a daily basis. The parent may also be the individual who accompanies his or her child to school; this is more common in early childhood settings, at the parent's request. Exhibit 19–11 lists some strategies for any individual accompanying a child to school.

Licensed or unlicensed assistive personnel who accompany the child to school may not always be a school employee. When this situation occurs, it is important for the parties involved to be a part of the educational planning team. In addition, it is important to consider the issues of confidentiality and of the documentation of care that is provided in school. The school nurse can play a pivotal role in the coordination of care and in communicating with the family, health care providers, other agencies, and the school. The school nurse is still responsible for the develop-

Exhibit 19–11 Strategies for Person Accompanying Child to School

---

Having an additional person accompanying the child in the classroom can affect the overall classroom environment and the child's ability to be viewed as a part of the classroom and the school environment. The following are a few effective strategies for paraprofessionals that may be useful for any individual accompanying a child to school:

- Stay in the background.

- The support should help the student gain independence and form relationships with peers. Overattachment can interfere with natural opportunities for friendship and support. To all children, relationships with peers are more important than those with adults.

- Contribute to the education of all the students in the class.

- Support the teacher and the entire class as well as the student with the disability.

- Be a team player.

- Paraprofessionals (and other assistive personnel) are valuable members of the educational team. Teachers, therapists, administrators, parents, and paraprofessionals must work together. All should be included in planning, delivering, and evaluating instruction.

- Develop a plan to fade support.

- Work directly with the classroom teacher to help the child participate in a variety of ways. Natural support from peers and other adults helps to increase the child's independence.

Source: Reprinted with permission from *Speak Out,* © 1996, Peak Parent Center, Inc.

---

ment of the individual health care plan for school, even though the care may be provided by personnel other than the school personnel. Roles and responsibilities of school personnel and assistive personnel should be documented. School staff should have access to information only on a need-to-know basis.

TRAINING, DELEGATION, AND SUPERVISION OF SPECIAL HEALTH CARE NEEDS

Schools and child care programs are faced with the challenge of providing education for children with special health needs that may require the performance of procedures, such as medication administration, gastrstomy tube feedings, catheterization, nebulizer treatments, or oxygen therapy, during school hours. These procedures are typically considered nursing tasks and require appropriately trained personnel to perform them. However, state laws such as the nurse practice acts, may complicate the issue by prohibiting delegation and supervision of the required tasks to unlicensed assistive personnel (Krajicek and Steinke 1995).

The provision of adequate services must be driven by the goals, objectives, and interventions included in the student's IEP. Students who are not enrolled in special education should have an individual health care plan as a part of their education programs. For children in child care centers, reasonable modifications in policies, practices, and procedures must be made to accommodate individuals with disabilities, based on the Americans with Disabilities Act.

Training, delegation, supervision, and support are essential elements of a program for children with special health care needs. Orientation and follow-up training for staff and classroom peers need to be individualized and should involve daily and emergency care (Caldwell, Todaro, and Gates 1989). The school could request support from hospitals, home health agencies, and health clinics to identify staff who are competent to provide specialized training for more complex health needs. The involvement of the family can help to ensure individualization of care (Caldwell and Sirvis 1991).

Children with special health care needs may be able to participate in sharing information with classroom peers. If the student participates in classroom-sharing activities, he or she should be prepared for questions that peers may ask and trained personnel should be available for support (Caldwell and Sirvis 1991).

The school nurse who is making the decision to delegate health procedures must be familiar with nursing standards for his or her role, his or her state's nurse practice act, and other state and federal rules, regulations, and legislation that may affect nursing practice.

Any task delegated by the school registered nurse should include the following:

- within the area of responsibility of the nurse delegating the task
- within the knowledge, skills, and ability of the nurse delegating the task
- of a routine, repetitive nature, not requiring nursing judgment or intervention
- a task that a reasonable and prudent nurse would find to be within generally accepted nursing practice
- an act consistent with the health and safety of the student
- limited to a specific student and within a specific time frame

The nurse needs to have knowledge and understanding of laws governing schools and nursing practice. The decision to delegate should be based on the school registered nurse's assessment of the following:

- student's health care needs including, but not limited to, the complexity and frequency of the nursing care, the stability of the student, and the degree of immediate risk if the task is not carried out
- health care needs of the school population
- school personnel's knowledge, skills, and abilities
- nature of tasks being delegated including, but not limited to, the degree of invasiveness, irreversibility, predictability of outcome, and the potential for harm
- available and accessible resources such as appropriate equipment, adequate supplies,

and other appropriate health care personnel to meet the student's nursing needs
- availability of the nurse for adequate supervision of school personnel providing care (Colorado Department of Education and Colorado Department of Public Health and Environment 1995; Luckenbill 1996)

When the decision has been made that a particular procedure may be delegated, then the final decision regarding delegation rests with delegate caregiver. In some states, the principal or administrator is sometimes defined by state education laws as the person with the authority to delegate or assign tasks (Luckenbill 1996). The following criteria should be used when making the choice of unlicensed assistive personnel:

- available staff
- assessment of the potential caregiver's competency
- consideration of the level of supervision available
- determination of the level and method of supervision required to ensure safe performance (Luckenbill 1996)

Care provided in the schools needs to be provided in the safest, most efficient, and cost-effective manner. The decision on how the care should be provided rests with the school nurse in consultation with the "team." The decision to delegate health care tasks that do not require nursing judgment is the nurse's sole responsibility.

Within the boundaries of state law, a school district's policies, procedures, and job descriptions can also affect the degree and type of delegation of nursing tasks. Additionally, collective bargaining agreements may guarantee paraprofessionals the right to refuse to perform health care procedures not listed in their job descriptions or for which they have not been trained (National Education Association n.d.).

The school registered nurse shall evaluate on an ongoing basis, including the following:

- the degree to which the student's health care needs are being met

- the delegate's performance of the delegated task
- the need for further instruction
- the need to withdraw delegation

The nurse must document the training, observations, and competence of the delegate and also keep the documentation available for legal protection (ANA 1995). The monitoring and supervision of the unlicensed assistive personnel must be documented in the personnel files of the unlicensed assistive personnel, according to school district policy (Luckenbill 1996).

The licensed nurse is responsible for evaluating student outcomes, documenting these in the student's health record, and altering the nursing care plan as necessary to achieve optimal results for the student. It is also the licensed nurse's responsibility to communicate with the family, the health care providers, and the school team regarding the student's progress. (Luckenbill 1996).

TRANSPORTATION

The two federal statutes, the Rehabilitation Act of 1973 (Section 504) and IDEA require schools to provide specialized transportation for certain students with disabilities. Transportation under Part H of IDEA includes the cost of travel and related costs necessary to enable the child and family to receive early intervention services.

Transportation, as a related service, becomes a requirement when it is specified in the student's IEP. Implementation of transportation services and fulfilling the requirement of service delivery in the least restrictive environment are challenging. Implementation of the least restrictive environment mandate requires the involvement of students, parents, administrators, and advocates.

When developing a school transportation plan, important information needs to be gathered, assessed, documented, and communicated to appropriately prepare for the transportation of a student with special health considerations. The IEP transportation plan can include information

that is important in assessing the child's health needs. (The information obtained must be kept confidential and provided only to those persons who need to know.) Including the child's health care providers in this assessment is critical. If transportation is listed as a related service, it is helpful to have a transportation representative participate in the development of the IEP.

Under IDEA, related service provisions transportation must be provided at no cost. Under Part H, parents may be required to assume some financial responsibility. A school district may choose to transport children younger than three years.

The school nurse and the transportation department must develop a transportation health care plan to ensure the safety of students and reduce the liability of school personnel and the school district. This plan incorporates the same information as the school health care plan but is modified to address special considerations specific to transportation. The names of the persons trained to carry out the health care plan should be included. Exhibit 19–12 lists information that may be useful in the development of the IEP transportation plan.

SPECIAL CONSIDERATIONS: DO NOT RESUSCITATE ORDERS AND THE SCHOOL

Advances in medical technology have enabled children with complex health needs to live longer and more active lives. However, this does not always mean that the child will live to an average adult life expectancy. A child may experience a life-threatening episode while he or she is attending school. In some instances, parents, with the support of health care providers, determine that it is in the best interest of the child to not intervene or provide treatment (Rushton, Will, and Murray 1994). Having a child in the school with a do not resuscitate (DNR) order brings about many ethical and legal considerations.

Health care professionals learn how to respond to DNR orders in their practice. They are

Exhibit 19–12 Useful Information for Development of IEP Transportation Plan

---

The following list shows information that may be useful in the development of the individual education plan (IEP) Transportation Plan:

- Can the student use regular transportation?
- Can the student walk to and from an established bus stop? Are there any limitations?
- What are the student's needs or conditions (behaviors, allergies, diseases, medications, medical devices and equipment, sensory assistive devices, emergency protocols, and do not resuscitate [DNR] orders)?
- Does the school district have adequate equipment to transport the student and any needed adaptive devices? If not, what alternative transportation exists?
- What is the maximum length of the bus ride ?
- Does the vehicle have a two-way radio in case of emergency?
- If special devices will be used on the bus, have therapists or others been made aware of the restriction or requirements that govern the transportation of students with special needs?
- Is the necessary training available to meet the student's needs?
- Will the monitor have first aid and cardiopulmonary resuscitation (CPR) certification?
- Has there been a discussion with the family regarding their role and responsibility in the transportation of their child?

Source: Adapted from IEP School Transportation Plan, *CDE Guidelines for Transporting Students with Disabilities*, Colorado Department of Education School Transportation Unit, 1996.

---

ferent from a health or medical setting. In school settings, educators and caregivers generally lack an understanding of the child's clinical condition, may not have the training to assess the child, and are not trained to determine if the situation is a DNR situation (Rushton, Will, and Murray 1994; Colorado Department of Public Health and Environment 1993).

Although many school districts honor requests to follow DNR orders, others have refused, and still others require parents to obtain a court order before honoring DNR orders (National Education Association 1994). It is important that school personnel develop guidelines to follow when a child with a DNR order attends school.

The National Education Association (NEA) (National Education Association 1994) developed guidelines for DNR orders in the schools, in the event a school district decides to honor a DNR order. This policy does not take a position on whether school districts should honor DNR orders.

The NEA suggested the following conditions *in the event a school board* decides to honor DNR orders:

- that the request should be submitted in writing and be accompanied by a written DNR order signed by the primary physician
- that the school establish a team, consisting of the parents or guardians, physician, school nurse, appropriate school personnel, and school superintendent, to consider the request and all available alternatives, and if no other alternatives are available, to develop a medical emergency plan
- that staff and students receive training and counseling (National Education Association 1994)

Upon receiving a written DNR order, an individual health care plan is developed for the student, which addresses the health needs related to the child's condition. Development of the health care plan can encourage school personnel, administrators, health care professionals, and par-

trained to make necessary judgments and to take the necessary actions. Parents also learn to accept the limitations of medical technology to sustain and restore life. A school setting is dif-

ents to pose important questions, voice concerns, share values, and participate in a team decision-making process regarding how certain situations should be handled. Many medical and legal issues need to be considered regarding the DNR order, including the following:

- the arrangements that will be made with the school, the physician, emergency medical services, and the local hospital
- the parents' rights in making the decision
- the child's rights
- if both parents signed the consent
- if schools should consider consulting with an attorney (Colorado Department of Public Health and Environment 1993)

In its statement, the NEA delineated the following elements of the medical emergency plan:

- It specifies what actions the school personnel should take if the student suffers a cardiac arrest or other life-threatening emergency.
- Other school employees who supervise students should be briefed regarding what procedures to follow in the event of an emergency.
- The student should wear an identification bracelet indicating that he or she is subject to a DNR order.
- The parents should execute a contract with the local emergency medical service and send a copy to the superintendent.
- The team should review the child's health condition and the plan annually (National Education Association, 1994).

Minimally, individual school districts should develop a school policy addressing DNR requests. School personnel can obtain additional support regarding these ethical and legal considerations from advisory boards. Community hospice programs can also be a supportive resource to the schools.

School personnel must examine their moral convictions and their public obligations regarding DNR orders. All involved must respect the choices of the parents, become knowledgeable about the child's condition and their responsibilities during a medical crisis, and consult with parents and health care professionals to work out a plan that addresses their concerns (Rushton, Will, and Murray 1994).

REIMBURSEMENT FOR SERVICES

Unfortunately, today's economic environment of health care limits options for health care services, especially for children with special needs. Families must be knowledgeable about their options and persistent when negotiating access to services. Payment for services that a child may need in the school setting depends on many factors. If the school district deems that services are health related, then the school district team will determine in the IEP what related services will be offered, the frequency of services, and who will provide those services. These health related services are funded through the school district. Occasionally, parents think that their child requires additional services or more frequent services than what the IEP offers. In this instance, parents must look beyond educational funding, unless they initiate an appeal or seek legal assistance.

When the school district determines that services are medically related, the family must pursue other options for payment and the provision of these services. Certified home health agencies provide skilled nursing, physical therapy, occupational therapy, and speech and language pathology services. Most agencies require a payment source. The family and/or home health agency can query the insurance company to determine coverage for requested services. Usually, the payer will authorize services for a specific time frame, often limited to a specific number of visits per year. Nursing services are provided in intermittent visits or hours of care. To qualify for hours of skilled nursing, often called "private duty nursing," the child's medical condition must require constant skilled nursing assessments and treatments in lieu of hospitalization.

Medicaid is a federal- and state-funded health insurance that is available for people with low incomes or for persons with disabilities and limited assets. Eligibility criteria vary from state to state. Medicaid services can include home nursing, inpatient and outpatient services, laboratory and radiograph services, physician and clinic services, and early and periodic screening, diagnostic, and treatment (EPSDT). EPSDT offers preventative care including well-child examinations, immunizations, dental care, and vision and hearing screens. If a condition is found on an EPSDT screen and the physician orders an intervention for the identified condition, Medicaid often is obligated to pay for that intervention. For example, if the physician determines that a child requires physical therapy services, then Medicaid must reimburse for that service.

Social security income (SSI) provides cash assistance to families of children with disabilities who are younger than 18 years and whose families have low income or limited resources. In most states, children receiving SSI benefits may qualify for Medicaid, which can offer access to services.

Many states offer extended care services through waivers and require that the child be dependent on technology such as a ventilator, tracheostomy, continuous infusions, or gastrostomy feedings or be diagnosed as HIV-positive. The waiver programs offer an option for working or insured parents to obtain Medicaid for their child with complex health needs and waive parental income eligibility. It is rare for managed care plans and health maintenance organizations (HMOs) to offer private duty nursing services unless these services will enable a child to leave the hospital earlier. Therefore, it is important to research the specific health care plans and policies carefully.

State health departments usually offer Title V Programs for Children with Special Needs (also known as Handicapped Children's Program or Health Care Program for Children with Special Needs). These public programs offer evaluation services and some inpatient care, outpatient services, and home care services such as short-term nursing or therapy visits within diagnostic eligibility criteria and as funding levels allow. Because funding is appropriated on a fiscal year beginning in July, it is best to seek reimbursement early in the fiscal year. Title V programs also offer case management services, which are invaluable for families attempting to negotiate the system.

Navigating the world of reimbursement and finance can be overwhelming. Resourceful and creative families and professionals help obtain support to pay for services and costs incurred. Various community organizations, private charities, special grants, and churches can be approached about the child's and family's individual needs that are not covered by federal, state, or insurance programs.

The population of children with special health care needs is expected to grow. In addition, the overall student enrollment of this population in schools is increasing. The growth in the special education population and costs, combined with limited resources, demand that accountability measures be implemented and evaluated. Collaboration among community agencies, state and federal agencies, public schools, and insurance companies can help consolidate costs, decrease fragmentation of care, and contribute to helping children and families make the best decisions in meeting their unique needs.

REFERENCES

American Nurses Association (ANA). 1995. *The ANA basic guide to safe delegation* (Item Number BGSD). Kearneysville, WV: American Nurses Publishing.

American Public Health Association and American Academy of Pediatrics. 1992. *Caring for our children national health and safety performance standards: Guide-*

lines for out-of-home child care programs. Washington DC: American Public Health Association.

Bailey, D.B., and M. Wolery. 1992. *Teaching infants and preschoolers with disabilities.* 2d ed. Columbus, OH: Merrill.

Bredekamp, S., ed. 1987. *Developmentally appropriate practice in early childhood programs serving children from birth through age 8.* Washington DC: National Association for the Education of Young Children.

Burt, C.J, et al. 1996. Preliminary development of the school health intensity rating scale. *Journal of School Health* 66:286–90.

Caldwell, T., and B. Sirvis. 1991. Students with special health conditions: An emerging population presents new challenges. *Preventing School Failure* 35, no. 3:13–18.

Caldwell, T.H., A. Todaro, and J. Gates. 1989. *Community providers' guide: An information outline for working with children with special health care needs in the community.* New Orleans: Children's Hospital/National Center for Training Caregivers.

Casey Foundation. 1996. *Kids count data book.* Baltimore: Annie E. Casey Foundation.

Children's Defense Fund. 1995. *The state of America's children yearbook.* Washington DC: Children's Defense Fund.

Colorado Department of Education and Colorado Department of Public Health and Environment. 1995. *Procedure guidelines for health care of students with special needs in the school setting.* Denver: Colorado Department of Education and Colorado Department of Public Health and Environment.

Colorado Department of Public Health and Environment, Family and Community Health Services Section. 1993. Information regarding do not resuscitate agreements (DNR). In *Procedure guidelines for health care of students with special needs in the school setting (Part I-17-18).* Denver: Colorado Department of Education and Colorado Department of Public Health and Environment.

Graff, J.C., and M.M. Ault. 1993. Guidelines for working with students having special health care needs. *Journal of School Health.* 63:335–38.

Haas, M.B., ed. 1993. *The school nurse's source book of individualized healthcare plans.* North Branch, MN: Sunrise River Press.

Helburn, S., et al. 1995. *Cost, quality, & child outcomes in child care centers, public report.* Denver: Economics Department, University of Colorado at Denver.

Igoe, J.B., and S. Speer. 1996. Community health nurse in the schools. In *Community health nursing: Process and practice for promoting health,* ed. M. Stanhope, and J. Lancaster, 879–906. St. Louis: Mosby–Year Book.

Ireys, H.T., H.A. Grason, and B. Guyer. 1996. Assuring quality of care for children with special needs in managed care organizations: Roles for pediatricians. *Pediatrics* 98:178–85.

Krajicek, M., and G. Steinke, eds. 1995. *Proceedings of the first national conference on developing policy and practice to implement IDEA related to invasive procedures for children with special health care needs.* Denver: University of Colorado Health Sciences Center, School of Nursing.

Krajicek, M., and G. Steinke. 1996. *The Project on Developing Policy and Practice to implement the Individuals with Disabilities Act (IDEA) related to invasive procedures for young children: Recommendations and conclusions.* Denver: University of Colorado Health Sciences Center, School of Nursing.

The Legal Center for People with Disabilities and Older People. 1993. *First steps to discovery.* Denver: The Legal Center.

The Legal Center for People with Disabilities and Older People. 1996. *Rights to special education in Colorado: A guide for parents.* Denver: The Legal Center.

Luckenbill, D.H. 1996. *The school nurse's role in delegation of care: Guidelines and compendium.* Scarborough, ME: National Association of School Nurses.

National Association of School Nurses. 1993. *Membership survey executive summary.* Scarborough, ME: National Association of School Nurses.

National Education Association: Executive Committee. June 1994. *Policy on do not resuscitate orders.* Washington, DC: National Education Association.

National Education Association Office of Educational Support Personnel and the National Center for Innovation. n.d. *Providing safe health care: The role of educational support personnel.* Washington, DC: National Education Association.

National Information Center for Children and Youth with Disabilities (NICHCY). 1995. *Disabilities that qualify children and youth for special education services under the Individuals with Disabilities Education Act (IDEA) (G3).* Washington DC.

National Information Center for Children and Youth with Disabilities (NICHCY). 1991. Related services for school-aged children with disabilities. *News Digest.* 1, no. 2:1–23.

Newacheck, P.W., and R.T. Taylor, 1992. Childhood chronic illness: Prevalence, severity, and impact. *American Journal of Public Health* 82:364–70.

Palfrey, J.S., et al. 1992. Project school care: Integrating children assisted by medical technology into educational settings. *Journal of School Health* 62:50–54.

Passarelli, C. 1994. School nursing: Trends for the future. *Journal of School Health* 64:141–46.

Perrin, J.M., M.W. Shayne, and S.R. Bloom. 1993. *Home and community care for chronically ill children.* New York: Oxford University Press.

Proctor, S.T., S.L. Lordi, and D.S. Zaiger. 1993. *School nursing practice: Roles and standards.* Scarborough, ME: National Association of School Nurses.

Rapport, M.J. 1996. Legal guidelines for the delivery of special health care services in schools. *Exceptional Children.* 62:537–49.

Rushton, C.H., J.C. Will, and M.G. Murray. 1994. To honor and obey—DNR orders and the school. *Pediatric Nursing.* 20:581–85.

Shriver, K. 1996. Providers find outreach is elementary. *Modern Healthcare,* 24 June, 140.

Small, M.L., et al. 1995. School health services. *Journal of School Health.* 65:319–26.

Swanson, J., M. Lerner, and L. Williams. 1995. More frequent diagnosis of attention deficit hyperactivity disorder. *New England Journal of Medicine* 333:944.

Task Force on Technology Dependent Children. 1988. *Fostering home and community based care for technology-dependent children.* Washington, DC: Department of

Health and Human Services, Health Care Financing Administration.

Urbano, M.T. 1992. *Preschool children with special health care needs.* San Diego: Singular Publishing Group, Inc.

U.S. Department of Health and Human Services, Public Health Services. 1995. *Child Health USA '94.* Maternal and Child Health Bureau, Health Resources and Services Administration. (DHHS Publication No. HRSA-MCH-95-1). Washington, DC: U.S. Government Printing Office.

Von Rembow, D., and W. Sciarillo, eds. 1993. *Nurses, physicians, psychologists and social workers within statewide early intervention systems: Clarifying roles under Part H of the Individuals with Disabilities Act.* Bethesda, MD: Association for the Care of Children's Health.

Wolery, M., et al. 1993. Research report. Mainstreaming in early childhood programs: Current status and relevant issues. *Young Children* 49, no. 1:79–84.

BIBLIOGRAPHY

Academy of Pediatrics: Committee on Children with Disabilities. 1993. Provision of related services for children with chronic disabilities. *Pediatrics* 92:879–81.

Academy of Pediatrics: Committee on Injury and Poison Prevention. 1994. School bus transportation of children with special needs. *Pediatrics* 93:129–30.

Boyle, C.B., DeCouflé, and M. Yeargin-Allsopp. 1994. Prevalence and health impact of developmental disabilities in U.S. children. *Pediatrics* 93:399–403.

Center for the Future of Children, the David and Lucille Packard Foundation. 1996. *The future of children: Special education for students with disabilities.* 6(1).

Clawson, J.A. 1996. A child with chronic illness and the process of family adaptation. *Journal of Pediatric Nursing* 11(1):52–61.

Collin, R.M. 1995. Nurses in early intervention. *Pediatric Nursing* 21:529–32.

Colorado Department of Education School Transportation Unit. 1996. *CDE guidelines for transporting students with disabilities.* Denver: Colorado Department of Education School Transportation Unit.

Haynie, M., J. Palfrey, and S. Porter. 1989. *Children assisted by medical technology in educational settings: Guidelines for care.* Boston: Project School Care, Children's Hospital.

Igoe, J.B. 1994. School nursing. *Nursing Clinics of North America* 29:443–58.

Joint Task Force for the Management of Children with Special Health Needs. 1990. *Guidelines for the delineation of roles and responsibilities for the safe delivery of spe-*

cialized health care in the educational setting. Reston, VA: Council for Exceptional Children.

Kohrman, A.F. 1992. Medical technology: Implications for health and social service providers. In *The medically complex child,* ed. N.J. Hochstadt, and D.M. Yost, 3–13. New York: Harwood Academic Publishers.

Krajicek, M., and G. Steinke, eds. 1996. *Proceedings of the Second National Conference on Developing Policy and Practice to Implement IDEA Related to Invasive Procedures for Children with Special Health Care Needs.* Denver: University of Colorado Health Sciences Center, School of Nursing.

Lehr, D.H., and P. McDaid. 1993. Opening the door further: Integrating students with complex health needs. *Focus on Exceptional Children* 25, no. 6:1–7.

Lilies, C. 1993. Serving children with special health care needs in school. *South Atlantic Regional Resource Center Newsletter* 3: 1–10.

Lynch, E.W., R.B. Lewis, and D.S. Murphy. 1993. Educational services for children with chronic illnesses: Perspectives of educators and families. *Exceptional Children* 59:210–20.

McGonigel, M.J., R.K. Kaufman, and B.H. Johnson, eds. 1991. *Guidelines and recommended practices for the individualized family service plan.* Bethesda, MD: Association for the Care of Children's Health.

National Information Center for Children and Youth with Disabilities NICHCY. 1991. The education of children and youth with special needs: What do the laws say? *News Digest* 1, no 1:1–16.

Osborne, A.G., and P. Dimattia. 1994. The IDEA's least restrictive environment mandate: Legal implications. *Exceptional Children* 61, no. 1:6–14.

Project School Care. 1992. *Working towards a balance in our lives*. Boston: Harvard University.

Shelton, T.L., and J.S. Stepanek. 1994. *Family centered care for children needing specialized health and developmental services*. Bethesda: Association for the Care of Children's Health.

Steele, S. 1991. Nurse case management in a rural parent infant enrichment program. *Issues in Comprehensive Pediatric Nursing* 14:259–66.

CHAPTER 20

The Parents' Perspective on Pediatric Home Care

Ruth Messinger and M. Katharine Dolan

Although many parents describe the birth of a child as one of the happiest events in their lives, parents who have a child with a serious illness or disability may not. They may describe getting a diagnosis of their child's serious illness or disability as the most devastating event in their lives (Brown, Goodman, and Kupper 1993). Thankfully, changes in medical technology, health care financing, and beliefs about what constitutes "best practice" have all influenced the tremendous growth in the development of a continuum of care for children in the past decade. With this expansion, there has been increasing attention to and implementation of pediatric home health care. For pediatric home health care providers to achieve success, they should have knowledge about family factors and seek parental input throughout the process. Caring for a child who is medically fragile in the home places tremendous physical, emotional, and financial demands on parents and families. Factors to consider include parental reactions, family-centered care, boundary issues, resiliency, and opportunities pediatric home care creates for professional helpfulness.

REACTIONS TO DIAGNOSIS OR CONDITION

The stage theory developed by Kubler-Ross (1972) for use with people who have terminal illness has been borrowed by the public to describe families' reactions to a diagnosis of seri-

ous illness or developmental disability. In this adaptation, when family members have a child with a serious illness or disability, they are supposed to move sequentially through stages or phases of denial, anger, bargaining, depression or guilt, and finally adaptation or acceptance. Family members or professionals may use this jargon when they say, for instance, "He's still in denial," or "I need to work through my anger."

In practice, the stage theory may be neither accurate nor helpful in describing families' reactions because families tell us that these stages are not linear, time bound, or even true for all family members. Other families object to use of the stage theory because they believe it tends to focus on negatives. Although these powerful emotions are a part of the adjustments of having a child with a serious medical condition or disability, most parents continue to have positive experiences with their children (Featherstone 1980).

With rare exception, no family asks to have a child who is medically fragile or has a chronic illness or developmental disability. Each family is different and reactions are frequently determined by past experience, cultural background, resources, and strengths. In addition, parents and other family members have unique ways of dealing with the challenges associated with a child who has special needs, so each family's reactions are an individualized matter.

Many family members do report that they are

on an emotional "roller coaster" with feelings that are associated with grief and loss (Moses 1987). After the diagnosis of serious illness or disability, families often grieve the loss of the child they envisioned and the life they had planned. These feelings may include a refusal to believe the diagnosis or prognosis, a sense of failure, fatigue including emotional and physical exhaustion, isolation, fear of the future, and being angry or overwhelmed by the burden of care. The professionals who plan for and engage in pediatric home care can assist parents by acknowledging the normalcy of all these feelings. For instance, more than one parent has been relieved to learn that dreaming about the death of the child is common and does not mean that he or she is "losing it," as one parent said, or a "bad" parent, as another interpreted it.

Regardless of whether a specific family experiences the progression of feelings described previously at the time of diagnosis, times of transition may trigger some recurrence of expression of grief. Transitions can be in the child's life or in the family's life cycle. The first time of transition, when parents begin to entertain the thought of home care, is often a major milestone, when the worry changes from "I'm afraid he'll die" to "How will we deal with his living?" Other transitions for the child can be discharge from hospital to home, readmission to the hospital, acute illness, secondary diagnosis, entering a special treatment protocol or program, birthdays and holidays, and the onset of adolescence. For example, one parent of a teenager has vivid memories of how overwhelmed she became by intense feelings of joy the first time her son rode the minibus to the first pre-school program he attended. Simultaneously, she experienced sadness as she was reminded of how different and "damaged" her child was, as symbolized by his inability to ride the regular school bus to a regular school.

Times of transition for the family include geographic relocation, the decision to get pregnant again or the birth of another child, another child leaving for school or camp or in some way surpassing the child receiving home care, divorce or parental separation, and illness or death of a close family member or friend.

FAMILY-CENTERED CARE

The concept of family-centered care (Shelton, Jepson, and Johnson 1987) is a new one to people who were taught that the unit of care is the diseased organ or the patient. Family-centered care acknowledges the centrality of the family, that the family is the basic unit of the child's world, and that professional caregivers come and go. "Family" can include parents, siblings, extended family, and even people who are not blood relatives.

For pediatric home care to be successful, families need to be an integral part of the team and have their voices heard. Those voices change over time. Families acknowledge that when they are first told of a diagnosis they may feel ignorant and totally reliant on the opinions and decisions of "the experts." As time progresses, families often become "the experts," knowing their children better than medical specialists and becoming more knowledgeable about negotiating with various bureaucracies, specialists, durable medical goods companies, and numerous "case managers" assigned to their cases.

Family-centered care reminds us of the importance of all family members. Siblings may become the neglected part of the family when parents' energy and time are devoted to the child with medical fragility. For instance, one parent recalled looking at a boy and thinking that his mother should have gotten him a haircut, only to realize that the boy was her own son, the sibling of her medically fragile toddler.

Even when parents do make a conscious effort to continue to address the needs of all their children, siblings sometimes feel that they are excluded from family secrets. Brothers and sisters will voice fears that they may have caused the medical problem or that they are afraid of catching "it." They may worry that the sick sibling is going to die or they may feel guilty about the jealousy associated with the sick child getting all the attention (Carlson, Leviton, and Mueller 1993). In some families, healthy children are reluctant to voice these concerns directly to their parents; it may feel safer to express these thoughts to a nonfamily member such as a home health care provider. When available, support groups for siblings help bring children with similar home situations together.

Despite families' geographic mobility and with extended families rarely living together, grandparents, aunts, and uncles can be invaluable sources of support or the opposite. In some cultures, a grandparent is the real decision maker in the family or "fictive kin," that is, nonblood relatives, may have significant authority about treatment decisions, including whether a child should be discharged to home for care at home (Westby 1995). Parents often wonder what information to share and how to share this information with family members or, conversely, have strong feelings against disclosure. One Tamil father, for example, requested that the team not tell his wife that their daughter's illness was terminal. The concept of family-centered care encourages home health care providers to recognize that who constitutes the family is defined by that particular family and to respect the importance of siblings and extended family members in making decisions and maintaining the general well-being in the family.

BOUNDARY ISSUES

The notion of boundaries is perhaps the most challenging dynamic for nurses, other home care providers, and families alike. Whereas in the hospital there is an established system of care, hierarchy of roles, and division of labor, in pediatric home care these boundary issues are subject to negotiation, based on the unique needs of and conditions in each family. Although nursing assistance is often a welcome relief, it is not without cost. Families open up their homes and lives to home care providers and lose a great deal of privacy in the process. Yet, home care providers can give much needed respite and support to parents regarding the care of their child and

bring some balance into the family's life so that they have time to sleep, relax, work, or take care of themselves, their spouses, or other children.

Finding out what works to everyone's satisfaction requires open, honest communication and being sure that everyone shares the same expectations about house rules, discipline of other children, roles, and division of labor. Such seemingly inconsequential things as use of the telephone, doing laundry, refrigerator use, and food consumption can become huge issues. For example, one nursing agency became angry when a family put signs on their telephones requesting that nonfamily users pay for each call. Conversely, a parent was aghast when a home health care nurse rearranged the furniture in the family room without requesting permission from the family. In this first example, the family did not wish to disclose to the nurses that because of dire financial circumstances, it used the telephone only in emergencies to avoid added charges. In the second example, the nurse moved the furniture for safety reasons but did not inform the family of his reason before or after.

Other issues, such as possible maltreatment (Benedict, Wulff, and White 1992), observed cultural differences in child-rearing practices, use of alternative health care practices (Pachter and Wellor 1993), substance use, or perceived neglect of siblings, are difficult to handle and may be best discussed with one's supervisor. When the home care provider is of a different cultural, ethnic, or linguistic background than the family, consultation with the agency supervisor or a surrogate can promote delivery of culturally competent services.

Whereas discussing a specific home care concern with one's supervisor at work is considered essential, sharing information about a family with others is not. Confidentiality, especially in the field of home care, is a fundamental element for demonstrating respect for the family unit.

RESILIENCY

Despite overwhelming challenges, many families are able to deal with the stress associated with having a child who requires pediatric home health care and to experience positive outcomes. Resiliency research in the last decade informs us that families who do well are those who learn to acquire necessary information and services, are flexible, can adjust their expectations, and are not isolated (Patterson 1991). Some families also believe in the value of humor and that to be able to laugh is an attribute they associate with resilience. Rather than focusing on the negative and the abnormality of the situation, the concept of resiliency is preferred by families and professionals because it is positive and, by extension, offers intervention suggestions for pediatric home care professionals to optimize the situation.

RECOMMENDATIONS FOR PROFESSIONALS

1. **Recognize that the family is the center of the child's care.**

   Pediatric home care providers can do much to promote family-centered care by finding out what each family values and wants, especially the less vocal family members. Continuous reassessment is necessary as families and children grow and as circumstances change. Different needs arise and altered behavior by home care providers may be required as parents acquire added skills and resources.

2. **View the family as expert and respect the choices it makes.**

   Sometimes parents make choices about their child's care that may not be what the home care provider would choose. These choices are often painful and difficult decisions that may be made when parents are attempting to balance the needs of the medically fragile child with those of other family members. Families may have strong feelings about choices for care or intervention, how they spend their time or other resources, and family rules. Respect

for the family's right to make these choices is a fundamental point of family-centered care.

3. **Communicate directly and clearly.**

   Understand family members' communication styles—how do members communicate to one another and to outsiders? Pediatric home care providers can serve as role models for direct communication that is not confrontational and conflict-resolution methods. Confidentiality is easily violated by discussing one family's business with another. Families deeply resent home care professionals discussing their personal lives with other families.

4. **Learn about available resources.**

   Even when the family is the expert, information and anticipatory guidance about barriers to care and service inadequacies from trusted professionals are appreciated. For instance, families unfamiliar with tertiary care centers may underestimate the time it takes for appointments or the cost and distance involved for parking. Or, families may not know that some programs have long waiting lists or specific geographic or financial eligibility criteria. When multiple treatment possibilities exist, families are empowered by knowing about those and having a choice of options.

5. **Focus on strengths.**

   To promote family competence and esteem, providers can note positives and strengths and celebrate successes especially when the child does well, a sibling achieves some milestone, or a parent finds his or her voice as advocate.

6. **Promote resilience by preventive intervention.**

   Before family members become isolated and overburdened, pediatric home care providers can suggest respite services and parent-to-parent support as two important forms of burnout prevention. Some parents have said that even a short period of respite makes an incredible difference in recharging emotional batteries. Others prefer the support that can come only from only other parents who have medically fragile children. One new way to obtain parent-to-parent support, particularly when child care is difficult to find and expensive, is to access the web sites on the Internet of families of children with chronic illnesses or disabilities. Computers offer many parents a rapid, comfortable (and anonymous) way to connect with other parents in similar situations but often separated by great distance.

7. **Model self-care of the caregiver.**
   Perhaps most important of all, pediatric home health care providers can model self-care and burnout prevention because home health care providers as well as families are at high risk for burnout. Symptoms such as depression, irritability, hopelessness, anger, and fatigue are all cause for concern. Because it is much easier to avoid burnout or take care of it early on, professionals need to use all the

preventive resources available to them. They can use their supervisors or managers for regular consultation before symptoms of burnout appear. They can also model self-care by respecting the family's boundaries and their own. They can seek out personally nourishing and nurturing activities for themselves, including use of stress management techniques, taking vacations, and doing work that advances their professional competence and growth.

Pediatric home care may not be easy, for the family or the home care professional. Success or failure in forming a satisfactory partnership depends on how home care providers view parents. The best equipment, knowledge, and skills combined will not guarantee a successful experience unless they are balanced by respect for and recognition of the important contributions parents and other family members make. When a satisfactory partnership is formed, challenges can be met and rewards and satisfaction exist for home care providers, the family, and the pediatric patient.

REFERENCES

Benedict, M.I., L.M. Wulff, and R.B. White. 1992. Current parental stress in maltreating and nonmaltreating families of children with multiple disabilities. *Child Abuse and Neglect* 16:155–63.

Brown, C., S. Goodman, and L. Kupper. 1993. *The unplanned journey: When you hear that your child has a disability.* Washington, DC: National Information Center for Children and Youth with Disabilities (NICHCY) 30:5–15.

Carlson, J., A. Leviton, and M. Mueller. 1993. Services to siblings: An important component of family-centered practice. *The ACCH Advocate* 1, no. 1:53–56.

Featherstone, H. 1980. *A difference in the family: Life with a disabled child.* New York: Basic Books.

Kubler-Ross, E. 1972. *On death and dying.* New York: Macmillan.

Moses, K. 1987. *Lost dreams and growth: Parents concerns.* Evanston, DE: Resource Network. Videotape.

Pachter, L.M., and S.C. Wellor. 1993. Acculturation and compliance with medical therapy. *Developmental and Behavioral Pediatrics* 14, no. 3:163–68.

Patterson, J. 1991. Family resilience to the challenge of a child's disability. *Pediatric Annals* 20:491–99.

Shelton, T.J., E.S. Jepson, and B.H. Johnson. 1987. *Family-centered care for children with special health care needs.* Washington, DC: Association for the Care of Children's Health.

Westby, C. 1995. *Developing cultural competence.* 3(1). (Part of University of New Mexico, Los Ninos Project.) 1–3.

CHAPTER 21

Stress Tolerance

Linda Gaudet

Serious illness in a child or adolescent is a significant and unusual family stressor. An understanding of the vast array of stressors that impact the family with a seriously ill child is essential for the professional working with these families. In this chapter, stress and coping in families with chronic pediatric illness are addressed, with the focus placed on the child receiving home nursing care. The term *child* refers to both children and adolescents throughout the chapter.

Family stressors are those life events or occurrences of sufficient magnitude to bring about change in the family system (Hill 1949). Baker (1969) defines a system as a set of units or elements that are actively interrelated and operate in some sense as a bounded unit. If this definition is considered within a family context, it is apparent that an understanding of family interactions and boundaries is vital to the successful provision of services to the ill child and his or her family, particularly in the home setting. In addition, the importance of establishing an initial positive rapport with the family system cannot be overstated. Therefore, the family system is examined in more detail to provide the nurse with a family framework rather than the more limited focus on the patient.

FAMILY SYSTEMS DEVELOPMENT

From a developmental perspective, family systems can be thought of as having lives of their own. In a manner similar to the way in which the individual child develops, family systems pass through predictable life stages (childbearing, latency, adolescence, launching), evolving new methods of taking care of themselves and coping with the demands of the external world (Carter and McGoldrick 1980). The concept of normative developmental tasks versus crises is important when considering the family system. All families can expect to experience normative developmental crises such as adolescence, the "empty nest" syndrome, and the midlife crisis. However, when a nonnormative event such as serious pediatric illness compounds these normal developmental crises, families are faced with the task of coping with an overwhelming degree of stress (Forman 1993; Philadelphia Child Guidance Center and Maguire 1993). Other factors to consider that may affect family functioning are the life stage of the family (as noted previously), the family structure (single-parent, two-parent, extended family, blended family), the family's emotional history, and the degree of pressure or support from the outside world.

Family interactions can be viewed on the following two levels: (1) the interactions within the family and (2) those between the family and the environment. The nurse entering the family system by working in the home setting must assess both the family's internal structure and where the family is in relation to its environment. An excellent means of making such an assessment is by examining boundaries. The clarity and flexibility of family boundaries, which are determined by the establishment of family rules and responsibilities, are useful parameters for evaluating family functioning.

Boundaries within the family structure may be examined in terms of being open or closed. Open boundaries provide good communication and interaction among family members. Closed boundaries imply little or no communication and interaction. The nurse can intervene with the family whose closed boundaries are interfering with optimal home care of the child by assisting the family in realigning its structure. In the case of a family in which the parents' reactions to their child's chronic illness has been to withdraw from each other, the simple task of assigning more parental responsibility and power in terms of both health care and family issues is often effective. The parental unit, whether single-parent or two-parent, must maintain the position of "head" of the family. Nurses can reinforce this role (thus, empowering parents), while mindful that although their clinical knowledge is critical to the family, the parents are the real experts on their child.

Boundaries can also be considered in terms of open or closed interactions between the family and its environment. Maintaining a balance between openness to the environment and shelter from it is a crucial aspect of family functioning. As a representative of both the health care team and society, the nurse has a unique opportunity to assist the family in developing a sense of openness and trust in relation to its environment. By clearly defining roles and expectations, in addition to conveying a willingness to advocate for the family, the nurse can enhance the family's sense of openness and trust.

FAMILY STRESSORS

There are many varied family stressors. The family with a chronically ill child is often characterized by strained family relationships. One often finds an over-involved relationship between the primary caregiver and the ill child, resulting in other family members feeling left out

and sibling competition increasing for parental time and attention. In addition, some scapegoating may be present in which parents blame each other for a current crisis or for the genetic responsibility for the child's condition. Another source of family stress involves the modifications the family must make in activities and goals that affect decisions concerning leisure time, career, and having additional children. Other family stressors include increased tasks and time commitments, social isolation, coordination of medical care, and the necessary grieving process for the loss of a normal childhood. And last, but certainly not least, is the overwhelming financial burden that the family may find that affects almost every area of life.

Indicators of family stress may be parental and sibling somatic complaints, parental medical noncompliance, parental depression, sibling depression or acting out, sibling school problems, and marital dysfunction. Marital tension may, in fact, result in one parent moving out of the home, either temporarily or permanently.

Within the family unit, stressors more specific to the chronically ill child may be frequent hospitalizations, school absences, separations from peers and family members, isolation from normal childhood activities and experiences, painful medical procedures, and, particularly for the adolescent, enforced dependency and loss of autonomy. Knowledge of the developmental tasks of childhood and adolescence is vital for the nurse to properly assess delays or regressions and their subsequent relation to stress. A helpful resource would be a book published by the well-known Philadelphia Child Guidance Center intended to help parents and professionals better understand normal versus problem behaviors resulting from stress (Philadelphia Child Guidance Center and Maguire 1993).

The nurse is in a primary position to recognize the indicators of stress for the ill child. Such indicators may be medical noncompliance, developmental regression, depression (may be "masked depression" in the form of acting-out behavior), self-consciousness, self-isolation, anxiety, helplessness, and school problems.

These family stressors are fairly common to all families experiencing chronic pediatric illness. The family who has the additional stress of caring for the child dependent on medical technology within the home setting must also contend with the constant disruption of normal family life and a lack of privacy due to the presence of health care professionals. Professionals in the home setting, who strive to provide optimal care for the patient and family, must be aware of stressors and alert to possible reactions to them. They must also strive to keep the focus of treatment on the child within the total family context.

No discussion of family stressors would be complete without considering the subject of abuse. The cumulative, complex, and chronic nature of stressors found in families experiencing pediatric chronic illness can lead to the extreme outcome of abuse. It is important to note that the most emotionally healthy of parents can be pushed to the emotional brink and lose control. The parent who brings to the experience of pediatric chronic illness a history of emotional problems, poor coping skills, or an already stressed marital relationship is at even higher risk for abusing the ill child. More specifically, families may be at high risk who have (1) poor communication skills; (2) poor physical, social, or psychological resources; (3) unresolved prior losses; and (4) poorly managed prior family illnesses.

Two categories of child and spousal abuse are considered in terms of indicators and interventions, with the primary focus being that of child abuse. For the purposes of this chapter, child abuse is defined as follows:

1. *Physical abuse:* The physical maltreatment of a child which either results in bruises, welts, or bleeding or surpasses socially acceptable standards of punishment or treatment.
2. *Emotional abuse:* Situations where a child subjected to ongoing parental rejecting, degrading, terrorizing, isolating, exploiting, ignoring, and/or failure to provide reliable and consistent parenting.

Although no one wants to think about the possibility of child abuse in the context of pediatric chronic illness, it behooves the health care professional to be aware of contributing factors and dynamics, as well as necessary and therapeutic steps to take if abuse is suspected. The first step in examining possible abuse, or even the potential for abuse, is to look for warning signs.

In terms of the child, indicators of abuse may be as follows:

1. decreased trust and increased fears
2. decreased concentration
3. increased regressive behaviors
4. exaggerated startle, hypervigilance, anxiety, irritability
5. increased tearfulness, depression, or other significant changes in mood
6. increased problems with sleep and decreased appetite
7. increased anger, acting out behaviors, increased passivity
8. unexplained marks or bruises

It is extremely important to note that the first seven indicators could also be due to the child's illness and required treatment or other factors. The health care professional should never, under any circumstances, accuse the parent of abuse solely on the basis of the previous indicators.

In terms of the parent, indicators of child abuse may be as follows:

1. decreased patience
2. decreased ability to control temper
3. harsh communication and/or "rough" handling of the child
4. decreased use of former problem-solving methods and coping strategies

In the event the health care professional observes the previous indicators and suspects possible emotional or physical abuse of the child, the following steps must be taken:

1. If unexplained marks, bruises, or bleeding are observed, a report to child protec-

tive services must be made and is required by law. It is usually helpful to talk with the parents first and explain the observations and the duty to report, engaging their cooperation if possible. Invite the parents to be present while the call is being made. It is important to explain that Child Protective Services can be an important resource for assistance and support (sometimes providing relief and help in the form of day care for other children or counseling), that is, its primary mission is to protect children and support the family's capacity to care for its children (in contrast to punishment).

2. If suspicions are substantial but no physical evidence exists, it is important to discuss concerns with the parents and give them resources for assistance from behavioral health specialists and community agencies. In addition, a "for information only" report can be made to child protective services of the concerns and suspicions, as well as a request for information on resources available to the family.
   Note: In many states, health care professionals are required to report even a suspicion of child abuse. Contact your local agency for specific information and requirements.

3. It is important to acknowledge and validate the significant stressors the family is attempting to cope with, while at the same time making it clear that emotional and/or physical abuse is never acceptable. What is acceptable and necessary is asking for and accepting help when necessary.

Spousal abuse involves similar dynamics as in the previous discussion of child abuse; however, the following two distinctions must be made:

1. There is no legal requirement to report (an adult is considered capable of and responsible for his or her own protection).

2. The abused spouse must be strongly encouraged to get professional help and support; if the abused spouse is unable to seek out or accept help, the ill child is likely at significant risk (physically and/or emotionally) and must be closely monitored and assessed for risk factors.

Whether the health care professional is dealing with child or spousal abuse, it is critical to consider that pediatric chronic illness itself is a form of trauma; abuse is an additional layer of trauma superimposed upon the illness and can be devastating for both child and family.

FAMILY COPING

Given the tremendous degree of stress that a family with a chronically ill child experiences, the question remains, "How can we as professionals better assist these families in the coping process?" In answer to this question, the coping process has been conceptualized by McCubbin and Patterson (1981) in an effort to find why some families grow and thrive in the face of multiple stressors and others grow weaker and possibly dissolve. Their Double ABCX Model of Family Adaptation presented in Figure 21–1 looks at family efforts over time to adapt to multiple stressors through the use of family resources and perceptual factors in an attempt to achieve family balance or bonadaptation.

Normally, when a family experiences a stressful event (a), the family draws on its resources (b), and its members have a perception of the event (c), each of which interact and result in stress. The stress may become a crisis (x) if the family is unable to use resources (b) and define the situation adequately (c).

In families experiencing pediatric chronic illness, however, not only are there normative stressors but often a "pileup" of stressors (A) as well. Coping for these families involves both their existing and new resources (B), in conjunction with their perceptions of the crisis (C), re-

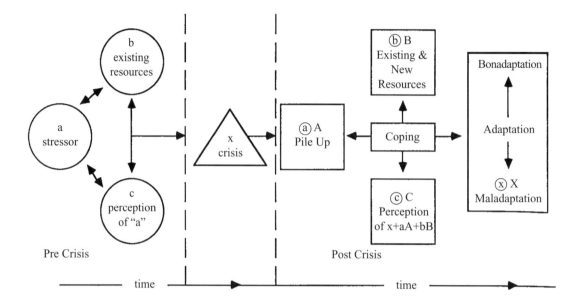

Figure 21–1 The Double ABCX Model of Family Adaptation. *Source:* Reprinted with permission from *Systematic Assessment of Family Stress, Resources, and Coping* by H.I. McCubbin and J. Patterson, Family Social Science, © 1981.

sulting in an adaptation (X). This adaptation may be a bonadaptation or a maladaptation.

Family stressors (A) have previously been examined. The three remaining components of the model are now examined in relation to the family with a chronically ill child.

Resources (B)

Often, it is the social worker and/or discharge planner who is exploring resources, both existing and new, to assist the family in coping with a chronically ill child during hospitalization. However, in the case of the pediatric nurse providing home care, it is the nurse who has most frequent contact with the family and, therefore, may become involved in assessing family resources and/or connecting the family with community resources. Nursing staff can provide an invaluable service to the family by making community resource referrals available to it.

Perception (C)

The family's perception of the crisis (diagnosis of the illness or subsequent crises) is critical in determining the kind of adaptation the family makes. If the family views the situation as hopeless, a maladaptation may occur, resulting in a dysfunctional family. If, on the other hand, the situation is viewed as a challenge, a bonadaptation, resulting in a functional family, is more likely. McCubbin and Patterson (1981) have found that the family's efforts to redefine a situation as a challenge, or as an opportunity for growth, appear to play an important role in facilitating family coping and eventually adaptation.

Several authors have suggested that parental attitudes have a strong influence on how well children with chronic illness adjust to their situations (Freeman 1968; Garrard and Richmond 1963; Mattson 1972). It would appear, therefore, that the nurse working in the home setting could play an important role by reframing the situation for the family in a positive context whenever possible (Exhibit 21–1). Consider the following example: Nurse M. is working with the Smith family and observes the family becoming more and more helpless in its attitude concerning the child's illness and care. The family's perception of the problem could be reframed by the nurse, noting the behavioral indicators of family strengths and new gains made. Nurse M. might also relay to the family observations made of the ill child's strengths and note opportunities for emotional and developmental growth.

Adaptation (X)

Before successful family adaptation can take place, parents must be able to face their problems with a minimum of stress so that their energies can be mobilized to meet the many future tasks. Families who do not adapt well to their children's chronic illness often view themselves as victims, powerless to fight the "system" or perhaps even supernatural forces.

Families who adapt well, on the other hand, often view themselves as activists. Many of these families become involved in efforts to "normalize" the child's life, to initiate aggressive searches of services for the child, and in some cases to bring about societal changes supportive of families with children who are chronically ill or have a disability. In meeting the challenges that their stressful situations impose, these families make bonadaptations, resulting in helping themselves and others.

It would appear useful, then, for nurses working with these families to assess, as early as possible, which families are dysfunctional as well as those that are at risk for becoming dysfunctional. One means of assessing parental coping patterns has been developed by McCubbin and colleagues (1983) and is titled CHIP—Coping Health Inventory for Parents. The CHIP was developed to record what parents find helpful or not helpful in the management of family life

Exhibit 21–1 Tips on Reframing the Crisis

The meaning that any event has depends on the "frame" in which it is perceived. Professionals can assist parents in changing the "frame" or meaning of a pediatric health crisis by doing the following:

- paying attention to the positive value of the family's behavior and views
- identifying the family's strengths and resources
- encouraging new skills and opportunities for emotional and developmental growth
- challenging generalizations, resistance, comparisons, and incomplete or inaccurate information
- asking reframing questions, such as "Compared with what?", "What would happen if . . . " and "What is the worst thing that could happen?"
- reframing the perceived problem within the family's frame of reference and as an opportunity for growth

when their child has a medical condition requiring continued care. The parent records how helpful each of 45 coping behaviors is to him or her on a scale ranging from not helpful to extremely helpful (Appendix 21–A). The CHIP assists parents in examining the need to balance the demands of caring for the ill child with their needs to (1) invest in themselves as individuals, (2) attend to the family unit, and (3) understand the medical situation.

The CHIP can easily and conveniently be used in the home setting. It is an excellent tool for determining differences in coping between mothers and fathers when administered to each parent separately, thus allowing the nurse to assist parents in better understanding each other's response to their child's illness. The reliability and validity of the CHIP have been noted by other researchers as well (Gaudet and Powers 1986, Powers et al. 1986; McCubbin and Patterson 1981).

Coping with Serious Illness

Forman (1993) presents an excellent discussion of the correlations between childhood stress and coping and physical health. Included are references for specific illnesses and their links to stressful events, as well as an extensive discussion of coping and coping skills.

The nurse is in an excellent position to facilitate the process of parents assisting their child in coping well with serious illness. The Philadelphia Child Guidance Center and Maguire (1993) assert that parents can best assist their ill child to cope with stress, depression, and other emotional turmoil that can accompany a serious illness by doing the following: (1) Ensuring both parents and child are as well informed as possible about the illness and what it means, (2) Avoiding making the child feel vulnerable or exceptional, (3) Encouraging the child to engage in activities that will develop self-confidence and self-esteem, and (4) Obtaining outside support for both parents and child.

INTERVENTIONS

Individual Therapy

The pediatric patient can benefit by numerous forms of psychotherapy. Forms of therapy that can be used by nurses are relaxation training, imagery, and hypnosis (Brett 1986; Dolgin and Jay 1989; Forman 1993; Garth 1992; Hilgard and LeBaron 1984; Mills and Crowley 1986; Murdock 1987; O'Grady 1991; Olness and Gardner 1988). These modalities can be extremely effective for pain management and as coping techniques.

Relaxation Therapy

The child can be taught progressive deep muscle relaxation according to his or her age and cognitive development. With the younger child or one with limited cognitive development, the nurse would begin by having the child close his or her eyes. The child would then be asked to take two deep breaths and very slowly let all the air out. The next step would be to ask that the child pretend he or she has two lemons, one in each hand; to squeeze those lemons as hard as possible; and then very slowly to let go of the lemons. Next the child is asked to pretend he or she is a very old person who is all wrinkled: "Wrinkle up your nose and face as hard as you can. Hold it for a minute, and now pretend those wrinkles just magically fall off your face, and your face is relaxed and smooth." The last step is to have the child squeeze his or her toes as tightly as possible. Then say, "Pretend those toes magically turn into soft, white fluffy marshmallows. Your marshmallows are beginning to melt into a white creamy puddle. And as those marshmallows just melt away, all your pain and tightness in your body will melt along with them, slowly leaving your body." The older child with a higher cognitive level can be taken through additional muscle groups beginning with the head and progressing down to the feet, requesting that he or she first tighten and then relax his or her muscles.

Imagery

Imagery is a powerful tool when time is a consideration and immediate results are desired. The child is asked to close his or her eyes and picture an object that is perceived as particularly pleasant. The nurse can help the child focus on the object by describing it in terms of all the child's senses—sight, hearing, smell, taste, and touch. The very young child responds well to visualizing food, such as an ice cream cone. The following imagery could be used: "Close your eyes and imagine a delicious ice cream cone. The cone holding the ice cream is dark brown and kind of bumpy. Your ice cream could be a dark brown chocolate, a pretty pink strawberry, or perhaps a cool white vanilla. I know that whatever flavor you choose, it will be your own very special flavor. Now just imagine that cold ice cream first touching your lips and tongue and then very slowly sliding down your throat. And now you can begin to bite into that crunchy cone. You might even hear the noise your cone makes as you slowly crunch every delicious bite. And when you are finished with your special cone, taking all the time you need, you may open your eyes, knowing you can bring your cone back in your mind any time you want and continue to taste, feel, and see your special treat."

The older child can be taken on a guided visual trip to a place that is very special to him or her. The first step is to gather information about the child's favorite places and experiences, either actual or desired. For instance, if the child describes having had pleasant experiences at the beach (or would like to), the following guided imagery might be developed: "Close your eyes and allow yourself to become very relaxed. Take two deep breaths and let go of your air very slowly. Now picture yourself standing on a cliff high over a beach. As you come closer to the edge of the cliff, you notice some stairs going down to the beach and the ocean beyond. You walk over to those stairs going down to the beach. You very carefully begin to walk down the steps. When you reach the bottom of the stairs, you decide to take off your shoes and allow your bare feet to feel the sand warmed by the sun. You begin walking across the sand toward the ocean, and suddenly a huge wave seems to come up out of nowhere. As the wave approaches the shore, you run up to it and catch the last part of it as it now gently rolls up to the shore's edge and in between your toes. The water is very cold, but it feels so good on your feet. As the water begins to go back out toward the ocean, you squish your toes even further into the wet sand and allow yourself to experience that cool, moist feeling. At the same time, you notice that the sun is warming your back and there is a cool mist on your face from the ocean spray. You may want to walk along the beach for a while, or perhaps you would like to sit down along the water's edge for a few moments, just allowing yourself to experience the beach and the ocean. When you are ready, you can walk back across the beach over to the stairs and slowly climb back up the cliff. Very slowly you may open your eyes and begin to stretch your arms, knowing that you may go back to your special place any time you wish." These types of guided imagery are effective for both the younger child and older child when attempting to divert the child's attention from pain or medical procedures.

Hypnosis

Hypnosis is another excellent therapeutic tool when working with the pediatric patient. The nurse can assist the child in accessing his or her inner resources, thus giving the child more control over his or her body and illness. For nurses desiring training in medical hypnosis, seminars are available for beginning through advanced training.

Play Therapy

Play therapy is one of the most effective and versatile means of working with the pediatric patient. Two excellent references for play therapy have been written by Landreth et al. (1996) and Oaklander (1978), who conceptualize the play therapy process as a way to enter the child's world in a nonthreatening manner. The therapy provides a means for the child to express feelings, arrive at closure, make choices, and lighten burdens. Various projective techniques are used, including drawing, storytelling, puppetry, and role playing.

An important point to remember is that the nurse need not purchase special play equipment (other than crayons, markers, and paper). The nurse also has the advantage of working in the child's home setting and may have a wealth of play material belonging to the child and his or her siblings. The nurse need only bring imagination and creativity, while using the child's own play resources. An example would be to use the child's play figures or animals and take a fantasy trip to the hospital. The nurse and child could experience the preparation and trip there, and once they arrived they could go through admitting, getting settled, and an explanation of routines and procedures. An excellent source of further information on play materials and ideas is the child life worker located in many hospital pediatric units.

Drawing Technique

The nurse could ask the child, first, to draw his or her pain; second, draw the pain looking all better; and, third, draw how the first picture could become the second picture. This process allows the child to develop some awareness of feelings and coping methods in relation to pain. The same procedure could be used with the child's actual illness or disability rather than pain. Another excellent drawing technique, which is simple yet effective, is to ask the child to draw a feeling, such as anger. By allowing the child to use any color or artistic means (for example, pencil, pen, crayon, or marker), the opportunity is provided for the development of awareness and emotional catharsis. The nurse need not interpret the drawing; the child can simply be asked to talk about the picture. The technique works equally well with preschoolers to adolescents.

Puppetry

Hand puppets are an excellent means of providing a nonthreatening way for the child and nurse to communicate. Children may express thoughts and feelings through puppets that they might never do in a more direct manner. Animal hand puppets work well, and it is useful to have one with a happy face and one with a sad face. Puppets dressed as nurses and physicians are also useful. The nurse and child can take turns using various hand puppets (stuffed animals and plastic figures will also work well), each responding spontaneously to the other.

Storytelling

Storytelling is an activity that most children are certain to enjoy. The nurse can assist the child in coping with illness by presenting a story that has a positive outcome. In the case of a terminal illness, positive ways can be provided in which both the child and the family are coping and assure the child that everyone will be all

right after the child's death. The knowledge that his or her family will be very sad but that they will feel better someday can be very reassuring to a child (this would be an excellent time to have the child draw the picture "sad").

Role Playing

Role playing is a fun and very useful way to allow the child to practice coping techniques and ways of relating to other individuals. For example, the nurse could take the role of a parent, allowing the child to practice expressing his or her feelings and concerns to parents.

When using play therapy, there are two important points to remember. The first is to always be mindful of the child's cognitive and developmental level of functioning. The second is to take the child's lead, allowing his or her needs and actions to serve as a guide. With these two points in mind, the nurse can then provide an experience that is both useful and mutually enjoyable for the child and nurse.

Behavior Therapy

Behavior therapy can be a useful technique for nurses involved in compliance issues with pediatric patients. The nurse providing home care has the advantage of observing the child in a natural setting. Ideally, there will be a mental health professional available to assist in developing a behavioral program. The focus would be on behavior rather than emotional or dynamic issues and would be aimed at providing concrete, direct, and rapid relief of the problem at hand (Gillmore 1986; Rimm and Masters 1979). The clinician typically would conceive of a hierarchy of reinforcers from primary (for example, food) to social behavior. The appropriate reinforcer would function either to increase or decrease behavior. It would be helpful to write down the program, either in chart form or as a contractual agreement. The child, family, and nurse would then be reasonably clear regarding expectations and consequences, leaving little room for misunderstanding. Bloomquist (1996) provides an excellent guidebook for both parents and professionals in behavioral skills training for children that includes numerous sample charts, contracts, and procedures for parents to implement in an easy-to-read format.

Learning "Feelings Talk"

Teaching the ill child "feelings talk" is possibly the most important and effective tool a parent or professional can provide. Sutton (n.d.) provides useful information and worksheets for working with children's feelings in general and specifically for working with denial, fear, anger, and depression. *Feelings: Everybody Has Them* is an excellent workbook that enables very young children to express their feelings and includes games, puzzles, and other fun activities (Neuman 1984). Bloomquist (1996) includes a feelings vocabulary chart that depicts various faces and includes a feelings vocabulary for the child to identify, allowing for a simple, fun, and nonthreatening way to begin feelings talk. The book also includes feelings worksheets and a feelings diary.

A simple and effective method for teaching feelings talk with both very young children and older children is cutting out and coloring "feelings faces" with children and requesting that they use the faces to identify their feelings. Children typically enjoy identifying the feelings of happy, sad, mad, scared, and confused in this manner. Most important, the child is given a lifelong skill to better cope with both normal and extreme stressors.

Family Therapy

Based on the systems perspective developed earlier in this chapter, it would appear that the most effective and efficient approach to treatment of the emotional and behavioral components of illness would be a family systems approach; therefore, the treatment of choice would be family therapy. A key difference in working with most families and those with chronic pediatric illness, however, is their reason for requiring family therapy. Rather than the existence of long-standing psychopathological processes, the family therapist would typically find a myriad of logistical difficulties (arranging home life around the care of the ill child) and prolonged developmental transitions (into school, adolescence, and adult life) that have left family structures rigid and obsolete (Mitchell and Rizzo 1985). Reactive versus proactive patterns are often found as a result of families dealing with repeated crises. These families, therefore, appear to respond more positively to treatment that is short term and oriented to problem solving and managing resources.

One short-term problem-solving approach used by the family therapist is in-home family therapy. The approach is based on the premise that the difficulty encountered in the family setting cannot be duplicated in an artificial setting. In the case of the pediatric patient receiving home care, it would seem more practical to observe the difficulties the family may encounter with other systems (such as nurses and other ancillary health care providers) and intervene appropriately in the family's natural setting. In addition, requiring a family with a chronically ill child to meet in an office setting is often difficult to achieve. Other advantages of in-home therapy are the increased likelihood of full compliance of all family members in the therapy process and the flexibility of hours necessary to meet the family's needs.

In addition to applying the problem-solving approach, which is primarily focused on the here and now, it can be extremely helpful to ascertain the transgenerational history of illness, loss, and crisis in the family, or, in other words, "What is the family's illness belief system?" (Rowland 1984). Some of the important areas that should be covered in the initial family session are (1) the family's understanding of the disease, including its progression and outcome; (2) the family's experience with crisis and how it was handled; and (3) the family's experience with and willingness to work with health care systems.

Family therapy is an essential component of services for families experiencing chronic pediatric illness. It is important to recognize, however, that current funding often does not provide for family therapy. Until increased funding becomes a reality, a good resource for families would be family counseling centers that offer sliding-fee scales. Many insurance plans also cover the cost of family therapy up to 80 percent.

Group Therapy

Group therapy occurs when individuals with similar situations gather together for the purpose of some type of therapeutic intervention. Increasingly, health care professionals have become aware of the many benefits of group therapy. The benefits of group therapy that are not available in a one-to-one approach are the following: (1) sharing of emotions, such as fear, anxiety, anger, and loneliness with a peer group; (2) gaining insight and a feeling of support without necessarily participating overtly; (3) allowing group members the valuable experience of helping each other therapeutically; and (4) sharing and receiving information vital to medical management and coping. The group modality is also important when working within a systems perspective, providing valuable interactional information.

Parent Groups

The primary interactional components of a parent group are education, support, self-help, and therapy. The group may deal primarily with one component or any combination of components. It is up to the group leader or leaders (it is helpful to have a coleader to assist with the group process) to evaluate the needs and desires of the group and choose the appropriate components.

The parent of a chronically ill child has many conflicting emotions to deal with on a personal level, yet the everyday needs and demands of the ill child are more often than not put above his or her own needs. The group is a place where parents can concentrate on their own needs, explore and clarify their emotions, and "let go" if necessary. The parent who can tend to his or her own needs in such a way is more likely to direct in-

creased energy into the care of his or her child in a focused manner.

Children's Groups

The primary goals of a group for children with chronic illness are to provide (1) the opportunity to normalize their situations and (2) the opportunity to openly express emotions with other children who are experiencing similar problems. If possible, the group should be divided into two sections—children aged 6 to 11 years and adolescents—thus allowing the adolescents to deal with their specific issues of independence, autonomy, dating, sexuality, marriage, and genetics as they pertain to their illnesses. The opportunity for both children and adolescents to deal openly with their feelings in a neutral, supportive environment can often result in their readiness to work cooperatively with their parents in managing home care and lessen the need for acting-out behavior in the home.

Sibling Groups

Siblings of children with chronic illness may have many different feelings about the patient, his or her illness, and the attention he or she receives. Sympathy, resentment, loneliness, misunderstanding concerning the illness, and a fear for their own health are typical feelings for siblings of the chronically ill child. The group setting for siblings can provide an opportunity to normalize the family situation and an opportunity to have their own time and attention, which is typically focused on the ill child.

Staff Groups

Personnel working with chronically ill children often receive little support or preparation for coping with the emotional demands of working with this group (Littlehales and Teyber 1981). Somehow we have developed the mistaken notion that to acknowledge feelings of fear, grief, sadness, and helplessness is incompatible with being competent, efficient, and effective.

A staff support group can provide opportunities to share common experiences, problem solve, and deal with feelings by ventilating, clarifying, and validating. The three major areas that would most likely be addressed in such a group are (1) patient care issues, (2) emotional needs of both the patient and the provider, and (3) interactions with the social system in which care is being provided (the family in the case of home care). The combined stress of dealing with these three areas often leads to exhaustion, more commonly referred to as "burnout." The group process is an excellent preventative measure to deal with this common problem.

Respite Care

Respite care is included as an intervention with the awareness that if it is not provided for the family, it is possible that other forms of intervention may be jeopardized. Respite care may be defined as the temporary relief of obligations and stress. Parents require occasional respite from the stress of caring for a chronically ill child in the home. An opportunity for parents to get away and attend to themselves and their marriage is essential for personal and marital health maintenance.

The child who is ill is also in need of occasional respite from his or her normal environment. For the mobile child, recreational camps and field trips with children with similar conditions can be an invaluable experience.

Genetic Counseling

Technology in the genetics field has been rapidly expanding; however, the developing social and psychological services for families with genetic disorders and birth defects are lagging. A genetic diagnosis can be potentially devastating, because it affects families over their life spans and is multigenerational. Genetic misinformation can be used as a weapon of attack, blame, and criticism within a troubled family (McCollum 1975). Accurate and properly transmitted genetic information, however, can be relieving.

Families require a specialized setting that provides the dual components of information and assistance. Large medical centers usually have genetic clinics with both geneticists and social workers available. The local March of Dimes is also a good resource and can provide families with information from the Birth Defect Information System in the form of a computer printout. Examples of diseases in which genetic counseling would be important are cystic fibrosis and hemophilia. In the case of hemophilia, female siblings have special concerns about being carriers; therefore, a special effort should be made to provide counseling to them as they approach childbearing age.

The Parent as Case Manager

Encouraging the parent to become his or her child's case manager can be extremely effective in fostering a parental sense of control, usefulness, and reduced anxiety. It also is an efficient means of coordinating an often vast array of services. A formal recordkeeping system can become a parent's "lifeline" to mastery of the "system" so that the parent does not become overwhelmed by it. The parent should be encouraged to keep records of all clinic visits (including treatments and medications given), the child's health (symptoms, fevers, and side effects, noting incident, date, time, and duration), conferences with medical staff, and all phone and written contacts (Exhibit 21–2).

In addition, the parent may find it helpful to prepare a background sheet for the child, including developmental milestones, health and medical history, and primary contacts with service providers. If the parent keeps a supply of these sheets available, there will be considerable time and effort saved when initiating a new service contact.

There are some specific methods the parent can implement in the home to ensure the smooth delivery of home nursing care. An equipment and supply inventory list is useful for identifying the quantity of supplies on hand and the need for reordering. Written nursing schedules should be

Exhibit 21–2 Contact Log Sheet

Person Contacted _____ Date _____

Organization _____ Telephone _____

Address _____

_____

Question/Information _____

_____

_____

_____

Outcome _____

_____

_____

Follow-Up—What do I do next?

Short Term: _____

_____

Long Term: _____

_____

required to be in place in the home at least two weeks ahead of time to allow for efficient planning and elimination of nursing coverage gaps. A bedside notebook containing sections on medical management, communication between nurses and the family, and a log for nurses to sign in and out would also be useful.

The parent using the previous examples of case management becomes the child's "frontline" case manager, assisted by a backup system of professionals for guidance and support. Some families will wish to assume responsibility for their children's case management as soon as possible, and others will prefer to rely on professional case management that allows for increasing parental responsibility on a gradual basis. Some excellent resources are available to assist parents in case management and coping with their child's chronic illness (Goldfarb et al. 1986; Gittler and Colton 1986; Kaufman and Lichtenstein n.d.) (see Chapter 1).

Coordination of Services

One of the biggest stressors many families find themselves facing is the lack of coordination of services. The parent attempting to take on the case management of a child often faces this immediate and sometimes overwhelming stressor. Therefore, coordination of services is included here as an important intervention.

Any discussion of coordination of services would be incomplete without mentioning the landmark Vanderbilt Study, officially titled "Public Policies Affecting Chronically Ill Children and Their Families" (Hobbs and Perrin 1985). This study has heightened awareness at a national level of (1) the need to coordinate services for the chronically ill child and his or her family and (2) the need for some type of national policy and federal funding. Vanderbilt University–sponsored state conferences have been conducted across the country and have served as the impetus for many state and local programs.

Examples of local efforts to coordinate services and provide direction and support for families are the Disability Helpline of Arizona (a statewide, bilingual database for comprehensive services for children and adults with disability or chronic illness) and SKIP (Sick Kids Need Involved People), which assists children dependent on medical technology. SKIP has developed into a national organization with many local chapters. Many additional efforts such as these are needed to assist families in dealing with the lack of coordination of services.

CASE STUDY: THE TAYLOR FAMILY

After examining various interventions designed to assist families coping with chronic pediatric illness, it may be useful now to examine a case study. We will consider what actually happened with this family and then examine what might have been done differently using some of the interventions previously mentioned.

The Taylors anxiously awaited the birth of their first child, full of hopes and dreams typical of a young expectant couple. Those dreams appeared to become reality when Mrs. Taylor delivered a seemingly healthy infant girl. However, the Taylors began having serious concerns about their daughter when the child, Jackie, was six months old and not developing normally. After completing a series of tests with several doctors, the Taylors received the devastating news that their daughter had an inherited enzyme deficiency that would eventually attack every part of her body. They were informed that Jackie would have multiple problems and would die before the age of nine years.

Initially, Mr. Taylor found it difficult to accept and deal with his only child's diagnosis of a fatal disease. There was no counseling or support group offered to the Taylors; therefore, they dealt with the shock and pain the best they knew how. Mrs. Taylor became totally involved with the demands of caring for her ill child; Mr. Taylor threw himself into his work and attempted to avoid his daughter and the reality of the home situation as much as possible.

The marital stress that followed was considerable. Mr. Taylor was unable to talk to his wife about their daughter, assist with physician appointments or other care, or support his wife in any other way. She had a need to talk; he had a need to keep it all inside. This situation continued for an entire year, until the family changed pediatricians. The new physician told Mrs. Taylor that she was on the verge of both physical and emotional exhaustion. He also informed her that he would not take her daughter as a patient unless Mr. Taylor came in to talk to him. In addition, the pediatrician indicated that the time had come for Mr. Taylor to come to terms with his daughter's illness. Mr. Taylor reluctantly agreed to talk with the pediatrician, and after that conversation, Mrs. Taylor described her husband as a new person. He became involved in Jackie's care and could enjoy her without dwelling on her diagnosis. He also became more supportive of his wife and they began talking about having another child.

One year later, with the help of a supportive physician and the results of an amniocentesis, their second child, Sandra, was born. The care required by both Jackie and their newborn daughter was constant and exhausting. The Taylors were able to support each other at this point; however, their sense of isolation was intense. The grandparents lived out of town and were dealing with their own pain to the extent that they were unable to give much support to the Taylors. In addition, the family had recently moved to a new city and had few acquaintances.

As far as Jackie's medical care was concerned, there was nothing the physicians could do for her other than keep her comfortable and treat her recurrent infections. Pain was a frequent and serious concern for the Taylors. Their primary goal was to provide care for Jackie in their home as long as possible while at the same time providing her with pain relief.

The final crisis in Jackie's short life lasted over two months. With increasing intracranial pressure came increased pain. Jackie was hospitalized at this point; however, the physicians resisted the Taylors' desire to increase her pain medication, fearing dangerous side effects. After one week in the hospital, the Taylors convinced the physicians to allow administration of a stronger pain medication in the home setting. The family arranged for 24-hour per day home care so that their daughter could die at home. The nurses caring for Jackie had pediatric intensive care experience and were highly efficient and supportive to the family. Jackie died peacefully and pain free at seven years of age.

A NEW ALTERNATIVE

The following treatment plan could have been more beneficial to this family.

As soon as the diagnosis was made, the physician would make a referral to an agency that would provide a case manager or advocate for the Taylor family. This individual would provide immediate supportive counseling and begin coordinating all necessary services. The Taylors would then be linked up with a support group consisting of families in similar situations.

The case manager would provide the Taylors with a computerized printout of all services and information pertinent to their situation and would also develop a treatment plan geared to their individual needs and desires, in this case a plan for home care. The next step would be to gather together the Taylors' closest relatives and friends (the significant others in their lives) and explain what they could expect and would need from each other, followed by an open dialogue encouraging the expression of feelings.

Once the family became somewhat stabilized, a regular system of respite care would be arranged so that the Taylors could regain some strength and refocus on their relationship (the Taylors did not have a vacation in seven years). In addition, in-home family therapy would be available to address current issues and prevent future problems.

The nurse would play a crucial role in assisting Jackie to cope with her painful and terminal illness. She would begin teaching Jackie some age-appropriate relaxation and imagery techniques to alleviate pain as soon as possible after home care was initiated. This could be followed by helping Jackie to adjust to her terminal illness by using a variety of play therapy techniques. Among them could be role playing using various methods of coping, expression of feelings by using hand puppets and drawings, and storytelling involving feelings and coping techniques. The nurse could also instruct Jackie's parents in these techniques, thus providing an opportunity for mutually satisfying parent-child interaction.

In summary, a true family systems perspective would be utilized, involving the patient, her family, and other significant areas of their lives. The developmental needs of both the patient and the family would be taken into account and every effort made to individualize treatment.

A natural question at this point might be "Where would the funding come for this 'ideal' treatment plan?" especially when traditional funding sources cannot provide this care. Components such as the support group and the case manager could be a volunteer effort. Private foundations and grants are a possibility, as is a national funding source as suggested by the Vanderbilt Study. Whatever treatment plan is used, it appears clear that the most helpful approach is a systematic one that meets the needs of the child and the family.

REFERENCES

Baker, F. 1969. Review of general systems concepts and their relevance for medical care. *Systemics* 7:209–29.

Bloomquist, M.L. 1996. *Skills training for children with behavior disorders: A parent and therapist guidebook.* New York: Guilford Press.

Brett, D. 1986. *Annie stories.* New York: Workman.

Carter, E., and M. McGoldrick. 1980. *The family life cycle.* New York: Gardner Press.

Dolgin, M.J. and S.M. Jay. 1989. Pain management in children. In *Treatment of childhood disorders*, ed. E.J. Mash and R.A. Barkley. New York: Guilford Press.

Forman, S. 1993. *Coping skills interventions for children and adolescents.* San Francisco: Jossey-Bass.

Freeman, R.D. 1968. Emotional reactions of handicapped children. In *Annual progress in child psychiatry and child development,* ed. S. Chess and A. Thomas. New York: Brunner/Mazel.

Garrard, S.D., and J.B. Richmond. 1963. Psychological aspects of the management of chronic disease and handicapping conditions in childhood. In *The psychological basis of medical practice,* ed. H.E. Leif, V.H. Leif, and N.R. Leif. New York: Harper & Row.

Garth, M. 1992. *Moonbeam: A book of meditations for children.* Australia: Collins Dove.

Gaudet, L.M., and G.M. Powers. 1986, July. *Differences in coping patterns in parents of chronically ill children.* Ann Arbor, MI: Educational Resources Information Center (ERIC) Clearinghouse for Counseling and Personnel Services, University of Michigan (Ann Arbor), and abstracted in Resources in Education, ERIC document reproduction No. ED 266-374, July.

Gillmore, J. 1986. Behavior therapy. In *Manual of clinical child psychiatry,* ed. K.S. Robson. Washington, DC: American Psychiatric Press.

Gittler, J., and M. Colton. 1986. *Community-based case management programs for children with special health care needs.* Prepared by National Maternal and Child Health Resource Center, grant #MCJ-193790-01, U.S. Department of Health and Human Services Public Health Service, HRSA, BHCDA, Division of Maternal and Child Health.

Goldfarb, L.A., et al. 1986. *Meeting the challenge of disability or chronic illness—A family guide.* Baltimore: Paul H. Brookes.

Hilgard, J.P., and S. LeBaron. 1984. *Hypnotherapy of pain in children with cancer.* Los Altos, CA: William Kaufman.

Hill, R. 1949. *Families under stress.* New York: Harper.

Hobbs, N., and J. Perrin. 1985. *Issues in the care of children with chronic illness.* San Francisco: Jossey-Bass.

Kaufman, J., and K.A. Lichtenstein. n.d. *The family as care manager: Home care coordination for medically fragile children.* Prepared by Georgetown University Child Development Center for the Division of Maternal and Child Health under grant #MCJ-113368.

Landreth, G.L., et al. 1996. *Play therapy interventions with children's problems.* Northvale, NJ: Jason Aaronson.

Littlehales, D.E., and E.C. Teyber. 1981. Coping with feelings: Seriously ill children, their families, and hospital staff. *Health and Social Work* 10:58–62.

Mattson, A. 1972. Long-term physical illness in childhood: A challenge to psychosocial adaptation. *Pediatrics* 50: 801–11.

McCollum, A.T. 1975. *The chronically ill child.* New Haven, CT: Yale University Press.

McCubbin, H.I., and J. Patterson. 1981. *Systematic assessment of family stress, resources, and coping.* St. Paul, MN: Family Social Science.

McCubbin, H.I., et al. 1983. *CHIP—Coping health inventory for parents.* Madison, WI: Family Stress, Coping, and Health Project, University of Wisconsin.

Mills, J.C., and R.J. Crowley. 1986. *Therapeutic metaphors for children and the child within.* New York: Brunner/Mazel.

Mitchell, W., and S.J. Rizzo. 1985. The adolescent with special needs. In *Adolescents and family therapy,* ed. M.P. Mirkin and S.L. Koman. New York: Gardner Press.

Murdock, M. 1987. *Spinning inward: Using guided imagery with children for learning, creativity, and relaxation.* Boston: Shambhala.

Neuman, S. 1984. *Feelings: Everybody has them.* Brecksville, OH: SNB Publishing, Inc.

Oaklander, V. 1978. *Windows to our children.* Moab, UT: Real People Press.

O'Grady, D.J. 1991. Hypnosis and pain management in children. In *Clinical hypnosis with children,* ed. W.C. Wester II and D.J. O'Grady. New York: Brunner/Mazel.

Olness, K., and G.G. Gardner. 1988. *Hypnosis and hypnotherapy with children.* Philadelphia: Grune & Stratton.

Philadelphia Child Guidance Center and J. Maguire. 1993. *Your child's emotional health.* New York: Macmillan.

Powers, G.M., L.M. Gaudet, and S. Powers. 1986. Coping patterns of parents of chronically ill children. *Psychological Reports* 59:519–22.

Rimm, D.C., and J.C. Masters. 1979. *Behavior therapy: Techniques and empirical findings.* New York: Academic Press.

Rowland, J.D. 1984. Toward a psychosocial typology of chronic and life-threatening illness. *Family Systems Medicine* 2:245–62.

Sutton, J.C. n.d. *Children of crisis, violence, and loss.* Pleasanton, TX: Friendly Oaks Publications.

CHIP—
Coping Health Inventory
for Parents
Family Health Program

PURPOSE

CHIP—The Coping–Health Inventory for Parents was developed to record what parents find helpful or not helpful to them in the management of family life when one or more of its members is ill for a brief period *or* has a medical condition which calls for continued medical care. Coping is defined as personal or collective (with other individuals, programs) efforts to manage the hardships associated with health problems in the family.

DIRECTIONS

- To complete this inventory you are asked to read the list of "Coping behaviors" below, one at a time.
- For each coping behavior you used, please record how helpful it was.
  HOW HELPFUL was this COPING BEHAVIOR to you and/or your family: Circle ONE number
    3 = *Extremely* Helpful
    2 = *Moderately* Helpful
    1 = *Minimally* Helpful
    0 = *Not* Helpful
- For each Coping Behavior you did *Not* use please record your "reason."
  Please *RECORD this* by *Checking* ☐ one of the reasons:
        Chose not to use it ✓   Not possible
              ☐   or   ☐
PLEASE BEGIN: Please read and record your decision for EACH and EVERY Coping Behavior listed below.

COMPUTER CODES: IID ☐☐☐☐   GID ☐☐☐   FAMID ☐☐☐☐

Source: © Hamilton I. McCubbin, 1983. Reprinted with permission from *Family Assessment Inventories for Research and Practice,* University of Wisconsin-Madison, 1987. (This inventory was written by Hamilton I. McCubbin, Marilyn A. McCubbin, Robert S. Nevin, and Elizabeth Cauble.)

COPING BEHAVIORS	Extremely Helpful	Moderately Helpful	Minimally Helpful	Not Helpful	I do not cope this way because:		For Computer Use Only		
					Chose Not To	Not Possible	F	S	M
1. Trying to maintain family stability	3	2	1	0	□	□ 12	○		□
2. Engaging in relationships and friendships which help me to feel important and appreciated	3	2	1	0	□	□	□	○	
3. Trusting my spouse (or former spouse) to help support me and my child(ren)	3	2	1	0	□	□	○	□	
4. Sleeping	3	2	1	0	□	□		○	□
5. Talking with the medical staff (nurses, social worker, etc.) when we visit the medical center	3	2	1	0	□	□		□	○
6. Believing that my child(ren) will get better*	3	2	1	0	□	□	○	□	
7. Working, outside employment	3	2	1	0	□	□	□	○	
8. Showing that I am strong	3	2	1	0	□	□	○		□
9. Purchasing gifts for myself and/or other family members	3	2	1	0	□	□	□	○	
10. Talking with other individuals/ parents in my same situation	3	2	1	0	□	□		□	○
11. Taking good care of all the medical equipment at home	3	2	1	0	□	□	○		□
12. Eating	3	2	1	0	□	□		○	□
13. Getting other members of the family to help with chores and tasks at home	3	2	1	0	□	□	○	□	
14. Getting away by myself	3	2	1	0	□	□	□	○	
15. Talking with the Doctor about my concerns about my child(ren) with the medical condition*	3	2	1	0	□	□	□		○
16. Believing that the medical center/ hospital has my family's best interest in mind	3	2	1	0	□	□	○	□	
17. Building close relationships with people	3	2	1	0	□	□	□	○	
18. Believing in God	3	2	1	0	□	□	○		□
19. Develop myself as a person	3	2	1	0	□	□	□	○	
20. Talking with other parents in the same type of situation and learning about their experiences	3	2	1	0	□	□		□	○

COPING BEHAVIORS	Extremely Helpful	Moderately Helpful	Minimally Helpful	Not Helpful	I do not cope this way because: Chose Not To	Not Possible	For Computer Use Only F	S	M
21. Doing things together as a family (involving all members of the family)	3	2	1	0	□	□	O	□	
22. Investing time and energy in my job	3	2	1	0	□	□		O	□
23. Believing that my child is getting the best medical care possible*	3	2	1	0	□	□ 34	O		□
24. Entertaining friends in our home	3	2	1	0	□	□ 35	□	O	
25. Reading about how other persons in my situation handle things	3	2	1	0	□	□		□	O
26. Doing things with family relatives	3	2	1	0	□	□	O	□	
27. Becoming more self-reliant and independent	3	2	1	0	□	□		O	□
28. Telling myself that I have many things I should be thankful for	3	2	1	0	□	□	O	□	
29. Concentrating on hobbies (art, music, jogging, etc.)	3	2	1	0	□	□	□	O	
30. Explaining our family situation to friends and neighbors so they will understand us	3	2	1	0	□	□		□	O
31. Encouraging child(ren) with medical condition to be more independent*	3	2	1	0	□	□	O	□	
32. Keeping myself in shape and well groomed	3	2	1	0	□	□		O	□
33. Involvement in social activities (parties, etc.) with friends	3	2	1	0	□	□	□	O	
34. Going out with my spouse on a regular basis	3	2	1	0	□	□	□	O	
35. Being sure prescribed medical treatments for child(ren) are carried out at home on a daily basis	3	2	1	0	□	□		□	O
36. Building a closer relationship with my spouse	3	2	1	0	□	□	O	□	
37. Allowing myself to get angry	3	2	1	0	□	□		O	□
38. Investing myself in my child(ren)	3	2	1	0	□	□	O		□

COPING BEHAVIORS	Extremely Helpful	Moderately Helpful	Minimally Helpful	Not Helpful	I do not cope this way because: Chose Not To	Not Possible	For Computer Use Only F	S	M
39. Talking to someone (not professional counselor/doctor) about how I feel	3	2	1	0	☐	☐	☐	○	
40. Reading more about the medical problem which concerns me	3	2	1	0	☐	☐		☐	○
41. Talking over personal feelings and concerns with spouse	3	2	1	0	☐	☐	○	☐	
42. Being able to get away from the home care tasks and responsibilities for some relief	3	2	1	0	☐	☐		○	☐
43. Having my child with the medical condition seen at the clinic/hospital on a regular basis*	3	2	1	0	☐	☐	○	☐	
44. Believing that things will always work out	3	2	1	0	☐	☐	○	☐	
45. Doing things with my children	3	2	1	0	☐	☐	○		☐

FAM ☐☐ 58

SUP ☐☐ 60

MED ☐☐ 62

PLEASE Check all 45 items to be sure you have either circled a number or checked a box for each one. This is important.

*Related to the eigenvalue for statistical analysis. For more information about scoring, write to the Family Stress Coping and Health Project, 1300 Linden Drive, University of Wisconsin at Madison, Madison, WI 53706.

Directory of Resources

The following are organizations that professionals and families can use to obtain information and support. This list is not comprehensive. Although it provides many major sources of information, there are other national organizations that are not listed that also provide services. In addition, information and support can be obtained through local community agencies such as United Way organizations, local community agencies, church organizations, hospitals, and other community groups.

ADVOCACY AND FINANCING

American Association for Continuity of Care
11250 Roger Bacon Drive
Suite 8
Reston, VA 22090-5202
Phone: 703-525-1191

American Association of University-Affiliated
  Programs
8630 Fenton Street
Suite 410
Silver Spring, MD 20910
Phone: 301-588-8252

Association for the Care of Children's Health
7910 Woodmont Avenue
Suite 300
Bethesda, MD 20814
Phone: 301-654-6549
        800-808-2224

Children's Defense Fund
25 E Street, N.W.
Washington, DC 20001
Phone: 202-628-8787

Council for Exceptional Children,
  Division of Early Childhood
1920 Association Drive
Reston, VA 22091-1589
Phone: 703-620-3660

Disability Rights Center, Inc.
2500 Q Street, N.W.
Suite 121
Washington, DC 20007
Phone: 202-337-4119

Federation for Children with Special Needs, Inc.
95 Berkeley Street
Suite 104
Boston, MA 02116
Phone: 617-482-2915

Kids Peace
5300 Kids Peace Drive
Orefield, PA 18069-9101
Phone: 215-799-8000

Make Today Count, Inc.
1235 E. Cherokee Street
Springfield, MO 65804-2203
Phone: 417-885-3324
(for parents of seriously ill children)

National Association for Home Care
519 C Street, N.E.
Stanton Park
Washington, DC 20002
Phone: 202-547-7424

National Association for Protection and
  Advocacy Services (NAPA)
900 2nd Street, N.E.
Suite 211
Washington, DC 20002
Phone: 202-408-9514

National Center for Child Advocacy
1625 K Street, N.W.
Suite 510
Washington, DC 20006
Phone: 202-828-6950

National Center for Education in Maternal and
  Child Health/National Maternal and Child
  Health Clearinghouse
38th and R Streets, N.W.
Washington, DC 20057
Phone: 202-625-8400

National Center for Youth with Disabilities
University of Minnesota
Box 721
420 Delaware Street, SE
Minneapolis, MN 55455–0392
Phone: 612-626-2825

National Education Association
Office of Educational Support Personnel
1201 16th Street, N.W.
Washington, DC 20036
Phone: 202-822-7570

National Information Center for Children and
  Youth with Disabilities (NICHCY)
1233 20th Street, N.W.
Suite 504
Washington, DC 20036
Phone: 800-695-0285

Parents Helping Parents
3041 Olcott Street
Santa Clara, CA 95054-3222
Phone: 408-727-5775

Pathfinders International
9 Galen Street
Suite 217
Watertown, MA 02172
Phone: 617-924-7200

SKIP (Sick Kids Need Involved People)
8360 Route 3
Millersville, MD 21108
Phone: 301-621-7830

Technical Assistance for Parents Programs
  (TAPP)
TAPP Central Office:
Federation for Children with Special Needs,
  Inc.
95 Berkeley Street
Suite 104
Boston, MA 02116
Phone: 617-482-2915

BIRTH DEFECTS/CHILDREN WITH DISABILITIES

Association of Birth Defect Children
Orlando Executive Park
5400 Diplomat Circle
Suite 270
Orlando, FL 32810
Phone: 407-629-1466

March of Dimes Birth Defects Foundation
1275 Mamaroneck Avenue
White Plains, NY 10650
Phone: 914-428-7100

National Birth Defects Center
30 Warren Street
Boston, MA 02135
Phone: 617-787-5958

National Network to Prevent Birth Defects
Box 15309, S.E. Station
Washington, DC 20003

CANCER

AMC Cancer Information Center
1600 Pierce Street
Lakewood, CO 80214
Phone: 800-525-3777

American Brain Tumor Association
3725 N. Talman Avenue
Chicago, IL 60618
Phone: 312-286-5571

American Cancer Society
46 Fifth Street, N.E.
Atlanta, GA 30308
Phone: 800-ACS-2345
        404-320-3333

Cancer Information Clearinghouse
National Cancer Institute
Office of Cancer Communications
9000 Rockville Pike
Building 31, Room 10A-18
Bethesda, MD 20892

Cancer Information Service
Phone: 800-422-6237
(Spanish language and materials
  available)

Candlelighters Childhood Cancer
  Foundation
7910 Woodmont Avenue
Suite 460
Bethesda, MD 20814–3015
Phone: 301-657-8401

Corporate Angel Network
Westchester County Airport
Building 1
White Plains, NY 10604
Phone: 914-328-1313

International Association of Cancer
  Victors and Friends
531 Main Street
Suite 1136
El Sugundo, CA 90245-3060
Phone: 310-822-5032

Leukemia Society of America, Inc.
600 3rd Avenue
New York, NY 10016
Phone: 212-573-8484

National Cancer Institute Cancer Information
Resource Branch
NCI/NIH
9000 Rockville Pike
Building 31, Room 10A-07
Bethesda, MD 20892
Phone: 800-4-CANCER
Fax: 301-402-0555

National Foundation for Cancer Research
800-321-CURE

CARDIAC/RESPIRATORY

American Academy of Allergy and
  Immunology
611 E. Wells Street
Milwaukee, WI 53202
Phone: 414-272-6071

American Heart Association
7272 Greenville Avenue
Dallas, TX 75231-4596
Phone: 214-373-6300

American Lung Association
1740 Broadway
New York, NY 10019-4374
Phone: 212-315-8700

American Sudden Infant Death Syndrome
  Institute
6065 Roswell Road
Suite 876
Atlanta, GA 30328
Phone: 404-843-1030

Asthma and Allergy Foundation of America
1125 15th Street, N.W.
Suite 502
Washington, DC 20005
Phone: 202-466-7643

Cystic Fibrosis Foundation
6931 Arlington Road
No. 200
Bethesda, MD 20814
Phone: 301-951-4422
        800-FIGHTCF

Central Hypoventilation Syndrome
    Parent Support Group
71 Maple Street
Oneonta, NY 13820

Mothers of Asthmatics
3554 Chain Bridge Road
Suite 200
Fairfax, VA 22030-2709
Phone: 703-385-4403

National Heart, Lung and Blood Institute
Building 31, Room 4A-21
9000 Rockville Pike
Bethesda, MD 20892
Phone: 301-496-5166

National Institute of Allergy and Infectious
    Disease
GRD
Building 31, Room 7A-32
9000 Rockville Pike
Bethesda, MD 20892
Phone: 301-496-5717

SKIP (Sick Kids Need Involved People)
8360 Route 3
Millersville, MD 21108
Phone: 301-621-7830

CHRONIC ILLNESS/GENETICS

Alliance of Genetic Support Groups
35 Wisconsin Circle, #440
Bethesda, MD 20815-7015
Phone: 800-336-GENE
        301-652-5553

FOCUS
(Families of Children Under Stress)
P.O. Box 1058
Conyers, GA 30207
Phone: 912-483-9845

National Foundation for Jewish Genetic
    Diseases
250 Park Avenue
Suite 1000
New York, NY 10177
Phone: 212-371-1030

Parents of Chronically Ill Children
1527 Maryland Street
Springfield, IL 62702
Phone: 217-522-6801

CRANIOFACIAL DISORDERS

American Cleft Palate–Craniofacial Associa-
    tion
American Cleft Palate Foundation
1218 Grandview Avenue
Pittsburgh, PA 15211
Phone: 800-24-CLEFT
        412-481-1376
        800-535-3643 (Spanish materials)

FACES
National Association for the Craniofacially
    Handicapped
P.O. Box 11082
Chattanooga, TN 37401
Phone: 800-332-2373

International Craniofacial Foundation
10210 North Central Expressway
Suite 230, LB37
Dallas, TX 75231
Phone: 800-535-3643
        214-368-3590

NFFR
(National Foundation for Facial
  Reconstruction)
c/o Arlyn Gardner
317 East 34th Street
Ninth Floor
New York, NY 10016
Phone: 800-422-FACE
          212-233-3503

DEVELOPMENTAL DISABILITIES/
LEARNING DISABILITIES

Administration on Developmental Disabilities
200 Independence Avenue, S.W.
349F Humphrey Building
Washington, DC 20201
Phone: 202-690-6590

American Association of University-
  Affiliated Programs for the
  Developmentally Disabled
8630 Fenton Street
Suite 410
Silver Spring, MD 20910
Phone: 301-588-8252

Council for Exceptional Children
  (Developmentally Delayed)
1920 Association Drive
Reston, VA 22091-1589
Phone: 703-620-3660

Learning Disabilities Association of America
c/o Jean Petersen
4156 Library Road
Pittsburgh, PA 15234
Phone: 412-341-1515
Fax: 412-341-8077

National Association of Developmental
  Disabilities Councils
1234 Massachusetts Avenue, N.W.
Suite 103
Washington, DC 20005
Phone: 202-347-1234

National Center for Learning Disabilities
99 Park Avenue
New York, NY 10016
Phone: 212-687-7211

National Information Center for Children and
  Youth with Disabilities (NICHCY)
1233 20th Street, N.W.
Suite 504
Washington, DC 20036
Phone: 800-695-0285

EDUCATION

Early Intervention and Child Care
First Start
University of Colorado Health Sciences
  Center
4200 E. 19th Avenue, Box C287
Denver, CO 80262
Phone: 303-315-8734
(Handbook for the Care of Infants, Toddlers
  and Young Children with Disabilities and
  Chronic Conditions [1996])

National Association for the Education of
  Young Children
1509 16th Street, N.W.
Washington, DC 20036-1426
Phone: 800-424-2460
          202-232-8777

National Association of Child Care Resource
  and Referral
13119 F Street, N.W.
Suite 810
Washington, DC 20004
Phone: 202-393-5501

National Early Childhood Technical Assistance
  System
NEC*TAS
Frank Porter Graham Child Development
  Center
University of North Carolina
137 E. Porter Street
Chapel Hill, NC 27514
Phone: 919-962-2001

National Education Association
Office of Educational Support Personnel
1201 16th Street, N.W.
Washington, DC 20036
Phone: 202-822-7570

National Resource Center for Health and Safety
  in Child Care
4200 E. Ninth Avenue, Box C–287
Denver, CO 80262
Phone: 800-598-KIDS (5437)
         303-315-8124

Zero to Three
National Center for Clinical Infant Program
  (NCCIP)
2000 14th Street, North
Suite 380
Arlington, VA 22201-2500
Phone: 703-528-4300
         800-899-4301 (Publications Phone)

ENDOCRINE/DIABETES

American Association of Diabetes Educators
444 North Michigan Avenue
Suite 1240
Chicago, IL 60611-3901
Phone: 312-644-2233

American Diabetes Association
1660 Duke Street
P.O. Box 25757
Alexandria, VA 22314
Phone: 703-549-1500

Human Growth Foundation
P.O. Box 3090
Falls Church, VA 22043
Phone: 800-451-6434
         703-883-1773

Juvenile Diabetes Foundation,
  International
432 Park Avenue South
New York, NY 10016-8013
Phone: 212-889-7575

GRIEF AND DYING

Compassionate Friends
P.O. Box 3696
Oakbrook, IL 60522-3696
Phone: 708-990-0010

International Association for Near-
  Death Studies
University of Connecticut
Box 520
East Window Hill, CT 06028
Phone: 203-528-5144

National Hospice Organization
1901 North Moore Street
Suite 901
Arlington, VA 22209
Phone: 703-243-5900
Fax: 703-525-5762

Shanti Project
1546 Market Street
San Francisco, CA 94102–6007
Phone: 415-777-CARE
Fax: 415-777-5152

HEMATOLOGY

Aplastic Anemia Foundation of America
P.O. Box 22689
Baltimore, MD 21203
Phone: 800-747-2820

Cooley's Anemia Foundation
129-09 26th Avenue
Flushing, NY 11354
Phone: 718-321-2873

National Association for Sickle Cell
  Disease, Inc.
200 Corporate Pointe
Suite 495
Culver City, CA 90230-7633
Phone: 310-216-6363

HIGH-RISK INFANT

American Sudden Infant Death Syndrome
  Institute
6065 Roswell Road
Suite 876
Atlanta, GA 30328
Phone: 404-843-1030

National Center for Clinical Infant Programs
200014th Street North
Suite 380
Arlington, VA 22201
Phone: 703-528-4300

National Council for Infant Survival
8178 Nadine River Circle
Fountain Valley, CA 92708
Phone: 800-247-4370

Parent Care, Inc.
9041 Colgate Street
Indianapolis, IN 46268-1210
Phone: 317-872-9913

Parents of Premature and High Risk Infants,
  International Inc.
9041 Colgate Street
Indianapolis, IN 46268-1210
Phone: 317-872-9913

Zero to Three
National Center for Clinical Infant Programs
  (NCCIP)
2000 14th Street, North
Suite 380
Arlington, VA 22201-2500
Phone: 703-528-4300
        800-899-4301 (Publications Phone)

IMMUNE DEFICIENCY/AIDS

AIDS Information
U.S. Public Health Service
Hubert Humphrey Building, Room #721-H
200 Independence Avenue, S.W.
Washington, DC 20201

Immune Deficiency Foundation
25 West Chesapeake Avenue
Towson, MD 21204
Phone: 410-321-6647

National AIDS Hotline
Phone: 800-342-2437
        800-344-7432 (Spanish speaking)

National AIDS Information Clearinghouse
P.O. Box 6003
Rockville, MD 20850

KIDNEY

American Kidney Fund
6110 Executive Boulevard, No. 1010
Rockville, MD 20852
Phone: 301-881-3052

National Association of Patients on
  Hemodialysis and Transplantation
211 East 43rd Street, No. 310
New York, NY 10017
Phone: 212-867-4486

National Kidney Foundation
2 Park Avenue
New York, NY 10016
Phone: 212-889-2210

MENTAL HEALTH

Federation of Families for Children's
  Mental Health
1021 Prince Street
Alexandria, VA 22314-2971
Phone: 703-684-7710

Make-A-Wish of America
100 West Clarendon Avenue
Suite 2200
2600 N. Central Avenue #936
Phoenix, AZ 85013
Phone: 800-722-9474

National Mental Health Association
1021 Prince Street
Alexandria, VA 22314-2971
Phone: 800-969-6642
        703-684-7722

MENTAL RETARDATION/DOWN
   SYNDROME

American Association on Mental Retardation
444 North Capitol Street, N.W.
Suite 846
Washington, DC 20001-1512
Phone: 202-387-1968

Association for Children with Down Syndrome
2616 Martin Avenue
Bellmore, NY 11710
Phone: 516-221-4700

Caring, Inc.
P.O. Box 400
Milton, WA 98354
Phone: 206-922-8607

Council for Exceptional Children
  (Developmentally Delayed)
1920 Association Drive
Reston, VA 22091-1589
Phone: 703-620-3660

National Association for Retarded Citizens
200 Varick Street
New York, NY 10014
Phone: 212-691-2100

National Down Syndrome Congress
1800 Dempster Street
Park Ridge, IL 60068-1146
Phone: 800-232-6372

National Down Syndrome Society
666 Broadway
Suite 810
New York, NY 10012
Phone: 800-221-4602
        212–460–9330

METABOLIC/GASTROINTESTINAL

American Liver Foundation
998 Pompton Avenue
Cedar Grove, NJ 07009
Phone: 800-223-0179

American Pseudo-obstruction and
  Hirschsprung's Society, Inc.
271 Spring Street
Suite 6
Medford, MA 02155
Phone: 617-395-4255

Children's Liver Foundation
14245 Ventura Boulevard
Suite 201
Sherman Oaks, CA 91423
Phone: 800-526-1593

Crohn's and Colitis Foundation of
  America, Inc. (CCFA)
444 Park Avenue, South
New York, NY 10016
Phone: 212-679-1570

Intestinal Disease Foundation, Inc.
1323 Forbes Avenue
Suite 200
Pittsburgh, PA 15219
Phone: 412-261-5888

The Oley Foundation for Home Parenteral and
  Enteral Nutrition
214 Hun Memorial
Albany Medical Center
Albany, NY 12208
Phone: 800-776-6539

United Ostomy Association
36 Executive Park
Suite 120
Irvine, CA 92714-6744
Phone: 714-660-8624

MISCELLANEOUS RESOURCES

Autism Society of America
8601 Georgia Avenue
Suite 503
Silver Spring, MD 20910
Phone: 301-565-0433

Disability Rights Center, Inc.
2500 Q Street, N.W.
Suite 121
Washington, DC 20007
Phone: 202-337-4119

Federation for Children with Special Needs,
   Inc.
95 Berkeley Street
Suite 104
Boston, MA 02116
Phone: 617-482-2915

Make-A-Wish of America
100 West Clarendon Avenue
Suite 2200
2600 N. Central Avenue #936
Phoenix, AZ 85013
Phone: 800-722-9474

March of Dimes Birth Defects Foundation
1275 Mamaroneck Avenue
White Plains, NY 10650
Phone: 914-428-7100

National Association for Protection and
   Advocacy Services (NAPA)
900 2nd Street, N.E.
Suite 211
Washington, DC 20002
Phone: 202-408-9514

National Association of Child Care Resource
   and Referral
13119 F Street, N.W.
Suite 810
Washington, DC 20004
Phone: 202-393-5501

National Epilepsy League
6 N. Michigan Avenue
Chicago, IL 60602

National Organization for Rare Disorders
P.O. Box 8923
New Fairfield, CT 06812-8923
Phone: 203-746-6518

National Resource Center for Health and Safety
   in Child Care
4200 E. Ninth Avenue, Box C-287
Denver, CO 80262
Phone: 800-598-KIDS (5437)
       303-315-8124

Parents of Chronically Ill Children
1527 Maryland Street
Springfield, IL 62702
Phone: 217-522-6801

Tay-Sachs Prevention Program
1100 Walnut Street
Medical Office Building, #413
Philadelphia, PA 19107
Phone: 215-955-8320

Technical Assistance for Parents
   Programs (TAPP)
TAPP Central Office:
Federation for Children with Special
   Needs, Inc.
95 Berkeley Street
Suite 104
Boston, MA 02116
Phone: 617-482-2915

MUSCULOSKELETAL

American Academy for Cerebral Palsy and
   Developmental Medicine
P.O. Box 11086
Richmond, VA 23230-1086
Phone: 804-282-0036

Arthritis Foundation
13 West Peachtree
Atlanta, GA 30309
Phone: 800-933-0032
     404-872-7100

Muscular Dystrophy Association
3300 E. Sunrise Drive
Tucson, AZ 85718-3208
Phone: 602-529-2000

Spina Bifida Association
4590 MacArthur Boulevard, N.W.
Suite 250
Washington, DC 20007-4226
Phone: 202-944-4226

United Cerebral Palsy Association
1522 K Street, N.W.
Suite 1112
Washington, DC 20005
Phone: 800-872-5827 (Community Service
   Division)
       800-872-1827
       202-842-1266

NEUROLOGIC DISORDERS

American Paralysis Association
500 Morris Avenue
Springfield, NJ 07081
Phone: 800-225-0292

Autism Society of America
8601 Georgia Avenue
Suite 503
Silver Spring, MD 20910
Phone: 301-565-0433

C.H.A.D.D.
(Children with Attention Deficit Disorder)
499 N.W. 70th Avenue
Suite 308
Plantation, FL 33317
Phone: 305-587-3700

Children's Brain Diseases Foundation
350 Parnassus Avenue
Suite 900
San Francisco, CA 94117
Phone: 415-565-6259

Epilepsy Foundation of America
4351 Garden City Drive
Landover, MD 20785-2267
Phone: 301-459-3700

National Society for Autistic Children
  (NSAC)
1234 Massachusetts Avenue, N.W.
Suite 1017
Washington, DC 20005
Phone: 202-783-0125

National Aphasia Association
P.O. Box 1887
Murray Hill Station
New York, NY 10156-0611
Phone: 212-263-6025

National Head Injury Foundation
1776 Massachusetts Avenue, N.W.
Suite 100
Washington, DC 20036-1904
Phone: 800-444-6443 (Family Helpline)
      202-296-6443

National Institute of Neurological Disorders
  and Stroke
9000 Rockville Pike
Building 31
Room 8A-16
Bethesda, MD 20892
Phone: 301-496-5751

National Stroke Association
8480 East Orchard Road
Suite 1000
Englewood, CO 80111-5051
Phone: 800-STROKES
      800-787-6537

PHYSICAL DISABILITY

American Academy for Cerebral Palsy
  and Developmental Medicine
P.O. Box 11086
Richmond, VA 23230-1086
Phone: 804-282-0036

Centers for Disease Control
Office of Public Inquiries
Birth Defects Branch
1600 Clifton Road, N.E.
Atlanta, GA 30330

Clearinghouse on the Handicapped
Office of Special Education and Rehabilitation
  Services
Department of Education
Switzer Building, Room 3119-S
Washington, DC 20202

Coordinating Council for Handicapped
  Children
20 East Jackson
Room 900
Chicago, IL 60604
Phone: 312-939-3613

Family Resource Center on Disability
20 E. Jackson Boulevard
#900
Chicago, IL 60604
Phone: 312-939-3513

Federation for Children with Special Needs
95 Berkeley Street
Suite 104
Boston, MA 02116
Phone: 617-482-2915

March of Dimes Birth Defects Foundation
1275 Mamaroneck Avenue
White Plains, NY 10605
Phone: 914-428-7100

Muscular Dystrophy Association
3300 E. Sunrise Drive
Tucson, AZ 85718-3208
Phone: 602-529-2000

National Easter Seal Society
230 W. Monroe Avenue, #1800
Chicago, IL 60606-4800
Phone: 312-726-6200

National Information Center for Children
  and Youth with Disabilities (NICHCY)
P.O. Box 1492
Washington, DC 20013-1492
Phone: 202-884-8200

Spina Bifida Association
4590 MacArthur Boulevard, N.W.
Suite 250
Washington, DC 20007-4226
Phone: 202-944-4226

SCHOOL HEALTH

Learner Managed Designs (Training
  Resources)
P.O. Box 3067
Lawrence, KS 66046
Phone: 913-842-9088

National Association of School Nurses
P.O. Box 1300
Scarborough, ME 04074

National Association of State School Nurse
  Consultants
Dorothy Cooper
Arizona Department of Health Services
411 North 24th Street
Phoenix, AZ 85008
Phone: 602-220-6550

Project Assist
University of Colorado Health
  Sciences Center
School of Nursing, Office of School
  Health
4200 E. Ninth Avenue, Box C-187
Denver, CO 80262
Phone: 800-669-9954
        303-315-4511 or 315-7435
(Unlicensed assistive personnel)

(A training manual for school nurses on the supervision of school health paraprofessionals [1997])

Project School Care
Children's Hospital
300 Longed Avenue
Gardner 610
Boston, MA 02115
Phone: 617-735-6714
(*Children and Youth Assisted by Medical Technology in Educational Setting: Guidelines for Care,* 2nd Edition [1997])

School Health Resource Services
University of Colorado
Office of School Health
4200 E. Ninth Avenue, Box C-287
Denver, CO 80262
Phone: 800-669-9954
     303-315-5990

School Nursing
American School Health Association
P.O. Box 708
Kent, OH 44240
Phone: 216-678-1601

The Children's Hospital
School Health Program
1056 East 19th Avenue
Box 215
Denver, CO 80218
Phone: 303-573-1234

SENSORY

ASDC
American Society for Deaf Children
814 Thayer Avenue
Silver Spring, MD 20910
Phone: 800-942-ASDC

ASHA
American Speech-Language-Hearing Association
10801 Rockville Pike
Rockville, MD 20852
Phone: 800-638-8255 (Voice/TDD)
    301-897-5700

American Foundation for the Blind
1110 Plaza Suite 300
New York, NY 10001
Phone: 800-232-5463

Auditory-Verbal International, Inc.
6 S. Third Street
Suite 305
Easton, PA 18042
Phone: 215-253-6616

International Hearing Society
20361 Middlebelt Road
Livonia, MI 48152
Phone: 800-521-5247
    313-478-2610

National Association for the Deaf
814 Thayer Avenue
Silver Spring, MD 20910
Phone: 301-587-1788
    301/587-1789 (TDD)

National Association for the Visually Handicapped
305 East 24th Street, Room 17-C
New York, NY 10010

National Library Service for the Blind and Physically Handicapped
The Library of Congress
Washington, DC 20442

TRANSPLANT

National Heart Assist and Transplant Fund
P.O. Box 163
Haverford, PA 19041
Phone: 215-527-5056

Transplant Recipient's International
  Organization
244 North Bellefield Avenue
Pittsburgh, PA 15312
Phone: 412-687-2210

United Network for Organ Sharing
3001 Hungary Spring Road
P.O. Box 28010
Richmond, VA 23228
Phone: 804-289-5380

Index

About the Editors

Wendy Votroubek, RN, MPH, is currently the pediatric pulmonary clinical nurse specialist at University Medical Center in Tucson, Arizona. She has presented extensively on the international, national, state, and local levels on care for the child with cystic fibrosis and asthma.

Wendy has worked for both the Visiting Nurses Association in Los Angeles as a pediatric home care nurse and Medical Personnel Pool as a pediatric home care supervisor. In her current position, she works closely with home care nurses regarding the care of her pediatric pulmonary patients.

Wendy was the coeditor of the original version of *Pediatric Home Care* and has published various articles on the care of children with various pediatric pulmonary conditions. Her latest project has been the adoption of her daughter Lila Grace Yuze Votroubek, from China.

Julie L. Townsend, RN, C, MS, attended St. Anthony's Hospital School of Nursing in Rockford, Illinois. She received her BSN and MS in nursing from the University of Missouri in Columbia. She is presently an instructor at the University of Arizona, College of Nursing, at Tucson. She teaches leadership and management to the seniors as well as teaches the accelerated pathways students. She was voted Undergraduate Teacher of the Year in 1996.

Julie has six years of clinical and management experience in maternal-pediatric home care. She has presented on the local, state, and national levels on issues ranging from care of the child with Type I diabetes, care of the terminally ill child, how to set up pediatric home care programs, and how to care for the caregiver.